Outline of ONCOLOGY Therapeutics

Outline of ONCOLOGY Therapeutics

Mark J. Ratain, M.D.
Chairman, Committee on Clinical Pharmacology
Professor of Medicine
The University of Chicago
Chicago, Illinois

Margaret Tempero, M.D.
Deputy Director, Comprehensive Cancer Center
Chief, Division of Medical Oncology
University of California, San Francisco
San Francisco, California

Consuelo Skosey, R.N., C.C.R.A.
Director, Clinical Trials Office
Division of the Biological Sciences
The University of Chicago
Chicago, Illinois

W.B. SAUNDERS COMPANY
A Harcourt Health Sciences Company
Philadelphia • London • New York • St. Louis • Sydney • Toronto

W.B. SAUNDERS COMPANY
A Harcourt Health Sciences Company
The Curtis Center
Independence Square West
Philadelphia, Pennsylvania 19106

Library of Congress Cataloging-in-Publication Data

Outline of oncology therapeutics / [edited by] Mark J. Ratain, Margaret Tempero, Consuelo Skosey.
p. cm.
ISBN 0-7216-8123-9
1. Antineoplastic agents. 2. Cancer—Chemotherapy. I. Ratain, Mark J. II. Tempero, Margaret. III. Skosey, Consuelo.
[DNLM: 1. Antineoplastic Agents. 2. Drug Therapy.
QV 269 O94 2001]
RC271.C5 O95 2001
616.99'4061—dc21 00-059064

Editor-in-Chief, Surgery: Richard H. Lampert
Senior Editorial Assistant: Beth LoGiudice

Outline of Oncology Therapeutics ISBN 0-7216-8123-9

Printed in the United States of America

Last digit is the print number: 9 8 7 6 5 4 3 2 1

CONTRIBUTORS

Michael L. Adler, M.D.
Clinical Instructor in Medicine, Cornell University, New York, New York; Attending Endocrinologist, Wilkes Barre General Hospital, Wilkes Barre, Pennsylvania
Hypercalcemia of Malignancy

Sanjiv S. Agarwala, M.D.
Assistant Professor of Medicine, University of Pittsburgh Cancer Institute, Pittsburgh, Pennsylvania
Cytokines
Interferon Alfa: Introduction

Frederick R. Ahmann, M.D.
Professor of Medicine and Surgery, Medical Oncology and Urology, University of Arizona College of Medicine and Arizona Cancer Center, Tucson, Arizona
Ketoconazole

Susan G. Arbuck, M.D.
Head, Developmental Chemotherapy Section, Cancer Therapy Evaluation Program, Division of Cancer Treatment and Diagnosis, National Cancer Institute, Bethesda, Maryland
Allergic Toxicity

Rashmi N. Aurora, M.D.
Fellow, Memorial Sloan-Kettering Cancer Center, New York, New York
Cytotoxic Pulmonary Injury

Jose Baselga, M.D.
Professor of Medicine, Universidad Vall d'Hebron de Barcelona; Chairman, Medical Oncology, Vall d'Hebron University Hospital, Barcelona, Spain
Tastuzumab

Patrick G. Beatty, M.D., Ph.D.
Professor of Medicine; Director, Blood and Marrow Transplant Program, University of Utah School of Medicine, Salt Lake City, Utah
Graft-versus-Host Disease (GVHD)

William T. Beck, Ph.D.
Professor, Department of Pharmaceutics and Pharmacodynamics, College of Pharmacy, University of Illinois at Chicago, Chicago, Illinois
Topoisomerase Inhibitors

Jos H. Beijnen, Ph.D.
Professor of Analytical Drug Toxicology, Department of Biomedical Analysis, Utrecht University, Utrecht, The Netherlands; Head, Department of Pharmacy and Pharmacology, Hospital Pharmicist/Clinical Pharmacologist, The Netherlands Cancer Institute/Slotervaart Hospital, Amsterdam, The Netherlands
Cisplatin
Topotecan

Mohamed Bekradda, M.D.
Oncologist Project Leader, Critovic et Associés Consultants, SA, Le Kremlin-Bicètre, France
Oxaliplatin
Vindesine

Deborah T. Berg, R.N., B.S.N.
Program Administrator/Clinical Trials Manager, Dana Farber Cancer Institute, Boston, Massachusetts
Actinomycin D
All-Trans Retinoic Acid
Busulfan
Epirubicin HCI
Irinotecan
Losoxantrone
Mitomycin C (Intrahepatic)
Mitroxantrone
Tumor Lysis Syndrome
Valspodar

Ellin Berman, M.D.
Member, Memorial Hospital, Memorial Sloan-Kettering Cancer Center, New York, New York
Daunorubicin
Idarubicin

Philip J. Bierman, M.D.
Associate Professor, University of Nebraska College of Medicine; Associate Professor, University of Nebraska Medical Center, Omaha, Nebraska
Tumor Lysis Syndrome

R. G. Bociek, M.D., M.Sc.
Assistant Professor, University of Nebraska Medical Center, Omaha, Nebraska
Myelosuppression

Susan C. Budds, R.N., M.S.N., O.C.N.
Oncology Case Manager, Oncology Clinical Nurse Specialist, Edward Hospital, Naperville, Illinois
Ambulatory Pumps: Introduction
Cisplatin (Intraperitoneal)
Elastomeric "Balloon" Ambulatory Pump
Intraperitoneal: Tenckhoff Catheter
Intraperitoneal: Implanted Ports
Peristaltic Ambulatory Pump
Syringe-driven Ambulatory Pump

Belinda Butler
Operations Manager, Southeast Cancer Control Consortium, Wake Forest University School of Medicine, Winston-Salem, North Carolina
9-Aminocamptothecin
Aminoglutethimide
2-Chlorodeoxyadenosine
Estramustine
Ifosfamide
Mechlorethamine
Medroxyprogesterone
Megestrol

Aman U. Buzdar, M.D.
Professor of Medicine, University of Texas M.D. Anderson Cancer Center, Houston, Texas
Anastrozole

Janine Caggiano, R.N., B.S.N.
Special Assistant for Patient Management, Office of the President, Memorial Sloan-Kettering Cancer Center, New York, New York
Bleomycin
Eniluracil
Goserelin
Isotretinoin
Leuprolide
Rituximab
Thiotepa

A. Hilary Calvert, M.D., M.Sc., F.R.C.P.
Professor of Medical Oncology and Director of Cancer Research, University of Newcastle upon Tyne; Consultant in Medical Oncology, Northern Centre for Cancer Treatment, Newcastle upon Tyne, England
Carboplatin

Robert L. Capizzi, M.D.
Magee Professor and Chairman, Department of Medicine, Jefferson Medical College, Thomas Jefferson University Hospital, Philadelphia, Pennsylvania
Cytarabine
Eniluracil
Goserelin
Isotretinoin
Leuprolide
Nephrotoxicity
Rituximab
Thiotepa
Toremifene

John T. Carpenter, Jr., M.D.
Professor of Medicine and Pathology, University of Alabama at Birmingham; Attending Physician, University Hospital, Birmingham, Alabama
Aminoglutethimide
Medroxyprogesterone Acetate
Megestrol

Bruce D. Cheson, M.D.
Clinical Professor of Medicine, Georgetown University School of Medicine, Lombardi Cancer Center, Washington, D.C.; Head, Medicine Section, Cancer Therapy Evaluation Program, Division of Cancer Treatment and Diagnosis, National Cancer Institute, Bethesda, Maryland
Fludarabine
Miscellaneous Cytotoxic and Modulating Agents: Introduction

Sreeni Chittoor, M.D.
Clinical Assistant Professor of Medicine, University of Texas Southwestern Medical Center, Dallas, Texas
Congestive Heart Failure

Esteban Cvitkovic, M.D.
Associate Professor, Faculté de Medecine, Université de Paris; Assistant Attending Physician, Service D'Oncologie Médicale, Hôpital Paul Brousse, Villejuif Cedex, France
Oxaliplatin
Vindesine

Erin P. Demakos, R.N.
Administrative Director, Data Management, Mount Sinai School of Medicine, New York, New York
Allergic Toxicity
L-Asparaginase
5-Azacytidine
Cytarabine
6-Mercaptopurine
Teniposide

Mark D. DeMario, M.D.
Instructor of Clinical Medicine, University of Chicago, Chicago, Illinois
JM-216
Liposome Encapsulated Daunorubicin

Hollie Devine, M.S.N., R.N., C.S., O.C.N.
Nurse Practitioner, Section of Bone Marrow Transplant and Cell Therapy, Rush-Presbyterian-St. Luke's Medical Center, Chicago, Illinois
Cisplatin (Intra-Arterial)
Daunorubicin
Doxorubicin
Graft-versus-Host Disease (GVHD)
Floxuridine (FUDR)
Idarubicin
Infusaid Pump
Intra-Arterial Chemotherapy: Introduction
SynchroMed Implanted Pump

Elisabeth G.E. deVries, M.D., Ph.D.
Professor Medical Oncology, University Hospital Groningen, Groningen, The Netherlands
Epirubicin HCI

M. Eileen Dolan, Ph.D.
Associate Professor of Medicine, University of Chicago, Chicago, Illinois
DNA-Binding Agents: Introduction

James H. Doroshow, M.D.
Chairman, Department of Medical Oncology, City of Hope Comprehensive Cancer Center, Duarte, California
Cardiotoxicity

Robert T. Dorr, Ph.D.
Professor of Pharmacology, Arizona Cancer Center, University of Arizona, Tucson, Arizona
Extravasation of Vesicant Anticancer Agents

J. Heidi Downey, R.N., B.S.N.
Thoracic Oncology Coordinator, Indiana/Ohio Cardiovascular and Thoracic Surgeons, Fort Wayne, Indiana
Adjuvant Devices for the Management of Advanced Thoracic Malignancies
Bleomycin (Intrapleural)
Pleural Access Port: Pleurx Pleural Catheter
Pleuroperitoneal Shunt
Thoracic Drainage Tubes/Chest Tubes

Anthony D. Elias, M.D.
Assistant Professor of Medicine, Harvard Medical School; Active Staff, Dana Farber Cancer Institute, Boston, Massachusetts
Cyclophosphamide
Ifosfamide

Dalila Essassi, Ph.D.
Critovic et Associés Consultants, SA, Le Kremlin-Bicètre, France
Oxaliplatin
Vindesine

Helen Evans, B.Sc. (Hons) Nursing
Oncology Service Manager, Charing Cross Hospital, Hammersmith, London, England
Temozolomide

Patricia Ferrill, R.N.
Oncology Nurse, Division of Medical Oncology, New York Presbyterian Hospital, New York, New York
Diarrhea

Robert A. Figlin, M.D.
Professor of Medicine, Johnsson Comprehensive Cancer Center, UCLA School of Medicine, Los Angeles, California
Aldesleukin

Gini F. Fleming, M.D.
Assistant Professor of Clinical Medicine, University of Chicago, Chicago, Illinois
Isotretinoin

Thomas J. Garrett, M.D.
Professor of Clinical Medicine, Columbia University, College of Physicians and Surgeons; Attending Physician, New York Presbyterian Hospital, New York, New York
Diarrhea

Janan B. Geick Miller, R.N., B.S.N.
Oncology Research Nurse, University of Iowa Hospitals and Clinics, Iowa City, Iowa
Antiemetics in Cancer Chemotherapy
Cachexia and Anorexia
Deoxycoformycin
Melphalan
Procarbazine
Raltitrexed

Donna Glover, M.D.
CCC Medical Group, Philadelphia, Pennsylvania
Neurotoxicity

Paula O. Goldfarb, R.N., O.C.N.
Nurse Coordinator, Bone Marrow Transplant Unit, Hematology/BMT; City of Hope National Medical Center, Duarte, California
Ambulatory Pumps: Introduction

William J. Gradishar, M.D.
Associate Professor of Medicine, Director, Breast Medical Oncology, Associate Director, Lynn Sage Breast Cancer Program, Robert H. Lurie Comprehensive Cancer Center, Northwestern University Chicago, Illinois
Tamoxifen
Torem

Richard J. Gralla, M.D.
Professor of Medicine; Director, Clinical Research and Solid Tumor Service; Associate Director, Herbert Irving Comprehensive Cancer Center, Columbia University, New York, New York
Antiemetics in Cancer Therapy

Michael R. Grever, M.D.
Division of Hematologic Malignancies, Johns Hopkins Oncology Center, Baltimore, Maryland
Deoxycoformycin

Louise B. Grochow, M.D.
Chief, Investigational Drug Branch, CTEP, DCTD, NCI, Visiting Associate Professor, Johns Hopkins University School of Medicine, Rockville, Maryland
Busulfan

Stuart A. Grossman, M.D.
Professor of Oncology, Medicine and Neurosurgery, The Johns Hopkins University School of Medicine; Director, Neuro-oncology, The Johns Hopkins Oncology Center, Baltimore, Maryland
Intrathecal/Intraventricular Therapy: Introduction
Methotrexate (Intraventricular)

Lisa F. Haser, R.N., B.S.N., O.C.N
Stem Cell Transplant Coordinator, Intermed Oncology Associates, Homewood, Illinois
Bladder Toxicity
Hypercalcemia of Malignancy

Corinne Haviley, M.S.-Oncology Nursing
Director, Ambulatory Oncology, Northwestern Memorial Hospital, Chicago, Illinois
Cytarabine
Methotrexate (Intraventricular)
Thiotepa (Intrathecal/Intraventricular)
Ventricular Reservoir

LuAnn Hestermann, Pharm.D.
Courtesy Faculty, University of Nebraska Medical Center; Clinical Staff Pharmacist, Oncology Hematology Service Line, Nebraska Health System, Omaha, Nebraska
Antiemetics in Cancer Chemotherapy
Neutropenic Fever

Gabriel N. Hortobagyi, M.D., F.A.C.P.
Professor of Medicine, Department of Breast Medical Oncology, The University of Texas M.D. Anderson Cancer Center; Internist, Chairman, Department of Breast Medical Oncology, Nellie B. Connally Chair in Breast Cancer, The University of Texas, M.D. Anderson Cancer Center, Houston, Texas
Osteoporosis/Osteopenia

Marianne Huml, R.N., M.S.
Clinical Ambulatory Nurse, University of Illinois at Chicago Hospital, Chicago, Illinois
Anastrozole
Chlorambucil
Diarrhea
Gemcitabine
Homoharringtonine
Tamoxifen
Topotecan

Barbara Jensen, R.N., B.S.N., O.C.N
Intermed Oncology Associates, Homewood, Illinois
Doxorubicin (Intravesical)
Mitomycin C (Intravesical)

Ellen Jessop, R.N., N.D., O.C.N.
Research Nurse, Stem Cell Transplant, Section of Hematology/Oncology, University of Illinois at Chicago Hospital, Chicago, Illinois
Ketoconazole
Pegasparaginase

Duncan I. Jodrell, D.M., M.Sc.
Reader, University of Edinburgh; Deputy Director, ICRF Medical Oncology Unit, Edinburgh, Scotland
Losoxantrone

Roy B. Jones, Ph.D., M.D.
Professor, University of Colorado Health Sciences Center; Director, Marrow Transplant, University of Colorado Hospital, Denver, Colorado
BCNU
Thiotepa

V. Craig Jordan, Ph.D., D.Sc.
Clinical Instructor, Northwestern University; Clinical Instructor, Northwestern Memorial Hospital, Chicago, Illinois
Antiestrogens and Related Drugs: Introduction

Ian Judson, M.D.
Reader in Clinical Pharmacology, CRC Centre for Cancer Therapeutics, The Institute of Cancer Research, Sutton, Surrey; Hon. Consultant Medical Oncologist, Royal Marsden (NHS Trust) Hospital, London, England
Raltitrexed

Nelson Kalil, M.D.
Clinical Associate, National Cancer Institute, Division of Clinical Sciences, Medicine Branch, Bethesda, Maryland
Allergic Toxicity

Gary Kalkut, M.D.
Associate Professor of Medicine, Albert Einstein College of Medicine; Montefiore Medical Center, Bronx, New York
Management of AIDS-Associated Malignancies

Barton A. Kamen, M.D., Ph.D
Professor of Pediatrics, American Cancer Society Clinical Research Professor, Cancer Institute of New Jersey, Robert Wood Johnson Medical School, New Brunswick New Jersey
Methotrexate
Trimetrexate

Catherine A. Kefer, R.N., M.J., O.C.N.
Nurse Associate, Northwest Oncology and Hematology, S.C., Elk Grove Village, Illinois
Butterfly, Angiocatheter, Midline
Extravasation
Groshong Catheter
Hickman and Broviac Catheters
Myelosuppression
Quinton, Subclavian, Pheresis

Nancy E. Kemeny, M.D.
Professor of Medicine, Weill Medical College of Cornell University, New York, New York; Attending Physician, Memorial Sloan-Kettering Cancer Center, New York, New York
Hepatic Arterial Chemotherapy (HAI): Introduction
Floxuridine (FUDR)
Mitomycin C (Intrahepatic)

Anne Kessinger, M.D.
Professor of Medicine, Chief, Oncology/Hematology Section, University of Nebraska Medical Center, Omaha, Nebraska
Myelosuppression

David Khayat, M.D., Ph.D.
Professor of Oncology, Pierre and Marie Curie University, Head, Department of Medical Oncology, Pitié-Salpetrière Hospital, Paris, France
Fotemustine
Dacarbazine

Hedy L. Kindler, M.D.
Assistant Professor, University of Chicago; Attending Physician, University of Chicago Medical Center, Chicago, Illinois
Mitomycin
MTA

John M. Kirkwood, M.D.
Professor and Vice Chairman for Clinical Research, Department of Medicine, University of Pittsburgh Medical Center; Director, Melanoma Center, University of Pittsburgh Cancer Institute, Pittsburgh, Pennsylvania
Cytokines: Introduction
Interferon Alpha

Ken Kobayashi, M.D.
Medical Officer, Division of Oncology Drug Products, U. S. Food and Drug Administration, Rockville, Maryland
Suramin

Timothy M. Kuzel, M.D.
Associate Professor of Medicine, Northwestern University Medical School; Northwestern Memorial Hospital; Chief, Section of Hematology/Oncology, Chicago VA Healthcare System-Lakeside Division, Chicago, Illinois
Denileukin diftitox

Richard A. Larson, M.D.
Professor of Medicine, The Pritzker School of Medicine, and Director, Leukemia Program, The University of Chicago, Chicago, Illinois
5-Azacytidine
L-Asparaginase
6-Mercaptopurine
Pegasparaginase

Yvonne Lassere, R.N., O.C.N., C.C.R.P.
Research Nurse Supervisor, The University of Texas M.D. Anderson Cancer Center, Houston, Texas
Capecitabine
S-1
Uracil/Tegafur

Allan Lipton, M.D.
Professor of Medicine and Oncology, M.S. Hershey Medical Center, Hershey, Pennsylvania
Letrozole

C.L. Loprinzi, M.D.
Professor and Chair, Medical Oncology, Mayo Medical School, Rochester, Minnesota
Chemotherapy-Induced Mucositis/Stomatitis

David G. Maloney, M.D., Ph.D.
Assistant Professor of Medicine, University of Washington; Assistant Member, Fred Hutchinson Cancer Research Center, Seattle, Washington
Monoclonal Antibodies and Fusion Proteins: Introduction
Rituximab

Mary Beth Mardjetko, R.N., M.S.N.
Lutheran General Hospital, Park Ridge, Illinois
JM-216
Etoposide
Vindesine
Vinorelbine

Maurie Markman, M.D.
Director, The Cleveland Clinic Taussig Cancer Center, Chairman, Department of Hematology and Medical Oncology, The Lee and Jerome Burkons Research Chair in Oncology, The Cleveland Clinic Foundation, Cleveland, Ohio
Cisplatin (Intraperitoneal)
Intraperitoneal Chemotherapy: Introduction

Spyros G.E. Mezitis, M.D., Ph.D.
Clinical Instructor, Division of Endocrinology, Diabetes, Metabolism, Weill Medical College of Cornell University; Attending Endocrinologist, The New York-Presbyterian Hospital, Lenox Hill Hospital, New York, New York
Hypercalcemia of Malignancy

Antonius A. Miller, M.D.
Professor of Medicine, Wake Forest University, Internal Medicine-Hematology/Oncology, Winston-Salem, North Carolina
Etoposide
Etoposide Phosphate

Jay M. Mirtallo, M.S., R.Ph.
Clinical Associate Professor, The Ohio State University, College of Pharmacy, Division of Pharmacy Practice; Specialty Practice Pharmacist, Nutrition Support/ Surgery, The Ohio State University Medical Center, Department of Pharmacy, Columbus, Ohio
Cachexia and Anorexia

Nancy P. Moldawer, R.N., M.S.N.
Clinical Nursing Coordinator, UCLA-Kidney Cancer Program, Jonsson Comprehensive Cancer Center, UCLA School of Medicine, Los Angeles, California
Aldesleukin

Malcolm J. Moore, M.D.
Associate Professor of Medicine and Pharmacology, Princess Margaret Hospital, University of Toronto, Toronto, Canada
Doxorubicin
Gemcitabine
Mitroxantrone

Michael J. Morris, M.D.
Instructor in Medicine, Joan and Sanford Weill Medical College of Cornell University; Clinical Assistant Physician, Memorial Sloan-Kettering Cancer Center, New York, New York
Bicalutamide
Flutamide
Nilutamide

Franco M. Muggia, M.D.
Professor of Medicine, New York University School of Medicine, New York, New York
Hexamethymelamine
Pegylated-Liposomal Doxorubicin (PLD)

James B. Nachman, M.D.
Professor of Clinical Pediatrics, The University of Chicago Pritzker School of Medicine, Chicago, Illinois
Actinomycin D

Edward S. Newlands, B.M., B.C.R., F.C.R.P., Ph.D.
Professor of Cancer Medicine, Imperial College School of Medicine, Kings School Bruton, Somerset; Charing Cross Hospital, London, England
Temozolomide

M. Kelly Nicholas, M.D., Ph.D.
Assistant Professor Neuro-Oncology, University of California, San Francisco, San Francisco, California
Lomustine
Procarbazine

Susan Noble-Kempin, R.N., M.S.
Director Research Administration, Salick Health Care, Los Angeles, California
Bicalutamide
Capecitabine
Cyclophosphamide
Dacarbazine
Liposome Encapsulated Daunorubicin
Lomustine
Osteoporosis/Osteopenia
Oxaliplatin
Pegylated-Liposomal Doxorubicin (PLD)
Vinblastine
Vincristine

Sheila M. O'Brien, R.N., M.S.
Clinical Oncology Manager, Aventis Pharmaceuticals, Forest Park, Illinois
Urinary Catheter

Susan O'Brien, M.D.
Professor of Medicine, University of Texas M. D. Anderson Cancer Center, Houston, Texas
Homoharringtonine

Scott H. Okuno, M.D.
Assistant Professor Medical Oncology, Mayo Medical School, Rochester, Minnesota
Chemotherapy-Induced Mucositis/Stomatitis

Karin B. Olson, M.S., Ph.D.
Physician Assistant, University of Michigan, Ann Arbor, Michigan
Estramustine

Ruth M. O'Regan
Clinical Instructor, Northwestern University; Clinical Instructor, Northwestern Memorial Hospital, Chicago, Illinois
Antiestrogens and Related Drugs: Introduction

Amita Patnaik, M.D.
Clinical Assistant Professor, Department of Medicine, University of Texas Health Science Center; Clinical Investigator, Institute for Drug Development, San Antonio, Texas
Doxorubicin
Gemcitabine
Mitoxantrone

Elizabeth L. Paxton, M.D.
Specialty Resident in Nutrition and Surgery, The Ohio State University Medical Center, Columbus, Ohio
Cachexia and Anorexia

Richard Pazdur, M.D.
Director, Division of Oncology Drug Products, Center for Drug Evaluation and Research, U.S. Food and Drug Administration, Rockville, Maryland
Capecitabine
S-1
Uracil/Tegafur

Kenneth J. Pienta, M.D.
Professor, University of Michigan, Ann Arbor, Michigan
Estramustine

Lawrence D. Piro, M.D.
Salick Healthcare, Los Angeles, California
2-Chlorodeoxyadenosine

Beth Popp, M.D.
Assistant Professor Medicine, State University of New York Health Sciences Center, Brooklyn, New York; Clinical Director, Palliative Medicine, St. Vincent's Hospital and Medical Center, New York, New York
Cancer Pain Management

Sandra Purl, R.N., M.S., A.O.C.N.
Clinical Nurse Specialist, Lutheran General Cancer Care Center, Park Ridge, Illinois
Ambulatory Pumps: Introduction
Elastomeric "Balloon" Ambulatory Pump
Peristaltic Ambulatory Pump
Syringe-driven Ambulatory Pump

Mark J. Ratain, M.D.
Professor of Medicine, Section of Hematology/Oncology; Chairman, Committee on Clinical Pharmacology, University of Chicago, Chicago, Illinois
Irinotecan
Vinblastine
Vincristine

Elizabeth Reed, M.D.
Associate Professor of Medicine; Director, Oncology/Hematology Special Care Unit; Director, Breast Center, University of Nebraska Medical Center, Omaha, Nebraska
Neutropenic Fever

R. J. Robbins, M.D.
Professor of Medicine, Weill Medical College at Cornell University, New York, New York; Attending Physician and Chief of Memorial Sloan-Kettering Cancer Center, New York, New York
Hypercalcemia of Malignancy

Kristine Rossof, R.N.
Nurse Manager, Inpatient Oncology/Hematology, Bone Marrow Transplant, Rush Medical Center, Chicago, Illinois
Hexamethylmelamine
Fotemustine

Eric K. Rowinsky, M.D.
Director, Clinical Research, Institute for Drug Development, Cancer Therapy and Research Center; Clinical Professor of Medicine, University of Texas Health Science Center, San Antonio, Texas
Antimicrotubule Agents: Introduction
Docetaxel
Paclitaxel

John C. Ruckdeschel, M.D.
Professor of Oncology and Medicine, University of South Florida College of Medicine; Director and CEO, H. Lee Moffitt Cancer Center and Research Institute, Tampa, Florida
Bleomycin (Intrapleural)
Intrapleural Therapy: Introduction

Ellen Samuelson, R.N., M.S.N.
G. D. Searle and Co., Skokie, Illinois
Denileukin diftitox

Jan H. M. Schellens, M.D., Ph.D.
Professor of Pharmacy, Pharmacy Faculty, Utrecht University, Utrecht; Medical Oncologist, Clinical Pharmacologist, Division of Medical Oncology, The Netherlands Cancer Institute, Amsterdam, The Netherlands
Cisplatin
Topotecan

Howard I. Scher, M.D.
Professor of Medicine, Weill Medical College of Cornell University, New York, New York; Chief, Genitourinary Oncology Service, Attending Physician, Memorial Sloan-Kettering Cancer Center, New York, New York
Bicalutamide
Flutamide
Nilutamide

Richard L. Schilsky, M.D.
Professor of Medicine and Associate Dean for Clinical Research, Biological Sciences Division, University of Chicago, Chicago, Illinois
Antimetabolites and Their Modulators: Introduction
Eniluracil
5-Fluorouracil
Folinic Acid

J. D. Shepherd, M.D., F.R.C.P.C.
Clinical Associate Professor, Department of Medicine, University of British Columbia; Member, Leukemia/Bone Marrow Transplant Program of British Columbia; Active Staff, British Columbia Cancer Agency, Vancouver Hospital, Vancouver, British Columbia, Canada
Bladder Toxicity

Branimir I. Sikic, M.D.
Professor of Medicine, Stanford University School of Medicine, Stanford, California
Valspodar

Consuelo Skosey, R.N., C.C.R.A.
Director, Clinical Trials Office, Division of the Biological Sciences, Pritzker School of Medicine, The University of Chicago, Chicago, Illinois
Access Devices and Pumps: Options in Administration: Introduction
Cancer Pain Management
Cytotoxic Pulmonary Injury
Myelosuppression
Mitomycin
MTA
Nephrotoxicity

Patricia A. Sorokin, R.N., B.S.N., O.C.N.
Research Nurse, Section of Hematology/Oncology, Department of Medicine, The University of Illinois at Chicago, Chicago, Illinois
Hickman and Broviac Catheters
Interferon Alpha
Peripherally Inserted Central Catheter: PICC
Port-A-Cath
Tastuzumab

Joseph A. Sparano, M.D.
Associate Professor of Medicine, Albert Einstein College of Medicine; Montefiore Medical Center, Bronx, New York
Management of AIDS-Associated Malignancies

Walter M. Stadler, M.D.
Assistant Professor of Medicine, Department of Medicine, Section of Hematology/Oncology, University of Chicago, Chicago, Illinois
Floxuridine

Victoria Staszak, M.S. (Business Administration), M.S. (Nursing)
Clinical Nurse Specialist, The University of Chicago Hospitals, Chicago, Illinois
Arsenic Trioxide
Letrozole
Nilutamide

Gary D. Steinberg, M.D., F.A.C.S.
Assistant Professor, Director of Urologic Oncology, University of Chicago; Department of Surgery, Section of Urology, University of Chicago Cancer Research Center, Chicago, Illinois
Bacillus Calmette-Guerin (BCG)
Doxorubicin (Intravesical)
Intravesical Therapy: Introduction
Mitomycin C (Intravesical)
Thiotepa (Triethylenethiophosphoramide) (Intravesical)

Clinton F. Stewart, Pharm. D.
Associate Professor, Department of Clinical Pharmacy, School of Pharmacy, University of Tennessee; Associate Member, Department of Pharmaceutical Sciences, St. Jude Children's Research Hospital, Memphis, Tennessee
Chronic Renal Insufficiency

Diane E. Stover, M.D.
Instructor, Clinical Medicine; Chief of Pulmonary Medicine, Head of General Medicine, Memorial Sloan-Kettering Cancer Center, New York, New York
Cytotoxic Pulmonary Injury

Howard Streicher, M.D.
Foundation for the Advancement of Education in Science; Warren G. Magnuson Clinical Center, Bethesda, Maryland
Allergic Toxicity

Sandra Swain, M.D.
Medicine Branch, Division of Clinical Sciences, National Cancer Institute, Bethesda, Maryland
Congestive Heart Failure

Chris H. Takimoto, M.D., Ph.D.
Senior Investigator, Medicine Branch, Division of Clinical Sciences, National Cancer Institute, Bethesda, Maryland
9-Aminocamptothecin

Kim Tanner, R.Ph., B.C.O.P.
Director of Pharmacy, Harold C. Simmons Comprehensive Cancer Center, University of Texas Southwestern Medical Center, Dallas, Texas
Methotrexate
Trimetrexate

Kelly R. Terrill, Pharm. D.
Clinical Pharmacist, Hematology/Oncology/Bone Marrow Transplant, Primary Children's Medical Center, Salt Lake City, Utah
Graft-versus-Host Disease (GVHD)

Richard L. Theriault, M.D.
Professor of Medicine, University of Texas M.D. Anderson Cancer Center, Houston, Texas
Osteoporosis/Osteopenia

Patricia Tiller, R.N., B.S.N.
Research Nurse Clinician, University of Illinois at Chicago, Chicago, Illinois
Bacillus Calmette-Guerin (BCG)
Cardiotoxicity
Thiotepa (Triethylenethiophosphoramide) (Intravesical)

Nancy Velez-Piñeiro, R.Ph.
Pain Management Specialist, New York Harbor Healthcare System-Brooklyn Campus, Brooklyn, New York
Cancer Pain Management

Alan P. Venook, M.D.
Associate Professor of Clinical Medicine, University of California, San Francisco, California
Liver Dysfunction

Joey Vitanza, M.S., R.Ph., B.C.P.S.
Affiliate Assistant Clinical Professor, St. John's University, Jamaica, New York; Clinical Pharmacist for Hematology/Oncology, New York Harbor Healthcare System-Brooklyn Campus, Brooklyn, New York
Cancer Pain Management

Nicholas J. Vogelzang, M.D.
Fred C. Buffett Professor of Medicine, Director of Genitourinary Oncology, Section of Hematology/Oncology, The University of Chicago Medical Center, Chicago, Illinois
Antiandrogens and Related Drugs: Introduction
Bleomycin
Goserelin
Leuprolide

Everett E. Vokes, M.D.
Professor of Medicine and Radiation Oncology, University of Chicago Pritzker School of Medicine; Director, Section of Hematology/Oncology, University of Chicago, Chicago, Illinois
Hydroxyurea
Vinorelbine

John H. Ward, M.D.
Professor of Medicine; Chief, Hematology/Oncology Division, University of Utah School of Medicine, Salt Lake City, Utah
Diabetes Mellitus

D.I. Warkentin, Pharm.D.
Clinical Assistant Professor, The University of British Columbia, Faculty of Pharmaceutical Sciences; Pharmacotherapeutic Specialist, Bone Marrow Transplant/Oncology, CSV Pharmaceutical Sciences, Vancouver Hospital and Health Sciences Center, North Vancouver, British Columbia, Canada
Bladder Toxicity

Raymond P. Warrell, Jr., M.D.
President and CEO, Genta Incorporated, Berkeley Heights, New Jersey
All-Trans Retinoic Acid
Arsenic Trioxide

Dolores Watts, R.N., B.S.N., M.H.A.
Clinical Nurse Consultant II/Oncology Research Nurse, Head and Neck, University of Illinois Hospital, Chicago, Illinois
Chemotherapy-Induced Mucositis/Stomatitis
Docetaxel
Etoposide Phosphate
Floxuridine
5-Fluorouracil
Hydroxyurea
Paclitaxel

Robert A. Weisman, M.D., F.A.C.S.
Clinical Professor of Surgery, University of California, San Diego School of Medicine; Attending Physician, University of California, San Diego Medical Center; Thornton Hospital; VA Medical Center
Intra-Arterial Chemotherapy: Introduction
Cisplatin (Intra-Arterial)

Brenda R. Werner, R.N.
Oncology Research Nurse, University of Iowa Hospitals and Clinics, Iowa City, Iowa
Carboplatin
Cisplatin
Folinic Acid
Flutamide
Methotrexate
Neutropenic Fever
Suramin
Trimetrexate

Naomi Winick, M.D.
Professor of Pediatrics, University of Texas Southwestern Medical Center, Dallas, Texas
Teniposide

Mohamed Yassine, M.D.
Senior Research Specialist, Bone Marrow Transplant Program, University of Illinois at Chicago, Chicago, Illinois
Surgical Considerations

Todd M. Zimmerman, M.D.
Assistant Professor of Medicine, University of Chicago, Chicago, Illinois
Chlorambucil
Melphalan
Mechlorethamine

PREFACE

The treatment of cancer usually involves the administration of multiple medications, which may include chemotherapeutic agents, antiemetics, analgesics, and growth factors. Patients may also receive antibiotics and a host of other supportive-care agents. These agents may be administered orally or parenterally, with the latter often involving one or more infusion devices.

Optimal care of such patients requires a carefully choreographed schedule involving physicians, nurses, and pharmacists. Our intention is to reach out to all three groups with this book, which provides rapid access to concise and critical information on all drugs used in the care of the cancer patient—not just the chemotherapeutic agents. This information should facilitate the use of these drugs by both experienced practitioners and trainees.

The first part of the book (Chapters 1–10) focuses on antineoplastic therapy, and is primarily organized by the class of the agent. We have attempted to include investigational agents that we believed were strong candidates for regulatory approval, as well as all approved agents (albeit some are only approved outside the United States). The second part (Chapters 11–13) focuses on agents used in supportive care of oncology patients and on points to consider in the treatment of cancer patients who also have certain chronic illnesses. We have tried to be inclusive here, and the chapters range from the commonly prescribed antiemetics to some infrequently prescribed antibiotics, as well as a host of newer medications aimed at preventing complications of disease or treatment. The final chapter is on devices, with a focus on venous access catheters. This part was written primarily by and for the oncology nurse. However, it should be noted that virtually all of the chapters include major nursing input, as evidenced by the "Nursing Considerations" and the nurse co-authors.

The editors greatly appreciate the efforts of our many authors, who were selected for their expertise with a particular agent or class of agents. We are particularly pleased that the majority of our contributions have senior oncologists or oncology nurses as the first author, which we believe greatly enhanced the quality of the contributions. We also appreciate the loyal assistance of Deborah Stoit, Lisa Stillahn, and Karen Soprych, as well as our Senior Medical Editor at W. B. Saunders Company, Richard Lampert.

NOTICE

Oncology is an ever-changing field. Standard safety precautions must be followed, but as new research and clinical experience broaden our knowledge, changes in treatment and drug therapy become necessary or appropriate. Readers are advised to check the product information currently provided by the manufacturer of each drug to be administered to verify the recommended dose, the method and duration of administration, and the contraindications. It is the responsibility of the treating physician, relying on experience and knowledge of the patient, to determine dosages and the best treatment for the patient. Neither the publisher nor the editor assumes any responsibility for any injury and/or damage to persons or property.

THE PUBLISHER

CONTENTS

CHAPTER 3 TOPOISOMERASE INHIBITORS

CHAPTER 4 ANTIMETABOLITES AND THEIR MODULATORS

CHAPTER 5 MISCELLANEOUS CYTOTOXIC AND MODULATING AGENTS

Chapter 1

DNA-BINDING AGENTS

Introduction

M. Eileen Dolan

USES

- Lymphomas, brain tumors, testicular cancer, breast cancer, ovarian cancer, melanoma, multiple myeloma, leukemias
- Effective combination chemotherapy includes one or more alkylating agents
- Effects may be additive or synergistic
- In high-dose protocols with bone marrow transplantation
- Original agents used in chemical warfare

BIOCHEMICAL PHARMACOLOGY

- Generation of a highly reactive intermediate that attacks nucleophilic sites on biologic molecules
- Spontaneous or enzymatic conversion to active species
- Mono-functional alkylating agents covalently bind to DNA
- Bifunctional alkylating agents cross-link DNA
- Binding of reactive molecules to cellular DNA results in lethal event
- Sites of alkylation
  - N-7, O^6, N-1 of guanine
  - N-7, N-3, N-1 of adenine
  - N-3 of cytosine
  - O^4 of thymine
- Selectivity of binding
  - specific base sequence
- Selectivity at level of DNA tertiary structure
- Inhibition of DNA replication and transcription

MECHANISMS OF RESISTANCE

- O^6-alkylguanine-DNA alkyltransferase (AGT)
  - repair of nitrosourea-induced O^6 lesions
- Inactivation of alkylating species by conjugation with glutathione
- Increased dehydrogenase results in resistance to cyclophosphamide
- Altered drug transport

MODULATORS OF DNA-BINDING AGENTS

- Inactivators of DNA repair proteins
- Inactivators of O^6-alkylguanine-DNA alkyltransferase
- Inactivators of mismatch repair
- Inactivators of excision repair
- Glutathione and related enzymes
- Topoisomerase inhibitors
- Mitochondrial toxins
- Inhibitors of endothelial cell proliferation (antiangiogenic and angiostatic agents)
- Intercellular signaling pathways
- Cyclo-oxygenase
- Lipoxygenase

TOXICITY

- Myelosuppression
- Alopecia
- Nausea and vomiting
- Pulmonary fibrosis
- Leukemogenesis
- Infertility
- Teratogenesis
- Nephrotoxicity and ototoxicity (cisplatin)

KEY REFERENCES

Berger NA: Alkylating agents. Cancer Chemother Biol Response Modif 1994; 15:32–43

Lawley PD, Phillips DH: DNA adducts from chemotherapeutic agents. Mutat Res 1996; 355(1–2):13–40

Penketh PG, Shyam K, Sartorelli AC: Mechanisms of resistance to alkylating agents. Cancer Treat Res 1996; 87:65–81

Drug: Cyclophosphamide

Anthony D. Elias and Susan Noble-Kempin

OTHER NAMES: CYTOXAN, CPA, CTX

USES

- FDA approved for malignant lymphomas, multiple myeloma, leukemias, mycoses fungoides, neuroblastoma, retinoblastoma, breast
- Also active in SCLC, ovarian, bladder, pediatric sarcomas

MECHANISM OF ACTION

- Alkylating agent
- Prodrug activated by P-450 in liver to 4-OH CPA
- Further metabolized to phosphoramide mustard
- A bifunctional alkylator and cross-linker, predominantly at the N-7 position of guanine

DOSING

- Administered IV as a 1 hr infusion, but for high-dose therapy can be given multiple boluses/day or by continuous infusion (CI) over multiple days
- Usually given with mesna if at high dose (> 3 g/m^2)
- Can be given orally over 14 days every month
- Schedules/doses
  - 600–1,200 mg/m^2 IV q3–4 wks in combination with other agents
  - 2,000–3,000 mg/m^2 IV single dose or 2,000–4,000 mg/m^2 IV in fractionated doses (daily or bid) with G-CSF or other cytokines for mobilization and collection of autologous stem cells (also combined with etoposide or paclitaxel)
  - 4,500–7,200 mg/m^2 total dose duration over 3–4 days by bolus or CI combined with other agents during stem cell–supported high-dose therapy
- Mesna or forced hydration/diuresis is given
- Commonly used combinations
  - 600–1,200 mg/m^2 given with doxorubicin 60 mg/m^2 IV q3wks in breast cancer (CA)
- CMF
  - 600 mg/m^2 IV with methotrexate (40 mg/m^2) + 5-FU 600 mg/m^2 for breast cancer q3wks
  - 600 mg/m^2 IV day 1, 8, methotrexate 40 mg/m^2 IV day 1, 8, and 5-FU 600 mg/m^2 IV day 1, 8 q4wks
  - 100 mg/m^2 po days 1–14 with methotrexate 40 mg/m^2 IV day 1, 8, and 5-FU 600 mg/m^2 IV day 1, 8
- CHOP
  - 600–1,000 mg/m^2 with doxorubicin, vincristine, prednisone in non-Hodgkin's lymphoma
- Transplant
  - 6,000 mg/m^2 IV with thiotepa 500 mg/m^2 IV and carboplatin 800 mg/m^2 IV (CTCb) by 96 hr CI for autotransplant for breast cancer
  - 120–200 mg/kg IV with TBI 1,200 Cby (CyTBI) or busulfan 16 mg/m^2 po (BuCy) with allogeneic or autologous stem cell support for hematologic malignancies

PHARMACOKINETICS

- Activated by CYP2B6 and CYP3A4 in liver to 4-OH CPA +4 aldo CPA
- Deactivated to inactive metabolites by aldehyde oxidase and by aldehyde dehydrogenase
- Activation induced by itself
- Potential effect of other agents not well studied
- Terminal half-life of 3–12 hrs
- 4% excreted unchanged in urine

TOXICITY

- Neutropenia common
- Nausea/vomiting common, but usually moderate, peaking 6–8 hrs after dose
- Hemorrhagic cystitis uncommon but requires adequate hydration (≥2 L hydration recommended)
- Cardiotoxicity (correlated with peak doses)
- Interstitial pneumonitis and veno-occlusive disease. Rare as single agent but more common when combined with busulfan, BCNU, or TBI
- Conjunctivitis/jaw pain
  - can be relieved by diphenhydramine
- Transient SIADH common at transplant dose

RECOMMENDATIONS FOR SUPPORTIVE CARE

- Antiemetic prophylaxis is recommended, although there is no standard regimen

PHARMACY ISSUES

- NS or D_5W

NURSING CONSIDERATIONS

- High-dose therapy requires administration of mesna; catheterization may be necessary if urine output cannot be monitored
- Medicate with antiemetics prior to and prophylactically for 24 hrs post treatment
- Assess
  - mucous membranes for stomatitis
  - hepatic dysfunction and renal impairment
  - signs and symptoms of cardiomyopathy in patients receiving high dose
  - for pulmonary dysfunction
- Teach patient
  - expected side effects and self-care measures
  - need for contraception; teratogenic effects
  - importance of adequate hydration (3 L/d) and need for frequent voiding to reduce risk of hemorrhagic cystitis
  - associated metallic taste with drug; may chew gum or eat hard candy to relieve

KEY REFERENCES

Antman K, Ayash L, Elias A, et al.: A phase II study of high dose cyclophosphamide, thiotepa, and carboplatin with autologous marrow support in women with measurable advanced breast cancer responding to standard dose therapy. J Clin Oncol 1992; 10:102–10

Fleming RA: An overview of cyclophosphamide and ifosfamide pharmacology. Pharmacotherapy 1997; 17:146S–54S

Lee CK, Harman GS, Hohl RJ, et al.: Fatal cyclophosphamide cardiomyopathy: its clinical course and treatment. Bone Marrow Transplant 1996; 18:573–7

Wood WC, Budman DR, Korzun AH, et al.: Dose and dose intensity of adjuvant chemotherapy for stage II, node positive breast cancer. N Engl J Med 1994; 330:1253–9

Drug: Ifosfamide

Anthony D. Elias and Belinda Butler

OTHER NAMES: IFEX, IFF

USES

- FDA approved for third-line therapy of germ cell testicular cancer
- Approved in Japan for relapsed ovarian cancer
- Also active in breast, SCLC, NSCLC, bladder, pediatric sarcoma, STS, lymphoma, cervix, head, and neck cancer

MECHANISM OF ACTION

- Alkylating agent
- Prodrug activated by P-450 enzymes (CYP3A4 and others) in liver to 4-OH IFF
- Subsequently metabolized to phosphoramide mustard, which cross-links DNA (at N-7 position of guanine)
- Deactivated by aldehyde oxidase and aldehyde dehydrogenase in peripheral tissues

DOSING

- Administered IV as 1 hr infusion usually as fractionated doses over 3–5 days
  - can be given as continuous IV infusion
  - given routinely with mesna
- Schedules/doses
  - 2,000–2,500 $mg/m^2/d$ for 3–4 days (total 8,000–10,000 mg/m^2)
  - 12,000–16,000 mg/m^2 over 4–6 days with G-CSF support
  - 10,000–21,000 mg/m^2 in transplant regimens
  - mesna given IV bolus at 20% of the dose at 0, 3, 6, 9, or 0, 4, 8 hrs after each dose of IFF
  - oral formulation of IFF appears to produce greater CNS toxicity
- Commonly used combinations
  - (VIP or EIP): IFF 1,200 $mg/m^2/d \times 5$ with carboplatin 20 $mg/m^2/d \times 5$ with either etoposide 80 $mg/m^2/d \times 5$ or vinblastine 0.11 mg/kg on day 1 and 2
  - (MAID): IFF 2,000–2,500 $mg/m^2/d \times 3$ with doxorubicin 20 $mg/m^2/d \times 3$ and DTIC 300 $mg/m^2/d \times 3$
  - (ICE): IFF 2,000 $mg/m^2/d \times 3$ with carboplatin targeted to AUC 5–6, and etoposide 75–100 $mg/m^2/d \times 3$

PHARMACOKINETICS

- Activated by P-450 CYP3A4 in liver to 4-OH IFF and 4-aldo IFF, fourfold more slowly than CPA
- Deactivated to inactive metabolites by aldehyde oxidase and ALDH in peripheral tissues and RBCs
- Dechloroethylation by P-450 CYP3A4 is also an important pathway (50% of parent drug)
- Produces chloroacetaldehyde thought to be an intoxicant producing toxic-metabolic encephalopathy
- Terminal half-life ~6–15 hrs
- Saturable clearance at >4 $g/m^2/d$
- Activation induced by itself
- Drug interactions poorly studied

TOXICITY

- Neutropenia common
- Nausea/vomiting common, but typically moderate
- Hemorrhagic cystitis in 5% without mesna, less common with adequate hydration/urinary output and with mesna
- Renal toxicity common and normally reversible
  - mostly renal tubular acidosis, electrolyte wasting (K^+, Mg^{++}), and occasionally Fanconi's syndrome and diabetes insipidus–like syndromes
  - more common with high dose rates
  - creatinine can rise by day 4 with peak typically by day 7
  - dose-limiting toxicity at transplant dose
  - avoid concurrent nephrotoxins
  - higher risk with concurrent cisplatin
- CNS toxicity is $\leq 5\%$
  - toxic metabolic encephalopathy: confusion, hallucination
  - elderly or those with renal toxicity at greatest risk
  - timing parallels renal toxicity
  - methylene blue reported as antidote
- Interstitial pneumonitis and cardiotoxicity rare
- Mucositis and diarrhea uncommon except at transplant doses

RECOMMENDATIONS FOR SUPPORTIVE CARE

- Antiemetic prophylaxis is recommended, although there is no standard regimen

PHARMACY ISSUES

- NS or D_5W

NURSING CONSIDERATIONS

- Determine renal function prior to each dose, monitor BUN, creatinine, and creatinine clearance
- Prevent hematuria/hemorrhagic cystitis by use in combination with mesna, vigorous hydration (oral/parenteral), dose fractionation
- Premedicate with antiemetics and continue prophylactically for 24 hrs
- Can be administered by IV bolus slowly over 30 min or continuous infusion for 5 days
- Patients who have received prior or concurrent radiotherapy or other antineoplastic agents are at increased risk for toxicities
- Assess
  - for alterations in urinary elimination; pattern changes, symptoms of hemorrhagic cystitis/hematuria (test urine for occult blood), prior to each dose
  - neurologic/mental status prior to and during therapy (somnolence, confusion, depressive psychosis, and/or hallucinations)
  - alterations in nutrition related to nausea and vomiting
  - serum transaminase and alkaline phosphatase; transient elevations may occur but resolve spontaneously
- Teach patient
  - measures to prevent hemorrhagic cystitis with frequent voiding and pre- and posthydration of 2 L a day
  - potential hazards to fetus or nursing infants and the need for contraception
  - potential for delayed wound healing
  - avoid OTC aspirin-containing medications
  - encourage small frequent feedings

KEY REFERENCES

Coiffier B: Ifosfamide in the treatment of lymphoma. Semin Oncol 1996; 23:2–7

Elias A, Ryan L, Sulkes A, et al.: Response to mesna, doxorubicin, ifosfamide and dacarbazine in 108 patients with metastatic or unresectable sarcoma and no prior chemotherapy. J Clin Oncol 1989; 7:1208–16

Loehrer PJ, Ansari R, Gonin R, et al.: Cisplatin plus etoposide with and without ifosfamide in extensive small-cell lung cancer: a Hoosier Oncology Group study. J Clin Oncol 1995; 13:2594–9

Loehrer PJ, Lauer R, Roth BJ, et al.: Salvage therapy with VP-16 or vinblastine plus ifosfamide plus cisplatin in recurrent germ cell tumors. Ann Intern Med 1988; 109:540–6

Drug: Melphalan

Todd M. Zimmerman and Janan B. Geick Miller

USES

- FDA-approved indications include the treatment of multiple myeloma and nonresectable epithelial ovarian tumors
- Also active in breast cancer, neuroblastoma, and rhabdomyosarcoma

MECHANISM OF ACTION

- Bifunctional alkylating agent similar to mechlorethamine
- Transfer of ethylamine groups to susceptible (nucleophilic) atoms in proteins and nucleic acids
- Rate of cross-link formation is slower than mechlorethamine

DOSING

- Most often administered po
- IV formulation available for patients who cannot tolerate oral therapy
  - melphalan IV 16 mg/m^2
  - also used in high dose (140–200 mg/m^2) with stem cell support
- Common combinations for the treatment of multiple myeloma
  - melphalan po (8 mg/m^2/d or 0.2 mg/kg/d) for 4 days with prednisone po (50–60 mg/m^2/d) for 4 days; repeat q28d
  - subsequent dose should be adjusted to achieve mild neutropenia or thrombocytopenia with each cycle of therapy
  - VBMCP (M2 regimen): vincristine 0.03 mg/kg (maximum 2 mg), day 1; carmustine IV 0.5 mg/kg, day 1; cyclophosphamide IV 10 mg/kg, day 1; melphalan po 0.25 mg/kg, days 1–4; prednisone po 40 mg days 1–7, then taper over 14 days
  - VMCP: vincristine IV 1 mg day 1, melphalan po 6 mg/m^2/d days 1–4, cyclophosphamide po 125 mg/m^2/d days 1–4, prednisone 60 mg/m^2/d days 1–4

PHARMACOKINETICS

- Plasma melphalan levels are highly variable after oral dosing
- Oral bioavailability decreases when taken with food
- Melphalan is eliminated from plasma primarily by hydrolysis to monohydroxy- and dihydroxymelphalan
- Renal elimination appears to be low, but a higher incidence of leukopenia has been noted in patients with renal insufficiency
- Although specific dosing guidelines are not available, melphalan should be used with caution in patients with renal insufficiency

TOXICITY

- Neutropenia and thrombocytopenia are common with a nadir at 14–21 days, respectively; the nadir may be extended in heavily pretreated patients
- Mucositis, which is rare at standard doses, is encountered at higher doses
- Rare incidence of pulmonary toxicity and hypersensitivity
- Secondary leukemias and myelodysplasia have been reported with prolonged exposure
- Nausea and vomiting are minimal at standard doses, moderately emetogenic at higher doses

RECOMMENDATIONS FOR SUPPORTIVE CARE

- No routine supportive care measures are recommended for standard dose melphalan
- Antiemetic prophylaxis is recommended for moderate/high-dose melphalan

PHARMACY ISSUES

- Protect from light; store at room temperature
- IV solution must be prepared fresh. Solution is stable for 1 hr after dilution and must be administered within that time

NURSING CONSIDERATIONS

- CBC and platelet count monitored frequently
- Premedicate with antiemetic 1 hr prior to dose
- Drug is an irritant; avoid extravasation
- Patients receiving prolonged therapy should be monitored for second malignancy
- Assess
  - for signs of anaphylaxis when given IV usually occurring in the first 15 min after administration
  - pulmonary status for signs of dysfunction; obtain periodic PFTs
  - skin integrity for maculopapular rash and urticaria
- Teach patient
  - signs of infection, and bleeding
  - take drug on an empty stomach to reduce nausea
  - potential for impaired fertility

KEY REFERENCES

Osterborg A, Ahre A, Bjorkholm M: Alternating combination chemotherapy (VMCP/VBAP) is not superior to melphalan/prednisone in the treatment of multiple myeloma patients stage III—a randomized study from MGCS. Eur J Haematol 1989; 43(1):54–62

Rivkin SE, Green S, Metch B, et al.: Adjuvant CMFVP versus melphalan for operable breast cancer with positive axillary nodes: 10-year results of a Southwest Oncology Group study. J Clin Oncol 1989; 7(9):1229–38

Samuels BL, Bitran JD: High-dose intravenous melphalan: a review. J Clin Oncol 1995; 13(7): 1786–99

Vesole DH, Barlogie B, Jagannath S: High-dose therapy for refractory multiple myeloma: improved prognosis with better supportive care and double transplants. Blood 1994; 84(3):950–6

Drug: Busulfan

Louise B. Grochow and Deborah T. Berg

OTHER NAMES: MYLERAN

USES

- Approved by the FDA for chronic myelogenous leukemia (CML)
- Used for myeloablation in bone marrow transplantation

MECHANISM OF ACTION

- Bifunctional alkylating agent
- Second alkylation proceeds slowly
- GST detoxification

DOSING

- Administered po or IV
- 0.7–1 mg/kg q6hrs for 2–4 days (120–160 mg/m^2/d in infants) for myeloablation
  - may be administered in a single daily dose of 4 mg/kg
  - administered with antiseizure medication to reduce risk
  - pharmacokinetic monitoring to adjust exposure after first dose
  - infrequently used as small daily dose (i.e., 4 mg) for CML
- Commonly used combinations
  - commonly combined in sequence with cyclophosphamide

PHARMACOKINETICS

- Metabolized in the liver through reaction with glutathione (mediated by GST) to noncytotoxic metabolites
- More rapid clearance in infants and toddlers than older children and adults
- Absorption half-life 20–40 min
- Variable lag time
  - absorption is near complete (bioavailability 80–120%)
- Clearance rate shows diurnal variation with more rapid clearance in the evening
- Half-life ~2.5 hrs (range 1–7 hrs)
- 1–5% of parent compound excreted by kidneys
- Crosses the blood-brain barrier; causes seizures but not delayed neurotoxicity
- Drug interactions: clearance increased by phenytoin, and increases phenytoin clearance

TOXICITY

- Pancytopenia proceeding to aplasia if not supported with bone marrow reinfusion
- Nausea and vomiting common but well controlled with Ativan
- Seizures
- Hepatic veno-occlusive disease occurs in 20% without dose adjustment
- Lethal in 50% when VOD develops
- Pulmonary toxicity (interstitial pneumonia and pulmonary fibrosis)
- Mucositis
- Cataracts
- Hyperpigmentation
- Infertility

RECOMMENDATIONS FOR SUPPORTIVE CARE

- Antiemetic prophylaxis
- Antiseizure prophylaxis

NURSING CONSIDERATIONS

- In CML dose is adjusted based on WBC, thus need to monitor CBC closely
- Severe myelosuppression is produced with high-dose therapy
- Hyperuricemia may develop in setting of hyperleucocytosis
- Assess
  - pulmonary status for signs and symptoms of pulmonary fibrosis
  - mucous membranes for signs and symptoms of stomatitis
  - liver injury tests and abdomen for signs and symptoms of liver dysfunction or veno-occlusive disease
  - neurologic status for signs and symptoms of seizure activity with high-dose busulfan therapy
- Teach patient
  - expected side effects and self-care measures
  - to avoid OTC aspirin-containing medications
  - potential of permanent sterility

KEY REFERENCES

Grochow LB: Busulfan disposition: the role of therapeutic monitoring in bone marrow transplantation induction regimens. Semin Oncol 1993; 20(4 suppl 4):18–25

Hassan M, Ljungman P, Bolme P, et al.: Busulfan bioavailability. Blood 1994; 84(7):2144–50

Hehlmann R, Heimpel H, Hasford, et al.: Randomized comparison of busulfan and hydroxyurea in chronic myelogenous leukemia: prolongation of survival by hydroxyurea. The German CML Study Group. Blood 1993; 82(2):398–407

Santos GW: The development of busulfan/cyclophosphamide preparative regimens. Semin Oncol 1993; 20(4 suppl 4):12–6, quiz 17

Drug: Chlorambucil

Todd M. Zimmerman and Marianne Huml

OTHER NAMES: LEUKERAN, CLB

USES

- FDA-approved indications include treatment of chronic lymphocytic leukemia, indolent non-Hodgkin's lymphoma, and Hodgkin's disease
- Also used in the palliative management of Waldenstrom's macroglobulinemia

MECHANISM OF ACTION

- Bifunctional alkylating agent of the nitrogen mustard type
- Interferes with DNA replication and RNA transcription by alkylation and cross-linking the strands of DNA

DOSING

- Administered orally
- Common combinations
  - chlorambucil 0.4 mg/kg day 1, prednisone 100 mg/d for days 1–2; repeat q4wks
  - chlorambucil 0.1–0.2 mg/kg/d; often administered in conjunction with prednisone
  - dose of chlorambucil should be increased to achieve maximal response or until toxicity ensues

PHARMACOKINETICS

- Oral bioavailability: 70–80%; food interferes with absorption resulting in 10–20% decrease in bioavailability
- Significant (99%) drug binding to plasma proteins occurs in vitro
- Metabolized in liver to phenyl acetic acid mustard, which is active
- Half-life: 90–120 min
- Elimination: 60% excreted in urine within 24 hrs, principally as metabolites

TOXICITY

- Neutropenia and thrombocytopenia are common, especially with prolonged dosing
  - irreversible bone marrow damage has been reported
- Nausea and vomiting is uncommon at standard doses
- Infertility, both reversible and irreversible, has been reported
- Secondary leukemias and myelodysplasia may occur, especially after prolonged exposure to chlorambucil
- Central nervous system toxicities have been encountered with larger doses
- Alveolar dysplasia and pulmonary fibrosis have been reported with long-term use

RECOMMENDATIONS FOR SUPPORTIVE CARE

- No specific supportive care measures are required for standard dose chlorambucil

PHARMACY ISSUES

- Available in 2 mg tablets
- Store at room temperature

NURSING CONSIDERATIONS

- Monitor CBC, differential; nadir occurs 10 days after dose
- Monitor PFTs periodically; pulmonary fibrosis is more likely to occur in patients receiving concurrent irradiation and cyclophosphamide therapy; preexisting lung disease; and cumulative dose at 1 g/m^2
- Increased toxicity may occur with prior barbiturate use
- Assess
  - baseline pulmonary status and prior to each dose
  - potential for sensory/perceptual alterations (e.g., ocular disturbances)
- Teach patient
  - expected signs and symptoms and self-care measures
  - need for contraception

KEY REFERENCES

Dighiero G, Maloum K, Desablens B, et al.: Chlorambucil in indolent chronic lymphocytic leukemia. The French Cooperative Group on Chronic Lymphocytic Leukemia. N Engl J Med 1998; 338(21):1506–14

A randomized clinical trial of chlorambucil versus COP in stage B chronic lymphocytic leukemia. The French Cooperative Group on Chronic Lymphocytic Leukemia. Blood 1990; 75(7):1422–5

Hartvig P, Simonsson B, Oberg G, et al.: Inter- and intraindividual differences in oral chlorambucil pharmacokinetics. Eur J Clin Pharmacol 1988; 35(5):551–4

Drug: Mechlorethamine

Todd M. Zimmerman and Belinda Butler

OTHER NAMES: MUSTARGEN, NITROGEN MUSTARD

USES

■ FDA-approved indications include treatment of Hodgkin's disease, chronic lymphocytic leukemia, chronic myeloid leukemia, polycythemia vera, mycosis fungoides, and bronchogenic carcinoma

■ Intrapleural, intraperitoneal, and intrapericardial infusions may be used for the treatment of malignant effusions

MECHANISM OF ACTION

■ Prototypical bifunctional alkylating agent

■ Inhibits DNA and RNA synthesis via formation of carbonium ions

■ Produces interstrand and intrastrand crosslinks in DNA resulting in miscoding, breakage, and failure of replication

DOSING

■ MOPP: mechlorethamine IV 6 mg/m^2/d day 1, 8; vincristine IV 1.4 mg/m^2 (maximum dose 2 mg) day 1; procarbazine po 100 mg/m^2/d days 1–14; prednisone 40 mg/m^2/d days 1–14; repeat cycle q28d

■ Mechlorethamine intracavitary, 10–20 mg diluted in 10 ml

■ Mechlorethamine 0.1 mg/ml topically to cutaneous lesions of mycosis fungoides

PHARMACOKINETICS

■ Drug undergoes rapid chemical transformation; unchanged drug is undetectable in the blood within a few minutes

TOXICITY

■ Highly emetogenic; nausea and vomiting occur in virtually 100% of patients wiithout antiemetic prophylaxis

■ Neutropenia is common, as is thrombocytopenia

■ Permanent infertility is frequently encountered

■ Potent vesicant; thrombophlebitis may occur

■ Secondary leukemias have been reported several years after therapy

RECOMMENDATIONS FOR SUPPORTIVE CARE

■ Aggressive antiemetics (including seratonin antagonists) should be administered to all patients prior to therapy

■ G-CSF or GM-CSF may be required to maintain dose intensification

■ Young males of childbearing potential should be counseled regarding sperm banking prior to beginning therapy

PHARMACY ISSUES

■ Store intact vials at room temperature

■ Solution is highly unstable and must be infused within 1 hr after preparation

NURSING CONSIDERATIONS

■ Aggressive antiemetics required (including sedatives, seratonin antagonists, and dexamethasone) and should be continued for 24 hrs

■ Patients having received extensive radiotherapy and chemotherapy are at risk for profound bone marrow depression; monitor counts carefully

■ If drug is administered as a central infusion, it must be given via a central line

■ Potent vesicant

■ Systemic toxic effects may occur with intracavitary drug administration

■ Potential for hyperuricemia, monitor uric acid, renal and hepatic function

■ Access
  - injection sites for thrombosis and/or thrombophlebitis
  - patients with hemorrhagic tendencies for vascular accidents due to strain from severe nausea and vomiting
  - nutritional status for symptoms of dehydration due to severe nausea and vomiting or diarrhea

■ Teach patient
  - risk of second malignancies
  - potential for permanent infertility; counsel on sperm banking
  - practice contraception
  - avoid OTC aspirin-containing medications
  - expected side effects and self-care measures

KEY REFERENCES

Connors JM, Klimo P, Adams G, et al.: Treatment of advanced Hodgkin's disease with chemotherapy—comparison of MOPP/ABV hybrid regimen with alternating courses of MOPP and ABVD: a report from the National Cancer Institute of Canada clinical trials group. J Clin Oncol 1997; 15(4):1638–45

Henkelmann GC, Hagemeister FM, Fuller LM, et al.: Two cycles of MOPP and radiotherapy for stage III1A and stage III1B Hodgkin's disease. J Clin Oncol 1988; 6(8):1293–1302

Longo DL, Young RC, Wesley M, et al.: Twenty years of MOPP therapy for Hodgkin's disease. J Clin Oncol 1986; 4(9):1295–1306

Vonderheid EC, Tan ET, Kantor AF, et al.: Long-term efficacy, curative potential, and carcinogenicity of topical mechlorethamine chemotherapy in cutaneous T cell lymphoma. J Am Acad Dermatol 1989; 20(3): 416–28

Drug: BCNU

Roy B. Jones and Susan Noble-Kempin

OTHER NAMES: CARMUSTINE, BCNU, 1,3-BIS (2-CHLOROETHYL)-1-NITROSOUREA

USES

- Approved by the FDA for
  - primary gliomas, ependymomas, medulloblastoma, and metastatic brain tumors
  - myeloma (with prednisone)
  - combination therapy for relapsed or refractory Hodgkins disease or lymphomas
- Single or combination therapy of high-risk or metastatic melanoma
- Also used extensively in combination high-dose alkylating agent therapy with marrow progenitor cell support for breast cancer, Hodgkins disease and lymphomas, and brain tumors

MECHANISM OF ACTION

- Single-strand DNA alkylation and double-strand cross-links
- Alkyltransferase can remove single-strand alkylation products by suicide inactivation and thus reduce biologic effects
- 2-chlorethylisocyanate produced by BCNU hydrolysis causes toxicity by protein cross-linking
- Not affected by multidrug resistance mechanisms
- Not cross-resistant with other alkylating agents

DOSING

- Generally used doses are 100–200 mg/m^2, with increases to 300–600 mg/m^2 with bone marrow transplant (BMT) regimens
- Usually administered no more often than q6wks
- Frequently used combination regimens
- BCVPP (BCNU, cyclophosphamide, vinblastine, procarbazine, prednisone) for lymphomas
- CBV (cyclophosphamide, BCNU, etoposide)
- CPB (STAMP I; cyclophosphamide, cisplatin, BCNU)
- BEAM (BCNU, etoposide, cytarabine, melphalan) for BMT programs

PHARMACOKINETICS

- Bioactivated by hydrolysis forming a 2-chloroethyl carbonium ion equivalent and 2-chloroethyl isocyanate
- Metabolized by P-450-mediated reductive denitrosation and glutathione conjugation
- Half-life: 20–25 min

TOXICITY

- Prolonged and severe myelosuppression lasting up to 6 wks and cumulative with repeated dosing
- Nausea and vomiting is common and frequently severe
- Hypotension frequently occurs with infusions at doses > 300 mg/m^2
- Pulmonary fibrosis occurs frequently when cumulative dose > 1,000 mg/m^2 using repeated lower dose cycles
- Previous smoking may exacerbate
- Steroid-responsive acute lung injury occurs in 20–50% of patients receiving higher single doses
- Extravascular infiltration produces local tissue necrosis
- Single doses > 300 mg/m^2 can produce hepatic veno-occlusive disease, cortical central nervous system injury, and ischemic retinal toxicity

RECOMMENDATIONS FOR SUPPORTIVE CARE

- Intensive antiemetic support
- Transfusion and anti-infective prophylaxis with high or repeated dosing
- Intensive hydration and occasionally vasopressor support with doses > 300 mg/m^2
- Steroid treatment for acute lung injury

PHARMACY ISSUES

- Formulate drug in 10% ethanol prior to dilution with aqueous media
- Use within 2 hrs of formulation
- Potent mutagen, teratogen, carcinogen

NURSING CONSIDERATIONS

- Administer antiemetic prior to therapy and continue prophylactically for 24 hrs posttreatment
- Administer slowly through a free-flowing IV to prevent burning along the vein during infusion; flush line with normal saline or D_5W before and after administration
- If local discomfort/pain occurs, slow the infusion rate, place ice pack above injection site
- Should be administered last if several drugs are being given
- Closely monitor patients receiving higher single (300 mg/m^2) or cumulative (1,000 mg/m^2) doses
- An oily film on the bottom of the vial is evidence of decomposition; if present, discard vial
- Do not place in polyvinyl chloride containers; potency is lost through adsorption
- Handle carefully; if drug comes in contact with skin, wash area immediately with soap and water to prevent burning and brown staining
- Monitor blood counts prior to drug administration
- Assess
  - for signs and symptoms of veno-occlusive disease
  - signs and symptoms of delayed myelosuppression
  - potential for impaired gas exchange related to pulmonary fibrosis
  - liver dysfunction
  - baseline renal function, and monitor BUN and creatinine prior to each dose
  - sensory or perceptual alterations related to ocular toxicity can occur with high doses
- Teach patient
  - report vomiting of > 24 hrs
  - signs and symptoms and prevention of infection and bleeding, and the importance of immediately contacting physician if symptoms develop
  - potential for teratogenic effects and hazards to an unborn child; emphasize the need for contraception throughout the treatment period

KEY REFERENCES

Levin VA, Wara WM, Davis RL, et al.: Phase III comparison of BCNU and the combination of procarbazine, CCNU, and vincristine administered after radiotherapy with hydroxyurea for malignant gliomas. J Neurosurg 1985; 63(2):218–23

Oken MM, Harrington DP, Abramson N, et al.: Comparison of melphalan and prednisone with vincristine, carmustine, melphalan, cyclophosphamide, and prednisone in the treatment of multiple myeloma: results of Eastern Cooperative Oncology Group Study E2479. Cancer 1997; 79(8):1561–7

Reece DE, Barnett MJ, Shepherd JD, et al.: High-dose cyclophosphamide, carmustine (BCNU), and etoposide (VP16–213) with or without cisplatin (CBV + /-P) and autologous transplantation for patients with Hodgkin's disease who fail to enter a complete remission after combination chemotherapy. Blood 1995; 86(2):451–6

Rusthoven JJ, Quirt IC, Iscoe NA, et al.: Randomized, double-blind, placebo-controlled trial comparing the response rates of carmustine, dacarbazine, and cisplatin with and without tamoxifen in patients with metastatic melanoma. J Clin Oncol 1996; 14(7):2083–90

Drug: Lomustine

M. Kelly Nicholas and Susan Noble-Kempin

OTHER NAMES: CCNU, CEENU

USES

- Approved by FDA for the treatment of primary and metastatic brain tumors following surgery and/or radiotherapy
- Approved by FDA for the treatment of primary and refractory Hodgkin's disease
- Occasionally used in advanced metastatic breast cancer and melanoma

MECHANISM OF ACTION

- Covalent DNA-binding drug, damaging the DNA template through alkylation
- May inhibit enzymatic processes via protein carbamoylation
- Elevated levels of O^6-alykylguanine DNA alkyltransferase may be associated with drug resistance

DOSING

- Administered orally
- Schedules/doses
  - 110 mg/m^2 on day 1 of PCV chemotherapy in combination with procarbazine 60 mg/m^2 on days 8–21 and vincristine 1.4 mg/m^2 (maximum 2 mg) IV day 8 and 29
    - □ conventionally repeated q6–8 wks as tolerated for 6 cycles in the treatment of primary brain tumors
  - 100 mg/m^2 on day 1 and 28 of B-CAVe chemotherapy in combination with bleomycin 5 U/m^2 IV on day 1, 28, and 35; doxorubicin 60 mg/m^2 IV on day 1 and 28, and vinblastine 5 mg/m^2 IV on day 1 and 28 in treatment of recurrent Hodgkin's disease
  - used in many other combined-treatment regimens for recurrent Hodgkin's disease, including ABDIC, Dexa-BEAM, CBVD, CEP, CEVD, and VABCD

PHARMACOKINETICS

- Rapidly absorbed following oral administration
- Parent compound is detectable in plasma after IV but not oral dosing
- The half-life of metabolites ranges from 16–48 hrs
- CSF concentrations of parent drug and metabolites exceed concurrent plasma concentrations by ≥50%, presumably due to high lipid solubility and low ionization at physiologic pH
- Some microsomal metabolism may occur

TOXICITY

- Delayed myelosuppression may be dose limiting
- Thrombocytopenia usually occurs 4 wks after drug administration
- Leukopenia may be delayed until 5–6 wks after drug administration
- Anemia may occur but is rare
- Pulmonary fibrosis may occur 6 mos or longer following treatment
- The risk for pulmonary toxicity is cumulative dose dependent, occurring more often after doses > 1,100 mg/m^2
- Nausea and vomiting commonly occur several hours after administration and usually last < 24 hrs
- Reversible hepatotoxicity is rarely reported
- Progressive renal dysfunction has been described following large cumulative doses

RECOMMENDATIONS FOR SUPPORTIVE CARE

- Antiemetic prophylaxis is recommended, but no standard regimen exists

PHARMACY ISSUES

- Supplied as 10 mg, 40 mg, and 100 mg capsules
- Should be taken on empty stomach

NURSING CONSIDERATIONS

- Do not administer concurrently with other emetogenic drugs. Premedicate with antiemetics prior to therapy and continue prophylactically for 24 hrs post treatment
- Review relevant lab values (i.e., CBC, WBC, platelets, BUN, and creatinine) prior to drug administration. (If abnormalities are noted, a creatinine clearance should be determined)
- Assess
  - altered urinary elimination
  - infection and bleeding related to myelosuppression
  - pulmonary function and signs of infection
- Teach patient
  - report signs/symptoms of unusual bleeding; avoid activities/procedures that could cause bleeding when thrombocytopenic
  - infection prevention measure; report signs/symptoms of infection
  - need for contraception because of potential for teratogenic effects and hazards to the unborn
  - suggest frequent and small feedings and importance of adequate hydration; discourage alcohol consumption after dosing
  - dosage may consist of two or more different-colored capsules; all capsules should be taken at one time
  - take on an empty stomach at bedtime

KEY REFERENCES

Cairncross JG, MacDonald DR, Ludwin S, et al.: Chemotherapy for anaplastic oligodendroglioma. J Clin Oncol 1994; 12:2013–21

Harker GW, Kushlan P, Rosenberg SA: Combination chemotherapy for advanced Hodgkin's disease after failure of MOPP: ABVD and B-CAVE. Ann Intern Med 1984; 101: 440–6

Levin VA, Silver P, Hannigan J, et al.: Superiority of post-radiotherapy adjuvant chemotherapy with CCNU, procarbazine and vincristine (PCV) over BCNU for anaplastic gliomas: NGOG 6G61 final report. Int J Radiat Oncol Biol Phys 1990; 18:321–4

Drug: Fotemustine

David Khayat and Kristine Rossof

OTHER NAMES: MUPHORAN

USES

- Metastatic malignant melanoma
- Metastatic non–small cell lung cancer
- Cerebral tumors
- This drug is not yet approved by the FDA in the US but is available in several countries in Europe, Asia, South Africa, and South America

MECHANISM OF ACTION

- Similar to other nitrosoureas
- Cytotoxicity primarily related to its alkylating activity
- Carbamoylation of cellular proteins may also be important
- Increased penetration across the blood-brain barrier may be due to presence in the molecule of an alanine amino acid
- Mechanism of resistance mainly due to O^6-alkylguanine-DNA-alkyltransferase

DOSING

- Administered IV as a 1 hr infusion
- Schedules/doses
  - 100 mg/m^2 weekly for 3 to 4 wks followed by a 4–5 wk rest period for induction; then, 100 mg/m^2 q3wks
- Commonly used combination
  - 100 mg/m^2 day 1, 8 in combination with dacarbazine 350 mg/m^2 day 1, 8 or day 1, 2 q3wks
- Hepatic intra-arterial administration of fotemustine at equivalent dose and schedule but as a 4 hr infusion

PHARMACOKINETICS

- Plasma protein binding is limited (25–30%)
- Penetrates significantly through the blood-brain barrier and can be found in the cerebrospinal fluid
- Short half-life of 30 min
- Rapidly metabolized to chloroethanol and diethyl-N-nitroso-1-imidazolidone ethyl phosphonate, which is then transformed into acetic acid
- Undergoes urinary excretion (50–60% of the administered dose) and fecal elimination

TOXICITY

- Delayed (days 42–46) thrombocytopenia and leukopenia (45%)
- Other toxicities include nausea, vomiting, and transient elevation of hepatic transaminases, alkaline phosphatases, and bilirubin without clinical consequences
- Rare toxicities include diarrhea, phlebitis, fever, abdominal pain, pruritus, transient and reversible neurologic symptoms (aguesia, paresthesia)

RECOMMENDATIONS FOR SUPPORTIVE CARE

- Antiemetic prophylaxis is recommended using a serotonin antagonist

PHARMACY ISSUES

- 5% dextrose is the preferred diluent
- Sodium chloride should not be used

NURSING CONSIDERATIONS

- Monitor CBC, platelets, hepatic transaminase, BUN, and creatinine
- Administered as an outpatient
- Toxicities moderate and manageable
- Hypersensitivity to other nitrosoureas
- Take precaution in patients with hepatic and renal disease
- Take precaution with doses higher than 100 mg/m^2
- Assess
  - hepatic dysfunction
  - renal impairment
  - pulmonary toxicity can present as pneumonia with sequential dacarbazine and fotemustine administration
- Teach patient
  - expected side effects and self-care measures

KEY REFERENCE

Jacquillat CL, Khayat D, et al.: Final report of the French multicenter phase II study of the nitrosourea fotemustine in 153 evaluable patients with disseminated malignant melanoma including patients with cerebral metastasis. Cancer 1990; 66:1873–8

Drug: Temozolomide

Edward S. Newlands and Helen Evans

OTHER NAMES: TEMODAL, CCRG 81045, M&B 39831, NSC 362856

USES

- Data to be submitted for licensing to the FDA in the US and EMEA in Europe for patients with malignant glioma and melanoma

MECHANISM OF ACTION

- DNA alkylator
- Prodrug spontaneously activating at physiologic pH to MTIC
- DNA methylating agent
- Cells that are mismatch repair deficient may be resistant
- Inhibition of alkyltransferase sensitizes cells to temozolomide

DOSING

- Orally bioavailable
- Schedules/doses
- 200 $mg/m^2 \times 5$ repeated q4wk
- Continuous administration over 7 wks (preliminary data indicates that 75 mg/m^2 daily for 7 wks can be administered safely)

PHARMACOKINETICS

- Ring spontaneously opens at physiologic pH to MTIC, which is the active form of the drug
- Peak plasma levels at 0.7 hrs after oral administration
- Half-life 1.8 hrs

TOXICITY

- Myelosuppression is dose limiting, affecting both neutrophils and platelets
- Nausea and vomiting is common but is usually controlled by serotonin antagonists
- Other toxicities are uncommon on the schedules identified here

RECOMMENDATIONS FOR SUPPORTIVE CARE

- Antiemetic prophylaxis with serotonin antagonists is recommended

PHARMACY ISSUES

- Temozolomide capsules are stable at room temperature

NURSING CONSIDERATIONS

- Premedication with administration of serotonin antagonist to decrease nausea and vomiting
- Myelosuppression is dose limiting
- No known adverse reactions with other drugs
- Assess
  - fatigue, particularly on days of administration of temozolomide
  - psychological support, particularly for neuro-oncology patients
  - skin changes (pigmentation)—in relation to sun exposure
- Teach patient
  - for neuro-oncology patients, the importance of repeated, clear, concise explanations of rationale and toxicity of treatment cannot be overstressed
  - to take drug at the same time daily
  - avoidance of sun to decrease pigmentation of skin
  - expected side effects and self-care measures in relation to neutropenia and thrombocytopenia

KEY REFERENCE

Newlands ES, et al.: Temozolomide: a review of its discovery, chemical properties, preclinical development and clinical trials. Cancer Treatment Reviews 1997; 23:35–81

Drug: Dacarbazine

David Khayat and Susan Noble-Kempin

OTHER NAMES: DTIC, DETICENE

USES

- Metastatic malignant melanoma
- Sarcoma
- Hodgkin's disease

MECHANISM OF ACTION

- Alkylating agent, monofunctional
- Must be activated through oxidative N-demethylation by liver enzymes to methyl diazonium, which methylates DNA
- Main mechanism of resistance is related to O^6-alkylguanine-DNA-alkyltransferases
- Presence of P-glycoprotein does not confer resistance

DOSING

- Administered IV as a 30 min infusion, protected from light
- Schedules/doses
  - 400–1,200 mg/m²/cycle divided into 1–5 daily doses
  - commonly used combinations
    - □ ABVD (Hodgkin's disease)
      - ▽ doxorubicin: 25 mg/m² day 1, 15
      - ▽ bleomycin: 10 U/m² day 1, 15
      - ▽ dacarbazine: 375 mg/m² day 1, 15
      - ▽ vinblastine: 6 mg/m² day 1, 15
    - □ CYVADIC (sarcoma)
      - ▽ cyclophosphamide: 500 mg/m² day 1
      - ▽ vincristine: 1 mg/m² day 1
      - ▽ doxorubicin: 50 mg/m² day 1
      - ▽ dacarbazine: 300 mg/m² day 1, 2, 3
    - □ DF (melanoma)
      - ▽ dacarbazine: 350 mg/m² day 1, 2
      - ▽ fotemustine—100 mg/m² day 1, 8
  - intra-arterial infusion for melanoma: 100 mg/m²/d for 5 days

PHARMACOKINETICS

- Biphasic with terminal half-life of 0.5 to 3 hrs
- Poor penetration into the spinal fluid
- Main site of metabolism is liver
- Variable renal excretion that decreases at higher doses

TOXICITY

- Nausea and vomiting are severe and frequent
- Leukopenia and, to a lesser extent, thrombocytopenia is moderate, dose dependent, and reversible
- More rarely, flulike syndrome with chills, malaise, dizziness
- Other rare toxicities include alopecia, transient hepatic liver dysfunction, eosinophilia, facial paresthesia
- Anaphylaxis occurs rarely

RECOMMENDATIONS FOR SUPPORTIVE CARE

- Antiemetics are necessary; neuroleptics, such as haloperidol, may be useful

PHARMACY ISSUES

- D_5W or sodium chloride can be used as diluent

NURSING CONSIDERATIONS

- Should not be administered before fotemustine (risk of ARDS)
- Generally administered in 250–500 mL over 15–30 min
- Use of hot packs or ice above injection site may decrease local pain, burning sensation, and irritation
- To minimize vein trauma when given peripherally, consider premedication with hydrocortisone IVP (DTIC forms precipitate with SoluCortef but not with hydrocortisone), lidocaine, or heparin
- A color change from pale yellow to pink is indicative of decomposition; discard solution
- Strong emetic potential; medicate with antiemetics and continue prophylactically for 24 hrs
- Evaluate blood counts and liver functions prior to administration
- Assess
  - potential for sensory/perceptual alterations related to facial paresthesia
  - hepatic dysfunction
  - blood counts
- Teach patient
  - avoid OTC aspirin-containing medications
  - regarding use of sunscreen and to avoid exposure to strong sunlight
  - suggest small feedings; importance of adequate hydration
  - need for contraception
  - signs, symptoms of infection, bleeding

KEY REFERENCES

Bonadonna G, et al: Combination chemotherapy of Hodgkin's disease with adriamycin, bleomycine, vinblastine and imidazole carboximide (ABVD) versus MOPP. Cancer 1975; 36:252–3

Buesa JM, Urrechaga E: Clinical pharmacokinetics of high-dose DTIC. Cancer Chemother Pharmacol 1991; 28:475–9

Drug: Thiotepa

Roy B. Jones and Janine Caggiano

OTHER NAMES: THIOPLEX

USES

- FDA approved for
  - breast carcinoma
  - ovarian carcinoma
  - intracavitary malignant effusions
  - superficial bladder tumors
  - lymphomas and Hodgkin's disease
  - also widely used in bone marrow transplant (BMT) regimens for breast cancer and hematologic malignancies and intrathecal treatment of meningeal carcinomatosis

MECHANISM OF ACTION

- DNA single- and double-strand alkylation
- Aziridine prodrug

DOSING

- 8–15 mg/m^2 at 3–4 wk intervals for standard IV regimens
- 10–15 mg for intrathecal use
- 500–1,000 mg/m^2 in BMT regimens
- Commonly used combinations
  - CTCb (cyclophosphamide, thiotepa, carboplatin), CT (cyclophosphamide, thiotepa) for BMT

PHARMACOKINETICS

- Extensively metabolized by P-450 enzymes
- TEPA metabolite is active but less so than thiotepa
- Deactivated by glutathione conjugation
- Half life: 1.5–4 hrs
  - Probably increases with increasing doses
- Concomitant administration of thiotepa and cyclophosphamide reduces formation of reactive cyclophosphamide metabolites

TOXICITY

- Dose-dependent myelosupression
- Nausea and vomiting (mild to moderate)
- BMT toxicities: mucositis, hepatic veno-occlusive disease, CNS

RECOMMENDATIONS FOR SUPPORTIVE CARE

- Antiemetic prophylaxis of intermediate intensity
- Antibacterial and antifungal prophylaxis directed at gastrointestinal organisms with BMT doses

PHARMACY ISSUES

- Use within 8 hrs of formulation
- Potent mutagen, teratogen, carcinogen

NURSING CONSIDERATIONS

- Standard chemotherapy handling precautions
- Double-verify BMT doses prior to administration
- Drug is an irritant; should be given through side arm of a running IV
- Premedicate with antiemetics and continue for at least 12 hrs after drug is given
- Monitor CBC, platelet count prior to drug administration
- Assess
  - for myelosuppression and prolonged thrombocytopenia
  - for rash and hives
  - potential for hypersensitivity reaction
  - for local irritation
- Teach patient
  - drug is mutagenic; sterility may be reversible; discuss strategies of sperm banking
  - risk of secondary malignancy and importance of health maintenance
  - instruct on neutropenic precautions and bleeding precautions

KEY REFERENCES

Antman K, Eder JP, Elias A, et al.: High-dose thiotepa alone and in combination regimens with bone marrow support. Semin Oncol 1990; 17(1 suppl 3):33–8

O'Dwyer PJ, LaCreta F, Engstrom PF, et al.: Phase I/pharmacokinetic reevaluation of thiotepa. Cancer Res 1991; 51(12):3171–6

Drug: Mitomycin

Hedy L. Kindler and Consuelo Skosey

OTHER NAMES: MITOMYCIN-C, MUTAMYCIN

USES

- Curative when used in combined-modality therapy of squamous cell carcinoma of the anal canal
- Also active in non–small cell lung cancer, gastric cancer, head and neck cancer, malignant mesothelioma, pancreatic cancer, esophageal cancer, breast cancer, and cervical cancer

MECHANISM OF ACTION

- Antitumor antibiotic derived from *Streptomyces*
- A bioreductive alkyalting agent preferentially activated under hypoxic conditions
- Alkylates DNA, inducing inter- and intrastrand cross-links and DNA adducts

DOSING

- Administered IV by slow push over 20 to 30 min or as a rapid infusion in the sidearm of a free-flowing IV line
- IV
  - 20 mg/m² q6wks as a single agent; 10 mg/m² q6wks when used in combination
- Commonly used combinations
  - FAM: 5-fluorouracil 600 mg/m² IV day 1, 8, 29, 36; doxorubicin 30 mg/m² IV day 1, 29; mitomycin 10 mg/m² IV on day 1
  - FM/RT: mitomycin 10 mg/m² IV on day 1, 43; continuous infusion 5-fluorouracil 1,000 mg/m²/d for 4 days × 2; radiotherapy 45–50 Gy
  - MV: mitomycin 10 mg/m² q4wks; vinblastine 6 mg/m² q2wks
  - MVP: vinblastine 4.5 mg/m² weekly, with half dose on day 8, or vindesine 3 mg/m² weekly; cisplatin 120 mg/m² day 1, 29 and q6wks; mitomycin 8 mg/m² with the first 3 doses of cisplatin only
  - MIC: mitomycin 6 mg/m²; ifosfamide 3 g/m²; cisplatin 100 mg/m² q4wks

PHARMACOKINETICS

- Cleared rapidly from the vascular compartment
- Terminal half-life 25–90 min
- Primarily hepatically metabolized, although metabolism also occurs in other tissues

TOXICITY

- Cumulative myelosuppression is dose limiting
- Neutropenia and thrombocytopenia can occur up to 8 wks after treatment
- Bronchospasm can develop when administered with vinca alkaloids
- Hemolytic uremic syndrome in 2–10% at cumulative doses > 50 mg/m²
- Pulmonary fibrosis, responsive to steroids
- Radiation recall
- Nausea in 10–30% of patients
- Stomatitis
- Mitomycin is a vesicant. Extravasation can produce severe cellulitis with ulceration

RECOMMENDATIONS FOR SUPPORTIVE CARE

- Prophylactic corticosteroids can prevent pulmonary toxicity but may affect efficacy

PHARMACY ISSUES

- Sterile water is the preferred diluent

NURSING CONSIDERATIONS

- The reconstituted solution requires protection from light if not used within 24 hrs
- Moderate emetic potential; provide antiemetic support
- Monitor renal and pulmonary function
- Assess
  - baseline pulmonary status and monitor during therapy for signs of pulmonary toxicity
  - evaluate relevant laboratory values prior to each dose (CBC, clotting tests, renal and liver functions)
  - observe site for signs of extravasation; delayed dermal reactions are possible
- Teach patient
  - report difficulty in breathing, swelling, burning, or pain at injection site, unusual bleeding or bruising
  - report painful or burning urination
  - may cause permanent sterility and birth defects
- Vesicant; take precautions to avoid extravasation

KEY REFERENCES

Flam M, John M, Pajak TF, et al.: Role of mitomycin in combination with fluorouracil and radiotherapy, and of salvage chemoradiation in the definitive nonsurgical treatment of epidermoid carcinoma of the anal canal: results of a phase III randomized intergroup study. J Clin Oncol 1996; 14(9):2527–39

Pisters KM, Kris MG, Gralla RJ, et al.: Pathologic complete response in advanced non-small-cell lung cancer following preoperative chemotherapy: implications for the design of future non-small-cell lung cancer combined modality trials. J Clin Oncol 1993; 11(9):1757–62

Drug: Hexamethylmelamine

Franco M. Muggia and Kristine Rossof

OTHER NAMES: ALTRETAMINE, HEXALEN, HMM

USES

- Approved by FDA for ovarian cancer failing first-line chemotherapy
- Antitumor activity in other solid tumors not determined by current criteria

MECHANISM OF ACTION

- Unknown, but hydroxylated metabolites likely form covalent bonds with DNA
- Needs microsomal activation for antitumor activity
- Not cross-resistant with classic alkylating agents
- Parent drug or metabolites do not yield nitrobenzyl piridine (NBP) reactive tests

DOSING

- Administered in daily oral schedules
- Most commonly used dose schedule is 180–260 mg/m^2/d × 14d q28d, in 4 divided doses
- Drug is most often given after meals and at bedtime, preceded by antiemetics
- Higher doses may be tolerable for shorter periods of time, but limited by nausea
- Most often used as single agent after failure of other drugs

PHARMACOKINETICS

- Microsomal metabolism removes methyl groups yielding various melamine derivatives and converted enzymatically to cytotoxic methylol derivatives
- Highly variable bioavailability because of variable first-pass metabolism in liver
- Half-life of the parent compound usually varies between 5 and 10 hrs

TOXICITY

- Nausea and vomiting is most prominent toxicity, related to dose and cumulative dose
- Peripheral neuropathy, both sensory and motor, may be ameliorated by pyridoxine
- Central nervous system toxicity: mood disorders, hallucinations, ataxia, vertigo
- Leukopenia and thrombocytopenia, with nadirs, usually at 3–4 wks
- Rarely: liver dysfunction, anemia, alopecia, skin rashes
- Toxicities are usually reversible upon discontinuation

RECOMMENDATIONS FOR SUPPORTIVE CARE

- Avoid concurrent administration of monoamine oxidase (MAO) inhibitors, which may cause orthostatic hypotension
- Antiemetics (dexamethasone, prochlorperazine, serotonin antagonists) may be helpful

PHARMACY ISSUES

- Supplied in 50 mg capsules, and stable at room temperature for 2 yrs

NURSING CONSIDERATIONS

- Leukopenia occurs end of first week of therapy; nadir occurs 3–4 wks post treatment; monitor CBC, WBC, differential and platelet count
- Can cause orthostatic hypotension if given concomitantly with MAO antidepressants
- May exacerbate neurotoxicities of other agents such as vinca alkaloids, cisplatin, paclitaxel; concurrent B6 (pyridoxine) may decrease neurotoxicity
- Assess
  - alterations in skin integrity
  - baseline neurologic status
  - alterations related to peripheral neuropathy and CNS effects
  - alterations in elimination and kidney dysfunction
- Teach patient
  - expected side effects and self-care measures
  - take 1–2 hrs after meals with antiemetic
  - use of preventative laxative
  - avoid alcohol and aspirin
  - consult with physician prior to dental work

KEY REFERENCE

Vergote I, et al.: Hexamethylmelamine as second-line therapy in platin-resistant ovarian cancer. Gyn Oncol 1992; 47:282–6

Drug: Procarbazine

M. Kelly Nicholas and Janan B. Geick Miller

OTHER NAMES: MATULANE

USES

- Used in combination chemotherapy for Hodgkin's lymphoma
- Used in combination chemotherapy or as a single agent in malignant glioma
- Also active in melanoma, small cell lung cancer, and non-Hodgkin's lymphoma

MECHANISM OF ACTION

- Methylation at O-6 and N-7 positions on guanine
- Oxidation to azoprocarbazine releases hydrogen peroxide affecting DNA–protein interactions via sulfhydryl groups
- Possible inhibition of t-RNA via inhibition of transmethylation

DOSING

- Administered orally
- Schedules/doses
  - administered at 50–100 mg/m^2 for 1–2 wks as part of many combination chemotherapy regimens for Hodgkin's lymphoma including BCVPP, ChlVPP, C-MOPP, MOPP, MVPP, and MVVPP
  - administered at 60 mg/m^2 for 2 wks on either days 1–14 or 8–21 as part of PCV chemotherapy for malignant glioma in conjunction with lomustine, 110 mg/m^2 on day 1 and vincristine, 1.4 mg/m^2 day 8, 29, repeated q6wks
  - administered at 50–150 mg/m^2 for 14–21 days as a single agent for malignant glioma, repeated q6wks

PHARMACOKINETICS

- Rapidly absorbed after oral administration with auto-oxidation to azoprocarbazine with subsequent metabolism via cytochrome P-450 to methylazoxyprocarbazine and benzylazoxyprocarbazine
- Half-life of parent compound 10 min, major metabolites 1 hr
- Crosses the blood-brain barrier efficiently, with rapid equilibration between plasma and cerebral spinal fluid

TOXICITY

- Leukopenia and thrombocytopenia, occurring 2–8 wks after initiating treatment
- Hemolysis in patients with G-6-PD deficiency
- Nausea and vomiting, often diminishing with ongoing treatment and lessened with stepwise increases in dose during the initiation of treatment and the use of standard antiemetic drugs
- Acute hypertensive reactions following coadministration of tricyclic antidepressants, sympathomimetic amines, or foods with a high tyramine content
- Altered mental status
- Rarely: psychotic reactions
- Paresthesias and peripheral neuropathy
- Arthralgias and myalgias
- Disulfuram-like reaction with ethanol coadministration
- Stomatitis
- Diarrhea

RECOMMENDATIONS FOR SUPPORTIVE CARE

- Antiemetic prophylaxis may be needed, especially during the initiation of treatment

PHARMACY ISSUES

- Supplied as 50 mg capsules

NURSING CONSIDERATIONS

- Patient education regarding dietary restrictions while taking procarbazine
- CBC and platelet count should be obtained and monitored closely
- Emetic potential moderately high; premedicate with antiemetic and use prophylactically
- Assess
  - neurologic status for alterations in perception and motor function
  - alteration in nutritional status
  - skin integrity for dermatitis reactions
- Teach patient
  - regarding food incompatibilities; avoidance of alcohol and foods high in tyramine (yogurt, ripe cheese, bananas)
  - to divide doses and take with meals to decrease GI toxicity
  - avoidance of antihistamines, barbiturates, and narcotics
  - impaired fertility

KEY REFERENCES

DeVita VT Jr, Serpick AA, Carbone PP: Combination chemotherapy in the treatment of advanced Hodgkin's disease. Ann Intern Med 1970; 73:881–95

Levin VA, Silver P, Hannigan J, et al.: Superiority of post-radiotherapy adjuvant chemotherapy with CCNU, procarbazine, and vincristine (PCV) over BCNU for anaplastic gliomas: NCOG 6G61 final report. Int J Radiat Oncol Biol Phys 1990; 18(2):321–4

Perry JR, Louis DN, Cairncross JG: Current treatment of oligodendrogliomas. Arch Neurol 1999; 56(4):429–33

Drug: Cisplatin

Jan H.M. Schellens, Jos H. Beijnen, and Brenda Werner

OTHER NAMES: PLATINOL, PLATINOL-AQ (USA), ABIPLATIN (CANADA)

USES

- Accepted indications are metastatic testicular cancer, ovarian cancer, transitional bladder cancer
- Also active and commonly used in head and neck cancer, non–small cell lung cancer, cervical cancer, endometrial cancer, gastric cancer, osteosarcoma, relapsing non-Hodgkin's lymphoma

MECHANISM OF ACTION

- Covalent binding to macromolecules such as DNA and RNA
- Four major intra- and interstrand DNA adducts are formed; the lethal lesion is not yet known
- Mechanisms of resistance include decreased intracellular accumulation, intracellular inactivation by glutathione or metallothioneins, mismatch repair deficiency, multidrug resistance protein (MRP) overexpression

DOSING

- Administered IV
- Infusion duration varies considerably, but most often 1–4 hrs
- Schedules/doses
  - many different schedules are used: once q3 or 4 wks, every week, daily × 5 q21d
- Commonly used combinations
  - BEP: bleomycin, etoposide, cisplatin; cisplatin 20 mg/m^2 × 5 q21d (testicular cancer)
  - MVP: mitomycin C, vinblastine, cisplatin; cisplatin 100 mg/m^2 q28d (NSCLC)
  - cisplatin/gemcitabine; cisplatin 75 or 100 mg/m^2 q21d (NSCLC)
  - cisplatin/paclitaxel; cisplatin 75 mg/m^2 (ovarian cancer)
  - MVAC: methotrexate, vinblastine, doxorubicin, cisplatin; cisplatin 70 mg/m^2 q28d (bladder cancer)

PHARMACOKINETICS

- Clearance of unbound drug by irreversible tissue and protein binding (major components) and by renal excretion
- Mostly mono-exponential decline of the plasma concentration time curve of unbound platinum
- Terminal half-life ~45 min
- Moderate interpatient variation in clearance
- Variation in creatinine clearance has only a moderate influence on exposure to cisplatin as measured in plasma
- Linear, but complex, pharmacokinetics
- Dose modifications in case of moderate renal dysfunction (creatinine clearance > 50 ml/min) are not recommended
- Important pharmacokinetic drug interactions include nephrotoxic and ototoxic medications (e.g., NSAIDs, aminoglycosides)
- Important pharmacodynamic drug interactions include bone marrow depressants, live virus vaccines, neurotoxic medications (e.g., paclitaxel)

TOXICITY

- The most important acute toxicities are nausea, vomiting, and renal dysfunction
- These toxicities are clearly dose related
- Vomiting may be acute (within 24 hrs post dosing) or delayed (later than 24 hrs post dosing)
- Renal dysfunction is related to hydration status (urine flow)
- Poor fluid intake due to delayed nausea and vomiting at home may substantially increase nephrotoxicity even up to several weeks after infusion
- Cumulative toxicities are hearing loss and peripheral neuropathy, which are both dose limiting
- These toxicities become manifest after cumulative doses of 300–400 mg/m^2
- Ototoxicity is irreversible; peripheral neuropathy is only partly reversible
- Severity of neurotoxicity may increase up to 6 mos post treatment
- Initial presentation is sensory neuropathy and paresthesias
- Followed by motor-neuron toxicity with muscle weakness; neurotoxicity develops initially in the distal parts of the extremities
- Hypersensitivity reactions may occur but are infrequent
- Dose-intensive weekly schedules may induce significant leukopenia and thrombocytopenia

RECOMMENDATIONS FOR SUPPORTIVE CARE

- Extensive pre- and posthydration, for example 1 L physiologic saline/dextrose pre- as well as postinfusion
- Urine flow should be close to a minimum of 100 ml/hr
- IV serotonin antagonists plus IV dexamethasone (e.g., 10 mg) prior to administration is considered standard
- Repeat dosing in case of failure of prophylaxis after 6 hrs
- Lorazepam could be added in case of vomiting within 6 hrs after start of the infusion
- Dexamethasone and metoclopramide can be effective in case of delayed vomiting

PHARMACY ISSUES

- Physiologic saline (0.9% sodium chloride) is the preferred diluent

NURSING CONSIDERATIONS

- CBC, platelet count, BUN, and creatinine should be checked prior to administration
- Administer antiemetics before dose then q2–4hrs for 3–5 doses
- Infuse over 1 hr to minimize emesis
- Mannitol or furosemide may be needed to assure urine output of 100–150 ml/hr
- Hydration should be maintained with 1–2 L of fluid for 8–12 hrs prior to dose
- Evaluate renal function prior to each dose
- Assess
  - baseline vital signs prior to and during infusion; assess for anaphylaxis
  - sensory/perceptual alterations related to neurologic toxicity
  - cardiopulmonary status, especially in patients with history of preexisting cardiac disease
  - vital signs prior to and during infusion for signs of hypersensitivity
- Teach patient
  - side effects of bleeding and infection
  - taste alterations
  - self-care measures

KEY REFERENCES

Cooley ME, Davis LE, DeStefano M, et al.: Cisplatin: a clinical review. Part I—current uses of cisplatin and administration guidelines. Cancer Nurs 1994; 17(3):173–84

Cooley ME, Davis LE, Abrahm J: Cisplatin: a clinical review. Part II—nursing assessment and management of side effects of cisplatin. Cancer Nurs 1994; 17(4):283–93

Saxman SB, Propert KJ, Einhorn LH: Long-term follow-up of a phase III intergroup study of cisplatin alone or in combination with methotrexate, vinblastine, and doxorubicin in patients with metastatic urothelial carcinoma: a cooperative group study. J Clin Oncol 1997; 15(7):2564–9

Schellens JH, Ma J, Planting AS: Relationship between the exposure to cisplatin, DNA-adduct formation in leukocytes and tumor response in patients with solid tumors. Br J Cancer 1996; 73(12):1569–75

Drug: Carboplatin

A. Hilary Calvert and Brenda Werner

OTHER NAMES: PARAPLATIN, JM8, CBDCA

USES

- Approved by FDA for first- and second-line ovarian cancer
- Also active in small cell and non–small cell lung cancer, seminoma, bladder cancer

MECHANISM OF ACTION

- Formation of DNA-platinum adducts in the form of intra- and inter-strand cross-links
- Presence of p-glycoprotein does not confer resistance
- Usually cross-resistant with cisplatin
- Possible processes implicated in resistance are cell membrane transport, intracellular glutathione metabolism, and DNA repair

DOSING

- Administered IV as an IV infusion over 30–60 min
- No significant oral bioavailability
- Schedule of doses
  - surface area dosing: 300 (in combination) or 400 mg/m^2 q3–4wks
  - formula dosing: dose (total mg) = AUC × (GFR + 25) when GFR is an estimate of the glomerular filtration rate
  - AUC (area under the curve) is 5 (in combination) to 7
  - formula dosing generally results in higher total doses but less unpredictable thrombocytopenia than surface area dosing
  - doses of up to 2,000 mg/m^2 or AUC 36 are used in high-dose transplant programs
- Commonly used combinations
  - AUC 5–7 + paclitaxel 175 mg/m^2 q3wks
  - AUC 5 + cyclophosphamide 600 mg/m^2

PHARMACOKINETICS

- ~70% of an administered dose is excreted intact in the urine
- Slow irreversible covalent binding to plasma and tissue proteins
- Half-life ~5 hrs
- Myelotoxicity related to free drug AUC, which is in turn related to renal function

TOXICITY

- Thrombocytopenia is dose limiting (33% grade 4 at AUC 6–7 in previously treated patients)
- Neutropenia: similar in incidence to thrombocytopenia
- Nausea and vomiting
- Allergic reactions (~2%)
- Other cisplatin-associated toxicities (renal toxicity, neurotoxicity, ototoxicity, and electrolyte disturbance) are rare or minimal at conventional doses

RECOMMENDATIONS FOR SUPPORTIVE CARE

- Antiemetic prophylaxis, normally with a serotonin antagonist
- Allergic reactions can be treated with epinephrine, antihistamines, and hydrocortisone
- Platelet transfusions in the event of severe thrombocytopenia; the use of G-CSF may alleviate neutropenia

PHARMACY ISSUES

- D_5W is the preferred diluent, since there is a theoretical possibility the use of saline would result in the displacement of cyclobutane dicarboxylate and the formation of cisplatin on storage

NURSING CONSIDERATIONS

- CBC, platelet count, and electrolytes should be validated prior to administration
- Dose should be reduced if creatinine clearance is < 60 cc/min
- Premedicate with antiemetics as delayed nausea and vomiting can occur 2–5 days after treatment
- Monitor fluid status and maintain adequate hydration
- Assess
  - mucous membranes
  - neurologic status for signs of peripheral neuropathy (sensory loss and coordination)
  - for hypersensitivity reactions
- Teach patient
  - expected side effects of infection and bleeding
  - self-care measures
  - importance of birth control measures

KEY REFERENCES

Calvert AH: A review of the pharmacokinetics and pharmacodynamics of combination carboplatin/paclitaxel. Semin Oncol 1997; 24(1 suppl 2):S2-85, S2-90

Calvert AH, Newell DR, Gumbrell LA, et al.: Carboplatin dosage: prospective evaluation of a simple formula based on renal function. J Clin Oncol 1989; 7(11):1748–56

Duffull SB, Robinson BA: Clinical pharmacokinetics and dose optimization of carboplatin. Clinical Pharmacokinetics 1997; 33(3): 161–83

Kearns CM, Egorin MJ: Considerations regarding the less-than-expected thrombocytopenia encountered with combination paclitaxel/carboplatin chemotherapy. Semin Oncol 1997; 24(1 suppl 2):S2-91, S2-96

Newell DR, Pearson AD, Balmanno K, et al.: Carboplatin pharmacokinetics in children: the development of a pediatric dosing formula. The United Kingdom Children's Cancer Study Group. J Clin Oncol 1993; 11(12):2314–23

Drug: Oxaliplatin

E. Cvitkovic, M. Bekradda, D. Essassi, and Susan Noble-Kempin

OTHER NAMES: ELOXATINE, L-OHP

USES

- Approved in Europe, alone or in combination with 5-FU, for the treatment of metastatic colorectal cancer (both previously untreated and pretreated/resistant to 5-FU)

MECHANISM OF ACTION

- Inter- and intrastrand DNA adducts/cross-links between two close or adjacent guanines (GG or GNG) or two adjacent guanine adenine (GA) base pairs
- Oxaliplatin-DNA binding is rapid and complete
- Inhibition of RNA replication
- Stereoselective reactivity of DACH-oxaliplatin with DNA
- Oxaliplatin Pt-DNA adducts have higher cytotoxic efficacy than cisplatin Pt-DNA adducts
- Partial or no cross-resistance with cisplatin and carboplatin, DNA mismatch repair complexes do not recognize DACH-Pt DNA adducts

DOSING

- Administered IV
- Schedule/doses
  - 130–135 mg/m² IV infusion over 2 hrs q3wks
  - 85 mg/m² oxaliplatin IV infusion over 2 hrs q2wks
- Commonly used combinations
  - FOLFOX 2 regimen: oxaliplatin 85–100 mg/m² IV infusion over 2 hrs on day 1 (q2wks), with folinic acid 200 mg/m² over 2 hrs and bolus 5-FU 400 mg/m² and 5-FU 600 mg/m² continuous IV infusion for 22 hrs on day 1 and day 2 q2wks
  - chronomodulated regimen: oxaliplatin 130 mg/m²/2–6 hrs (day 1 and day 22), with chronomodulated folinic acid
  - oxaliplatin 300 mg/m²/d for 5 days and 5-FU 700 mg/m²/d for 5 days
  - oxaliplatin 85 mg/m² IV infusion over 2 hrs followed after 1 hr interval by CPT-11 200 mg/m² IV infusion over 30 min, or CTP-11 150 mg/m² (q2wks)

PHARMACOKINETICS

- Oxaliplatin undergoes spontaneous nonenzymatic conversions
- Several transient reactive species are formed including chlorinated and aquated species that complex with amino acids, proteins, and other macromolecules in plasma and tissues
- No evidence of cytochrome P-450-mediated metabolism using human liver microsomes in vitro; the ability of oxaliplatin to induce or inhibit human CYP isoenzymes is unknown
- Oxaliplatin undergoes extensive biotransformation
  - at the end of 2 hrs infusion, oxaliplatin was below the limit of detection in plasma and urine
  - up to 11 platinum-containing products were observed in the plasma ultrafiltrate (the major one was monochloro-DACH-platin)
- Up to 17 platinum-containing products were resolved by HPLC in urine
- Rapid distribution phase followed by an elimination phase with a terminal half-life of 24 hrs
- Terminal half-life of 240 hrs
- Linear pharmacokinetics over the range of studied doses (30–200 mg/m²)
- No significant changes in half-life or in total drug concentration in impaired renal function patients (20–60 ml/min creatinine clearance)

TOXICITY

- Neurosensory toxicities (acute and chronic), dose dependent with cumulative characteristics
- The acute toxicities are characterized by paresthesias and dysesthesias, often triggered or enhanced by cold, reversible on discontinuation
- Nausea and vomiting, severe in 1% of patients, reduced by an appropriate prophylactic antiemetic treatment
- Diarrhea less frequent and rarely severe (4% of patients grade 3–4)
- Minor hematologic toxicity

RECOMMENDATIONS FOR SUPPORTIVE CARE

- With serotonin antagonists the incidence of vomiting grade 3–4 is < 5%

PHARMACY ISSUES

- 5% dextrose, avoid aluminum surfaces, never mix with saline solution

NURSING CONSIDERATIONS

- Neurotoxicity regresses and may be completely reversible on cessation of therapy
- Administer antiemetic prior to therapy and continue prophylactically for 24 hrs post treatment
- Monitor CBC, WBC, differential, and platelet count prior to administration
- Assess
  - concurrent use of medications that may be associated with effects on the neurologic system
  - baseline neurologic status and periodically thereafter. A neurotoxicity scale that evaluates symptoms of both intensity and duration should be used.
  - pulmonary dysfunction
- Teach patient
  - avoid exposure to cold to prevent triggering or worsening of neurotoxicity that may also be manifested in the perioral area and as a transient laryngospasm-like syndrome
  - particularly the elderly, who may be more susceptible, regarding symptoms of neurotoxicity and self-care measures to prevent complications (e.g., urinary retention, constipation, burns, and falls)
  - signs and symptoms of infection and bleeding and measures to prevent them
  - to immediately report development of dyspnea and cough
  - maintain adequate hydration, report

KEY REFERENCE

Cvitkovic E, Chaney S, eds: Oxaliplatin: a new option for the treatment of colorectal cancer. Sem in Oncol 1998; 25(2 suppl 5)

Wasserman E, Cuvier C, Lokiec F, et al. Combination of oxaliplatin plus irinotecan in patients with gastrointestinal tumors: results of two independent phase I studies with pharmacokinetics. J Clin Oncol 1999; 17:1751–9

Drug: JM-216 (Bis-Acetato-Ammine-Dichloro-Cyclohexylamine-Platinum IV)

Mark D. DeMario and Mary Beth Mardjetko

USES

- US phase II trials have shown activity in hormone-refractory prostate cancer and small cell lung cancer

MECHANISM OF ACTION

- Platinum analogue with oral bioavailability
- Forms inter- and intrastrand DNA cross-links
- In preclinical models, JM-216 exhibits cytotoxicity equivalent to cisplatin and carboplatin
- JM-216 has demonstrated activity (non-cross-resistance) in cisplatin-resistant xenografts

DOSING

- JM-216 has been administered on a daily × 5 schedule, q21–28d. Dosages of 120 mg/m^2/d and 100 mg/m^2/d have been recommended for untreated and previously treated patients, respectively
- An investigation using a 14 consecutive day schedule noted 40 mg/m^2/d as the maximum tolerated dose

PHARMACOKINETICS

- JM-216 is rapidly transformed following oral administration into at least 6 species
- JM-118 has been identified as the major cytotoxic species in preclinical models
- Following biotransformation, the terminal half-life of platinum in ultrafiltrate is 6–8 hrs
- Urinary platinum recovery accounts for < 10% of the total JM-216 dose
- JM-216 displays linear pharmacokinetics at doses < 120 mg/m^2
- At doses > 200 mg/m^2, C_{max} and AUC increased less than proportionally to dose
- Pharmacokinetic studies of daily × 5 administration schedules suggest accumulation of protein-bound platinum and platinum in ultrafiltrate with repetitive daily dosing
- JM-216 is unique among platinum drugs for its schedule dependency
- In preclinical models, optimal antitumor activity has been demonstrated with a daily × 5 schedule

TOXICITY

- JM-216 lacks the nephrotoxicity and neurotoxicity frequently observed with cisplatin
- Dose-limiting toxicities are neutropenia and thrombocytopenia
  - cytopenias may be delayed (median neutrophil and platelet nadirs 21 and 17 days, respectively, in one phase I study—daily × 5 schedule)
- Nausea and emesis (very common)
  - severe (> grade 3) nausea or emesis was noted in ~10% of these treatment courses
- Diarrhea, rarely exceeding grade 2 severity, occurred in 20% of treatment courses in one large phase I study

RECOMMENDATIONS FOR SUPPORTIVE CARE

- Antiemetic prophylaxis is necessary
  - there is no standard antiemetic regimen
  - phase I and II studies have utilized daily ondansetron or a combination of ondansetron and oral dexamethasone

PHARMACY ISSUES

- JM-216 formulated as 5, 10, 50, and 200 mg gelatin capsules
- JM-216 is stored in light-resistant packaging and is stable at temperatures to 30–50°C
- AM administration with liquid on an empty stomach at least 1 hr prior to the first meal

NURSING CONSIDERATIONS

- Antiemetic regimen is recommended for acute and delayed nausea
- Myelosuppression is dose limiting; monitor blood counts before and during treatment cycles
- Monitor kidney function, although nephrotoxicity is not significant
- Assess
  - ototoxicity is not significant
  - baseline neurologic status; neurotoxicity does not appear to be significant
- Teach patient
  - signs and symptoms of infection and bleeding
  - side effects and self-care

KEY REFERENCE

McKeage MJ, Raynaud F, Ward J, et al.: Phase I and pharmacokinetic study of an oral platinum complex given daily for 5 days in patients with cancer. J Clin Oncol 1997; 15:2691–2700

Chapter 2

ANTIMICROTUBULE AGENTS

Introduction

Eric K. Rowinsky

APPROVED AGENTS AND SOURCES

- Structure
  - complex, bulky alkaloids derived from trees and plants
- Vinca alkaloids: naturally occurring and semisynthetic nitrogenous bases found in the pink periwinkle plant *Catharanthus roseus* G. Don
  - vincristine
  - vinblastine
  - vinorelbine
  - vindesine
- Taxanes: naturally occurring and semisynthetic alkaloid esters derived from several *taxus* species of trees and plants
  - paclitaxel
  - docetaxel

MECHANISM OF ACTION

- Although the antimicrotubule agents bind to different binding sites and differentially affect microtubules, the end results with regard to the effects on cellular processes are very similar
- Principal target: microtubules
  - polymers of tubulin heterodimers composed of alpha and beta subunits
  - microtubules and tubulin heterodimers are in dynamic equilibrium
  - microtubule assembly and disassembly effects
    - □ mitotic spindle apparatus
      - ▽ functions to pull apart the divided chromosomes during cell division
    - □ microtubule cytoskeleton
      - ▽ functions in maintaining cellular structure and scaffolding, solute transport, and growth signal transmission
  - tubulin polymerization and depolymerization are affected by chemical (calcium, magnesium, guanosine triphosphate) and cellular (cyclins, signal-transducing proteins) mediators
  - although known largely as "antimitotic" drugs, interphase processes are also affected
- Vinca alkaloids
  - inhibit microtubule assembly, principally affecting the mitotic spindle apparatus in rapidly dividing cells
- Taxanes
  - inhibit microtubule disassembly, principally affecting the mitotic spindle apparatus in rapidly dividing cells
  - demonstrated to induce cytokines, mediate production of tumor necrosis factor, affect signal transduction pathways
  - cause phosphorylation of the antiapoptotic proteins Bcl-2 and $Bclx_L$, as well as Raf, although the significance of these effects are unknown
  - Antiangiogenic effects in preclinical studies

MECHANISMS OF RESISTANCE

- Multidrug resistance
  - both Vinca alkaloids and taxanes are substrates for membrane P-glycoprotein membrane transporter proteins
- Tubulin mutations
  - mutations resulting in excessively stable microtubules are associated with resistance to the Vinca alkaloids
  - mutations resulting in intrinsically unstable microtubules are associated with resistance to taxanes

PHARMACODYNAMICS

- Duration of cellular exposure is the principal determinant of drug action and cytotoxicity in vitro, with drug concentration being less important
- However, relationships between the duration of drug infusion and antitumor activity do not appear as strong in vivo, since these agents distribute widely and bind avidly to peripheral tissues and tumors

KEY REFERENCES

Rowinsky EK: The development and clinical utility of the taxane class of antimicrotubule chemotherapy agents. Annu Rev Med 1997; 48:353–74

Rowinsky EK, Donehower RC: The clinical pharmacology and use of antimicrotubule agents in cancer chemotherapeutics. Pharmacol Ther 1991; 52(1):35–84

Drug: Vincristine

Mark J. Ratain and Susan Noble-Kempin

OTHER NAMES: ONCOVIN

USES

- Approved by FDA for acute leukemia, Hodgkin's disease, non-Hodgkin's lymphoma, rhabdomyosarcoma, neuroblastoma, and Wilms' tumor
- Also active in multiple myeloma, small cell lung cancer, breast cancer, malignant glioma, Kaposi's sarcoma, and soft tissue sarcoma

MECHANISM OF ACTION

- Antimitotic agent
- Binds to tubulin and inhibits microtubule assembly
- Overexpression of P-glycoprotein confers resistance
- Resistance may also occur secondary to alterations in tubulin proteins

DOSING

- Administered IV as a bolus or continuous infusion
- Continuous infusion probably confers no advantage over bolus administration because of long half-life
- Schedules/doses
  - maximum single dose of 1.4 mg/m^2 in adults and 2.0 mg/m^2 in children
  - commonly used combinations
    - □ 2 mg/m^2 (maximum dose of 2 mg) weekly + prednisone 60 mg/m^2 every day (VP for acute lymphoblastic leukemia)
  - more intensive combinations incorporate daunorubicin and L-asparaginase
    - □ 1.4 mg/m^2 (maximum dose of 2.5 mg; day 1, 8) + mechlorethamine 6 mg/m^2 (day 1, 8) + procarbazine 100 mg/m^2 (days 1–14) + prednisone 40 mg/m^2 (days 1–14) (MOPP for Hodgkin's disease)
    - □ 1.4 mg/m^2 (maximum dose of 2 mg; day 1) + cyclophosphamide 750 mg/m^2 (day 1) + doxorubicin 50 mg/m^2 (day 1) + prednisone 100 mg (days 1–5) (CHOP for non-Hodgkin's lymphoma)
    - □ 0.4 mg/d (days 1–4 by infusion) + doxorubicin 9 mg/m^2 (days 1–4 by infusion) + dexamethasone 40 mg (days 1–4, 9–12, 17–20) (VAD for multiple myeloma)

PHARMACOKINETICS

- Extensively metabolized by CYP3A4
- Also undergoes biliary excretion
- Terminal half-life usually > 72 hrs

TOXICITY

- Peripheral neurotoxicity is dose limiting
- Myelosuppression is uncommon
- Nausea and vomiting are minimal
- Alopecia is common
- Vesicant if extravasated
- Inhibitors of CYP3A4 and/or biliary excretion (i.e., cyclosporine) will inhibit drug clearance and enhance toxicity

RECOMMENDATIONS FOR SUPPORTIVE CARE

- Antiemetic prophylaxis should be directed at more emetogenic agents in the combination
- Stool softeners should be administered prophylactically

PHARMACY ISSUES

- Normal saline is the preferred diluent

NURSING CONSIDERATIONS

- When given in combination with L-asparaginase administer vincristine 2–24 hrs prior to L-asparaginase to prevent hepatic toxicity
- Administer through free-flowing IV, flush with saline or D_5W after administration; if extravasation occurs stop infusion and aspirate residual drug before removing IV line; circumferential injections of hyaluronidase is recommended
- Should not be administered to patients receiving radiation therapy to ports that include the liver
- Label syringes "Fatal if given intrathecally. For IV use only"
- Assess
  - for signs and symptoms of neurotoxicity; may be more frequent or severe in patients with underlying neurologic problems and in the elderly
  - concurrent use of medications that may be associated with effects on neurologic system
  - for signs and symptoms of uric acid nephropathy
- Teach patient
  - with leukemia and lymphoma importance of taking allopurinol and maintenance of hydration (3 L/day) to increase urine output
  - expected side effects and self-care measures (e.g., urinary retention, constipation, burns, and falls)
  - teratogenic effects and need for contraception

KEY REFERENCE

Zhou XJ, Rahmani R: Preclinical and clinical pharmacology of vinca alkaloids. Drugs 1992; 44(suppl 4):1–16

Drug: Vinblastine

Mark J. Ratain and Susan Noble-Kempin

OTHER NAMES: VELBAN

USES

- Approved by FDA for Hodgkin's disease, non-Hodgkin's lymphoma, testis cancer, Kaposi's sarcoma, histiocytosis X, choriocarcinoma, and breast cancer
- Also active in bladder cancer, non–small cell lung cancer, and prostate cancer

MECHANISM OF ACTION

- Antimitotic agent
- Binds to tubulin and inhibits microtubule assembly
- Overexpression of P-glycoprotein confers resistance
- Resistance may also occur secondary to alterations in tubulin proteins

DOSING

- Administered IV as a bolus or continuous infusion
- Schedules/doses
  - single agent
    - □ 3 mg/m² or 0.15 mg/kg weekly
    - □ 0.11 mg/kg every day × 2 or 6 mg/m² q3wks
    - □ 1.5–2.0 mg/m²/d for 96 hr continuous infusion
  - commonly used combinations
    - □ 6 mg/m² + mitomycin 12 mg/m² (for breast cancer)
    - □ 6 mg/m² + mitomycin 10 mg/m² + cisplatin 100 mg/m² (MVP for non–small cell lung cancer)
    - □ 3 mg/m² (day 2, 15) + methotrexate 30 mg/m² (day 1, 15) + doxorubicin 30 mg/m² (day 2) + cisplatin 70 mg/m² (MVAC for bladder cancer)

PHARMACOKINETICS

- Extensively metabolized by CYP3A4
- Also undergoes biliary excretion
- Half-life of ~24 hrs

TOXICITY

- Neutropenia is dose limiting
- Thrombocytopenia is uncommon
- Nausea and vomiting are minimal
- Peripheral and autonomic neuropathies (constipation) may limit cumulative dose
- Alopecia is common
- Vesicant if extravasated
- Inhibitors of CYP3A4 and/or biliary excretion (i.e., cyclosporine) inhibit drug clearance and enhance toxicity

RECOMMENDATIONS FOR SUPPORTIVE CARE

- Antiemetic prophylaxis should be directed at more emetogenic agents in the combination
- Stool softeners should be administered prophylactically

PHARMACY ISSUES

- Normal saline is the preferred diluent

NURSING CONSIDERATIONS

- Vesicant; administer through free-flowing IV; flush line with normal saline or D_5W after administration; if extravasation occurs stop infusion and aspirate residual before removing IV line; the manufacturer recommends circumferential injections of hyaluronidase
- Label syringes "Fatal if given intrathecally. For IV use only"
- Assess
  - for signs and symptoms of neurotoxicity
  - for hepatic dysfunction
  - for myelasuppression
- Teach patient
  - expected side effects and self-care measures (sensory and perceptual changes)
  - need for contraception
  - infection preventive measures and signs and symptoms of infection to report

KEY REFERENCE

Zhou XJ, Rahmani R: Preclinical and clinical pharmacology of vinca alkaloids. Drugs 1992; 44(suppl 4):1–16

Drug: Vindesine

E. Cvitkovic, M. Bekradda, D. Essassi, and Mary Beth Mardjetko

OTHER NAMES: ELDISINE

USES

- Approved in Europe and Japan for the treatment of lymphoblastic leukemia and lymphomas refractory to chemotherapy, and other solid tumors
- Breast, esophageal, head, and neck cancer
- Also active in carcinomas of various primary sites, mainly lung (NSCLC)

MECHANISM OF ACTION

- After active transport by a transmembrane carrier, vindesine binds to tubulin and inhibits tubulin polymerization
- Main mechanism of resistance is P-glycoprotein mediated
- Resistance to vindesine may be associated with resistance to other drugs such as anthracyclines and actinomycin D (modifications of membrane components involved in the transmembrane transport of the drugs)
- In solid tumors, the spectrum of antitumor activity is similar, but not identical to that of vinblastine and vincristine

DOSING

- Strictly IV injection at weekly intervals
- Schedules/doses
  - 3–4 mg/m² every wk
- Commonly used combinations
  - active in childhood acute lymphoblastic leukemia in combination with L-asparaginase, prednisolone, and doxorubicin
  - combination of vindesine, cyclophosphamide, doxorubicin, and prednisone is active in refractory myeloma (CAPE regimen)
  - in NSCLC
    - □ vindesine and cisplatin
    - □ vindesine, cisplatin, and mitomycin C
    - □ vindesine, cisplatin, and ifosfamide
  - vindesine, VP-16, and ifosfamide in SCLC
  - in head and neck cancers:
    - □ vindesine, cisplatin, and mitomycin C
    - □ vindesine and cisplatin
    - □ vindesine, cisplatin, bleomycin, mitomycin, and methylprednisolone
    - □ vindesine, cisplatin, and 5-fluorouracil
    - □ vindesine, methotrexate, and bleomycin
  - vindesine, cyclophosphamide, cisplatin, and adriamycin (DECAV regimen) in soft tissue sarcoma
  - vindesine, bleomycin, mitomycin C, and cisplatin (BEMP regimen) in cervical squamous carcinoma

PHARMACOKINETICS

- Triexponential plasma decay has been reported with terminal half-life of 20 hrs
- 10–15% renal excretion
- Relative extent of biliary excretion and hepatic metabolism unknown

TOXICITY

- Main dose-limiting toxicity: dose-related myelosuppression (predominantly granulocytes) with recovery within 8–10 days
- More myelotoxic than vincristine and less than vinblastine
- Other dose-limiting toxicity
  - neurotoxicity
    - □ peripheral neuropathy (less than vincristine), not cumulative, appeared to be dose related
- Constipation (mild)
- Alopecia (>25% hair loss) was common
- Fever within 48 hrs of treatment (38–39°C, sporadic)

RECOMMENDATIONS FOR SUPPORTIVE CARE

- Antiemetics recommended in combination with more emetogenic agents

PHARMACY ISSUES

- Sterile water, isotonic saline, or glucose after dissolution in any solvent
- The drug becomes unstable and must be used immediately

NURSING CONSIDERATIONS

- Drug is a vesicant; take precautions to avoid extravasation (e.g., appropriate vein selection; assure catheter is properly placed); if extravasation occurs, stop infusion, follow institutional procedures
- Flush line with at least 100 cc of IV solution after drug infusion
- Leukopenia is dose-limiting; monitor blood counts before and during treatment cycles
- Assess
  - observe site of infusion vigilantly during drug administration
  - baseline neurologic status and during treatment; assess bowel elimination pattern; implement interventions as appropriate
- Teach patient
  - signs and symptoms of infection
  - report peripheral paresthesias, muscle weakness, myalgias, headache, and constipation
  - alopecia occurs in 80–90%; instruct regarding options (wigs, hats, short haircuts) and scalp care
  - use of stool softeners and high-fiber foods

KEY REFERENCES

Cvitkovic E, Wasserman E: Role of vindesine as neoadjuvant chemotherapy for non–small cell lung and head and neck cancers. Anticancer Drugs 1997; 8:734–45

Gokbuget N, Hoelzer D: Vindesine in the treatment of leukemia. Leuk Lymphoma 1997; 26:497–506

Vansteenkiste JF, DeLeyn PR, Deneffe GJ, et al.: Vindesine-ifosfamide-platinum (VIP) induction chemotherapy in surgically staged IIIA-N2 non–small cell lung cancer: a prospective study. Leuven Lung Cancer Group. Ann Oncol 1998; 9:261–7

Drug: Vinorelbine

Everett E. Vokes and Mary Beth Mardjetko

OTHER NAME: NAVELBINE

USES

- Approved by FDA for advanced non–small cell lung cancer as single agent and in combination with cisplatin
- Also active in breast cancer, prostate cancer, and ovarian cancer

MECHANISM OF ACTION

- Semisynthetic vinca alkaloid that has been structurally modified on the catharanthine nucleus
- Inhibition of assembly of mitotic spindle
- Binds to tubulin (basic protein subunit of microtubules) resulting in inhibition of tubulin polymerization and microtubule assembly
- Inhibition of mitosis at metaphase
- Cell cycle phase-specific antimitotic agent
- In vitro studies suggest increased specificity for mitotic microtubules and a lesser effect on axonal microtubules than other vinca alkaloids

DOSING

- Administered IV as a 10 min infusion
- Oral formulation in development
- Schedules
  - 25–30 mg/m^2 weekly as single agent or in combination with cisplatin at 100 mg/m^2 q4wks, or 120 mg/m^2 q6wks
  - has also been administered as 96 h continuous infusion (8 mg/m^2 IV over 5 min on day 1 followed immediately by a 96 h continuous infusion of 5.5 or 8 mg/m^2/d)
  - 30 mg/m^2 for 3 consecutive days with ifosfamide 1.6 gm/m^2 for 3 consecutive days followed by the administration of G-CSF on days 5–12

PHARMACOKINETICS

- Terminal half-life ranges from 28–44 hrs
- Rapidly and extensively distributed into tissues
- Penetrates the blood-brain barrier with a ratio of 20%
- Metabolism in the liver (by CYP3A4) and excretion primarily in the bile

TOXICITY

- Neutropenia
  - occurs 7–10 days after a dose
- Mild to moderate peripheral neuropathy is the most frequently reported neurologic toxicity
- Occasional alopecia
- Mild to moderate nausea
- Transient elevations of liver enzymes
- Chest pain
- Other toxicities include jaw pain, myalgia, arthralgia, and tumor pain
- Systemic allergic reactions have been reported

RECOMMENDATIONS FOR SUPPORTIVE CARE

- Antiemetic prophylaxis is recommended, although there is no standard regimen

PHARMACY ISSUES

- D_5W is the preferred diluent

NURSING CONSIDERATIONS

- Leukopenia is dose limiting; monitor blood counts before and during treatment cycles
- Drug is a vesicant; take precautions to avoid extravasation (e.g., appropriate vein selection; assure IV catheter is properly placed); if extravasation occurs, stop infusion, follow institutional procedures
- Injection site reactions may occur during or a few days after treatment; diluted vinorelbine should be infused over 6–10 min, into a sidearm port closest to the IV bag, not the patient
- After drug infusion, flush vein with at least 100 cc of IV solution instructing patient to report pain or stinging at site of administration
- Shortness of breath and bronchospasm has been reported, most commonly when used in combinations with mitomycin; assure emergency measures are available
- Radiation recall may occur
- Pretreatment with antiemetics
- Assess
  - monitor patient during drug infusion
  - observe site of infusion vigilantly during drug administration
  - pain syndrome may occur; can be reported in jaw or tumor site; analgesics prior to or after administration may be helpful
  - baseline neruologic status and prior to each treatment; implement interventions as appropriate
- Teach patient
  - signs and symptoms of infection
  - report peripheral paresthesias, muscle weakness, myalgias, headache, or constipation
  - avoid OTC aspirin-containing medications
  - side effects and self-care measures

KEY REFERENCES

Le Chevalier T, Brisgand D, Douillard J-Y, et al.: Randomized study of vinorelbine and cisplatin versus vindesine and cisplatin versus vinorelbine alone in advanced non-small-cell lung cancer: results of a European multicenter trial including 612 patients. J Clin Oncol 1994; 12:360–7

Vokes EE: Integration of vinorelbine into current chemotherapy strategies for advanced non–small cell lung cancer. Oncol 1995; 9:565–77

Wozniak AJ, Crowley JJ, Balcerzak SP, Livingston RB: Randomized trial comparing cisplatin with cisplatin plus vinorelbine in the treatment of advanced non–small-cell lung cancer: a Southwest Oncology Group study. J Clin Oncol 1998; 16(7):2459–65

Drug: Estramustine

Kenneth J. Pienta, Karin B. Olson, and Belinda Butler

OTHER NAMES: EMCYT, EMP

USES

- Metastatic and/or progressive androgen-independent prostate cancer

MECHANISM OF ACTION

- Conjugate of estradiol and nornitrogen mustard with antimitotic properties preferentially taken up by prostate epithelial cells
- Binds to microtubule-associated proteins, tubulin, and proteins of the nuclear matrix
- Arrests cells in G2/M phase

DOSING

- 280 mg tid (or 140 mg tid in elderly, debilitated patients or those who have difficulty tolerating 280 mg tid)
- Commonly used combinations
  - 280 mg tid for 21 of every 28 days with etoposide 50 mg po bid
  - 280 mg tid for 5 days with paclitaxel 135 mg/m^2 IV on day 3 q3wks
  - 140–280 mg tid for 3 days with paclitaxel 100 mg/m^2 IV on day 2 weekly for 6 wks
  - 280 mg tid for 42 days with vinblastine 4 mg/m^2 IV weekly for 6 wks
  - 280 mg tid for 5 days with docetaxel 40–60 mg/m^2 on day 3

PHARMACOKINETICS

- After dephosphorylation, oxidation of hydroxyl at C17 of estramustine results in estromustine
- Plasma half-life is 10–20 hrs

TOXICITY

- Primary toxicity is nausea
- Diarrhea and gastrointestinal upset may also occur
- Mild–moderate breast enlargement and tenderness commonly seen
- Fluid retention, most often manifest as peripheral edema is also common
- May also cause or exacerbate hypertension and/or exacerbate reexisting CHF
- Use with caution in patients with known CHF
- May decrease glucose tolerance
- Castrate levels of serum testosterone after 1 mo of daily dosing at 540 mg/d
- May increase LDH and/or SGOT
- Use with caution in patients with impaired liver function
- Occasional leukopenia and/or thrombocytopenia
- This risk is increased when used in combination with other chemotherapeutic agents
- May increase risk of thromobembolism
  - use with caution with patients with history of thrombosis, thrombophlebitis, thromboembolic disease, coronary artery disease, or history of cerebral vascular accident

RECOMMENDATIONS FOR SUPPORTIVE CARE

- Phenothiazine antiemetics
- Treat mild peripheral edema with HCTZ/triamterene

PHARMACY ISSUES

- Available in 140 mg oral capsules
- May be taken with food to decrease nausea
- Patients should be instructed to avoid calcium/dairy products 1 hr before to 1 hr after dosing

NURSING CONSIDERATIONS

- Monitor liver, renal, and endocrine function tests
- WBC and platelets should be monitored closely if given with other chemotherapeutic agents
- Diabetic patients should be observed for decreased glucose tolerance
- To be used cautiously in patients with thrombophlebitis, thromboembolic disorders, or coronary artery disease; drug may worsen CHF
- Available for IV administration (investigational use only); IV preparation is a vesicant
- Assess
  - alterations in tissue perfusion related to thrombophlebitis or thrombosis, obtain baseline cardiac and peripheral vascular status including signs of CHF; obtain weekly weights and observe for fluid retention during therapy
  - baseline LFTs and calcium; observe for signs of hypercalcemia and renal insufficiency
  - blood pressure and glucose tolerance during therapy
- Teach patient
  - take with water 1 hr before or 2 hrs after meals (as recommended by manufacturer)
  - avoid calcium-rich foods and drugs 1 hr before and 1 hr after administration
  - practice contraception
  - transient paresthesias of mouth, perineal itching, and pain may occur after IV administration (investigational)
  - expected side effects and self-care measures

KEY REFERENCES

Hudes G: Estramustine-based chemotherapy. Seminars Urologic Oncol 1997; 15:13–19

Perry CM, McTavish D: Estramustine phosphate sodium. A review of its pharmacodynamic and pharmacokinetic properties, and therapeutic efficacy in prostate cancer. Drugs Aging 1995; 7(1):49–74

Pienta KJ, Redman B, Hussain M: Phase II evaluation of oral estramustine and oral etoposide in hormone-refractory adenocarcinoma of the prostate. J Clin Oncol 1994; 12(10):2005–12

Drug: Paclitaxel

Eric K. Rowinsky and Dolores Watts

OTHER NAMES: TAXOL, ANZATAX, PAXENE

USES

- Approved by the FDA (Taxol only)
  - epithelial ovarian cancer after failure of first-line or subsequent chemotherapy
  - metastatic breast cancer after failure of combination chemotherapy or relapse within 6 mos of adjuvant chemotherapy (prior therapy should have included an anthracycline)
  - non–small cell lung cancer with cisplatin in previously untreated advanced disease
  - Adjuvant therapy in early-stage high-risk breast cancer
  - Kaposi's sarcoma
- Consistently notable antitumor activity demonstrated
  - advanced small cell lung cancer, bladder, endometrial, esophageal, testicular, and head and neck carcinomas
- Modest antitumor activity in cervical, prostate, and gastric carcinomas, and lymphoma

MECHANISM OF ACTION

- Antimicrotubule agent inhibiting disassembly of tubulin polymers (microtubules) and tubulin dimers
- Mitotitic block at the metaphase-anaphase boundary
- Inhibits malignant angiogenesis
- Induces apoptosis
- Cytotoxic activity correlated with presence of mutated or deficient p53 suppressor oncogene
- Resistance conferred by P-glycoprotein and multidrug resistance–associated protein in vitro, and tubulin mutations; however, the clinical role of these mechanisms in conferring resistance is uncertain

DOSING

- Approved at a dose of 175 mg/m^2 as a 3 hr IV infusion (recurrent and refractory breast and ovarian cancer) or 135 mg/m^2 as a 24 hr IV infusion q3wks
- Although there does not appear to be any increased benefit for higher doses as a 24 hr infusion, higher paclitaxel doses on the 3 hr infusion schedule may result in greater benefit
- Approved for Kaposi's sarcoma as a 3 hr IV infusion at a dose of 135 mg/m^2
- Other schedules
  - 1 hr IV infusion at doses of 200–250 mg/m^2 q3wks
  - 96 hr IV infusion at a total dose of 140 mg/m^2 q3wks
  - 1 hr IV infusion weekly at a dose of 80–100 mg/m^2, which has been associated with prominent antitumor activity with less toxicity, particularly myelosuppression, compared to less frequent schedules
  - well tolerated in patients with severe renal impairment, and dose modifications are not required
  - dose reductions of at least 50% are recommended for patients with a moderate hepatic excretory dysfunction (e.g., moderate hyperbilirubinemia) and moderate to severe elevations in hepatic transaminases

PHARMACOKINETICS

- Nonlinear pharmacokinetics, particularly evident on short infusion schedules
- Half-life range of 6–14 hrs with clinically relevant dosing schedules
- High protein binding (> 90%) in plasma
- Large volume of distribution with extensive tissue binding
- Predominantly eliminated as inactive hydroxylated metabolites in the bile and feces
- Moderate metabolism primarily by CYP2C8 and CYP3A4
- Prolonged (24 hr) infusions associated with sequence-dependent toxicologic and pharmacologic effects with cisplatin and doxorubicin
- Inhibits clearance of cisplatin and doxorubicin when administered first
- Paclitaxel and/or its Cremophor EL (polyoxyethylated castor oil) formulation vehicle modifies the pharmacologic behavior of doxorubicin, such as reducing its clearance
- The administration of paclitaxel, particularly on shorter (3 hr) schedules with doxorubicin, enhances the cardiotoxic effects of doxorubicin and decreases the cumulative doses associated with congestive cardiotoxicity

TOXICITY

- Neutropenia is the principal dose-limiting toxicity when administered as a continuous IV infusion over 1–96 hrs q3wks
  - brief and noncumulative
  - more prominent with prolonged infusion durations
- Anemia and thrombocytopenia are rarely clinically significant
- Alopecia of the scalp and total body are common
- Peripheral neurotoxicity, particularly neurosensory toxicity, with cumulative dosing
  - shorter infusions appear to be associated with a higher incidence of peripheral neurotoxicity, particularly in combination with a platinum compound
  - patients with underlying peripheral neuropathies due to diabetes mellitus or chronic alcoholism are at high risk for peripheral neurotoxicity
- Myalgias in the peritreatment period are related to dose and appear to be more common with shorter infusions
  - prophylaxis with analgesic medications is often effective
- Acute hypersensitivity reactions, most likely due to histamine release secondary to either Cremophor EL (polyoxyethylated castor oil) formulation vehicle and/or the taxane moiety, appeared to be more common with shorter infusion schedules in early studies
  - reactions typically occur during the first several minutes of course 1 or 2
- Asymptomatic bradycardia is common
  - other intrinsic cardiac rhythm disturbances, including Mobitz I (Wenckeback syndrome), Mobitz II, and third-degree heart block, are rare
  - these disturbances have rarely been associated with hemodynamic effects
- Mucositis is generally noted with prolonged infusion (e.g., 96 hr) schedules
- Other gastrointestinal toxicities, including nausea, vomiting, and diarrhea, are uncommon
- Inflammation may occur at the injection site, along the course of an injected vein, and in areas of previous drug extravasation; inflammatory skin reactions over previously irradiated sites (radiation recall) have been reported
- Nail disorders with weekly treatment

RECOMMENDATIONS FOR SUPPORTIVE CARE

- Premedication regimen used for prevention of acute hypersensitivity reactions most likely due to histamine release secondary to the Cremophor EL (polyoxyethylated castor oil) formulation vehicle and/or the taxane moiety
- Most common premedication regimen is dexamethasone 8 mg po 12 and 6 hrs before treatment and diphenhydramine 50 mg IV and either cimetidine 300 mg IV, rantidine 50 mg IV, or famotidine 20 mg IV 30 min before treatment
- Acute hypersensitivity reactions are optimally managed by promptly discontinuing the infusion
- Diphenhydramine 50 mg IV should be administered immediately if manifestations persist or worsen
- For acute bronchospasm, epinephrine and/or nebulized bronchodilators should be considered
- Patients who have experienced acute hypersensitivity reactions have been successfully rechallenged with paclitaxel
- The most common procedure involves dexamethasone 20 mg IV q6hrs for 4 doses followed by the same dose of paclitaxel set to be administered over 96 hrs, with a progressive increase in the rate to the original rate over the course of the infusion
- Routine administration of narcotic and other analgesics are effective prophylaxis in the peritreatment for patients who have experienced severe myalgia and/or acute exacerbation of neurosensory toxicity

Drug: Paclitaxel *(Continued)*

■ Antihistamine, antidepressant, and anti-inflammatory agents have been used to prevent acute exacerbation of neurotoxicity and/or severe myalgia, as well as to manage these toxicities; however, the success of these maneuvers is largely anecdotal

■ Routine prophylaxis with antiemetics is generally not required because paclitaxel is not highly emetogenic

■ Granulocyte-colony stimulating factor (G-CSF) 5 μg/kg/d, starting 24 hrs after treatment and continuing until the resolution of neutropenia, is an effective means to ameliorate neutropenia and neutropenic complications in high-risk patients

PHARMACY ISSUES

■ May be diluted in either 0.9% sodium chloride, USP, 5% dextrose injection, USP, 5% dextrose and 0.9% sodium chloride injection, USP, or 5% dextrose in Ringer's lactate injection, USP

■ Physically and chemically stable at 0.3–1.2 mg/ml for up to 27 hrs at room temperature after final dilution

■ Only glass or polyolefin containers and nitroglycerin tubing (polyethylene lined) are recommended for administration because significant amounts of the plasticizer diethylhexylphthalate (DEHP) may be leached from PVC-containing plastic solution bags after contact with Cremophor EL

■ Upon preparation, solutions may be hazy, which has been attributed to the formulation vehicle

■ Should be administered through an in-line filter not greater than 0.22 μg

NURSING CONSIDERATIONS

■ Prior to treatment verify patient has received premedication with corticosteroids, diphenhydramine, and H2 antagonist according to prescribed regimen and schedule

■ Potential for hypersensitivity during the first 10 min of infusion; emergency drugs and equipment should be accessible

■ Administer paclitaxel first when given in combinations with cisplatin or carboplatin

■ ANC should be $>1{,}500/mm^3$ prior to initial or subsequent doses

■ Access
- baseline neurologic status; monitor for peripheral neuropathy during treatment
- baseline cardiac status; monitor changes in rhythm
- for myalgia and arthralgia, which begins 2–3 days after therapy

■ Teach patient
- signs and symptoms of infection
- to follow an oral hygiene regime
- report sensory and perceptual changes during infusion
- review safety intervention issues for patients with sensory deficits; avoid use of sharp objects and avoid extreme hot or cold temperatures
- avoid OTC aspirin-containing medications

KEY REFERENCES

Rowinsky EK, Donehower RC: Paclitaxel (taxol). N Engl J Med 1995; 332(15):1004–14

Venook AP, Egorin MJ, Rosner GL, et al.: Phase I and pharmacokinetic trial of paclitaxel in patients with hepatic dysfunction: Cancer and Leukemia Group B9264. J Clin Oncol 1998; 16:1811–19

Drug: Docetaxel

Eric K. Rowinsky and Dolores Watts

OTHER NAMES: TAXOTERE

USES

- Approved by the FDA for patients with metastatic breast cancer who have progressed or relapsed following first-line treatment
- Approved by the FDA for patients with non–small cell lung cancer with recurrent disease after first-line chemotherapy
- Registered in many other countries for treatment of patients with advanced breast and non–small cell lung cancer
- Consistently notable antitumor activity demonstrated for docetaxel as a single agent in previously treated patients with head and neck cancer, bladder cancer, esophageal cancer, and small cell lung cancer
- Modest antitumor activity in cervical, prostate, and gastric cancers, and lymphoma
- Although there have been reports of responses to docetaxel in patients whose disease had progressed following treatment with paclitaxel, it is unclear whether this phenomenon represents partial cross-resistance between the agents or reflects differences in aggressiveness between the taxane dose schedules

MECHANISM OF ACTION

- Antimicrotubule agent inhibiting disassembly of tubulin polymers (microtubules) and tubulin dimers
- ~ two- to threefold more potent than paclitaxel at inhibiting tubulin polymerization and inducing cytotoxicity in vitro
- Cellular uptake and retention appears to be greater than paclitaxel
- Mitotitic block at the metaphase-anaphase boundary
- Inhibits malignant angiogenesis
- Induces apoptosis
- Cytotoxic activity related to presence of mutated or deficient p53 suppressor oncogene
- Resistance conferred by P-glycoprotein and multidrug resistance–associated protein in vitro, and rarely by tubulin mutations; however, the clinical role of these mechanisms in conferring resistance is uncertain

DOSING

- Results of nonrandomized studies indicate the possibility of a dose-response relationship in the range of 60–100 mg/m² in lung and breast cancers
- Docetaxel appears to be well tolerated in patients with severe renal impairment, and dose modifications do not appear to be required
- Patients with liver metastases with and without elevations in plasma levels of hepatocellular enzymes and/or alkaline phosphatase have reduced docetaxel clearance
- Predisposing these patients to more severe neutropenia, mucositis, and rashes than patients with or without liver metastases and no liver function test abnormalities
- Reduce doses by 25% in patients with elevations in both plasma concentrations of hepatic transaminases (≥1.5-fold) and alkaline phosphatase (≥2.5-fold)
- Preliminary prospective data involving patients with mild or moderate elevations in serum bilirubin indicate that the dose should be reduced at least by 50%
- Schedules/doses
  - in other tumor types and in treatment settings involving less heavily pretreated patients, docetaxel has most commonly been administered at 75–100 mg/m² as a 1 hr infusion q3wks
  - also can be given weekly at a dose of 36–45 mg/m², which has been associated with prominent antitumor activity with less toxicity, particularly myelosuppression, compared to less frequent schedules

PHARMACOKINETICS

- Linear pharmacokinetics in the clinically relevant dosing range
- Nonlinear pharmacokinetics have been noted at much higher doses and in patients with hepatic impairment, particularly patients with hyperbilirubinemia
- Triexponential disposition in plasma with a terminal half-life range of 11–14 hrs
- High protein binding (>90%) in plasma
- Large volume of distribution with extensive tissue binding
- Predominantly eliminated as inactive metabolites in the bile and feces, with renal disposition of parent compound accounting for 5–10% of administered drug
- Moderate metabolism by CYP3A4
- Significant sequence-dependent toxicologic and pharmacologic effects between docetaxel and either cisplatin and doxorubicin have not been observed

TOXICITY

- Neutropenia is the principal dose-limiting toxicity of docetaxel administered as a 1 hr IV infusion q3wks
  - brief and noncumulative
- Anemia and thrombocytopenia common
  - rarely clinically significant
- Alopecia of the scalp and total body are common
- Skin toxicity, consisting of erythema, dryness, desquamation, and/or maculopapular rash that principally affects the forearms, hands, and feet, occurs in the majority of patients
- Nails of patients undergoing repeated courses may show progressive thickening, discoloration, and even loss in some individuals; worse with weekly administration
- The incidence of a syndrome of cumulative fluid retention, characterized by the progressive development of peripheral edema and occasionally with pleural and pericardial effusions, is cumulative and increases with repeated treatment
  - progressively increases as the cumulative dose of docetaxel exceeds 400 mg/m²
  - co-medication with corticosteroids has been demonsrated to reduce the severity and incidence of fluid retention and to delay its onset
- Although neuromuscular toxicities are noted with docetaxel, the incidences of both acute myalgias in the peritreatment period and cumulative, clinically relevant peripheral neurosensory toxicity are low
- Asthenia or malaise occur are common in patients receiving repeated doses of docetaxel, particularly on weekly schedules
- Hypersensitivity reactions have been observed with docetaxel, particularly during the first several minutes of the first two courses
  - severe reactions are rare
  - most hypersensitivity reactions have been subacute
  - overall incidence of both acute and subacute hypersensitivity reactions have been substantially lower following the advent of premedication
- The incidence of mucositis appears to be higher with docetaxel than with paclitaxel, but is generally noted with prolonged infusion (e.g., 96 hr) schedules
- Other gastrointestinal toxicities, including nausea, vomiting, and diarrhea, are uncommon
- Inflammation may occur at the injection site, along the course of an injected vein, and in areas of previous drug extravasation; inflammatory skin reactions over previously irradiated sites (radiation recall) have been reported
- Hyperlacrimination may occur with chronic weekly treatment

RECOMMENDATIONS FOR SUPPORTIVE CARE

- Premedication with corticosteroids with or without H1 and H2 histamine antagonists does reduce the incidence and median number of courses before the onset of this toxicity
  - dexamethasone 8 mg po twice daily for 5 days beginning 1 day before docetaxel administration
  - dexamethasone 8 mg po twice daily for 3 days beginning 1 day before the docetaxel infusion
- The use of a premedication regimen to prevent hypersensitivity reactions is recommended
  - diphenhydramine 50 mg IV and either cimetidine 300 mg IV, ranitidine 50 mg IV, or famotidine 20 mg IV 30 min before treatment

Drug: Docetaxel *(Continued)*

■ Palmar-plantar erthrodysesthesia that occurs despite prophylaxis may respond to administration of pyridoxine 50 mg orally three times each day
■ Routine administration of narcotic and other analgesics is effective prophylaxis in the peritreatment for patients who have previously experienced severe myalgia and/or acute exacerbation of neurosensory toxicity
■ G-CSF 5 μg/kg/d, starting 24 hrs after treatment and continuing until the resolution of neutropenia, is an effective means to ameliorate neutropenia and neutropenic complications in high-risk patients
■ Routine prophylaxis with antiemetics is generally not required, since docetaxel is not highly emetogenic
■ For clinically significant hyperlacrimation, consider withholding docetaxel for 2 wks, reinstituting on a weekly × 3 q4wk schedule, and using corticosteroid opthalmic solution 2 gtts q12hrs for 3 d; if no history of herpetic eye disease

PHARMACY ISSUES

■ Strengths available: 20 mg per 0.5 ml (single dosing vial) [docetaxel (polysorbate 80: 1,040 mg per ml)]; and 80 mg per 2 ml (single dosing vial) [docetaxel (polysorbate 80: 1,040 mg per ml)]
■ Product is packaged together with accompanying diluent (0.5 ml for the 20-mg-per-0.5-ml vial; 2 ml for the 80 mg-per-2-ml vial)
■ The diluent contains 13% alcohol
■ The vials contain overfills of docetaxel and diluent to allow for loss due to foaming, adhesion to the vial walls, and dead space during initial dilution of the concentrate
■ Recommended infusates for dilution include 0.9% sodium chloride injection, USP, and 5% dextrose injection, USP
■ It is recommended that the required quantity of the premix solution be diluted into 250 ml of the infusate to achieve a final concentration of 0.3–0.9 mg per ml
■ If a dose >240 mg of docetaxel is required, a larger volume of vehicle should be used so the concentration does not exceed 0.9 mg per ml
■ The premix solution is stable for up to 8 hrs at room temperature (15–25°C [59–77°F]) or in a refrigerator (2–8°C [26–46°F])
■ However, it is recommended that the solution be used as soon as possible
■ Contact of undiluted docetaxel with plasticized polyvinyl equipment is not recommended because such contact may cause leaching of the plasticizer, diethylhexylphthalate (DEHP)
■ It is recommended that glass bottles or polypropylene or polyolefin plastic products be used for preparation and storage of the infusion, and that the infusion be administered through polyethylene-lined administration sets

NURSING CONSIDERATIONS

■ Administration of antidiuretic therapy may be helpful in managing fluid retention
■ Administration of corticosteroids regime, such as dexamethasone, can reduce incidence and severity of fluid retention and severity of hypersensitivity reactions; premedicate for 3–5 d beginning 1 day prior to docetaxel administration (see supportive care)
■ Incidence and severity of fluid retention increases sharply at cumulative doses of 400 mg/m^2
■ Neutropenia is dose limiting on most schedules; monitor blood counts prior to and weekly during treatment
■ Patients that have received prior cisplatin, or with existing neuropathies (ethanol and diabetes mellitus related), are at higher risk for neurotoxicity
■ Estravasation may produce localized pain and discoloration without necrosis; erythema with peeling may occur 6 wks after
■ Solution should be mixed in a glass bottle or plastic bag (polypropylene/polyolefin) with either 0.9% sodium chloride or 5% dextrose for a concentration of 0.3–0.9 mg/ml; once solution is prepared it should be given as soon as possible over 1 hr
■ Assess
- alterations in fluid balance related to fluid retention
- patients with preexisting effusions should be monitored for possible exacerbation of the effusion with chronic treatment
- baseline neurologic status and monitor for neuromotor and neurosensory deficits during treatment
- impairment in skin integrity; oncholysis (partial separation of nail plate from nail bed), hyper/hypopigmentation, and calcification of nail beds; evidence of mucositis/stomatitis

■ Teach patient
- report evidence of rash, erythema that may occur on hands, feet, neck, upper chest, and arms
- importance of rest periods in management of fatigue
- side effects and self-care measures

KEY REFERENCES

Dieras V, Chevallier B, Kerbrat P, et al.: A multicentre phase II study of docetaxel 75 mg/m^2 as first-line chemotherapy for patients with advanced breast cancer: report of the Clinical Screening Group of the EORTC, European Organization for Research and Treatment of Cancer. Br J Cancer 1996; 74:650–6

Piccart MJ, Klijn J, Paridaens R, et al.: Corticosteroids significantly delay the onset of docetaxel-induced fluid retention: final results of a randomized study of the European Organization for Research and Treatment of Cancer Investigational Drug Branch for Breast Cancer. J Clin Oncol 1997; 15:3149–55

Chapter 3

TOPOISOMERASE INHIBITORS

Introduction

William T. Beck

BIOCHEMICAL PHARMACOLOGY

- Inhibitors of DNA synthesis
- Act by inhibiting DNA topoisomerases
- Mammalian cells have two forms of topoisomerases
  - type I (topoisomerase I)
    - □ Mr 100,000 kD
    - □ relieves torsional stress on DNA
    - □ involved in transcription
  - type II (topoisomerase II)
    - □ two forms in mammalian cells: alpha, Mr 170,000 kD; beta, Mr 180,000 kD; separate gene products
    - □ alpha appears to be regulated through the cell cycle; beta is not
    - □ catalyzes double-strand passage through covalent linkage to DNA, formation of transient strand breaks, passage of transfer strand, and reannealing of broken strand
    - □ requires ATP
    - □ involved in replication, transcription, recombination, chromatin assembly, possibly repair
    - □ structural component of nuclear matrix
- Two mechanisms of topoisomerase II inhibition
  - *complex-stabilizing:* stabilizing cleaved complexes (prevent religation of broken DNA)
    - □ drug examples: anthracyclines (doxorubicin, daunorubicin), epipodophyllotoxins (etoposide, teniposide), aminoacridines (amsacrine)
    - □ anthracenediones (mitoxantrone)
    - □ anthracyclines are DNA intercalators; cause single- and double-stranded breaks
  - *catalytic inhibition:* inhibition of enzyme function (locking enzyme on DNA in a "closed clamp" conformation)
    - □ drug examples: bisdioxopiperazines (ICRF-187), merbarone, aclarubicin
  - block cells in G_2/M phase of cell cycle
  - inhibition of topo II by complex-stabilizing topo II inhibitors leads to induction of programmed cell death pathways
- Mechanisms of tumor cell resistance to
  - topoisomerase II inhibitors—complex-stabilizing
    - □ MDR/Pgp, MRP/Mrp, mutation in topo II, decreased amount of topo II
  - topoisomerase II inhibitors—catalytic inhibitors
    - □ increased topo II, others to be defined
  - topoisomerase I inhibitors
    - □ MDR/Pgp, mutation in topo I, decreased amount of topo I
- Structural features: diverse, but with common elements
  - natural products or their semisynthetic derivatives
  - inhibitors of DNA topoisomerase II
  - planar polar compounds
  - aromatic heterocycles
    - □ anthracyclines (daunorubicin, doxorubicin, idarubicin, epirubicin)
    - □ epipodophyllotoxins (etoposide [VP-16], teniposide [VM-26])
    - □ aminoacridines (amsacrine [m-AMSA])
    - □ anthracenediones (mitoxantrone)
    - □ ellipticines (elliptinium [NMHE])
- Inhibitors of DNA topoisomerase I
  - major agents are derivatives of camptothecin, an extract of the Camptotheca acuminata plant
    - □ topotecan, irinotecan (CPT-11)

KEY REFERENCES

Gerrits CJ, de Jonge MJ, Schellens JH, et al.: Topoisomerase I inhibitors: the relevance of prolonged exposure for present clinical development. Br J Cancer 1997; 76(7): 952–62

Nitiss JL, Beck WT: Antitopoisomerase drug action and resistance. Eur J Cancer 1996; 32A(6):958–66

Ratain MJ, Rowley JD: Therapy-related acute myeloid leukemia secondary to inhibitors of topoisomerase II: from the bedside to the target genes. Ann Oncol 1992; 3(2):107–11

Rothenberg ML: Topoisomerase I inhibitors: review and update. Ann Oncol 1997; 8(9):837–55

Stewart CF, Zamboni WC, Crom WR, et al.: Topoisomerase I interactive drugs in children with cancer. Invest New Drugs 1996; 14(1):37–47

Drug: Etoposide

Antonius A. Miller and Mary Beth Mardjetko

OTHER NAMES: VP-16, VP-16-213, VEPESID

USES

- Approved by FDA for testicular tumors and small cell lung cancer
- Also active in non–small cell lung cancer, lymphoma, Hodgkin's disease, acute myelogenous leukemia, gestational trophoblastic tumors, pediatric sarcomas

MECHANISM OF ACTION

- Interference with the scission-reunion reaction of the enzyme DNA topoisomerase II and stabilization of the enzyme-DNA cleavable complex
- Inhibition of the DNA "strand-passing" activity of topoisomerase II
- Accumulation of cells in late S and early G_2 phase of the cell cycle
- Presence of P-glycoprotein confers resistance
- Decreased topoisomerase II expression results in resistance
- Other possible mechanisms of resistance include alteration in formation or repair of DNA strand breaks and structural alterations of topoisomerase II

DOSING

- Administered IV as a 30–60-min infusion (do not give by rapid IV injection)
- Oral formulation available as 50 mg capsules
- Schedules/doses
  - testicular cancer: 50–100 mg/m²/d IV daily for 5 days or 100 mg/m²/d on day 1, 3, and 5
  - small cell lung cancer: 35–50 mg/m²/d IV daily for 4 or 5 days or 80–100 mg/m²/d IV daily for 3 days; oral dose is generally twice the IV dose rounded to the nearest 50 mg
  - commonly used combinations
    - □ BEP for testicular cancer: bleomycin 30 U IV day 2, 9, 16; etoposide 100 mg/m²/d IV days 1–5; cisplatin 20 mg/m²/d IV days 1–5
    - □ small cell lung cancer: cisplatin 80 mg/m²/d IV day 1; etoposide 80 mg/m²/d IV days 1–3
  - the use of G-CSF as an adjunct to chemotherapy in patients with small cell lung cancer led to reductions in the incidence, duration, and severity of grade IV neutropenia and reduction in the incidence of febrile neutropenia

PHARMACOKINETICS

- 50 mg oral etoposide has bioavailability of 66%
- Biphasic plasma disposition with terminal half-life 3–11 hrs
- Drug elimination is by urinary excretion (~40–50%), hepatic metabolism, and minor component of biliary excretion
- ~94% protein bound, mostly to albumin
- Decreased albumin and/or increased bilirubin results in higher free fraction
- Does not accumulate with daily IV or po dosing
- Does not penetrate effectively into the cerebrospinal fluid

TOXICITY

- Myelosuppression is dose limiting; recovery by day 21
- Neutropenia is common with nadir occurring 7–14 days after drug administration
- Thrombocytopenia is less common
- Nausea and vomiting occur in ~30–40% of patients and are usually mild to moderate
- Mucositis may occur at higher doses
- Hypotension may occur following rapid IV administration
- Hypersensitivity reactions including fever, chills, tachycardia, bronchospasm, dyspnea, and hypotension occur in ~1–2% of patients
- Alopecia is common and reversible
- Other dermatologic toxicities (hyperpigmentation, pruritus, radiation recall dermatitis, Stevens-Johnson syndrome) are rare
- Peripheral neuropathy is unusual
- Optic neuritis and transient cortical blindness are very rare
- Reversible hepatotoxicity at very high doses with autologous bone marrow rescue has been reported
- Secondary acute myeloid leukemia (see Pui et al.)

RECOMMENDATIONS FOR SUPPORTIVE CARE

- Antiemetic prophylaxis is recommended, although there is no standard regimen
- If hypotension occurs stop infusion, administer IV fluid, restart etoposide at slower infusion rate

PHARMACY ISSUES

- IV formulation should be diluted with either 5% dextrose or 0.9% sodium chloride to give final concentration of 0.2–0.4 mg/ml

NURSING CONSIDERATIONS

- Leukopenia is dose limiting; monitor blood counts before and during treatment cycles
- Administer over 30–60 min
- Transient hypotension may occur and is rate related; stop infusion, administer IV fluids, and restart at a slower rate after recovery of blood pressure
- Anaphylactic reactions are more common during initial infusion; assure emergency measures are available
- Assess
  - patient for signs of anaphylaxis during the first 15 min of the infusion (chills, rigors, tachycardia, hypotension, bronchospasm, and dyspnea); rechallenge can be successful with histamine blockers and a slower rate; *but* if bronchospasm or laryngospasm is present rechallenge is *not* recommended
  - injection sites for signs of phlebitis and pain
  - alterations in nutritional status related to nausea, vomiting, and stomatitis (more often seen in patients receiving the oral form or higher IV doses)
- Teach patient
  - signs and symptoms of infection
  - report sensory and perceptual changes while receiving infusion
  - hard candy/gum lessen metallic taste associated with drug
  - drug is teratogenic and mutagenic

KEY REFERENCES

Hainsworth JD, Greco FA: Etoposide: twenty years later. Ann Oncol 1995; 6(4):325–41

Joel S: The clinical pharmacology of etoposide: an update. Cancer Treat Rev 1996; 22(3):179–221

Lowis SP, Newell DR: Etoposide for the treatment of pediatric tumors: what is the best way to give it? Eur J Cancer 1996; 32A(13): 2291–7

Miller AA, Tolley EA, Niell HB, et al.: Pharmacodynamics of prolonged oral etoposide in patients with advanced non–small cell lung cancer. J Clin Oncol 1993; 11(6):1179–88

Pui CH, Ribeiro RC, Hancock ML, et al.: Acute myeloid leukemia in children treated with epipodophyllotoxins for acute lymphoblastic leukemia. N Engl J Med 1991; 325:1682–7

Stewart CF: Use of etoposide in patients with organ dysfunction: pharmacokinetic and pharmacodynamic considerations. Cancer Chemother Pharmacol 1994; 34(suppl): S76–83

Drug: Etoposide Phosphate (Also See Etoposide)

Antonius A. Miller and Dolores Watts

OTHER NAMES: ETOPOPHOS

USES

- Approved by FDA for testicular tumors and small cell lung cancer
- Other uses same as for etoposide
- Mechanism of Action
- Water-soluble prodrug of etoposide
- Mechanism of action same as for etoposide

DOSING

- Administered IV as a 5 min or longer infusion
- Oral formulation not available in US
- Schedules/doses
  - etoposide phosphate doses are calculated as molar equivalents of etoposide (113.6 mg etoposide phosphate is the molar equivalent of 100 mg etoposide)

PHARMACOKINETICS

- Rapid in vivo conversion of etoposide phosphate to etoposide
- After conversion same pharmacokinetic profile as equimolar dose of etoposide

TOXICITY

- Etoposide phosphate has the same toxicity profile as equimolar dose of etoposide

RECOMMENDATIONS FOR SUPPORTIVE CARE

- Antiemetic prophylaxis is recommended, although there is no standard regimen

PHARMACY ISSUES

- Supplied as single-dose vials with white flip-off seals containing etoposide phosphate equivalent to 100 mg etoposide
- Etoposide phosphate is water soluble and can be prepared at high concentrations and may be given by bolus injection

NURSING CONSIDERATIONS

- Dose modifications should be made in patients with impaired renal function, those previously treated with chemotherapy or radiation therapy who may have compromised bone marrow reserve
- Monitor blood counts to assure adequate bone marrow recovery with subsequent cycles
- Patients with low serum albumin may be at increased risk for toxicities
- Potential for anaphylaxis during infusion; assure emergency measures are available
- Assess
  - oral cavity for signs of ulceration
  - for clinical signs of hypersensitivity reaction/anaphylaxis during drug infusion; monitor blood pressure prior to, during, and after infusion
- Teach patient
  - report sensory/perceptual changes while receiving infusion
  - to follow an oral hygiene regimen to reduce secondary infections and stomatitis
  - side effects and self-care measures

KEY REFERENCES

Budman DR, Igwemezie LN, Kaul S, et al.: Phase I evaluation of a water-soluble etoposide prodrug, etoposide phosphate, given as a 5-minute infusion on days 1, 3, and 5 in patients with solid tumors. J Clin Oncol 1994; 12(9):1902–9

Hainsworth JD, Levitan N, Wampler GL, et al.: Phase II randomized study of cisplatin plus etoposide phosphate or etoposide in the treatment of small-cell lung cancer. J Clin Oncol 1995; 13:1436–42

Thompson DS, Greco FA, Miller AA, et al.: A phase I study of etoposide phosphate administered as a daily 30 minute infusion for 5 days. Clin Pharmacol Ther 1995; 57:499–507

Drug: Teniposide

Naomi Winick and Erin P. Demakos

OTHER NAMES: VM-26, VEHEM, VUMON

USES

- Approved by FDA for refractory leukemia
- Also active in Hodgkin's and non-Hodgkin's lymphomas, germ cell tumors, small cell lung carcinoma, CNS malignancies, bladder carcinoma, and neuroblastoma

MECHANISM OF ACTION

- Topoisomerase II inhibitor
- Induces formation of a covalent bond between DNA repair enzyme topoisomerase II and DNA
- Reversibly inhibits nucleoside transport across the plasma membrane
- May undergo activation to form free radicals
- Presence of P-glycoprotein confers resistance
- Atypical multidrug resistance is associated with altered topoisomerase II and leads to reduced formation of drug-induced cleaveable complexes
- Clinical reports suggest a lack of complete cross-resistance with etoposide
- Synergistic in vitro with cytosine arabinoside, carmustine, hexamethylmelamine, and methotrexate

DOSING

- Administered IV as a 45–60 min infusion
- Has been given po with a 41% mean bioavailability
- Local bladder installation may be used for superficial bladder malignancies
- Schedules/doses
  - 60–90 mg/m^2 weekly for solid tumors
  - 60 mg/m^2/d as a 5 day continuous infusion has been well tolerated
  - commonly used combinations
    - □ 150–200 mg/m^2 twice weekly for 4–8 doses in combination with cytosine arabinoside for refractory leukemias

PHARMACOKINETICS

- Extensively metabolized with the glucuronidated aglycone having cytotoxic activity
- Extensively protein bound; > 99%
- Half-life of ~ 6–10 hrs
- 0–10% eliminated via biliary excretion

TOXICITY

- Primarily leukopenia with thrombocytopenia less common
- Grade 1–2 nausea and vomiting
- Reversible alopecia
- The epipodophyllotoxins have been associated with a distinct form of secondary AML characterized by a short latency, the absence of a preceding myelodysplastic phase, FAB M4 or M5 morphology, and abnormalities of 11q23
  - the incidence of secondary AML is significantly dependent on the schedule of epipodophyllotoxin administration and to a lesser extent on total cumulative dose
- Hypersensitivity reactions may be more common in adults with brain tumors
- Rapid infusion may be associated with hypotension with or without fever, chills, bronchospasm, chest pain, urticaria, and flushing
- Usually self-limited and may be caused by the polyoxyethylated caster oil diluent used to increase drug solubility
- Diphenhydramine and hydrocortisone have been used to treat the hypersensitivity reactions with inconsistent results
- Rarely pulmonary toxicity may occur

RECOMMENDATIONS FOR SUPPORTIVE CARE

- Antiemetic prophylaxis is recommended, although there is no standard regimen
- When given in multiple doses combined with other agents, support with G-CSF may be indicated, though there is no standard recommendation

PHARMACY ISSUES

- Isotonic, sodium chloride, or D_5W can be used as diluents
- Maximal stability is achieved with a final drug concentration of 0.2 mg/ml; concentrations of 0.4 and 1.0 mg/ml are stable for ~ 4 hrs and are associated with a decrease in stability

NURSING CONSIDERATIONS

- Do not administer if precipitate is seen; chemical phlebitis can occur if not diluted properly
- Rapid infusion may cause hypotension
- Ensure proper placement of IV catheter; drug is an irritant and extravasation could result in tissue necrosis
- Premedicate with diphenhydramine and hydrocortisone
- Implement special precautions regarding hypersensitivity
- Mild increases in LFTs may occur; monitor LFTs prior to and during drug administration
- Assess
  - cardiac status prior to and during drug administration; obtain baseline vital signs prior to and 30 min after initiation of drug administration; if systolic drops below 90 mm Hg, stop infusion and notify physician
  - for signs of myelosuppression
  - baseline neurologic status
- Teach patient
  - report untoward symptoms immediately while receiving drug infusion
  - avoid OTC aspirin-containing medications
  - practice contraception
  - potential for second malignancy

KEY REFERENCES

Muggia FM: Teniposide: overview of its therapeutic potential in adult cancers. Cancer Chemother Pharmacol 1994; 34:S127–33

Rodman JH, Furman WL, Sunderland M, et al.: Escalating teniposide systemic exposure to increase dose intensity for pediatric cancer patients. J Clin Oncol 1993; 11(2):271–8

Drug: Doxorubicin

Malcolm Moore, Amita Patnaik, and Hollie Devine

OTHER NAMES: ADRIAMYCIN, HYDROXYDAUNORUBICIN, HYDROXYDAUNOMYCIN, RUBEX

USES

- Approved for use
  - adjuvant and metastatic breast cancer regimens
  - Hodgkin's and non-Hodgkin's lymphoma
- Also active in other solid tumors, including ovary, lung, transitional cell carcinoma

MECHANISM OF ACTION

- Topoisomerase II inhibitor
- Induces formation of covalent topo II-DNA complexes
  - preventing the enzyme from completing the religation portion of the ligation-religation reaction
- DNA intercalation
  - causing single- and double-stranded breaks
- Free radical formation causing oxidative damage to cellular proteins
- Alters cell membranes
- Stimulation of apoptosis
- Cell cycle-phase nonspecific
- Increased expression of P-glycoprotein confers resistance
- Other mechanisms of resistance
  - overexpression of MRP (multidrug resistance–associated protein)
  - altered topoisomerase II activity and expression
  - enhanced antioxidant defense
  - enhanced DNA repair
  - overexpression of bcl-2
  - mutations in p53

DOSING

- Administered slowly through a running IV line over 2–5 min using extravasation precautions, or continuously infused through a central line
- Rapid administration may cause arrhythmias, flushing, or syncope
- Protect drug from sunlight
- Schedules/doses
  - 45–60 mg/m² IV bolus or continuous infusion over 2–4 days q3–4wks
  - 10–20 mg/m² IV weekly
  - 30 mg/m² IV daily for three days q3–4wks
- Commonly used combinations
  - adjuvant therapy for breast cancer: 30 mg/m² given IV on day 1, 8 in combination with 5-fluorouracil 500 mg/m² IV day 1, 8 and cyclophosphamide 100 mg/m² po daily for 14 days
  - treatment of advanced breast cancer: 50 mg/m² IV in combination with 5-fluorouracil 500 mg/m² IV and cyclophosphamide 500 mg/m² IV q3wks
  - treatment of non-Hodgkin's lymphoma: 50 mg/m² IV in combination with cyclophosphamide 750 mg/m² IV, vincristine 2 mg, prednisone 100 mg for 5 days, q3wks (CHOP)
  - treatment of Hodgkin's disease: 25 mg/m² IV in combination with bleomycin 10 mg/m² IV, vinblastine 6 mg/m² IV, DTIC 375 mg/m² IV q14d (ABVD)

PHARMACOKINETICS

- Widely distributed throughout body
- 70% protein bound
- Distributes in high concentrations into certain tissues (heart, liver, kidneys)
- Terminal half-life of 30–50 hrs
- Rapidly metabolized in the liver to one active (doxorubicinol) and several noncytotoxic metabolites
- Dose reductions required for hyperbilirubinemia or impaired liver function
  - no precise guidelines exist

TOXICITY

- Dose limiting
  - myelosuppression, especially leukopenia, with a nadir at 10–15 days and recovery within 21 days
- Cardiotoxicity
  - acute: nonspecific EKG changes during or immediately after infusion, pericarditis-myocarditis syndrome
  - chronic: dose-dependent congestive cardiomyopathy
    - □ total cumulative dose should not exceed 450–500 mg/m² as the risk of clinical cardiac toxicity rises rapidly beyond this dose
    - □ threshold for cardiotoxicity is lower in patients with preexisting cardiac dysfunction
    - □ using more prolonged administration schedules with lower peak concentrations of doxorubicin also reduces the risk of cardiomyopathy
    - □ prior cardiac radiation exposure (2000 cGy in 200 cGy/d fractions) doubles the rate at which cardiac toxicity occurs, so cumulative doxorubicin dose should not exceed 250 mg/m²
- Common
  - alopecia
  - nausea and vomiting
  - mucositis
  - severe local tissue damage from drug extravasation
  - radiation sensitizer
- Occasional
  - diarrhea
  - hyperpigmentation of nail beds, dermal creases, facial flush, skin rash, conjunctivitis
  - red-colored urine

RECOMMENDATIONS FOR SUPPORTIVE CARE

- Antiemetic prophylaxis with 5-HT3 antagonists and steroids, both pretreatment and postchemotherapy for 24–48 hrs
- Monitoring of cardiac function using gated nuclear angiogram to assess; ejection fraction can detect impairments prior to the development of clinical signs of heart failure

NURSING CONSIDERATIONS

- Drug is a vesicant; administer through a running IV; avoid extravasation; if it occurs stop infusion and follow institutional procedures
- Myelosuppression is major dose-limiting side effect; monitor CBC, WBC, differential, and platelet count prior to drug administration
- Patients with previous history of mediastinal RT, coronary, valvular, or myocardial heart disease, hypertension, and > 70 yrs of age are at higher risk for cardiotoxicity
- Premedicate with antiemetics
- Assess
  - cardiac function prior to and during chemotherapy with EKG, MUGA, and/or echocardiogram
  - accurately document each dose: cumulative anthracycline dose should include administration of concurrent and prior doxorubicin and daunorubicin compounds
  - skin for signs of radiation recall: treat symptomatically with cool compresses, emollients, antimicrobial ointment, and topical steroids
  - for GI toxicities: stomatitis, esophagitis
  - for flare reaction: if it occurs consider reconstituting drug in an isotonic medium or administer systemic antihistamines or corticosteroids as premedication prior to doxorubicin
  - inspect injection sites for signs of extravasation
- Teach patient
  - if given by continuous infusion via ambulatory pump, provide instructions regarding regulation of pump and management of chemotherapy spills at home
  - urine may appear pink after treatment; encourage fluids
  - alopecia is reversible
  - drug is teratogenic, mutagenic, and carcinogenic

KEY REFERENCES

Bielack SS, Erttmann R, Kempf-Bielack B, et al.: Impact of scheduling on toxicity and clinical efficacy of doxorubicin: what do we know in the mid-nineties? Eur J Cancer 1996; 32A(10):1652–60

Bristow MR, Lopez MB, Mason JW, et al.: Efficacy and cost of cardiac monitoring in patients receiving doxorubicin. Cancer 1982; 50:32–41

Curran CF, Luce JK, Page JA: Doxorubicin-associated flare reactions. Oncol Nursing Forum 1990; 17(3):387–9

Gianni L, Munzone E, Capri G, et al.: Paclitaxel by 3 hour infusion in combination with bolus doxorubicin in women with untreated metastatic breast cancer: high antitumor efficacy and cardiac effects in a dose-finding and sequence-finding study. J Clin Oncol 1995; 13(11):2688–99

Launchbury AP, Habboubi N: Epirubicin and doxorubicin: a comparison of their characteristics, therapeutic activity and toxicity. Cancer Treat Rev 1993; 19(3):197–228

Drug: Daunorubicin

Ellin Berman and Hollie Devine

OTHER NAMES: DAUNOMYCIN, CERUBIDINE, RUBIDOMYCIN

USES

- Standard component of many initial induction regimens in adult and pediatric acute myelogenous and acute lymphoblastic leukemia

MECHANISM OF ACTION

- Intercalates between DNA base pairs interfering with action of topoisomerase II
  - this causes strand breakage and interference with strand elongation
- Causes free radical formation
- Does not cross blood-brain barrier
- Presence of P-glycoprotein confers resistance

DOSING

- Administered through a free-flowing IV line in either normal saline or D_5W over 10–15 min
- No oral formulation
- Commonly used combinations
  - 45–60 mg/m^2/d for 3 days in combination with other antileukemic agents

PHARMACOKINETICS

- Extensively metabolized by the liver with rapid formation of active metabolite daunorubicinol
- Elimination half-life for parent compound is 14–20 hrs; for metabolite, 23–40 hrs
- Primarily excreted by the bile; small amount of urinary excretion

TOXICITY

- Dose-related marrow suppression
- Dose-related cardiotoxicity with nonreversible cardiac failure seen at doses exceeding 350 mg/m^2
  - also causes EKG abnormalities, arrythmias, conduction disturbances
  - incidence of congestive failure may be reduced by use of dezriazoxane
- Gastrointestinal effects
  - nausea, vomiting, mucositis, diarrhea, abnormalities in liver function tests
- Urine may turn orange after drug administration
- Alopecia
- Can cause severe extravasation reactions

RECOMMENDATIONS FOR SUPPORTIVE CARE

- Antiemetic prophylaxis required
- Use of myeloid growth factor such as G-CSF or GM-CSF depending on clinical setting

PHARMACY ISSUES

- Diluent: either normal saline or D_5W

NURSING CONSIDERATIONS

- Drug is a vesicant; administer through a running IV; avoid extravasation; if it occurs stop infusion and follow institutional procedures
- Patients with previous history of mediastinal RT, coronary, valvular, or myocardial heart disease, hypertension, and >70 yrs of age are at higher risk for cardiotoxicity
- Pericarditis more likely to result with daunorubicin than with doxorubicin
- Monitor CBC, WBC, differential, and platelet count following drug administration
- Monitor renal and liver function; dose adjustment if hepatic dysfunction
- Assess
  - cardiac function prior to chemotherapy with EKG, MUGA, and/or echocardiogram
  - accurately document each dose
  - for hypersensitivity reaction; urticaria, pruritis, dyspnea, angioedema, bronchospasm, and hypotension; consider premedication with antihistamines and steroids (rare)
  - GI toxicities; nausea and vomiting and stomatitis
  - skin for signs of radiation recall or flare reaction
- Teach patient
  - report signs and symptoms of infection and extravasation
  - report irregular heartbeat, shortness of breath, and swelling of lower extremities
  - urine may be orange for several days after therapy
  - alopecia is reversible
  - drug is mutagenic and teratogenic

KEY REFERENCES

Berman E, Heller G, Santorsa J, et al.: Results of a randomized trial comparing idarubicin and cytosine arabinoside with daunorubicin and cytosine arabinoside in adult patients with newly diagnosed acute myelogenous leukemia. Blood 1991; 77(8):1666–74

Berman E, Wiernik P, Vogler R, et al.: Long-term follow-up of three randomized trials comparing idarubicin and daunorubicin as induction therapies for patients with untreated acute myeloid leukemia. Cancer 1997; 80(11 Suppl): 2181–5

Usui N, Dobashi N, Kobayashi T, et al.: Role of daunorubicin in the induction therapy for adult acute myeloid leukemia. J Clin Oncol 1998; 16(6):2086–92

Drug: Epirubicin HCl

Elisabeth G.E. de Vries and Deborah T. Berg

OTHER NAMES: 4′-EPIADRIAMYCIN HYDROCHLORIDE, 4′-EPIDOXORUBICIN HYDROCHLORIDE, 4′-EPIADRIAMYCIN, PIDORUBICIN HYDROCHLORIDE

USES

- Worldwide (except US) registered for breast carcinoma, ovarian carcinoma, lung carcinoma, gastric carcinoma, bladder cancer, soft tissue/osteosarcoma, non-Hodgkin's lymphoma, and Hodgkin's disease
- Registered in US for adjuvant therapy in patients with evidence of axillary node tumor involvement following resection of primary breast cancer
- Also active in leukemias, multiple myeloma

MECHANISMS OF ACTION

- Intercalation between DNA base pairs
- Inhibits DNA and RNA synthesis
- Topoisomerase II inhibitor
- Generation of free radicals
- Most active in S and G_2 phase cell cycle
- Presence of the pumps: P-glycoprotein and MRP1 does confer resistance, decreased topoisomerase II expression results in resistance, and resistance may occur due to blockade of the apoptotic pathway (e.g., by aberrant p53 expression)

DOSING

- Administered IV as slow (e.g., 15 min) infusion
- Conventional dose 75–100 mg/m^2 q3wks
- In combination regimens 50–75 mg/m^2 q3wks
- Increasingly used at higher doses, 100–120 mg/m^2 q3wks
- Higher doses (> 120 mg/m^2) have been used with hematopoietic growth factors or as part of high-dose chemotherapy regimen followed by hematopoietic stem cell support
- Dosage reduction of 50% is recommended in patients with moderately impaired liver function
- Withhold drug in patients with severe liver impairment
- The drug has been administered intravesically for bladder carcinoma, intra-arterial and continuously IV through a central venous catheter

PHARMACOKINETICS

- > 90% protein binding
- Terminal half-life 18–54 hrs
- Large volume of distribution
- Extensive hepatic metabolism to epirubicinol and aglycone and glucuronide metabolites
- 6–13% renal excretion, 35% biliary excretion
- Reduced plasma clearance in patients with hepatic dysfunction

TOXICITY

- Nausea, vomiting
- Bone marrow depression consisting of thrombocytopenia, anemia but especially leucocytopenia
- Leukocyte nadir occurs 10–14 days after treatment
- Irreversible cardiac toxicity can occur if cumulative dose approaches 900 mg/m^2
- Cardiac toxicity can develop earlier in case of prior anthracycline, age < 15 yrs, mitomycin C therapy, mediastinal radiotherapy, or cardiac disease
- Hair loss
- Diarrhea can take place
- Mucositis can occur 5–10 days after administration
- Recall of skin reaction due to prior radiotherapy can appear
- Irritating effect at site of drug administration
- Local tissue necrosis if extravasated during IV administration
- Mutagenic, carcinogenic
- Similar treatment efficacy as doxorubicin and moderately less toxic concerning immediate and delayed side effects (< hematologic and cardiac toxicity)
- Doxorubicin 90 mg/m^2 is comparable to epirubicin 120 mg/m^2

RECOMMENDATION FOR SUPPORTIVE CARE

- Antiemetic prophylaxis
- Contraception

PHARMACY ISSUES

- Epirubicin is incompatible with heparin, fluorouracil, and alkali
- The lyophilized formulation is stable for 3 yrs at room temperature; the reconstituted solution of this formulation is 24 hrs stable
- Photodegeneration may occur at lower concentrations (< 500 μg/ml)
- Epirubicin hydrochloride is administered IV in 0.9% sodium chloride or as small volume in water for injection into fast-running infusion 0.9% sodium chloride or 5% glucose

NURSING CONSIDERATIONS

- Dose modification based on WBC, platelet count, and LFTs
- Reduce dose if patient received prior chest irradiation or anthracyclines
- If extravasation occurs, immediately stop infusion and follow hospital policy
- Cumulative lifetime dose is 900 mg/m^2
- Premedicate with antiemetics and continue for 1–2 days
- Assess
  - cardiac function should be assessed for signs and symptoms of cardiomyopathy; CHF and EKG changes and MUGA or cardiac echography in patients receiving large cumulative doses
- Teach patients
  - expected side effects and self-care measures
  - inform patient that urine will turn reddish orange
- Contraindicated in patients with neutropenia, severe myocardial insufficiency, recent MI, severe renal or hepatic dysfunction, or those who have received maximum doses of other anthracyclines
- Dose modifications based on absolute neutrophil count, platelet count, and LFTs
- Monitor LVEF at initiation of epirubicin and periodically during therapy to avoid potential cardiac impairment
- Carefully monitor geriatric patients, especially elderly (≥70 yr old) women

KEY REFERENCES

Bonadonna G, Gianni L, Santora A, Bonfante V, Bidoli P, Casali P, DeMiceli R, Valagussa P: Drugs ten years later: Epirubicin. Ann Oncol 1993; 4:359–69

Loukell AJ, Faulds D: Epirubicin. An updated review of its pharmacodynamic and pharmacokinetic properties and therapeutic efficacy in the management of breast cancer. Drugs 1997; 53: 453–82

Drug: Idarubicin

Ellin Berman and Hollie Devine

OTHER NAMES: 4-DEMETHOXYDAUNORUBICIN

USES

- Approved by FDA for use in acute myelogenous leukemia; activity also demonstrated in acute lymphoblastic leukemia
- The drug is usually combined with other agents for induction chemotherapy
- Preliminary data suggest activity in lymphoma
- Limited activity in solid tumors

MECHANISM OF ACTION

- Intercalates between DNA base pairs, interfering with strand elongation
- Changes in DNA configuration also interfere with topoisomerase II activity causing DNA strand breaks
- Causes free radical formation
- Preclinical data suggest that the drug is less susceptible to overexpression of P-glycoprotein

DOSING

- Administered through a free-flowing IV line in either normal saline or D_5W over 10–15 min
- Commonly used combinations
  - 10–12 mg/m^2 daily for 3 days in combination with other antileukemic agents
  - oral formulation not yet available for use in the US

PHARMACOKINETICS

- Metabolism occurs primarily in the liver
- Undergoes biliary excretion with some renal excretion noted
- Parent compound converted to active metabolite, idarubinol
- Metabolite appears much more potent than other anthracycline metabolites
- Both parent drug and metabolite cross blood-brain barrier
- Half-life of idarubicin is ~22 hrs
- Half-life of idarubicinol >45 hrs

TOXICITY

- Dose-related marrow suppression
- Dose-related cardiotoxicity with nonreversible cardiac failure; assuming 5:1 potency ratio compared to daunorubicin, dose-limiting cardiotoxicty is in the range of 84 mg/m^2
  - also causes EKG abnormalities, arrythmias, conduction disturbances
  - no data exist for cardioprotective effect of dezrazoxane
- Gastrointestinal effects
  - nausea, vomiting, mucositis, diarrhea, abnormalities in liver function tests
- Urine may turn orange after drug administration
- Alopecia
- Can cause severe extravasation reaction

RECOMMENDATIONS FOR SUPPORTIVE CARE

- Antiemetic prophylaxis required
- Use of myeloid growth factor depending on clinical setting

PHARMACY ISSUES

- Diluent: either normal saline or D_5W

NURSING CONSIDERATIONS

- Drug is four to five times more potent than doxorubicin
- Drug is a vesicant; administer through a running IV; avoid extravasation; if it occurs stop infusion and follow institutional procedures
- Incompatible with heparin; causes a precipitate
- Patients with impaired renal and hepatic dysfunction are at increased risk for toxic effects; dose reductions recommended for increased bilirubin; monitor kidney and liver functions
- Maintain accurate records of total dose; cardiotoxicity increases as cumulative dose exceeds 70 mg/m^2
- Myelosuppression is dose-limiting effect; monitor CBC and platelet count
- Assess
  - cardiac function prior to each dose; document each dose accurately; cardiotoxicity increases as the cumulative dose approaches 84 mg/m^2
  - for GI toxicities: mucositis, stomatitis, diarrhea, nausea, and vomiting
- Teach patient
  - urine may appear orange for up to 48 hrs after administration
  - encourage fluids to promote urination
  - to report irregular heartbeat, chest pain, shortness of breath, pain at injection site
  - side effects and self-care measures
  - alopecia is reversible

KEY REFERENCES

Berman E, Heller G, Santorsa J, et al.: Results of a randomized trial comparing idarubicin and cytosine arabinoside with daunorubicin and cytosine arabinoside in adult patients with newly diagnosed acute myelogenous leukemia. Blood 1991; 77(8):1666–74

Berman E, Wiernik P, Vogler R, et al.: Long-term follow-up of three randomized trials comparing idarubicin and daunorubicin as induction therapies for patients with untreated acute myeloid leukemia. Cancer 1997; 80(11 suppl):2181–5

Buckley MM, Lamb HM: Oral idarubicin. A review of its pharmacological properties and clinical efficacy in the treatment of hematological malignancies and advanced breast cancer. Drugs Aging 1997; 11(1):61–86

Parker JE, Pagliuca A, Mijovic A, et al.: Fludarabine, cytarabine, G-CSF and idarubicin (FLAG-IDA) for the treatment of poor-risk myelodysplastic syndromes and acute myeloid leukemia. Br J Haematol 1997; 99(4):939–44

Drug: Pegylated-Liposomal Doxorubicin (PLD)

Franco M. Muggia and Susan Noble-Kempin

OTHER NAMES: DOXIL, CAELYX, PLD

USES

- Approved by FDA for AIDS-related Kaposi's sarcoma (KS) and for platinum- and paclitaxel-refractory ovarian cancer
- Active against breast cancer previously untreated with anthracyclines

MECHANISM OF ACTION

- Actions are related to release of doxorubicin in the extracellular fluid of tumors
- Long circulation of the liposomes and leaky vasculature in tumors contribute to preferential localization in tumors
- Once in tumors, doxorubicin exerts antitumor effects through DNA interaction and topoisomerase II inhibition, leading to apoptosis
- Presumably same mechanisms of resistance as doxorubicin

DOSING

- After reconstitution, the drug is administered IV at a rate of 1–2 mg/min
- Administration is often slower during the first 10 min, to avoid pseudo-allergic reactions
- Schedule/doses
  - for Kaposi's sarcoma, 20 mg/m^2 q2–3wks
  - for solid tumors, 40–50 mg/m^2 q4wks
  - in drug combinations (with 80 mg/m^2/wk short infusion of paclitaxel, or with 50 mg/m^2 of cisplatin) doses of 30–40 mg/m^2 q3–4 wks are used

PHARMACOKINETICS

- Clearance occurs by uptake of circulating liposomes by reticuloendothelial cells, and by removal of the liposomes in areas where leaky tumor vasculature exists
- One-third of the injected dose is cleared in 1–3 hrs
- The remainder is cleared with a half-life exceeding 42 hrs, and as high as 72 hrs
- Volume of distribution at steady state is similar to the blood volume
- Pharmacokinetics for total and liposome-associated doxorubicin are nearly identical
- Radio-labeled pegylated liposomes preferentially are retained by solid tumors
- Concentrations of doxorubicin in KS lesions are higher after PLD than free drug

TOXICITY

- Common toxicities (incidence > 15%)
  - palmar-plantar erythrodysesthesia (hand-foot syndrome)
  - stomatitis
  - neutropenia
- Nausea and vomiting, alopecia, fever are distinctly uncommon
- Cardiac toxicity and extravasation necrosis do not occur following PLD, although greater experience and endomyocardial biopsy studies are awaited
- Acute reactions during the first minutes of an infusion (flushing, dyspnea, facial swelling, back pain) occur in ~10–30%, probably from complement activation
- Grade 4 toxicities occur in < 2% of patients receiving 40 mg/m^2 q4wks

RECOMMENDATIONS FOR SUPPORTIVE CARE

- Antiemetic prophylaxis is not needed
- Dexamethasone IV may prevent pseudo-allergic reactions
- Pyridoxine has been claimed to improve skin manifestations
- Avoidance of trauma to feet and avoidance of hot beverages 3 days after drug are reasonable precautions

PHARMACY ISSUES

- The drug is available in 25 mg vials that are stable when stored at room temperature
- Reconstitution is with either D_5W or NS to a volume from 100–250 ml

NURSING CONSIDERATIONS

- Rapid infusion increases risk of infusion-related reaction; do not administer as a bolus injection; do not flush infustion line at or near end of administration
- Acute infusion reactions tend to occur immediately with the first dose and rarely after
- Stop infusion and administer antihistamines and/or corticosteroids
- Reinstitute at a slower rate
- Premedicate to avoid future hypersensitivity reactions
- Patients with a history of asthma or other allergies are prone to infusion reactions
- Administer infusion in view of a nurse
- Avoid in-line filters for administration
- Use of bacteriostatic agents or diluent other than D_5W may cause a precipitate
- Avoid extravasation; stop infusion and follow institutional policies
- Assess
  - cardiac function prior to chemotherapy; cumulative anthracycline dose should include administration of concurrent and prior doxorubicin and daunorubicin compounds
  - skin integrity with each treatment; topical anesthetics of diphenhydramine-containing creams may exacerbate skin toxicity
  - mucous membranes for stomatitis
  - blood counts
- Teach patient
  - avoid use of tape on skin, tight clothing pressure friction on skin, hot water, sun exposure, vigorous activities, and leaning on bony prominences for 3 days after drug administration
  - emphasize avoidance of hot baths/showers for 24 hrs prior to and 72 hrs after administration; vigorous washing and drying of skin (pat dry)
  - good oral hygiene; avoidance of alcohol-containing mouth wash; infection control measures

KEY REFERENCES

Markman M, guest ed: Disease management of solid tumors and the emerging role of pegylated liposomal doxorubicin. Drugs 1997; 54(suppl 4):1–35

Porche DJ: Liposomal doxorubicin (Doxil). J Assoc Nurses Aids Care 1996; 7(2):55–9

Drug: Liposome Encapsulated Daunorubicin

Mark D. DeMario and Susan Noble-Kempin

OTHER NAMES: DAUNOXOME

USES

■ Approved by FDA for treatment of advanced HIV-associated Kaposi's sarcoma

MECHANISM OF ACTION

■ The anthracycline antibiotic daunorubicin is encapsulated within lipid vesicles (liposomes), which are composed of a lipid bilayer of distearoylphosphatidylcholine and cholesterol in a 2:1 molar ratio

■ In the circulation, liposome encapsulation protects daunorubicin from enzymatic degradation and protein binding

■ Liposomal encapsulation enhances drug delivery to neoplastic tissues

■ This specificity is likely conferred by increased permeability of tumor vasculature

■ Once in the tumor interstitium, the liposomes release daunorubicin over time

DOSING

- Administer IV as a 60 min infusion
- Schedules/doses
  - 50–60 mg/m² q2wks
- Commonly used combinations
  - combination therapy with liposomal daunorubicin is investigational at this time

PHARMACOKINETICS

■ Following IV infusion, plasma clearance demonstrates monoexponential decline

■ Mean total body clearance range 3–7% that of free daunorubicin

■ Elimination half-life is ~4 hrs

TOXICITY

■ Myelosuppression, primarily granulocytic series, is common (20% incidence grade 3 or greater)

■ One study demonstrated 9–20% LVEF reduction in 3 of 13 patients

■ This finding was not dose related, nor was it associated with clinical CHF

■ Another study demonstrated no evidence of cardiotoxicity by LVEF at cumulative doses > 1,000 mg/m²

■ Infusion reactions consisting of back pain, flushing, and chest tightness occur within minutes of the start of infusion in ~10% of patients

■ Symptoms resolve when infusion is stopped

■ Reinitiating infusion at a lower rate generally prevents recurrence

■ Potential hepatotoxicity (transaminase elevation)

- Low-grade fever (> 25%)
- Mild/moderate nausea is common
- Diarrhea: 10%
- Mild alopecia

RECOMMENDATIONS FOR SUPPORTIVE CARE

■ Patient monitoring is required during infusion time due to potential for infusion reactions

■ Monitoring of hematologic, hepatic, and renal function is indicated prior to each treatment course

■ Hold treatment for absolute granulocyte count < 750/mm³
  - reduce dose by 50% for serum bilirubin > 3 mg/dl or serum creatinine > 3 mg/dl

PHARMACY ISSUES

- Dilute 1:1 with 5% dextrose
- Stability: refrigerate at 2–8°C (36–46°F)

■ Reconstituted solution is stable for 6 hrs and should be protected from light

NURSING CONSIDERATIONS

■ Rapid infusion increases risk of infusion-related reacton; do not administer as a bolus injection; do not flush infusion line at or near the end of administration

■ Acute infusion reactions tend to occur with first dose; stop infusion and administer antihistamines and/or corticosteroids; reinstitute infusion at slower rate; premedicate to avoid future hypersensitivity reactions

■ Use of bacteriostatic agents or diluent other than D_5W may cause a precipitate

■ Do not use in-line filters for administration

■ Take precautions to avoid extravasation; stop infusion and follow institutional procedures

- Assess
  - monitor patient during infusion for signs of hypersensitivity
  - cardiac function prior to chemotherapy; cumulative anthracycline dose should include administration of concurrent and prior doxorubicin and daunorubicin compounds
- Teach patient
  - report dyspnea, palpitations, and peripheral edema
  - infection prevention measures; signs and symptoms to report

KEY REFERENCES

Gill PS, et al.: Phase I/II clinical and pharmacokinetic evaluation of liposomal daunorubicin. J Clin Oncol 1995; 13:996

Guaglianone P, et al.: Phase I and pharmacologic study of liposomal daunorubicin (DaunoXome). Investigational New Drugs 1994; 12:103

Tupule A, et al.: Phase II trial of liposomal daunorubicin in the treatment of AIDS-related pulmonary Kaposi's sarcoma. J Clin Oncol 1998; 16:3369

Drug: Mitoxantrone

Malcolm J. Moore, Amita Patnaik, and Deborah T. Berg

OTHER NAMES: NOVANTRONE, DIHYDROXYANTHRACENEDIONE, DHAD

USES

- Breast cancer, lymphoma, acute leukemia, prostate cancer

MECHANISM OF ACTION

- Inhibition of topoisomerase II is likely main mechanism of cytotoxicity
- DNA intercalation
- Single-stranded and double-stranded DNA breakage
- Unlike doxorubicin there is little or no free radical formation
- Increased P-glycoprotein levels associated with resistance
- Overexpression of MRP may also confer resistance

DOSING

- Administered IV as a 30 min infusion
- Should not be administered in solutions containing heparin
- Schedule/doses
  - 12–14 mg/m^2 once q3wks for patients with solid tumors
  - 12 mg/m^2/d for 3 days for the treatment of AML
- Commonly used combinations
  - induction therapy for AML: 12 mg/m^2 IV days 1–3 in combination with cytosine arabinoside 100–200 mg/m^2 by continuous IV infusion days 1–7
  - for prostate cancer 12–14 mg/m^2 IV day 1, prednisone 10 mg po every day; cycles repeated q21d

PHARMACOKINETICS

- Highly protein bound
- Metabolized in the liver to inactive carboxylic acid derivatives and excreted in bile and urine as metabolites and unchanged drug
- Renal clearance accounts for ~10% of total body clearance
- Elimination may be impaired in patients with liver dysfunction
- Terminal half-life of 23–42 hrs

TOXICITY

- Myelosuppression
- Dose limiting
  - primarily neutropenia
  - common but rarely severe using doses of 12–14 mg/m^2
  - severe thrombocytopenia is uncommon (< 5%)
- Cardiac toxicity
  - although considered less cardiotoxic than anthracyclines such as doxorubicin, a dose-dependent cumulative cardiomyopathy occurs
  - total dose of mitoxantrone given should not exceed 180 mg/m^2
  - lower total dose (120–140 mg/m^2) in patients with prior cardiac problems
- Other common toxicities
  - mild nausea and vomiting
  - alopecia (mild; seen in 20–30%)
  - blue discoloration of urine, sclerae, and fingernails
- Occasional/rare toxicities
  - mucositis
  - jaundice, seizures, and pulmonary toxicity

RECOMMENDATIONS FOR SUPPORTIVE CARE

- Antiemetic prophylaxis for low emetogenic potential agents (e.g., steroids plus prochlorperazine)

NURSING CONSIDERATIONS

- Dose modifications are based on WBC and platelet count, thus need to closely monitor CBC
- Nonvesicant
- Blue-green coloration of the urine for 1–2 days after administration
- Premedication with antiemetic regimen indicated as is continuation of antiemetics for 1–2 days
- Assess
  - cardiac function for signs and symptoms of cardiomyopathy and other cardiac toxicities (dyspnea, edema, or arthopnea)
  - vital signs and patient's general status prior to and during administration for signs and symptoms of hypersensitivity reaction
- Teach patient
  - expected side effects and self-care measures
  - encourage small, frequent feedings of cool, bland foods
  - potential of permanent sterility

KEY REFERENCES

Dunn CJ, Goa KL: Mitoxantrone: a review of its pharmacological properties and use in acute nonlymphoblastic leukemia. Drugs & Aging 1996; 9(2):122–47

Lowenberg B, Suciu S, Archimbaud E, et al.: Mitoxantrone versus daunorubicin in induction-consolidation chemotherapy—the value of low-dose cytarabine for maintenance of remission, and an assessment of prognostic factors in acute myeloid leukemia in the elderly: final report European Organization for the Research and Treatment of Cancer and the Dutch Belgian Hemato-Oncology Cooperative Hovon Group. J Clin Oncol 1998; 16(3):872–81

Moore MJ, Osoba D, Murphy K, et al.: Use of palliative end points to evaluate the effects of mitoxantrone and low-dose prednisone in patients with hormonally resistant prostate cancer. J Clin Oncol 1994; 12(4):689–94

Tannock IF, Osoba D, Stockler MR, et al.: Chemotherapy with mitoxantrone plus prednisone or prednisone alone for symptomatic hormone-resistant prostate cancer: a Canadian randomized trial with palliative end points. J Clin Oncol 1996; 14(6):1756–64

Wiseman LR, Spencer CM: Mitoxantrone: a review of its pharmacology and clinical efficacy in the management of hormone resistant advanced prostate cancer. Drugs & Aging 1997; 10: 473–85

Drug: Losoxantrone

Duncan I. Jodrell and Deborah T. Berg

OTHER NAMES: BIANTRAZOLE, CI-941, DUP-941

USES

- Approved by the Canadian regulatory authorities for breast cancer

MECHANISM OF ACTION

- Anthrapyrazole
- Inhibitor of DNA topoisomerase II

DOSING

- IV slow bolus
- Schedule: 50 mg/m^2 q3wks

PHARMACOKINETICS

- Primarily eliminated by biliary excretion
- Terminal half-life, 21 ± 9 hrs

TOXICITY

- Neutropenia is dose limiting
- Nausea and vomiting, mucositis, alopecia, and skin discoloration also noted
- Possibility of drug-related cardiotoxicity has been reported, but not fully defined

RECOMMENDATIONS FOR SUPPORTIVE CARE

- Prophylactic antiemetics (no standard approach)

PHARMACY ISSUES

- Lyophilized powder for reconstitution in water for injection

NURSING CONSIDERATIONS

- Dose modifications are based on WBC and platelet count; monitor closely
- Nonvesicant
- Premedication with antiemetic regimen is indicated and should be continued for 1–2 days
- Assess
  - cardiac function for signs and symptoms of cardiomyopathy or other cardiac toxicities
- Teach patient
  - expected side effects and self-care measures
  - potential for permanent sterility

KEY REFERENCE

Talbot DC, Smith IE, Mansi JL, et al.: Anthrapyrazole CI941: a highly active new agent in the treatment of advanced breast cancer. J Clin Oncol 1991; 12:2141–7

Drug: Actinomycin D

James B. Nachman and Deborah T. Berg

OTHER NAMES: DACTINOMYCIN, COSMAGEN

USES

- First-line therapy in Wilms' tumor, rhabdomyosarcoma, and Ewing's sarcoma
- Second-line therapy in germ cell tumors

MECHANISM OF ACTION

- Intercalates with DNA, inhibiting DNA-dependent RNA polymerase
- Phase specific, primarily G and S phase
- Causes topoisomerase-mediated single- and double-strand breaks in DNA
- Enters cells by passive diffusion; agents such as amphotericin B may facilitate uptake

DOSING

- Always given as an IV push injection
- Standard dosing has been 0.015 mg/kg/d for 5 days with a maximum dose of 0.5 mg/d
- Courses repeated at 3 wk intervals
- Current Wilms' dosing is 0.045 mg/kg IV push for patients < 30 kg; for patients > 30 kg, 1.35 mg/m^2 with a maximum dose of 2.3 mg
- Usually administered with vincristine and cytoxan (VAC) or vincristine and ifosfamide (VAI)

PHARMACOKINETICS

- Avidly binds to tissues
- Terminal half-life of 36 hrs
- Eliminated by renal and biliary excretion (primarily biliary)
- Only a small fraction of dose appears to be metabolized

TOXICITY

- Severe tissue damage if drug is extravasated
- Myelosuppression
- Mucositis (may involve entire GI tract)
- Severe skin sensitivity in previously radiated areas (radiation recall)
- Hepatic toxicity (particularly in patients receiving radiation to abdominal structures)
  - hepatomegaly, ascites, LFT abnormalities
- Diarrhea

RECOMMENDATIONS FOR SUPPORTIVE CARE

- Highly emetogenic; recommend serotonin receptor antagonist and dexamethasone prophylaxis

PHARMACY ISSUES

- Reconstitute 500 mcg vial with 1.1 ml sterile water without preservative

NURSING CONSIDERATIONS

- Closely monitor CBC, WBC, platelet count, LFTs, BUN, and creatinine
- Vesicant; if extravasation occurs, immediately stop infusion and follow hospital policy
- Assess
  - skin for signs of radiation recall, rash, or discoloration along vein
  - mucous membranes for signs of stomatitis
  - general status for signs and symptoms of fatigue, malaise, or depression
- Teach patient
  - expected side effects and self-care measures
  - avoid OTC aspirin-containing medications
  - potential of permanent sterility

KEY REFERENCE

Green D, et al.: Comparison between single dose and divided dose administration of dactinomycin and doxorubicin for patients with Wilms' tumor: A report from the National Wilms' Tumor Study Group. J Clin Oncol 1997; 16:237–45

Drug: Topotecan

Jan H.M. Schellens, Jos H. Beijnen, and Marianne Huml

OTHER NAMES: HYCAMTIN

USES

- Approved by the FDA for second-line platinum-resistant ovarian cancer
- Also active in small cell lung cancer

MECHANISM OF ACTION

- Topoisomerase I inhibitor
- Reversible pH-dependent topotecan lactone ring opening results in loss of activity
- At physiologic pH the inactive form predominates
- P-glycoprotein overexpression does not confer resistance
- Other mechanisms of resistance include decreased topoisomerase I expression, presence of topotecan-resistant forms of topoisomerase I, subnuclear distribution of topoisomerase I, overexpression of breast cancer resistance protein (BCRP) or cMOAT (MRP2), reduced intracellular accumulation of topotecan

DOSING

- Administered IV as a 30-min infusion
- Oral formulation in development
- Most commonly used schedule is 1.5 mg/m^2 every day × 5
- Combination chemotherapy regimens are in development

PHARMACOKINETICS

- Primarily renal elimination of topotecan lactone and ring-opened inactive carboxylate form
- N-demethylation is a minor metabolic pathway
- Linear pharmacokinetics
- The terminal half-life is 3–4 hrs
- Renal dysfunction results in substantially increased systemic exposure (see toxicity)
- Important pharmacokinetic interactions with cisplatin in the sequence cisplatin–topotecan
- Important pharmacodynamic interactions with bone marrow depressants, live virus vaccinations

TOXICITY

- Neutropenia common and may result in fever and hospitalization
- Clearly related with exposure (see Pharmacokinetics)
- Renal dysfunction necessitates dose adjustment
- Mild nausea and vomiting common
- Alopecia is common
- Fatigue is disabling and only partly associated with anemia

RECOMMENDATIONS FOR SUPPORTIVE CARE

- prophylactic antiemetics (metoclopramide or serotonin antagonists) may reduce nausea and vomiting
- G-CSF is not recommended for prophylaxis of neutropenia

PHARMACY ISSUES

- Topotecan is reconstituted in sterile water and diluted in an infusion fluid (0.9% sodium chloride)

NURSING CONSIDERATIONS

- Review relevant lab values prior to administration (i.e., BUN, creatinine, LFTs, and platelets)
- Premedicate with serotonin antagonist, and continue for 24 hrs
- Assess
  - for signs of infection and bleeding
  - for symptoms of fluid and electrolyte imbalance: monitor I/O and daily weights
  - for signs and symptoms of hepatotoxicity
- Teach patient
  - report stomatitis and diarrhea
  - encourage adequate hydration
  - expected side effects and self-care measures

KEY REFERENCES

Berg DT: New chemotherapy treatment options and implications for nursing care [published erratum appears in Oncol Nurs Forum 1992; 24(3):442]

Herben VMM, ten Bokkel Huinink WW, Beijnen JH: Clinical pharmacokinetics of topotecan. Clin Pharmacokinet 1996; 31: 85–102

Maliepaard M, et al: Subcellular localization and tissue distribution of the BCRP transporter in normal human tissue. Amer Assoc Cancer Res 91st Annual Meeting, April 1–5, 2000

Schellens JHM, Pronk LC, Verweij J: Emerging drug treatments for solid tumors. Drugs 1996; 51: 45–72

Drug: Irinotecan

Mark J. Ratain and Deborah T. Berg

OTHER NAMES: CPT-11, CAMPTOSAR, CAMPTO

USES

- Approved for metastatic colorectal cancer refractory to 5-fluorouracil (approval pending for first-line therapy)
- Also active in non–small cell lung cancer, gastric cancer, cervical cancer, and lymphoma

MECHANISM OF ACTION

- Topoisomerase I inhibitor
- Prodrug requiring activation by carboxylesterases to SN-38
- Presence of P-glycoprotein does not confer resistance
- Decreased topoisomerase I expression results in resistance
- Other possible mechanisms of resistance include decreased carboxylesterase, increased UGT1A1, and increased multidrug resistance–associated protein (MRP)

DOSING

- Administered IV as a 90-min infusion
- Oral formulation in development
- Schedules/doses
  - 125 mg/m^2 weekly for 4 wks followed by 2 wks of rest (recommended weekly dose in Japan is 100 mg/m^2) or 350 mg/m^2 q3wks
  - administration on weekly schedule with G-CSF only allows modest dose escalation (to 145 mg/m^2); has been given at doses up to 600 mg/m^2 q3wks
- Commonly used combinations
  - 125 mg/m^2 weekly in combination with 5-fluorouracil 500 mg/m^2 and leucovorin 20 mg/m^2

PHARMACOKINETICS

- Extensively metabolized by carboxylesterases (activation to SN-38) and CYP3A4 (detoxification)
- Also undergoes biliary excretion
- Half-life of ~9 hrs
- SN-38 is metabolized to SN-38 glucuronide (detoxification) by UGT1A1
- SN-38 glucuronide can be reactivated to SN-38 by bacterial beta-glucuronidases in lumen of intestine
- Screening for genetic mutations in either UGT1A1 promoter (Gilbert's) or coding region may eventually permit individualization of dosing

TOXICITY

- Neutropenia common (20% incidence of grade 3–4 leukopenia) but rarely dose limiting
- Nausea and vomiting common but usually grade 1–2
- Delayed diarrhea (generally peaking around day 10 from the start of treatment) is very common and is severe to life threatening (cholera-like) in up to 30% of patients treated at standard doses
- Its severity may be reduced by aggressive use of loperamide at the earliest signs of diarrhea
- An acute cholinergic syndrome may also occur and atropine appears to be effective for treatment or prophylaxis
- Pulmonary toxicity may also occur
- Some studies have suggested that older patients are at increased risk for toxicity
- Gilbert's syndrome appears to be a major risk factor for toxicity
- Inducers of glucuronidation (i.e., phenobarbital) or inhibitors of SN-38 biliary excretion (i.e., cyclosporine) may reduce toxicity
- Concomitant administration of inhibitors of glucuronidation (i.e., valproate) may result in excessive toxicity

RECOMMENDATIONS FOR SUPPORTIVE CARE

- Antiemetic prophylaxis is recommended, although there is no standard regimen
- Loperamide should be administered q2hrs once significant diarrhea occurs

PHARMACY ISSUES

- D_5W is the preferred diluent

NURSING CONSIDERATIONS

- Nonvesicant; may cause irritation. If extravasation occurs, stop infusion, flush IV site with sterile water, and apply ice
- Dose is based on level of neutropenia and severity of diarrhea; monitor CBC and bowel function
- Atropine 0.25–1 mg IV or SubQ is recommended for early cholinergic syndrome
- Do not use loperamide prophylactically. Administer 4 mg initially, followed by 2 mg q2hrs until diarrhea free for 12 hrs; 4 mg q4hrs may be taken during the night
- Assess
  - bowel function
  - for alteration in nutritional status resulting from nausea and vomiting or diarrhea
  - monitor patients carefully after drug administration for toxicities
- Teach patient
  - give written and verbal details of intensive loperamide schedule (as indicated above) for delayed diarrhea
  - loperamide tablets purchased at local pharmacy/grocery store *do not* contain dosage as recommended by the physician to treat irinotecan-induced diarrhea
  - importance of communication with physician or nurse regarding vomiting, fevers, or if diarrhea persists for 2 or more days
  - avoid OTC aspirin-containing medications
  - importance of compliance with self-care measures

KEY REFERENCES

Berg DT: Irinotecan (CPT-11): drug profile and nursing implications of topoisomerase I inhibitor in advanced colorectal cancer patients. Oncol Nurs Forum 1998; 25:535–43

Iyer L, King CD, Whitington PF, et al.: Genetic predisposition to the metabolism of irinotecan (CPT-11): role of uridine diphosphate glucuronosyltransferase isoform 1A1 in the glucuronidation of its active metabolite (SN-38) in human liver microsomes. J Clin Invest 1998; 101, 847–54

Rothenberg ML: Topoisomerase I inhibitors: review and update. Ann Oncol 1997; 8:837–55

Drug: 9-Aminocamptothecin

Chris H. Takimoto and Belinda Butler

OTHER NAMES: 9-AC

USES

- Investigational anticancer agent
- Responses seen in phase I/II trials in ovarian, bladder, colon, and non–small cell lung cancer

MECHANISM OF ACTION

- Topoisomerase I poison
- P-glycoprotein does not confer resistance
- Decreased topoisomerase I expression results in resistance
- Other possible mechanisms of resistance include mutations in topoisomerase I and decreased uptake and retention of drug within cells

DOSING

- Administered as IV infusion in a colloidal dispersion formulation
- Schedules/doses
  - 35 mcg/m^2/hr (0.84 mg/m^2/d) over 72 hrs q2wks
  - 45 mcg/m^2/hr (1.1 mg/m^2/d) over 72 hrs q2wks plus G-CSF
  - 25 mcg/m^2/hr (0.6 mg/m^2/d) over 120 hrs weekly for 2 of q3wks
  - 18.8 mcg/m^2/hr (0.45 mg/m^2/d) daily for 14 days or 21 days continuous IV infusion
  - 1.1 mg/m^2/d over 30 min daily × 5 q3wks
  - 1.65 mg/m^2 over 24 hrs weekly for 4 of 5 wks
- Oral formulation in development

PHARMACOKINETICS

- Rapid hydrolysis of terminal lactone ring to the carboxylate form
- No plasma or urinary metabolites identified
- Half-life of total plasma 9-AC of 8 hrs
- Potential drug interaction with anticonvulsants such as phenytoin and phenobarbital leading to decreased drug toxicity and possible increased drug clearance

TOXICITY

- Neutropenia most common dose-limiting toxicity
- Thrombocytopenia and anemia are less common
- Mild-to-moderate fatigue
- Mild nausea and vomiting
- Mild diarrhea
- Mild alopecia

RECOMMENDATIONS FOR SUPPORTIVE CARE

- Antiemetic prophylaxis recommended, but no standard regimens
- Monitor blood counts

PHARMACY ISSUES

- Colloidal dispersion formulation prepared in $D_{50}W$
- 9-aminocamptothecin lactone stable as colloidal dispersion for at least 1 wk

NURSING CONSIDERATIONS

- Neutropenia is dose limiting; monitor CBC, WBC, and platelets
- Consider dose interruption/reduction if ANC is $< 1{,}000/mm^3$ or platelet count $< 75{,}000/mm^3$
- Premedicate with antiemetics; for severe nausea and vomiting consider combinations including ondansetron or granisetron
- Investigational agent; adhere to specific research protocol requirements
- Assess
  - alterations in nutrition secondary to diarrhea, mucositis, nausea, vomiting, abdominal cramps, and fatigue
- Teach patient
  - avoid OTC aspirin-containing medications
  - expected side effects and self-care measures

KEY REFERENCE

Dahut W, Harold N, Takimoto C, et al.: Phase I and pharmacologic study of 9-aminocamptothecin given by 72-hour infusion in adult cancer patients. J Clin Oncol 1996; 14:1236–44

Chapter 4

ANTIMETABOLITES AND THEIR MODULATORS

Introduction

Richard L. Schilsky

BIOCHEMICAL PHARMACOLOGY

- Inhibitors of DNA synthesis
- Act by enzyme inhibition or misincorporation into nucleic acids
- Structurally similar to endogenous compounds (e.g., pyrimidine/purine bases or folates)
- Compete with endogenous substrates for cell membrane transport and/or target enzyme binding
- Require intracellular activation (e.g., phosphorylation or polyglutamation)
- Cell cycle and S-phase specific

CLINICAL PHARMACOLOGY

- Cytotoxicity is dose and time dependent
- Often more effective when given by prolonged infusion
- Pharmacokinetics may be nonlinear
- Rapid plasma disappearance
- Polymorphisms of drug-metabolizing enzymes may influence clearance and, therefore, toxicity
- Toxicity usually limited to rapidly dividing tissues (e.g., GI mucosa and bone marrow)
- Multiple drug interactions among members of this class, often sequence dependent

KEY ENZYMES IN ANTIMETABOLITE ACTIVITY

- Dihydrofolate reductase (DHFR)
  - catalyzes reduction of dihydrofolate to tetrahydrofolate, a carbon donor required for purine and pyrimidine synthesis
  - target of methotrexate, trimetrexate, and other antifolates
  - inhibition results in depletion of reduced folates and increase in dihydrofolate polyglutamates, which directly inhibit purine synthetic enzymes
  - overexpression results in drug resistance
- Thymidylate synthase (TS)
  - catalyzes reductive methylation of deoxyuridine to thymidine
  - target of fluoropyrimidines (5-fluorouracil, UFT, fluorodeoxyuridine, capecitabine, and S1) and direct TS inhibitors such as raltitrexed
  - inhibition results in thymidine depletion
  - overexpression results in drug resistance
- Ribonucleotide reductase
  - catalyzes conversion of ribonucleotide diphosphates to deoxyribonucleotide diphosphates
  - target of hydroxyurea; also inhibited by intermediate metabolite of gemcitabine (difluorodeoxycytidine diphosphate)
  - inhibition results in depletion of purine and pyrimidine nucleotides necessary for DNA synthesis
- Hypoxanthine-guanine phosphoribosyl transferase
  - necessary for activation of 6-mercaptopurine (6-MP) and 6-thioguanine (6-TG) to active nucleotide forms
  - incorporation of 6-MP and 6-TG nucleotides into DNA correlates with cytotoxicity
- Thiopurine methyl transferase (TPMT)
  - key enzyme involved in degradation of thiopurines such as 6-thioguanine and 6-mercaptopurine
  - 1 in 300 of general population is TPMT deficient and 11% have reduced enzyme activity
  - deficient patients at risk of severe toxicity if given full dose 6-TG, 6-MP, or azathioprine
- Dihydropyrimidine dehydrogenase (DPD)
  - catalyzes initial and rate-limiting step in catabolism of uracil and 5-fluorouracil
  - 2–5% of population estimated to be partially DPD deficient
  - deficient patients at risk for severe 5-FU toxicity following administration of conventional drug doses
  - overexpression of DPD in tumors confers relative 5-FU resistance
  - specific DPD inhibitors, such as eniluracil, improve oral bioavailability of 5-FU and may improve the therapeutic index of the drug
- DNA polymerase alpha
  - catalyzes incorporation of deoxynucleotide triphosphates into DNA
  - competitively inhibited by ara C triphosphate resulting in premature termination of DNA strand elongation
  - extent of ara CTP incorporation in DNA related to cytotoxicity and remission duration in AML

KEY REFERENCES

Fleming GF, Schilsky RL: Antifolates: the next generation. Semin Oncol 1992; 19(6):707–19

Kobayashi K, Schilsky RL: Update on biochemical modulation of chemotherapeutic agents. Oncology-Huntingt 1993; 7(5):99–106, 109; discussion 110–14, 117

Rustum YM, Harstrick A, Cao S, et al.: Thymidylate synthase inhibitors in cancer therapy: direct and indirect inhibitors. J Clin Oncol 1997; 15(1):389–400

Spears CP: Clinical resistance to antimetabolites. Hematol Oncol Clin North Am 1995; 9(2):397–413

Drug: Cytarabine

Robert L. Capizzi and Erin P. Demakos

OTHER NAMES: ARA-C, CYTOSINE ARABINOSIDE, CYTOSAR

USES

- Approved by the FDA for the treatment of acute myeloid and lymphocytic leukemia in adults and children typically used in combination with an anthracycline antibiotic; also approved for the treatment of blast phase of chronic granulocytic leukemia
- Has also been used in the treatment of non-Hodgkin's lymphoma and myelodysplastic syndromes

MECHANISM OF ACTION

- Cytarabine is an analogue of deoxytidine
- It is successively phosphorylated to the mono-(ara-CMP), di-(ara-CDP), and triphosphate (ara-CTP)
- Ara-CTP is incorporated into DNA and causes chain termination
- Also inhibits DNA polymerase
- Most active in S phase of the cell cycle
- The specific activity of the enzyme, deoxycytidine kinase, is the rate-limiting step in the anabolism of ara-C
- Catabolized by cytidine deaminase to ara-U and by deoxycytidylate deaminase to ara-UMP
- Both catabolites are inactive
- Low anabolic activity and high catabolic activity of leukemia cells contribute to drug resistance

DOSING

- For induction of complete remission, ara-C is used in 2 different dosing regimens
  - standard dose (i.e., 100–200 mg/m^2/d as a continuous IV infusion for 7 days)
  - high dose (i.e., 1–3 g/m^2 as a 3 hr infusion q12hrs for 6–8 doses)
- For intensification or consolidation following the attainment of a complete remission, 4 courses of high-dose ara-C (1–3 g/m^2 as a 3 hr infusion q12hrs on day 1, 3, 5) are given at 4–6 wk intervals
- Marrow hypoplasia and pancytopenia ensue after each course, necessitating close observation of the patient and use of supportive care measures with antibiotics and blood products as needed
- Schedules/doses
  - Commonly used combinations
    - □ ara-C 100 mg/m^2/d by continuous infusion for 7 days with
      - ▽ daunorubicin 50 mg/m^2 every day × 3 or
      - ▽ mitoxantrone 12 mg/m^2 every day × 3 or
      - ▽ idarubicin 12 mg/m^2 every day × 3
    - □ ara-C 200 mg/m^2 every day × 4, BCNU 300 mg/m^2, VP-16 400 mg/m^2 every day × 3, melphalan 140 mg/m^2 (BEAM for NHL)
    - □ ara-C 2 g/m^2, VP-16 240 mg/m^2, methylprednisolone 500 mg/d, cisplatin 100 mg/m^2 (ESHAP for NHL)

PHARMACOKINETICS

- Ara-C is not orally bioavailable due to rapid catabolism to the inactive uracil arabinoside (ara-U)
- The major mechanism for systemic clearance is via hepatic metabolism by cytidine deaminase forming the inactive nucleoside, ara-U
- Evidence exists for dose-dependent pharmacokinetics

MECHANISM OF ACTION

- Membrane translocation of ara-C by the nucleoside transporter, anabolism and retention of the triphosphate nucleoside, ara-CTP, and its incorporation into DNA are cellular pharmacologic parameters of ara-C critical to its cytotoxic effect

SIDE EFFECTS

- Extravasation does not cause tissue irritation
- Hematologic suppression with profound pancytopenia is expected and is the goal of induction therapy for acute leukemia
- Therefore, infectious disease precautions and surveillance with prompt initiation of antibiotics is essential
- Likewise bleeding precautions and usage of blood products as clinically indicated is essential
- Nausea and vomiting are a function of dose and duration of infusion
- Diarrhea is a function of dose and duration of infusion
- Side effects unique to high-dose ara-C
  - conjunctivitis
  - maculopapular skin rash
  - palmar and plantar eyrthema
  - polyserositis (sterile pleuritis, peritonitis)
  - bilateral pulmonary infiltrates with signs and symptoms resembling ARDS
  - cerebellar toxicity
  - peripheral neuropathy
  - hepatic toxicity with associated cholestatic jaundice

NURSING CONSIDERATIONS

- Diluent provided in the container *should not* be used (it is benzyl alcohol preserved); use sodium chloride USP (unpreserved) or Ringer's injection USP (unpreserved)
- Avoid contamination; use strict aseptic technique
- Risk of serious neurologic toxicity is less with cytarabine than with methotrexate
- Assess
  - baseline neurologic status
  - for acute arachnoiditis (most common toxic reaction); headaches, back pain, nuchal rigidity, and fever
  - assessment of access site for signs of infection
- Teach patient
  - to remain supine for 30 min following the procedure
  - acute complications, which could include nausea, vomiting, fever, headache, and rigidity of neck; usually they subside within 72 hrs
  - report unusual symptoms

KEY REFERENCES

Capizzi RL: Curative chemotherapy for acute myeloid leukemia: the development of high-dose ara-C from the laboratory to bedside. Invest New Drugs 1996; 14(3):249–56

Mills W, Chopra R, McMillan A, et al.: BEAM chemotherapy and autologous bone marrow transplantation for patients with relapsed or refractory non-Hodgkin's lymphoma. J Clin Oncol 1995; 13(3):588–95

Priesler HD, Davis RB, Kirshner J, et al.: Cancer and Leukemia Group B: Comparison of three remission induction regimens and two postinduction strategies for the treatment of acute nonlymphocytic leukemia. N Eng J Med 1994; 331:896–903

Rubin EH, Andersen JW, Berg DT, et al.: Risk factors for high-dose cytarabine neurotoxicity: an analysis of a cancer and leukemia group B trial in patients with acute myeloid leukemia. J Clin Oncol 1992; 10(6):948–53

Velasquez WS, McLaughlin P, Tucker S, et al.: ESHAP—an effective chemotherapy regimen in refractory and relapsing lymphoma: a 4 year follow-up study. J Clin Oncol 1994; 12(6):1169–76

Drug: Gemcitabine

Malcolm Moore, Amita Patnaik, and Marianne Huml

OTHER NAMES: GEMZAR, 2′, 2′-DIFLUORODEOXYCYTIDINE, DFDC

USES

- Approved by FDA for use in advanced pancreatic cancer
- Also active in non–small cell lung cancer, breast cancer, transitional cell cancer, and ovarian cancer

MECHANISM OF ACTION

- A deoxycytidine analogue (similar to cytosine arabinoside)
- Much broader range of activity than cytosine arabinoside likely due to differences in intracellular pharmacology
- Activated through phosphorylation by cellular kinases
- Inhibits ribonucleotide reductase resulting in depletion of nucleotide pools
- Metabolites incorporated into DNA resulting in chain termination
- Resistant to excision resulting in a longer intracellular half-life than cytosine arabinoside
- Potent radiosensitizer
- Deoxycytidine kinase deficiency results in resistance to gemcitabine
- Other potential mechanisms of resistance include increased levels of deoxycytidine deaminase, mutated DNA polymerase, increased DNA excision/repair, and decreased membrane transport

DOSING

- Administered IV as a 30-min infusion
- Schedules/doses
  - 1,000 mg/m^2 weekly for 3 wks q28d
  - for pancreatic cancer initial dose is 1,000 mg/m^2 weekly × 7
- Commonly used combinations
  - 1,000 mg/m^2 IV weekly for 3 wks in combination with cisplatin 70–100 mg/m^2 IV day 1 q28d (for non–small cell lung cancer)

PHARMACOKINETICS

- Rapidly eliminated from plasma by deamination to inactive uracil derivative difluorodeoxyuridine
- Protein binding negligible
- Terminal half-life for 30 min infusion is 45–75 min
- Almost all drug/metabolites recovered in urine

TOXICITY

- Side effects vary dramatically according to schedule of administration
- Dose-limiting toxicity is myelosuppression
- Other toxicities
  - abnormalities of liver enzymes
  - nausea and vomiting
  - mild proteinuria and hematuria
  - skin rash
  - fever/flulike syndrome
  - peripheral edema
- Less common toxicities
  - transient dyspnea
  - alopecia
  - somnolence
  - diarrhea
  - constipation
  - mucositis
- Rarely
  - bronchospasm
  - hemolytic-uremic syndrome
- Cumulative organ toxicity not reported, although hematologic toxicity may become more pronounced with repeated cycles of the drug

RECOMMENDATIONS FOR SUPPORTIVE CARE

- Antiemetic prophylaxis for low emetogenic potential agents (e.g., steroids plus prochlorperazine)
- Use of acetaminophen or low-dose steroids for 24–48 hrs after administration if fever, flu-like syndrome occurs

NURSING CONSIDERATIONS

- Lower doses are given in patients receiving concomitant radiation therapy
- Dose is based on CBC to avoid neutropenia/thrombocytopenia. Monitor counts, differential, and platelet count prior to administration
- Recovery from neutropenia usually occurs by withholding only one dose
- Administered on an outpatient basis
- Obtain baseline BUN, creatinine, and LFTs prior to initiation of therapy and monitor periodically thereafter
- Assess
  - alterations in nutrition related to nausea and vomiting, diarrhea, and stomatitis
  - skin integrity for finely maculopapular pruritic rashes involving trunk and extremities
  - liver dysfunction and renal impairment
- Teach patient
  - expected side effects and self-care measures

KEY REFERENCE

Noble S, Goa K: Gemcitabine: A review of its pharmacology and clinical potential. Drugs 1997; 54:447–72

Drug: 5-Fluorouracil

Richard L. Schilsky and Dolores Watts

OTHER NAMES: 5-FU, ADRUCIL

USES

- Approved by FDA as treatment for carcinomas of the colon, rectum, stomach, pancreas, breast
- Also commonly used for treatment of head and neck cancer, anal carcinoma, gallbladder carcinoma, and other solid tumors

MECHANISM OF ACTION

- Pyrimidine antimetabolite
- Converted intracellularly to active nucleotide derivatives 5-fluorouracil triphosphate (5-FUTP), 5-fluorodeoxyuridine monophosphate (5-FdUMP), and 5-fluorodeoxyuridine triphosphate (5-FdUTP)
- Primary mechanism of action believed to be inhibition of thymidylate synthase (TS) by 5-FdUMP resulting in thymidine depletion and apoptosis
- Other effects include inhibition of RNA processing and function by 5-FUTP and production of DNA strand breaks by 5-FdUTP
- Resistance is multifactorial
  - increased expression of TS
  - increased expression of dihydropyrimidine dehydrogenase (DPD)
  - depletion of intracellular reduced folates
  - decreased activation of 5-FU to nucleotide derivatives

DOSING

- Administered IV as IV bolus or continuous IV infusion
- Oral administration not recommended due to variable and erratic oral bioavailability; however, oral bioavailability is 100% when 5-FU is co-administered with eniluracil (see eniluracil)
- Schedules/doses
  - single agent given by IV bolus
    - □ doses range from 300–500 mg/m²/d for 5 days q28d or 600–750 mg/m² weekly
  - IV infusion
    - □ 5 day infusion of 1,000 mg/m²/d repeated q3–4wks or as a continuous IV infusion of 300 mg/m²/d indefinitely with duration of infusion dependent on patient tolerance
- Commonly used regimens given with leucovorin include
  - 5-FU 425 mg/m² IV bolus plus leucovorin 20 mg/m² IV bolus daily × 5
    - □ repeat q28d or
  - 5-FU 500 mg/m² IV over 15–30 min leucovorin 500 mg/m² IV over 2 hrs weekly for 6 wks
    - □ repeat q8wks

PHARMACOKINETICS

- Extensively metabolized by DPD to inactive metabolites that are excreted in the urine
- 10–20% of administered dose excreted in urine as unchanged 5-FU
- Half-life 8–20 min depending on dose and schedule of administration
- Pharmacokinetics are nonlinear
- Clearance falls with increasing dose rate due to saturation of DPD
- ~2% of general population are probably partially DPD deficient (may be as high as 5% of women with breast cancer)
- Such individuals have reduced 5-FU clearance and are at risk for increased toxicity following administration of standard doses

TOXICITY

- Varies with dose and schedule of administration
- Neutropenia, mucositis, diarrhea most common
  - mucositis and neutropenia most common with daily × 5 schedule
  - diarrhea and mucositis most common with weekly schedule
- Hand-foot syndrome most common with continuous IV infusion
- Other toxicities
  - tear duct fibrosis resulting in increased lacrimation
  - cerebellar ataxia
  - coronary artery spasm and cardiac ischemia (with infusional regimens)
  - skin hyperpigmentation
  - photosensitivity
  - nail changes; nausea; vomiting; rash
- Neutropenia, mucositis, diarrhea may all be increased when 5-FU is co-administered with leucovorin
- If 5-FU is co-administered with eniluracil, the 5-FU dose must be markedly reduced (see eniluracil) to prevent life-threatening toxicity

RECOMMENDATIONS FOR SUPPORTIVE CARE

- Antiemetic prophylaxis may be necessary for some patients
- If severe diarrhea occurs, administer loperamide and push oral fluids; hospitalization for IV fluids is recommended for severe diarrhea in elderly patients
- Oral pyridoxine (50–100 mg/d) may ameliorate hand-foot syndrome

PHARMACY ISSUES

- Store intact vials at room temperature and protect from light
- May be further diluted in D_5W or NS for injection
- Precipitation may occur if mixed with leucovorin

NURSING CONSIDERATIONS

- Patients who have had adrenalectomy may need higher doses of prednisone while receiving 5-FU
- Dose should be reduced in patients with compromised bone marrow function and malnutrition
- Monitor blood counts to ensure adequate bone marrow recovery before each treatment
- Diarrhea can be severe; obtain stool culture to rule out pathogen-induced diarrhea
- Assess
  - IV site for patency and signs of infiltration; 5-FU is an irritant
  - skin integrity; changes in nails, skin, and oral mucosa; erythema of hands and soles of feet
  - alterations in nutritional status related to stomatitis or diarrhea
  - baseline neurologic status; assess for evidence of unsteady gait, ataxia, slurred speech, coarse nystagmus indicating acute cerebellar syndrome
- Teach patient
  - hyperpigmentation of skin will subside at completion of therapy
  - avoid OTC aspirin-containing medications
  - avoid prolonged exposure to sunlight; use sunglasses and sunblock
  - to follow an oral hygiene regime; avoid use of commercial mouthwashes that can irritate oral mucosa

KEY REFERENCES

Cameron DA, Gabra H, Leonard RC: Continuous 5-fluorouracil in the treatment of breast cancer. Br J Cancer 1994; 70(1):120–4

Machover D: A comprehensive review of 5-fluorouracil and leucovorin in patients with metastatic colorectal carcinoma. Cancer 1997; 80(7):1179–87

Ross PJ, Webb A, Cunningham D, et al.: Infusional 5-fluorouracil in the treatment of gastrointestinal cancers: the Royal Marsden Hospital experience. Ann Oncol 1997; 8(2):111–15

Rustum YM, Cao S, Zhang Z: Rationale for treatment design: biochemical modulation of 5-fluorouracil by leucovorin. Cancer J Sci Am 1998; 4(1):12–18

Sobrero, A, Aschele, C, Bertino, JR: Fluorouracil in colorectal cancer—a tale of two drugs: implications for biochemical modulation. J Clin Oncol 1997; 15:368–81

Drug: Floxuridine

Walter M. Stadler and Dolores Watts

OTHER NAMES: FUDR, FLUORODEOXYURIDINE

USES

■ Systemic infusion for gastrointestinal malignancies as an alternative to 5-FU
■ Therapy of gastrointestinal metastases to the liver via hepatic artery infusion

MECHANISM OF ACTION

■ Converted to 5-fluoro-2′-deoxyuridine monophosphate (FdUMP) by thymidine kinase
■ FdUMP, in conjunction with reduced folate, is a potent inhibitor of thymidylate synthase (TS)
■ FdUMP can also be converted to FdUTP, and inhibit DNA replication by misincorporation
■ TS mutations or increased expression may lead to resistance
■ Decreased reduced folate pools decreases efficacy

DOSING

- Systemic administration
  - 0.5–1 mg/kg/d by continuous infusion for 1–2 wks q4wks
- Hepatic artery infusion
  - 0.15–0.18 mg/kg/d by continuous infusion via arterial catheter or pump for 14 days q28d
  - dose may be combined with leucovorin and also dexamethasone

PHARMACOKINETICS

■ Systemic administration leads to rapid conversion to 5-FU by thymidine phosphorylase and subsequent inactivation to dihydrofluorouracil by dihydropyrimidine dehydrogenase (DPD)
■ First-pass extraction by normal liver parenchyma ~95% and thus hepatic arterial infusion associated with minimal systemic toxicities
■ Hepatic arterial infusion favors activation (to FdUMP) over metabolism to 5-FU

TOXICITY

- Typical systemic infusion toxicities include
  - stomatitis, esophagitis, diarrhea
  - hand-foot syndrome, dermatitis, increased skin toxicity from radiation

RECOMMENDATIONS FOR SUPPORTIVE CARE

■ Ice chips may decrease incidence of mucositis
■ Loperamide may control mild diarrhea; more severe diarrhea or gastrointestinal bleeding is an indication for holding therapy

PHARMACY ISSUES

■ Should be reconstituted in sterile water and diluted in D_5W or normal saline

NURSING CONSIDERATIONS

- Assess
  - skin integrity for evidence of hand and foot syndrome
  - catheter prior to each cycle for position, signs, and symptoms of infection and patency; do not force flushing solution
  - nutritional status; ensure adequate hydration
- Teach patient
  - to follow an oral hygiene regime to decrease infection and stomatitis
  - report rash and erythema on palms of hands or soles of feet
  - expected side effects and self-care measures

KEY REFERENCES

Hohn DC, Stagg RJ, Friedman MA: A randomized trial of continuous intravenous versus hepatic intraarterial floxuridine in patients with colorectal cancer metastatic to the liver: the Northern California Oncology Group trial. J Clin Oncol 1989; 7(11):1646–54

Levin RD, Gordon JH: Fluorodeoxyuridine with continuous leucovorin infusion. A phase II clinical trial in patients with metastatic colorectal cancer. Cancer 1993; 72(10):2895–901

Drug: Uracil/Tegafur

Richard Pazdur and Yvonne Lassere

OTHER NAMES: UFT, ORZEL

USES

■ Approved in Japan and some European and South American countries for the treatment of colorectal, breast, stomach, head and neck, liver, gallbladder, bile duct, pancreas, prostate, bladder, and cervix cancers

MECHANISM OF ACTION

■ UFT is comprised of tegafur and uracil (1:4 molar ratio)
■ Tegafur is metabolized to 5-fluorouracil (5-FU) by CYP2A6
■ Uracil inhibits dihydropyrimidine dehydrogenase (DPD), the primary catabolic enzyme of 5-FU
■ Competitive inhibition of DPD by uracil results in elevated plasma concentrations of 5-FU, derived from tegafur, and higher intratumoral exposure to 5-FU anabolites compared to tegafur alone
■ Oral calcium leucovorin (when used with UFT) biochemically modulates the 5-FU generated from tegafur
■ Administration of leucovorin enhances the DNA-directed effects of 5-FU

DOSING

■ Administered po
■ Dose: 300 mg/m^2/d po
  - daily dose is divided into 3 doses (higher dose in AM)
  - each dose is given q8hrs (at least 1 hr before or after a meal) for 28 days, followed by 1 wk of rest
■ Leucovorin 75–90 mg/d po divided into 3 doses usually administered with UFT
■ Dosing delays and/or modifications may be necessary

PHARMACOKINETICS

■ Peak plasma concentrations of tegafur, uracil, and 5-FU were achieved in < 2 hrs
■ 5-FU peak plasma concentrations are between 150–200 ng/ml and remain detectable for the 8-hr dosing interval
■ Plasma concentrations were highest for tegafur, followed by uracil and 5-FU
■ Steady-state plasma concentration data for uracil, tegafur, and 5-FU showed a consistent peak and trough appearance during each dosing interval with no evidence of accumulation

TOXICITY

■ Diarrhea
  - most common toxicity
  - dose-limiting toxicity
  - hold therapy for grade 2 diarrhea; resume therapy upon resolution of diarrhea
  - hold therapy for grade 3 diarrhea; resume therapy with dose reduction upon resolution of diarrhea
  - intensive use of antidiarrhea medications may be necessary
■ Nausea and vomiting usually mild
■ Fatigue
■ Skin rash
■ Excessive lacrimation
■ Transient hyperbilirubinemia

RECOMMENDATIONS FOR SUPPORTIVE CARE

■ Intensive use of antidiarrhea medications (e.g., loperamide) recommended for treatment of diarrhea

PHARMACY ISSUES

■ UFT capsules: 100 mg
  - daily dose of UFT rounded to nearest 100 mg and divided into 3 separate doses given q8hrs
■ Course of treatment not extended for missed doses
■ Halogenated antiviral agents must not be used when taking UFT-containing regimens
■ UFT may increase phenytoin levels
■ UFT may interact with coumadin and prolong bleeding time

NURSING CONSIDERATIONS

■ Patient education of dosing schedule and management of toxic effects is of utmost importance
■ Dosing issues
  - doses taken with 6–8 ounces of water q8hrs (at least 1 hr before or 1 hr after a meal) for 28 days, followed by 7 days of rest
  - UFT treatment stops at day 28 regardless of number of doses missed
■ Side effects
  - instruct patients to stop UFT immediately and notify physician if
    □ more than 4 BMs in 24 hrs
    □ any grade 2 toxicity
  - dose of UFT may need to be modified before resuming
  - side effects can become severe if UFT is not held and prolonged hospitalizations can occur

KEY REFERENCES

Pazdur R, Lassere Y, Diaz-Canton E, Bready B, Ho DH: Phase I trial of uracil-tegafur (UFT) plus oral leucovorin: 28-day schedule. Cancer Invest 1998; 20:573–6

Pazdur R, Lassere Y, Rhodes V, et al.: Phase II trial of uracil and tegafur plus oral leucovorin. An effective oral regimen in the treatment of metastatic colorectal carcinoma. J Clin Oncol 1994; 2296–300

Sulkes A, Benner SE, Canetta RM: Uracil-ftorafur: an oral fluoropyrimidine active in colorectal cancer. J Clin Oncol 1998; 16(10):3461–75

Takiuchi H, Ajani JA: Uracil-tegafur in gastric carcinoma: a comprehensive review. J Clin Oncol 1998; 16(8):2877–85

Note: The views expressed are the result of independent work and do not represent the views of the U.S. Food and Drug Administration or the United States government. Work described herein was performed while Richard Pazdur was an employee of The University of Texas M. D. Anderson Cancer Center.

Drug: Capecitabine

Richard Pazdur, Yvonne Lassere, and Susan Noble-Kempin

OTHER NAMES: XELODA

USES

- Approved by the FDA for the treatment of patients with metastatic breast cancer who are resistant to both paclitaxel and an anthracycline-containing regimen or resistant to paclitaxel and for whom further anthracycline-containing therapy may be contraindicated
- Has demonstrated activity in metastatic colorectal cancer

MECHANISM OF ACTION

- Rationally designed oral fluoropyrimidine carbamate developed to generate 5-fluorouracil (5-FU) in tumors through three sequential enzyme reactions
  - transformed to 5′-deoxy-5-fluorocytidine (5′-DFCR) by hepatic carboxylase
  - 5′-DFCR converted to 5′-deoxy-5-fluorouridine (5′-DFUR) (doxifluridine) by cytidine deaminase
  - 5′-DFUR converted to 5-FU by thymidine phosphorylase, an enzyme found in higher concentrations in tumors than in normal tissues

DOSING

- Administered po
- Dose: 2,500 mg/m^2/d po every day
  - daily dose is divided between 2 doses given 12 hrs apart, within 30 min of a meal
  - course of treatment is 14 days of capecitabine followed by 1 wk of rest
- Dose delays and/or modifications may be necessary

PHARMACOKINETICS

- Gastrointestinal absorption of orally administered capecitabine has been shown to be at least 70% (CV 30%)
- With short half-lives (<1 hr), capecitabine, 5′-DFCR, and 5′-DFUR do not accumulate in plasma after chronic dosing
- Following administration of capecitabine to colorectal cancer patients, concentrations of 5-FU were approximately 3 times greater in primary colorectal tumor than in adjacent healthy tissue

TOXICITY

- Diarrhea (13% incidence of grade 3–4)
  - dose limiting
  - hold therapy for grade 2 diarrhea
- Hand-foot syndrome (13% incidence of grade 3)
  - hold for grade 2 hand-foot syndrome
- Stomatitis (4% incidence of grade 3)
- Fatigue (5% incidence of grade 3)
- Nausea/vomiting (3–4% incidence of grade 3)
- Skin rash
- Hematology: neutropenia (5% incidence of grade 3–4), thrombocytopenia (2% incidence of grade 3–4)
- Transient hyperbilirubinemia

RECOMMENDATIONS FOR SUPPORTIVE CARE

- Intensive use of antidiarrheal medications recommended

PHARMACY ISSUES

- Capsules
  - 500 mg, 150 mg
- Course of treatment not extended for missed doses
- If antacids are administered, must be given 2 hrs after capecitabine administration
- May interact with coumadin and prolong bleeding time

NURSING CONSIDERATIONS

- Doses should be taken with water within 30 min of a meal q12hrs
- Elderly patients with mild to moderate hepatic dysfunction due to liver metastases may be more sensitive to the effects of the drug and should be monitored closely
- Contraindicated in patients with hypersensitivity to 5-fluorouracil
- Patients receive a combination of 500 mg and 150 mg capsules for 14 days, followed by 7 days of rest
- Capecitabine treatment stops at day 14 regardless of number of doses missed
- Assess
  - for hand-foot syndrome
  - mucous membranes for signs of stomatitis
  - alteration in nutritional status due to GI toxicities; may require fluid and electrolyte replacement
- Teach patient
  - notify physician if
    - □ >4 BMs in 24 hrs
    - □ pain, swelling, or redness of hands or feet
    - □ vomiting for >24 hrs
    - □ fever
  - expected side effects and self-care measures
  - to correctly identify tablets for each dose to prevent under- or overdosing
  - not to take a missed dose or double up on the next dose
  - avoid multiple vitamins that contain folic acid
  - need for contraception

KEY REFERENCES

Budman DR, Meropol NJ, Reigner B, et al.: Preliminary studies of a novel oral fluoropyrimidine carbamate: Capecitabine. J Clin Oncol 1998; 16:1803–10

Mackeran MJ, Planting AS, Twelves C, et al.: A phase I and pharmacological study of intermittent twice daily oral therapy with capecitabine in patients with advanced and/or metastatic cancer. J Clin Oncol 1998; 16(9):2977–85

Note: The views expressed are the result of independent work and do not represent the views of the U.S. Food and Drug Administration or the United States government. Work described herein was performed while Richard Pazdur was an employee of The University of Texas M. D. Anderson Cancer Center.

Drug: Eniluracil

Richard L. Schilsky and Janine Caggiano

OTHER NAMES: 776C85, 5-ETHYNYLURACIL

USES

- Investigational agent
- To enhance the oral bioavailability and improve the therapeutic index of 5-fluorouracil and related fluoropyrimidines

MECHANISM OF ACTION

- Irreversible inactivator of dihydropyrimidine dehydrogenase
- Results in inhibition of 5-FU catabolism, prolonged 5-FU clearance, absence of 5-FU catabolites
- Enhanced renal excretion of unchanged 5-FU
- Prolongation of 5-FU half-life to 4–5 hrs
- 100% oral bioavailability of 5-FU

DOSING

- IV and po formulations available for investigational use
- po administration preferred
- Schedules/doses
  - administered po at doses of 20–50 mg/d in combination with oral 5-fluorouarcil
  - regimens currently being tested in clinical trials include
    - □ eniluracil 50 mg/d po for 7 days plus 5-fluorouracil 20 mg/m^2/d po during days 2–5 of eniluracil administration; repeat q28d
    - □ eniluracil 11.5 mg/m^2 twice daily po for 28 days plus 5-fluorouracil 1.15 mg/m^2 twice daily po for 28 days; repeat q35d

PHARMACOKINETICS

- Half-life of eniluracil ~4 hrs
- Doses of >10 mg inactivate DPD in ~1 hr and produce sustained DPD inhibition in peripheral blood mononuclear cells for 12–24 hrs

TOXICITY

- Has no significant clinical toxicity
- Significantly increases the toxicity of 5-fluorouracil
- Conventional doses of 5-FU must not be administered to patients who have received eniluracil or within 60 days of a dose of eniluracil
- Fatal toxicity could occur if conventional doses of 5-FU are administered with eniluracil
- The co-administration of eniluracil with 5-fluorouracil markedly increases the renal elimination of 5-FU
- Therefore, patients with impaired renal function (creatinine clearance <50 ml/min) may not be appropriate for treatment with this regimen

RECOMMENDATIONS FOR SUPPORTIVE CARE

- No supportive care measures are necessary for administration of eniluracil alone
- Supportive care measures for 5-fluorouracil are described under the listing for that drug

PHARMACY ISSUES

- Eniluracil is an investigational agent and should be handled as such in the pharmacy
- Eniluracil is available as 1 mg and 5 mg round white tablets and as 10 mg round off-white tablets
- Should be stored at room temperature in a dry place, protected from light

NURSING CONSIDERATIONS

- Obtain accurate history of dates and doses of eniluracil and 5-FU administration to avoid toxicity due to combination therapy with nonreduced doses of 5-FU
- Monitor for enhanced 5-FU toxicity including bone marrow suppression, diarrhea, and mucositis; obtain results of creatinine clearance prior to administration; eniluracil increases renal elimination of 5-FU
- Use cautiously in patients with impaired renal function; these patients may not be candidates for combination therapy with 5-FU and eniluracil
- Assess
  - renal function: baseline and during therapy
  - alterations in nutrition as a result of diarrhea
- Teach patient
  - to follow an oral hygiene regime to prevent and treat stomatitis
  - management of diarrhea
  - expected side effects and self-care measures

KEY REFERENCES

Baker SD, Khor SP, Adjei A, Doucette M, Spector T, Donehower RC, Grochow LB, Sartorius SE, Noe DA, Hohneker JA, Rowinsky EK: Pharmacokinetic, oral bioavailability and safety study of fluorouracil in patients treated with 776C85, an inactivator of dihydropyrimidine dehydrogenase. J Clin Oncol 1996; 14:3085–96

Schilsky RL, Hohneker J, Ratain MJ, Janisch L, Smetzer L, Lucas VS, Khor SP, Diasio R, VonHoff DD, Burris H: Phase I clinical and pharmacologic study of eniluracil plus 5-fluorouracil in patients with advanced cancer. J Clin Oncol 1998; 16:1450–7

Drug: S-1 (Combination of Tegafur, 5-Chloro-2,4-Dihydroxypyridine, Potassium Oxonate)

Richard Pazdur and Yvonne Lassere

OTHER NAMES: BMS247616

USES

- Investigational use only
- Japanese clinical trials have described activity in gastric cancer, breast cancer, head and neck cancer, colorectal cancer, and non–small cell lung cancer

MECHANISM OF ACTION

- S-1 is composed of tegafur, 5-chloro-2,4-dihydroxypyridine (CDHP), and potassium oxonate in a 1:0.4:1 molar ratio
- Tegafur is metabolized to 5-fluorouracil (5-FU) by CYP2A6
- CDHP is a potent inhibitor of dihydropyrimidine dehydrogenase (DPD), the primary catabolic enzyme of 5-FU
  - 200-fold more potent than uracil in inhibiting DPD
- Leads to sustained 5-FU levels
- Potassium oxonate inhibits the phosphorylation of 5-FU by orotate phosphoribosyl transferase
  - selectively inhibits the phosphorylation of 5-FU in normal gastrointestinal tissues while minimizing its inhibition in tumor tissues

DOSING

- Administered orally
- Clinical trials are ongoing to determine optimal dose and schedule
- Japanese trials have used an every 12 hr administration for 28 days, followed by 1 wk rest

PHARMACOKINETICS

- Peak plasma concentrations of tegafur, CDHP, and potassium oxonate were achieved in 2–3 hrs; 5-FU in 3–4 hrs
- 5-FU peak plasma concentrations are between 90–170 ng/ml and remain >50 ng/ml for 6 hrs
- Plasma concentration data for 5-FU showed a consistent peak and trough appearance during administration for 28 consecutive days with no evidence of accumulation

TOXICITY

- Diarrhea
  - dose-limiting toxicity in European clinical trial
  - hold S-1 for grade 2 diarrhea and resume therapy after resolution of toxicity
  - hold S-1 for grade 3 diarrhea and resume therapy with dose reduction after resolution of toxicity
  - intensive use of antidiarrheal medications may be necessary
- Mucositis
- Nausea/vomiting
- Excessive lacrimation
- Skin rash
- Fatigue, anemia, anorexia
- Leukopenia and thrombocytopenia
  - dose-limiting toxicities in Japanese clinical trials
- Transient hyperbilirubinemia

RECOMMENDATIONS FOR SUPPORTIVE CARE

- Intensive use of antidiarrheal medications

PHARMACY ISSUES

- Concomitant medications to avoid while receiving S-1
  - sorivudine, uracil, dipyridamole (enhances S-1 activity)
  - allopurinol (diminishes S-1 activity)
  - phenytoin (S-1 enhances phenytoin activity)
  - flucytosine, a fluorinated pyrimidine antifungal agent (enhances S-1 activity)
- Current capsules
  - 20 mg, 25 mg
  - round dose to nearest 5 mg
- Course of treatment not extended for missed doses
- May interact with coumadin and prolong bleeding time

NURSING CONSIDERATIONS

- Patient education of dosing schedules and management of toxic effects is of utmost importance
- Dosing issues
  - doses are to be taken within 1 hr after meals
  - patients could receive a combination of 20 mg and 25 mg capsules
  - S-1 treatment stops at day 28 regardless of number of doses missed
- Side effects
  - instruct patients to stop S-1 immediately and notify physician if
    - more than 4 BMs in 24 hrs
    - any grade 2 toxicity
- Dose of S-1 may need to be modified before resuming
- Side effects can become severe if S-1 is not held, and prolonged hospitalizations can occur

KEY REFERENCES

Horikoshi N, Aiba K, Nakano Y, et al.: Pharmacokinetic study of S-1, a new oral fluoropyrimidine consisting of DPD inhibitor and GI protector. Proc Am Soc Clin Oncol 1998; 17:234a (abst #899)

Ohtsu A, Sakata Y, Horikoshi Y, Mitachi K, Sugimachi K, Taguchi T: A phase II study of S-1 in patients with advanced gastric cancer. Proc Am Soc Clin Oncol 1998; 17:262a (abst. #1005)

Shirasaka T, Shimamato Y, Ohsimo H, et al.: Development of a novel form of oral 5-fluorouracil derivative (S-1) directed to the potentiation of the tumor selective cytotoxicity of 5-fluorouracil by two biochemical modulators. Anticancer Drugs 1996; 7(5): 548–57

Note: The views expressed are the result of independent work and do not represent the views of the U.S. Food and Drug Administration or the United States government. Work described herein was performed while Richard Pazdur was an employee of The University of Texas M. D. Anderson Cancer Center.

Drug: 5-Azacytidine

Richard A. Larson and Erin P. Demakos

OTHER NAMES: 5-AZACITIDINE; 5-AZC, 5-AZA-C (NSC #102816)

USES

- Investigational agent for myelodysplastic syndromes and acute myeloid leukemia
- Has been shown to increase hemoglobin F synthesis in sickle-cell disease and thalassemia

MECHANISM OF ACTION

- Ring analogue of the pyrimidine nucleoside cytidine
- Enters cells by facilitated nucleoside transport mechanism
- The triphosphate competes with CTP for incorporation into RNA, resulting in disassembly of polyribosomes, inhibition of RNA processing and function, and marked inhibition of protein synthesis
- There is lesser incorporation into DNA
- Greatest cytotoxic effect in S phase
- Competitive inhibitor of uridine kinase and orotidylate decarboxylase
- Inhibits DNA methyltransferase, leading to hypomethylation of DNA, and thereby to enhanced expression of a variety of genes and to cellular differentiation
- Resistance occurs through depletion of the activating enzyme uridine-cytidine kinase

DOSING

- Administered SubQ or IV
- Schedules/doses
  - for MDS: 75 mg/m^2/d SubQ for 7 days; repeated q4wks
  - if the volume is >4 ml, split dose and inject SubQ at 2 sites
  - for AML: 150–200 mg/m^2/d IV for 5 days. Usually given as continuous IV infusion to lessen GI toxicity
  - repeat after 14–28 days depending on the response

PHARMACOKINETICS

- When given IV, the t 1/2 is 3.5 hrs
- 90% of the drug is excreted in urine within 24 hours

TOXICITY

- Myelosuppression is dose related and may be severe
- Renal dysfunction is common at higher doses and renal tubular acidosis may occur with hypokalemia, hypophosphatemia, hyponatremia, and elevated serum creatinine
- Nausea is common with SubQ doses; vomiting can occur
- Continuous IV infusion markedly decreases the vomiting that follows IV bolus injections
- Diarrhea, fever, myalgia, fatigue, anorexia, paresthesias, and drowsiness may occur
- Hepatotoxicity and neuromuscular toxicity may occur
- Erythema occurs frequently at the injection site, sometimes with tenderness, but usually resolves within 24–72 hrs

RECOMMENDATIONS FOR SUPPORTIVE CARE

- Monitor WBC and platelets
- Monitor serum electrolytes, bicarbonate, BUN, and creatinine
- Reduce dosage by 50% if serum bicarbonate falls to <19 mEq/L
- Antiemetic prophylaxis may be necessary

PHARMACY ISSUES

- Supplied by the NCI as a powder in 100 mg vials with 100 mg of mannitol
- Dissolve the contents of each vial in 4 ml sterile water
- Inject dose SubQ as a slurry immediately
- Store vials at 2–8°C
- Due to spontaneous chemical instability, the drug becomes inactive after several hours in D_5W or NS
- In buffered solutions such as Ringer's lactate and at acidic pH, stability improves with a t 1/2 of 65 hrs at 25°C and 94 hrs at 20°C

NURSING CONSIDERATIONS

- Use cautiously in patients with hepatic metastasis; monitor LFTs
- Do not reconstitute with 5% dextrose
- Antiemetic strongly recommended 1 hr postinjection (5HT3 antagonist)
- Assess
  - baseline neurologic status and subsequently for sensory/perceptual alterations
  - potential for thromboembolic phenomena
  - pain and erythema at injection site can be treated with alternating warm and cold compresses
- Teach patient
  - proper injection technique for SubQ administration; provide adequate time for patient to return demonstration; provide written instructions
  - side effects and self-care measures to minimize risk of infection and bleeding
  - avoid OTC aspirin-containing medications

KEY REFERENCES

Kornblith AB, Herndon JE, Silverman LR, Demakos EP, Reissig R, Holland JF, Cooper MR, Crawford J, Seagren SL, Larson R, Schiffer C, Holland JF. Impact of 5-Azacytidine on the quality of life of myelodysplastic syndrome patients treated in a randomized phase III trial of the cancer leukemia group B (BALGB). Proc Am Soc Clin Oncol 1998; 17:49a

Silverman LR, Demakos EP, Peterson B, Odchimar-Reissig R, Nelson D, Kornblith AB, Stone R, Holland JC, Powell BL, DeCastro C, Ellerton J, Larson RA, Schiffer CA, Holland JF. Subcutaneous azacitidine compared to supportive care in patients with the myelodysplastic syndrome: A study of the cancer and leukemia group B (CALGB). Cancer Investigation 1998; 17(suppl 1):4

Pinto A, Zagonel V: 5-Aza-2′-deoxycytidine (Decitabine) and 5-azactytidine in the treatment of acute myeloid leukemias and myelodysplastic syndromes: past, present and future trends. Leukemia 1993; 7(suppl 1):51–60

Von Hoff D, Slavik M, Muggia FM: 5-azacytidine, a new anti-cancer drug with effectiveness in acute myelogenous leukemia. Ann Intern Med 1976; 85:237–45

Drug: Methotrexate

Kim Tanner, Barton A. Kamen, and Brenda Werner

OTHER NAMES: NSC-740, MTX, AMETHOPTERIN, SODIUM METHOTREXATE, FOLEX, RHEUMATREX, METHOTREXATE PF SOLUTION, METHOTREXATE TABLETS, METHOTREXATE LPF, FOLEX PFS

USES

- Acute lymphocytic leukemia, meningeal leukemia, gestational trophoblastic diseases, breast cancer, head and neck cancer, mycosis fungoides, squamous and small cell lung cancer, advanced non-Hodgkin's lymphoma, Burkitt's lymphoma, transitional cell carcinoma of the urothelium, osteosarcoma

MECHANISM OF ACTION

- Classical folate antagonist; arrests cellular protein synthesis, DNA and RNA production, and cellular replication by binding to dihydrofolate reductase (DHFR)
- DHFR is necessary in the reduction of dihydrofolate to tetrahydrofolic acid, the active form of folic acid; tetrahydrofolic acid is the one-carbon donor in thymidine, purine, and amino acid synthesis
- Cellular resistance to methotrexate develops as a result of increased or mutated DHFR or decreased cellular uptake or metabolism of methotrexate by malignant cells

DOSING

- Most common regimen dosing is 40 mg/m^2/wk (acute leukemia)
- Drug can be administered po, by IV infusion, IV push, intrathecally (preservative-free formulations only), intra-arterially, or IM
- Leucovorin rescue is employed in high-dose regimens to reduce toxic effects of methotrexate; leucovorin calcium is initiated 24 hrs after methotrexate dose and is dosed q6hrs for up to 12 doses
- Methotrexate is rarely used as a single-agent cytotoxic treatment when treating various neoplastic diseases, but is usually part of a combination chemotherapy regimen
- Dosage reduction is necessary in patients with renal impairment
- Methotrexate accumulates in third space effusions resulting in an increased half-life; thus either leucovorin must be used or the effusions drained prior to treatment

PHARMACOKINETICS

- ~50% protein bound; widely distributed in tissues
- Oral bioavailability is dose dependent; at standard doses about 30–50% is absorbed
- Metabolized to a polyglutamate form that increases intracellular retention; polyglutamates may be converted back to methotrexate and released from stores such as red cell and liver
- Half-life ranges from 2–10 hrs depending on route of administration and dosage
- At conventional doses (< 100 mg/m^2) primarily renally excreted unchanged with $< 10\%$ excreted in bile; at higher doses may be metabolized by liver to 7-OH methotrexate

TOXICITY

- Gastrointestinal: vomiting, diarrhea, stomatitis of the mouth or ulcerations of any portion of the gastrointestinal mucosa
- Myelosuppression 7–10 days
- Mucositis 5–7 days
- Hematologic-anemia, leukopenia, or thrombocytopenia may occur; counts recover rapidly
- Chronic or acute hepatotoxicity: usually occurs after prolonged use (years); risk enhanced by predisposing conditions
- Pulmonary toxicity: potentially fatal, may at occur at any dosage, can progress rapidly; consider if patient presents with pulmonary symptoms such as dyspnea and dry, unproductive cough during treatment
- Dermatologic reaction: ranging from rash, photosensitivity, or dermatitis to severe, fatal cutaneous or sensitivity reactions such as exfoliative dermatitis and Stevens-Johnson syndrome; alopecia may occur with recovery after discontinuance of drug
- Nephrotoxicity: usually a result of methotrexate precipitation in the renal tubules; ensure adequate hydration and alkalinization of urine and monitor renal function
- Neurotoxicity: may be acute or delayed; symptoms of acute neurotoxicity may appear within 1 day up to 2 wks after methotrexate administration and may include dizziness, malaise, blurred vision, headache, nausea, emesis, or seizure. Delayed neurologic symptoms may occur weeks to months after methotrexate exposure as leukoencephalopathy

RECOMMENDATIONS FOR SUPPORTIVE CARE

- Emetogenic potential of methotrexate increases with dose increase; antiemetic prophylaxis is recommended for doses > 250 mg/m^2
- Methotrexate is insoluble in acidic urine; precipitation of MTX in renal tubules may occur; for doses greater than 1 g/m^2 patient should be hydrated with an alkaline solution (sodium bicarbonate) to maintain a urine pH of at least 7.0
- MTX increases homocysteine and adenosine levels. These substances appear to contribute to MTX-induced neurotoxicity. Methylxanthines, such as aminophyllin and caffeine, and dextromethorphan have been useful in resolving some acute neurotoxic effects related to MTX administration
- For inadvertent overdose or delayed clearance, carboxypeptidase G_2 should be used to enzymatically degrade MTX

PHARMACY ISSUES

- Only preservative-free preparations should be used for intrathecal and high-dose IV administrations (> 1 g/m^2)
- Leucovorin rescue should be ordered in regimens using MTX 500 mg/m^2 or higher
- Methotrexate may be displaced from serum albumin by other highly protein bound drugs resulting in increased toxicity. Methotrexate toxicity may be increased by salicylates, phenylbutazone, phenytoin, and sulfonamides, penicillins, probenecid, omeprazole, NSAIDs. Methotrexate may decrease the clearance of theophylline. Folic acid–containing vitamins may decrease the effectiveness of methotrexate

NURSING CONSIDERATIONS

- Proper hydration and alkalinization of urine must be maintained in patients receiving 1 g/m^2 or greater
- Leukopenia, thrombocytopenia, and anemia can occur quickly
- High-dose methotrexate must be given with leucovorin rescue
- Premedicate with antiemetics as indicated and continue for 24 hrs
- Methotrexate serum levels may be critical and should be monitored carefully
- Evaluate BUN, creatinine, and LFTs prior to administration
- Assess
  - signs and symptoms of pulmonary dysfunction
  - for hepatotoxicity and gastrointestinal toxicity
- Teach patient
  - expected side effects and self-care measures
  - may cause permanent sterility
  - avoid alcohol and prolonged exposure to sun (use of sunscreen)

KEY REFERENCES

Ackland SP, Schilsky RL: High-dose methotrexate: a critical reappraisal. J Clin Oncol 1987; 5(12):2017–31

Quinn CT, Kamen BA: A biochemical perspective of methotrexate neurotoxicity with insight on nonfolate rescue modalities. J Invest Med 1996; 44:522–30

Drug: Trimetrexate

Kim Tanner, Barton Kamen, and Brenda Werner

OTHER NAMES: NSC-352122, TRIMETREXATE GLUCURONATE, TMTX

USES

- FDA orphan drug designation, indicated for treatment of moderate to severe *Pneumocystis carinii* pneumonia in immunosuppressed patients, including AIDS; used in co-trimoxazole refractory PCP and in cases where co-trimoxazole is contraindicated
- In phase II trials trimetrexate exhibited activity in breast, non–small cell lung and head and neck cancer, stomach, colon, prostate, bladder, and renal cell carcinoma

MECHANISM OF ACTION

- Nonclassical folate antagonist; inhibits the action of dihydrofolate reductase leading to depletion of reduced folates, resulting in inhibition of DNA and RNA synthesis in sensitive cells
- Enters cells by passive diffusion
- Activity of trimetrexate may be reversed by thymidine or leucovorin, depending on dose of trimetrexate
- Cellular resistance may develop through changes in the DHFR enzyme or by enhanced drug efflux via multidrug resistance (MDR) by overexpression of p-glycoprotein, a multidrug resistance gene product

DOSING

- Phase I and II clinical trials have used many different dosing schedules
  - 10 mg/m^2 q14–21d
  - 10 mg/m^2/d by 24 hr continuous infusion
  - 0.5–15 mg/m^2/d for 5 days q3wks
  - 1 mg/m^2/d by continuous infusion for 5 days
  - 35 mg/m^2/d weekly × 3
- Combination chemotherapy with trimetrexate, fluorouracil, and leucovorin (LV) for colorectal cancer has demonstrated superior response rates to 5-FU and LV alone (based on phase II trials)
  - trimetrexate 110 mg/m^2/wk

PHARMACOKINETICS

- Terminal half-life: ~12 hrs
- Mean bioavailability of oral TMTX is 44%
- Metabolized by liver; 10–20% excreted by kidneys
- Trimetrexate does not undergo polyglutamation and therefore rapidly exits cells
- Two possibly active metabolites have been identified that are O-demethylated glucuronide conjugates

TOXICITY

- Hematologic: rapidly reversible granulocytopenia and thrombocytopenia; most common, dose-limiting toxic effect
- Dermatologic: pruritic rash, local reactions, hyperpigmentation, maculopapular rash
- Gastrointestinal: mucositis, stomatitis, nausea, vomiting
- Severe diarrhea has occurred with TMTX + 5-FU + LV combination
- Hypersensitivity reactions, including anaphylactic shock (rarely)
- TMTX is an inhibitor of histamine methyltransferase enzyme responsible for histamine metabolism, which may result in histamine-mediated reactions
- Other: transient elevations in liver enzymes or serum creatinine, flulike symptoms

RECOMMENDATIONS FOR SUPPORTIVE CARE

- In cases of severe mucositis, trimetrexate dose should be held and leucovorin dosing continued

PHARMACY ISSUES

- Drug interactions may occur with other highly protein-bound drugs or other drugs metabolized by cytochrome P-450 enzymes
- Trimetrexate will precipitate in the presence of chloride ion; dilute in 5% dextrose solution only
- After reconstitution, filter with a 0.22 micron filter into the final 5% dextrose solution
- 0.25–2 mg/ml solution is stable for 24 hrs at room temperature or refrigerated

NURSING CONSIDERATIONS

- Monitor CBC and platelet counts
- Premedicate with antiemetics and continue for 24 hrs
- Use only D_5W for IV infusion; drug is incompatible with chloride-containing solutions and leucovorin
- Trimetrexate clearance is decreased and toxicity increased in patients with serum albumin of <3.5 g/dl
- For treatment of PCP, give with leucovorin
- Assess
  - pulmonary status
  - renal and hepatic function in patients receiving higher doses
  - mucous membranes for signs of stomatitis
  - skin integrity for dermatologic reactions
- Teach patient
  - expected side effects and self-care measures
  - ensure adequate hydration
  - report new onset or worsening of dyspnea

KEY REFERENCES

Blanke CD, Messenger M, Taplin SC: Trimetrexate: review and current clinical experience in advanced colorectal cancer. Semin Oncol 1997; 24(5 suppl 18):S18-57–S18-63

Lin JT, Bertino JR: Trimetrexate: a second generation folate antagonist in clinical trial. J Clin Oncol 1987; 5:2032–40

Drug: Raltitrexed

Ian Judson and Janan B. Geick Miller

OTHER NAMES: TOMUDEX, ZD1694

USES

- Approved in UK and certain other European countries as a single agent for treatment of advanced colorectal cancer where 5-fluorouracil and folinic acid–based regimens are either not tolerated or inappropriate
- Demonstrated equivalent response rate, progression free, and overall survival, compared with different 5-fluorouracil plus leucovorin regimens, in 2 out of 3 multicenter randomized trials
- Caused less neutropenia and stomatitis, similar nausea and vomiting, slightly more asthenia and anemia and reversible liver toxicity
- Was significantly easier to administer, which may be associated with overall cost savings

MECHANISM OF ACTION

- Specific inhibitor of thymidylate synthase (TS)
- Rapidly and extensively polyglutamated by folyl polyglutamate synthetase (FPGS)
- Actively taken up into cells by the reduced folate carrier (RFC)
- Resistance could occur due to overexpression of TS, downregulation of the RFC or FPGS, or upregulation of gamma-glutamyl hydrolase

DOSING

- Recommended dose 3 mg/m^2 by 15 min IV infusion in 50–250 ml 0.9% saline or 5% dextrose, q3wks
- Renal impairment: reduce dose by 50% and increase dose interval to 4 wks if creatinine clearance 25–65 ml/min (1.5–3.9 L/hr)
- Do not give if creatinine clearance <25 ml/min (1.5 L/hr)
- Reduce dose by 25% for grade 3 myelosuppression or grade 2 gastrointestinal (GI) toxicity (diarrhea or mucositis), reduce by 50% for grade 4 myelosuppression or grade 3 GI toxicity and delay retreatment until toxicity resolved
- Stop treatment for grade 4 GI toxicity or a combination of grade 3 GI toxicity and grade 4 myelosuppression and give intensive supportive care (i.e., IV hydration and bone marrow support). May be helpful to administer folinic acid 25 mg/m^2 q6hrs
- No dose modifications required for mild to moderate hepatic impairment

PHARMACOKINETICS

- Marked interpatient variability in clearance
- Linear increase in C_{max} and AUC with increasing dose
- Prolonged terminal elimination half-life of 100–140 hrs reported in various studies
- Mean terminal elimination half-life increased from 140–274 hrs in patients with mild to moderate renal impairment (creatinine clearance 25–65 ml/min) compared with patients with clearance >65 ml/min
- 93% protein bound
- May be secreted by renal tubules
- NSAIDs inhibit renal clearance

TOXICITY

- Asthenia, with GI and hematologic toxicities was dose limiting in phase I trials
- GI: diarrhea, nausea, and vomiting may be grade 3 or 4 in 10–15%
- Hematologic: grade 3 or 4 neutropenia may occur up to 20%
- Stomatitis is rare
- Grade 3 or 4 reversible elevations in liver transaminase plasma levels are common (25%) but do not delay treatment and do not appear to have any serious sequelae
- Maculopapular rash may occur but is rarely serious

RECOMMENDATIONS FOR SUPPORTIVE CARE

- IV hydration and bone marrow support in case of grade 3 or 4 GI toxicity

PHARMACY ISSUES

- Provided in 5 ml glass ampules containing 2 mg raltitrexed as lyophilized powder
- Store at 2–8°C protected from light
- Reconstitute with 4 ml sterile water
- Dilute with 5–250 ml 5% dextrose or 0.9% saline for infusion; once diluted is stable for 24 hrs at room temperature exposed to light, no preservative added
- Take usual precautions for preparation of cytotoxics

NURSING CONSIDERATIONS

- Increases in transaminase may occur
- Monitor CBC, differential, and blood chemistries closely
- Premedicate with antiemetics and use prophylactically
- Assess
  - alterations in nutrition due to diarrhea, nausea, and vomiting, and stomatitis
  - skin integrity for rashes
  - for signs of asthenia
- Teach patient
  - signs of infection, bleeding, and anemia
  - self-care measures

KEY REFERENCE

Zalcberg JR, Cunningham D, van Cutsem E, et al.: ZD1694: a novel thymidylate synthase inhibitor with substantial activity in the treatment of patients with advanced colorectal cancer. J Clin Oncol 1996; 14:716–21

Drug: Folinic Acid

Richard L. Schilsky and Brenda Werner

OTHER NAMES: LEUCOVORIN, CITROVORUM FACTOR, 5-FORMYL TETRAHYDROFOLATE, WELLCOVORIN

USES

- To prevent severe toxicity following administration of methotrexate
- To enhance efficacy of 5-fluorouracil treatment of colorectal cancer and other tumors

MECHANISM OF ACTION

- Reduced folate
- Repletes/increases intracellular reduced folate pools that are depleted when dihydrofolate reductase is inhibited by methotrexate
- Competes with methotrexate for transport into cells and conversion to polyglutamate forms
- Expands intracellular pools of 5-10-methylene tetrahydrofolate, a key cofactor necessary to optimize binding of 5-fluorodeoxyuridine monophosphate to thymidylate synthase

DOSING

- As an antidote to methotrexate, usual dosage is 10–20 mg/m^2 IV or po q6hrs beginning within 24 hrs following methotrexate dose and continuing until serum methotrexate level is < 0.05 μM
- If methotrexate clearance is delayed (estimated half-life > 10–12 hrs) or if renal dysfunction develops, increase leucovorin dose to 50–100 mg/m^2 IV q4–6hrs until serum methotrexate level is < 0.05 μM
- When administered with 5-fluorouracil, usually given IV in doses of 20 mg/m^2 daily × 5, 200 mg/m^2 daily × 5, or 500 mg/m^2 weekly, depending on the specific chemotherapy regimen employed
- Low-dose leucovorin with 5-FU produces similar antitumor efficacy as high-dose leucovorin with 5-FU in patients with colorectal cancer
- Oral formulation available

PHARMACOKINETICS

- Commonly used formulation is a racemic mixture of stereoisomers of which the biologically active isomer is l (6S) leucovorin
- Following IV or po administration, l-leucovorin is rapidly converted to 5-methyl tetrahydrofolate, a biologically active reduced folate
- D-leucovorin is slowly eliminated by renal excretion
- Because d-leucovorin is biologically inert, there is no pharmacological or clinical advantage to administration of pure "l" leucovorin

TOXICITY

- Toxicity is rare following administration of leucovorin alone
- Toxic effects reported in < 1% of patients include rash, pruritus, and anaphylactic reactions
- Leucovorin may enhance the toxicities of 5-fluorouracil

RECOMMENDATIONS FOR SUPPORTIVE CARE

- Supportive care not required

PHARMACY ISSUES

- Store at room temperature protected from light
- Reconstitute with bacteriostatic Water for Injection, USP, and dilute in D_5W
- Incompatible if mixed with 5-fluorouracil (precipitation occurs)

NURSING CONSIDERATIONS

- Do not administer simultaneously with systemic methotrexate (time intervals range from 0–72 hrs)
- Assess
  - hypersensitivity reactions (dermatologic reactions)
- Teach patient
  - take exactly as directed at evenly spaced times
  - take with antacids, milk, or juice

KEY REFERENCES

Scheithauer W, Kornek G, Marczell A, et al.: Fluorouracil plus racemic leucovorin versus fluorouracil combined with pure 1-isomer of leucovorin for the treatment of advanced colorectal cancer: a randomized phase III study. J Clin Oncol 1997; 15:908–14

Schilsky RL, Ratain MJ: Clinical pharmacokinetics of high dose leucovorin calcium after intravenous and oral administration. J Natl Cancer Inst 1990; 82:1411–15

Drug: 6-Mercaptopurine

Richard A. Larson and Erin P. Demakos

OTHER NAMES: 6-MP, PURINETHOL

USES

- Approved by FDA for treatment of acute lymphoblastic leukemia in children and adults
- Marginal activity in myeloid leukemias (AML or CML)

MECHANISM OF ACTION

- 6-thio derivative of hypoxanthine, a pro-drug that must be converted to 6-MP-ribose-phosphate intracellularly by hypoxanthine: guanine phosphoribosyl transferase (HGPRT)
- Conversion to the ribonucleotide derivative is a prerequisite for activity
- Inhibits the first step of purine biosynthesis de novo by inhibiting the enzyme glutamine-5-phoosphoribosyl pyrophosphate (PRPP) amido-transferase
- Synergistic with methotrexate in inhibiting purine biosynthesis
- Inhibits conversion of IMP to AMP
- Inhibits the conversion of IMP to XMP and then to GMP
- Inhibits the exonuclease repair activity of DNA polymerase
- Triphosphorylated nucleotide metabolites are incorporated into DNA leading to DNA strand breaks, but this has questionable significance
- Cell cycle S phase specific
- Resistance occurs from absence of HGPRT or increased concentrations of a membrane-bound alkaline phosphatase or a conjugating enzyme, 6-thiopurine methyltransferase
- Cross-resistant to 6-TG

DOSING

- IV formulation is investigational
- For maintenance therapy of ALL: 50–60 mg/m^2/d po
- Can be continued for months
- For remission induction of leukemia: 100–200 mg/m^2/d po until response occurs, or alternatively 500–700 mg/m^2/d po for 5 days

PHARMACOKINETICS

- Incompletely and erratically absorbed after oral administration (average, 20–50% of the administered dose)
- Peak plasma levels are attained in 2 hrs
- Plasma t $^1/_2$ is about 90 min
- No drug is detectable after 8 hrs
- Extensively metabolized in the liver
- Patients deficient in thiopurine methyl-transferase (10%) are at increased risk of toxicity
- 50% of the drug and major metabolites excreted in the urine in 24 hrs
- Low protein binding
- Low penetrance into CSF

TOXICITY

- DLT is bone marrow depression
  - gradual in onset but may persist for several days
- Anorexia, nausea, and vomiting are usually mild
- Diarrhea and oral stomatitis may occur
- Hepatic dysfunction occurs in one-third of adults but less frequently in children
  - cholestasis is most common but is reversible
- Immunosuppressive

RECOMMENDATIONS FOR SUPPORTIVE CARE

- Dose must be reduced by one-third to one-half if allopurinol is used concomitantly for hyperuricemia because 6-MP is metabolized by xanthine oxidase to 6-thiouric acid
- Monitor CBC

PHARMACY ISSUES

- Available as an oral 50 mg tablet
- Food intake and co-trimoxazole reduce absorption

NURSING CONSIDERATIONS

- Coumadin can decrease or increase PT
- Cholestatic jaundice, clay-colored stools, frothy dark urine may develop after 2–5 mos of treatment; hepatic dysfunction is reversible; monitor LFTs
- Reduce dose in cases of hepatic or renal dysfunction
- Elevations in serum glucose and uric acid possibly related to effects of medication
- Assess
  - skin integrity; skin eruptions and rash may occur
  - notify physician if patient complains of hepatic tenderness; stop drug
  - for signs of myelosuppression
- Teach patient
  - encourage adequate fluid intake (1–3 L)
  - report GI side effects that could be related to hepatotoxicity
  - side effects and self-care measures

KEY REFERENCES

Camitta B, Mahoney D, Leventhal B, et al.: Intensive intravenous methotrexate and mercaptopurine treatment of higher-risk non-T, non-B acute lymphocytic leukemia: A Pediatric Oncology Group study. J Clin Oncol 1994; 12(7):1383–9

Koren G, Ferrazini G, Sulh H, et al.: Systemic exposure to mercaptopurine as a prognostic factor in acute lymphocytic leukemia in children. N Engl J Med 1990; 323(1):17–21

Lennard L: The clinical pharmacology of 6-mercaptupurein. Eur J Clin Pharmacol 1992; 43(4):329–39

Drug: 6-Thioguanine

Richard A. Larson and Erin P. Demakos

OTHER NAMES: 6-TG

USES

- Used for treatment of acute myeloid leukemia, usually in combination with other drugs
- Also used in ALL and CML in blast phase

MECHANISM OF ACTION

- 6-thio analogue of guanine, a prodrug that must be converted to 6-TG-ribose-phosphate intracellularly by hypoxanthine:guanine phosphoribosyl transferase (HGPRT)
- Conversion to the ribonucleotide derivative is a prerequisite for activity
- Inhibits the first step of purine biosynthesis de novo by inhibiting the enzyme glutamine-5-phoosphoribosyl pyrophosphate (PRPP) amidotransferase
- Inhibits conversion of inosinic acid to guanylic acid (GMP) and of GMP to GDP
- Triphosphorylated deoxynucleotide metabolites are incorporated into DNA leading to DNA strand breaks, but this has questionable significance
- Cell cycle S phase specific
- Resistance occurs from absence of HGPRT or increased concentrations of a membrane-bound alkaline phosphatase or conjugating enzyme, 6-thiopurine methyltransferase
- Cross-resistant to 6-MP

DOSING

- For remission induction of AML together with cytarabine and daunorubicin: 100 mg/m^2 po q12hrs for 7 days
- For chronic suppression of leukemia: 80 mg/m^2/d po and titrate against the response

PHARMACOKINETICS

- Incompletely absorbed after oral administration (average, 30% of the administered dose)
- Peak plasma levels are attained in 2–4 hrs
- Mean plasma t $^1/_2$ is ~90 min
- Extensively metabolized and inactivated in the liver
- Patients deficient in thiopurine methyltransferase (10%) are at increased risk of toxicity
- 6-TG is not extensively deaminated and only a small amount is converted to thiouric acid by xanthine oxidase
- A dose reduction is not required in the presence of allopurinol
- 25–50% of the drug is excreted as metabolites in the urine in 24 hrs
- Low protein binding
- Low penetrance into CSF

TOXICITY

- DLT is bone marrow depression
  - gradual in onset but may persist for several days
- Anorexia, nausea, and vomiting are usually mild
- Diarrhea and oral stomatitis may occur
- Hepatic dysfunction with cholestasis may occur but is reversible
- Immunosuppressive

RECOMMENDATIONS FOR SUPPORTIVE CARE

- Dose does not need to be reduced if allopurinol is used concomitantly for hyperuricemia
- Monitor CBC

PHARMACY ISSUES

- Available as an oral 40 mg tablet

NURSING CONSIDERATIONS

- Can be given full dose with allopurinol
- Hepatotoxicity rare but may be associated with hepatic veno-occlusive disease, jaundice, clay-colored stools and frothy urine; monitor LFTs
- Monitor serum uric acid levels; increasing urine alkalization and administration with allopurinol can minimize hyperuricemia
- Oral dose should be taken on an empty stomach to facilitate absorption
- Assess
  - notify physician if patient complains of hepatic tenderness; stop drug
  - potential for sensory/perceptual alterations; assess vibratory sensation and gait before each dose and between treatments
- Teach patient
  - to take dose on an empty stomach between meals
  - report early stomatitis
  - side effects and self-care measures

KEY REFERENCES

Evans WE, Relling MV: Mercaptopurine vs thioguanine for the treatment of acute lymphoblastic leukemia. Leuk Res 1994; 18(11):811–14

Lancaster DL, Lennard L, Rowland K, et al.: Thioguanine versus mercaptopurine for therapy of childhood lymphoblastic leukemia: a comparison of hematological toxicity and drug metabolite concentrations. Br J Haematol 1998; 102(2):439–43

Lennard L, Davies HA, Lilleyman JS: Is 6-thioguanine more appropriate than 6-mercaptopurine for children with acute lymphoblastic leukemia? Br J Cancer 1993; 68(1):186–90

Drug: Hydroxyurea

Everett E. Vokes and Dolores Watts

OTHER NAME: HYDREA

USES

- Approved by FDA for use with concomitant radiation therapy in squamous cell carcinomas of the head and neck excluding the lip
- Responses have also been demonstrated in melanoma, chronic myelocytic leukemia, and recurrent metastatic or inoperable carcinoma of the ovary

MECHANISM OF ACTION

- Causes inhibition of DNA synthesis
- Inhibits the enzyme ribonucleotide reductase
- Interaction with radiotherapy may be due to eradication of normally radiation-resistant S-phase cells and cell cycle arrest in the G_1-S cell cycle phase when cells are more susceptible to the effects of radiation
- Also inhibits the normal repair process of cells damaged but not killed by irradiation

DOSING

- Concomitant therapy with radiation
  - 80 mg/kg administered po as a single dose every third day
- Administration at 1 g po every day or twice per day with careful monitoring of hematologic toxicities
- Higher doses are used in chronic myelogenous leukemia (20–30 mg/kg daily)

PHARMACOKINETICS

- Bioavailability: 100%
- Half-life: 2–3 hrs
- Renal clearance linear
- ~40% total clearance
- Also undergoes metabolism that is nonlinear

TOXICITY

- Common
  - leukopenia, anemia, and occasionally thrombocytopenia
- Less common
  - stomatitis, anorexia, nausea, vomiting, diarrhea
- Dermatologic reactions (maculopapular rash, skin ulceration, and facial erythema)
- Rare neurologic disturbances include headaches, dizziness, disorientation, hallucination, and convulsions
- Concomitant use with radiation results in exacerbated radiotherapy reactions, including dermatitis, mucositis, esophagitis, diarrhea, gastric irritation depending on the specific site of radiotherapy

RECOMMENDATIONS FOR SUPPORTIVE CARE

- Antiemetic prophylaxis may be necessary

PHARMACY ISSUES

- Supplied as 500 mg capsules

NURSING CONSIDERATIONS

- Dose must be reduced in patients with renal dysfunction
- Dermatologic radiation recall may occur
- Potential to dramatically lower WBC (24–48 hrs); monitor counts frequently
- Assess
  - alterations in LFTs and kidney functions
  - drug crosses blood-brain barrier; assess for CNS effects
- Teach patient
  - expected side effects
  - contents can be emptied in a glass of water and taken immediately (a powder residue may still exist once dissolved); avoid skin contact
  - discuss possibility of drowsiness in patients receiving high doses; avoid operating vehicles or machinery requiring mental alertness
  - to follow an oral regimen to decrease stomatitis
  - monitor temperature daily
  - avoid OTC aspirin-containing medications

KEY REFERENCES

Gale RP, Hehlmann R, Zhang MJ, et al.: Survival with bone marrow transplantation versus hydroxyurea or interferon for chronic myelogenous leukemia. The German CML Study Group. Blood 1998; 91(5):1810–19

Stehman FB, Bundy BN, Keys H, et al.: A randomized trial of hydroxyurea versus misonidazole adjunct to radiation therapy in carcinoma of the cervix. A preliminary report of a Gynecologic Oncology Group study. Am J Obstet Gynecol 1988; 159(1):87–94

Tracewell WG, Trump DL, Vaughan WP, et al.: Population pharmacokinetics of hydroxyurea in cancer patients. Cancer Chemother Pharmacol 1995; 35(5):417–22

Vokes EE, Haraf DJ, Panje WR, et al.: Hydroxyurea with concomitant radiotherapy for locally advanced head and neck cancer. Semin Oncol 1992; 19(3 suppl 9):53–8

Drug: MTA

Hedy L. Kindler and Consuelo Skosey

OTHER NAMES: MULTITARGETED ANTIFOLATE, LY231514

USES

- Active in non–small cell lung cancer, malignant mesothelioma, and cancers of the head and neck, pancreas, breast, bladder, cervix, and colon

MECHANISM OF ACTION

- A pyrrolo-pyrimidine-based antifolate antimetabolite
- Transported via the reduced folate carrier
- A substrate for folypoly-γ-glutamate synthetase, resulting in extensive intracellular polyglutamation, prolonged intracellular retention, and greater affinity for its target enzymes
- MTA and its polyglutamated metabolites inhibit multiple folate-dependent enzymes thereby inhibiting de novo purine and thymidine synthesis including
  - thymidylate synthase (TS)
  - dihydrofolate reductase (DHFR)
  - glycinamide ribonucleotide formyltransferase (GARFT)
  - aminoimidazole carboxamide ribonucleotide formyltransferase (AICARFT)

DOSING

- Administered IV over 10 min
- Schedules/doses
  - MTA 500 or 600 mg/m^2 q21d
  - Commonly used combinations
    - □ MTA 500 or 600 mg/m^2 and cisplatin 75 mg/m^2 q3wks
    - □ gemcitabine 1,000 mg/m^2 day 1, 8 and MTA 500 mg/m^2 day 8 of a 21-day cycle

PHARMACOKINETICS

- Mean half-life of 3.1 hrs
- Renally excreted
- 80% protein bound
- Linear pharmacokinetics

TOXICITY

- Neutropenia and thrombocytopenia are dose limiting
- Fatigue
- Erythematous maculopapular rash
- Mucositis
- Reversible elevations in hepatic transaminases
- Nausea
- Diarrhea
- Elevated pretreatment homocysteine levels correlate with grades 3 and 4 hematologic and nonhematologic toxicity

RECOMMENDATIONS FOR SUPPORTIVE CARE

- Prophylactic corticosteroids can prevent or ameliorate the rash (dexamethasone 4 mg po bid for 3 days, starting the day before MTA therapy)
- It is recommended that patients discontinue the use of NSAIDs, which are known to decrease the renal clearance of methotrexate and may decrease the clearance of MTA
- Leucovorin rescue may reverse MTA toxicity

PHARMACY ISSUES

- Sterile normal saline or Water for Injection are the preferred diluents

NURSING CONSIDERATIONS

- Monitor liver functions for elevations in transaminase
- Monitor blood counts
- Assess
  - skin for signs of rash, which can be ameliorated with prophylactic dexamethasone
- Teach patient
  - report mucositis, skin rash, diarrhea, nausea, and vomiting
  - self-care measures

KEY REFERENCES

Calvert AH, Walling JM: Clinical studies with MTA. Br J Cancer 1998; 78(suppl 3):35–40

Cripps MC, Burnell M, Jolivet J, et al.: Phase III study of a multi-targeted antifolate (LY231514) (MTA) as first line therapy in patients with locally advanced or metastatic colorectal cancer (MCC). Proc Am Soc Clin Oncol 1997; 16:A949

O'Dwyer PJ, Nelson K, Thornton DE: Overview of phase II trials of MTA in solid tumors. Sem Oncol 1999; 26(2)(suppl 6):99–104

Thodtmann R, Depenbrock H, Dumez H, et al. Clinical and pharmacokinetic phase I study of multitargeted antifolate (LY231514) in combination with cisplatin. J Clin Oncol 1999; 17(10):3009–16

Chapter 5

MISCELLANEOUS CYTOTOXIC AND MODULATING AGENTS

Introduction

Bruce Cheson

DRUG CLASSES

- Retinoids
- Nucleoside analogues
- Enzyme/growth factor/protein inhibitors
- DNA inhibitors
- Reversal of P-gp-mediated mdr-1
- Differentiation agents

BIOCHEMICAL PHARMACOLOGY

- Retinoids
  - interact with cellular receptors leading to dimerization of nuclear proteins, binding of the complex to DNA, and activational transcription of target genes
- Arsenic trioxide
  - induces cellular differentiation
  - induces apoptosis
- Nucleoside analogues
  - fludarabine and cladribine require intracellular activation by deoxycytidine kinase
  - inhibit enzymes required for DNA replication and repair
  - inhibit RNA and protein synthesis
  - induce apoptosis
- Suramin
  - inhibits a wide range of growth factors
  - dissociates growth factors from their receptors
  - interferes with glycosaminoglycan metabolism
- Homoharringtonine
  - inhibits protein synthesis
  - interferes with cell cycle progression
- Bleomycin
  - induces single- and double-strand DNA breaks
- L-asparaginase, PEG-L-asparaginase
  - catalyze conversion of L-asparagine to aspartic acid, which cannot be converted to asparagine by cancer cells
- PSC-833
  - reverses P-gp-mediated drug resistance

Drug: All-*Trans* Retinoic Acid

Raymond P. Warrell, Jr. and Deborah T. Berg

OTHER NAMES: VESANOID, ATRA, ATRAGEN (LIPOSOMALLY ENCAPSULATED FORMULATION)

USES

- Approved by FDA for induction therapy of relapsed acute promyelocytic leukemia (APL)
- Drug is now standard of care for newly diagnosed patients with APL
- Investigational use: maintenance therapy of APL

MECHANISM OF ACTION

- Cytodifferentiation, followed by apoptosis

DOSING

- Administered po on once or twice per day schedule
- Schedules/doses
  - induction therapy of APL: 45 mg/m^2/d as single dose or in two equally divided doses. Doses as low as 15 mg/m^2/d have also proved effective and can be considered for patients who are intolerant of higher doses (e.g., children with headache)
  - postremission (maintenance) therapy: 45 mg/m^2/d as single dose or in two equally divided doses
  - no treatment courses are standard
  - schedules that have been used are generally intermittent (e.g., 14 days of treatment once every 3 mos, etc.)
  - maximum duration of 1–2 yrs
- Other schedules: under investigation; no published experience
- IV use: liposomal formulation (Atragen) only

PHARMACOKINETICS

- Primarily biliary excretion
- Plasma half-life ~10 hrs
- Autoinduction of catabolism
- Broad-spectrum cytochrome P-450 inhibitors (e.g., ketoconazole) increase plasma levels

TOXICITY

- Headache
  - worse in children
  - may progress to frank pseudotumor cerebri, requiring lumbar puncture and corticosteroids for management
- Facial flushing
- Musculoskeletal pain
- "Retinoic acid syndrome" (in patients with acute promyelocytic leukemia only): characterized by hectic fever, dyspnea, weight gain, fluid retention
  - prophylactic therapy with high-dose corticosteroids mandatory at earliest manifestation of syndrome
  - extremely difficult to reverse once established
- Leukocytosis (~70% of leukemia patients): usually requires no specific therapy
- However, specialists differ on need for concurrent cytotoxic therapy to "control" leukocytosis (e.g., hydroxyurea, full-dose chemotherapy, etc.)
  - common practice is to administer drug with full dose of chemotherapy (i.e., anthracycline plus cytosine arabinoside) for patients who present with initial leukocyte count >10,000 cells/cu mm
- Skin reactions: dryness; flaking; peeling, especially palms and soles; cheilitis; scrotal or vulvar ulcerations
- Hypertriglyceridemia (less commonly hypercholesterolemia)
- Hepatotoxicity (usually mild elevation of hepatic enzymes only)
- Highly teratogenic, especially in first trimester
- Nausea: uncommon

RECOMMENDATIONS FOR SUPPORTIVE CARE

- Observation related to induction therapy for leukemia: retinoic acid syndrome, exacerbation of disseminated intravascular coagulopathy

PHARMACY ISSUES

- Supplied as 10 mg gelatin-filled capsules
- Protect from direct light
- Atragen: supplied on investigational basis only from the manufacturer (Aronex Pharmaceuticals, Inc., Houston, TX)

NURSING CONSIDERATIONS

- Use cautiously in patients with known elevated cholesterol as may cause increases in triglycerides and cholesterol
- Headaches are common and are treated symptomatically
- Assess
  - skin integrity (e.g., redness, dryness, vesicles, and peeling of skin on palms of hands and soles of feet, and pruritis of skin and mucous membranes)
  - for retinoic acid syndrome as evidenced by hyperleukocytosis, thrombocytosis, fever, dyspnea on exertion, pulmonary edema, and diffuse interstitial infiltrates
- Teach patient
  - expected side effects and self-care measures
  - mechanism of action of tretinoin: not a cytotoxic agent but a differentiating agent
  - regarding use of sunscreen and to avoid being in the sun

KEY REFERENCES

Stanley R, Frankel MD, Eardley E, et al.: The retinoic acid syndrome in acute promyelocytic leukemia. Ann Intern Med 1992; 117(4):292–6

Warrell RP Jr., et al.: Acute promyelocytic leukemia. N Engl J Med 1993; 329:177–89

Drug: Isotretinoin

Gini F. Fleming and Janine Caggiano

OTHER NAMES: 13-CIS-RETINOIC ACID, ACCUTANE

USES

- Approved by FDA for use in severe recalcitrant nodular acne
- Modest single agent activity in cutaneous T-cell lymphomas
- High-dose therapy reverses oral leukoplakia
- Randomized trials suggest benefit in prevention of secondary primaries in patients with head and neck cancer, and prevention of skin cancers in patients with xeroderma pigmentosum
- One randomized study shows that maintenance isotretinoin improves event-free survival in neuroblastoma patients

MECHANISM OF ACTION

- Induces cellular differentiation or suppresses proliferation in a number of cell lines
- Possesses some anti-inflammatory activity
- Binds to intracellular retinoic acid receptors (RARs) that dimerize and bind to specific DNA segments in retinoid target genes, thereby regulating their transcription

DOSING

- Administered po, usually in 2 doses daily
- Dosage for acne is 0.5–2 mg/kg given in two divided doses daily for 15 to 20 wks; similar dose ranges have been used in many cancer-related trials

PHARMACOKINETICS

- Following oral administration peak levels occur at about 3 hrs
- The terminal half-life averages 10–20 hrs
- Administration with food or milk maximizes bioavailability
- Metabolized in liver to 4-oxo-isotretinoin, which has a half-life of 20–30 hrs
- The drug and its metabolites are excreted in urine and feces
- 99% bound in plasma, mostly to albumin

TOXICITY

- Similar toxicities to those seen with vitamin A overdose
- Exceedingly teratogenic; exposed fetuses have shown CNS abnormalities such as microcephaly, ear and eye abnormalities including micropinna and microphthalmia, cardiovascular abnormalities and facial dysmorphia
- Mild to moderate dry skin, cheilitis, and conjunctivitis are very common
- Hypertriglyceridemia is common (25% of patients)
- Triglyceride levels should be monitored on therapy
- Myalgias and arthralgias occur fairly often
- Skeletal hyperostosis has been observed
- Lethargy, fatigue, and headaches may occur
- Pseudotumor cerebri has been reported
- Decreased night vision, cataracts, and corneal opacities can be seen
- Occasional mild increases in alkaline phosphatase and transaminases
- Mild decreases in leucocycte and erythrocyte values may be seen

RECOMMENDATIONS FOR SUPPORTIVE CARE

- Women of childbearing potential must use adequate contraception
- Patients should avoid vitamin supplements with vitamin A to prevent additive toxicity
- Hypertriglyceridemia should be controlled by restriction of dietary fat and alcohol and, if needed, lipid-lowering agents

PHARMACY ISSUES

- 10 mg, 20 mg, and 40 mg capsules available
- Capsules should be stored at room temperature and protected from light

NURSING CONSIDERATIONS

- Elevations in liver enzyme, typically alkaline phosphatase and aspartate aminotransferase, have been noted; monitor triglycerides
- Capsules should be protected from light and stored at room temperature
- Assess
  - for central nervous system side effects; baseline neurologic function and frequent assessment during treatment
  - for signs of xerostomia, mucositis, and cheilitis
  - for signs of skin toxicity
- Teach patient
  - teratogenic potential; avoid pregnancy while on treatment and avoid becoming pregnant for 3 mos once off treatment to allow clearance of drug and metabolites
  - report dizziness or visual disturbances
  - to follow an oral hygiene regimen that includes lubrication of lips
  - avoid sun exposure

KEY REFERENCE

Hong WK, Lippman SM, Itri LM, et al.: Prevention of second primary tumors with isotretinoin in squamous-cell carcinoma of the head and neck. N Engl J Med 1990; 323:795–801

Drug: Fludarabine

Bruce D. Cheson and Erin P. Demakos

OTHER NAMES: FLUDARA, FAMP, FLUDARABINE MONOPHOSPHATE

USES

- Approved by FDA for chronic lymphocytic leukemia resistant to alkylating agents
- Also active in prolymphocytic leukemia, indolent non-Hodgkin's lymphomas, including Waldenström's macroglobulinemia, and cutaneous T-cell lymphomas

MECHANISM OF ACTION

- Purine nucleoside analogue
- Rapidly dephosphorylated after IV injection
- Enters cells by nucleoside carrier transport mechanism
- Rephosphorylated to F-ara-ATP via deoxycytidine kinase
- Triphosphate incorporated into DNA
- Inhibits ribonucleotide reductase, DNA polymerase, DNA primase, DNA ligase
- Induces apoptosis

DOSING

- Administered IV as a 30 min infusion
- No premedication for nausea/vomiting or hydration necessary
- Oral formulation in development
- Schedules/doses
  - 25 mg/m^2 for 5 consecutive days q28d
  - alternatives include 30 mg/m^2 for 5 consecutive days q28d, and 30 mg/m^2 for 3 consecutive days
  - commonly used combinations
    - □ 30 mg/m^2 for 3 days in combination with mitoxantrone at 10 mg/m^2 IV on day 1 and dexamethasone mg po days 1–5, repeated q28d
    - □ at a dose of 20 mg/m^2 days 1–5 in combination with cyclophosphamide 600–1,000 mg/m^2 day 1
    - □ at 30 mg/m^2 days 1–3 and cyclophosphamide 350 mg/m^2 days 1–3
  - administration in combination with G-CSF has not shown consistent reduction in infection

PHARMACOKINETICS

- Poorly water soluble, thus all pharmacokinetic studies describe the kinetics of F-ara-AMP
- Most studies suggest biphasic decay curve
  - rapid dephosphorylation (< 5 min) to F-ara-A following IV injection
  - terminal half-life of 10–33 hrs

TOXICITY

- Neutropenia and thrombocytopenia common and may be cumulative, but generally not dose limiting
  - febrile neutropenia in 20% of patients
- Hemolytic anemia uncommon but may be severe
- Profound lymphocytopenia, particularly CD4 cells, which may persist for a year or longer
  - opportunistic infections including *Herpes zoster, Herpes simplex, Pneumocystis carinii,* candida, aspergillus, and others
- Severe, life-threatening, and fatal neurotoxicity when administered at higher than recommended doses
  - neurotoxicity in 15% of patients at standard doses, mostly grade I–II, rarely severe
- Tumor lysis syndrome in < 0.5%, but may be fatal and not preventable with allopurinol and/or hydration
- Nonhematologic toxicities (e.g., nausea, vomiting, alopecia) are uncommon
- Toxicities may be greater in patients who are older or poorly responsive to therapy

RECOMMENDATIONS FOR SUPPORTIVE CARE

- Trimethoprim/sulfamethoxasole if concurrent steroids are necessary
- Prophylactic antimicrobials or myeloid growth factors generally not routinely indicated

PHARMACY ISSUES

- Reconstituted with 2 ml of sterile water
- D_5W or normal saline can be used as diluents

NURSING CONSIDERATIONS

- Generally administered on an outpatient basis
- Do not administer drug in combination with pentostatin
- Administer cautiously in patients with renal insufficiency
- Evaluate BUN, creatinine, and LFTs prior to administration
- Assess
  - liver dysfunction and renal impairment
- Teach patient
  - avoidance of OTC aspirin-containing medications
  - signs and symptoms of anemia and thrombocytopenia and the potential for blood support
  - potential for tumor lysis syndrome and importance to maintain hydration
  - expected side effects and self-care measures

KEY REFERENCES

Adkins JC, Peters DH, Markham A: Fludarabine. An update of its pharmacology and use in the treatment of hematological malignancies. Drugs 1997; 53(6):1005–37

Cheson BD, Frame JN, Vena D, et al.: Tumor lysis syndrome: an uncommon complication of fludarabine therapy of chronic lymphocytic leukemia. J Clin Oncol 1998; 16(7):2313–20

Decaudin D, Bosq J, Tertian G, et al.: Phase II trial of fludarabine monophosphate in patients with mantle-cell lymphomas. J Clin Oncol 1998; 26(2):579–83

Sorensen JM, Vena DA, Fallavollita A, et al.: Treatment of refractory chronic lymphocytic leukemia with fludarabine phosphate via the group C protocol mechanism of the National Cancer Institute: five-year follow-up report. J Clin Oncol 1997; 15(2):458–65

Zinzani PL, Bendandi M, Magagnoli M, et al.: Fludarabine mitoxantrone combination containing regimen in recurrent low-grade non-Hodgkin's lymphoma. Ann Oncol 1997; 8(4):379–83

Drug: Deoxycoformycin

Michael R. Grever and Janan B. Geick Miller

OTHER NAMES: PENTOSTATIN, NIPENT, DCF

USES

- FDA approved for treatment of patients with hairy cell leukemia
- Also active in chronic lymphocytic leukemia, cutaneous T-cell lymphoma, and some indolent lymphomas

MECHANISM OF ACTION

- Potent transition state inhibitor of adenosine deaminase
- May induce tumor cell apoptosis in presence of intracellular accumulation of dATP
- May enhance DNA damage by other chemotherapeutic agents, but exact mechanism of this effect is unknown

DOSING

- Administered IV by bolus or short infusion over 20–30 min diluted in a larger volume
- Patients should have a creatinine clearance > 50–60 ml/min to receive the standard dose of the drug
- The standard dose of this agent for hairy cell leukemia is 4 mg/m^2 IV q14d
- Dose modification must be made for renal insufficiency
- In those patients with renal insufficiency, caution must be exercised
- DCF should be held in the face of active infection that requires treatment
- Optimal duration of therapy for hairy cell leukemia is unknown, but it usually is best given until the patient is in remission
- There is no known advantage to continuing treatment beyond attainment of a complete remission

PHARMACOKINETICS

- Primary route of elimination is renal
- Half-life in patients with renal insufficiency is markedly prolonged

TOXICITY

- Nausea, vomiting, and skin rash are frequent side effects, and the skin rash may necessitate stopping the drug
- Patients may have myelosuppression, keratoconjunctivitis, or renal insufficiency, which necessitate holding the drug until safe to resume at lower doses
- Increased risk of infection in particular if administered in close proximity to other potentially immunosuppressive agents

RECOMMENDATIONS FOR SUPPORTIVE CARE

- Hydration is important
- Antiemetics are required, but avoidance of unnecessary exposure to corticosteroids is prudent
- Prophylaxis for pneumocystis should be considered in patients receiving other immunosuppressive agents in conjunction with DCF
- Prompt use of antiviral therapy for early onset of herpetic disease is recommended
- IV fluids are recommended both before and after drug administration. In fact, this can be accomplished as an outpatient with the total fluid administration being in the range of 500–1,000 ml. While fluid administration is proceeding, renal function studies should be checked before each dose of the drug

PHARMACY ISSUES

- May be diluted either with D_5W or 0.9% sodium chloride injection USP

NURSING CONSIDERATIONS

- Obtain complete CBC with differential
- Vesicant; use caution when administering
- Prophylactic use of antiemetic
- Evaluate renal function prior to administration
- Assess
  - signs of immunosuppression manifested by herpes simplex and herpes zoster
  - neurologic status
  - pulmonary status (i.e., lung sounds). Obtain periodic PFTs
- Teach patient
  - expected side effects and self-care measures
  - to report signs of lethargy and fatigue
  - Importance of hydration (3 L/d)

KEY REFERENCES

Grever MR, Kopecky K, Foucar MK, et al.: Randomized comparison of pentostatin versus interferon alpha-2a in previously untreated patients with hairy cell leukemia: an intergroup study. J Clin Oncol 1995; 13:974–82

Malspeis L, et al.: Clinical pharmacokinetics of deoxycoformycin. Cancer Treatment Symposia 1984; 2:43–9

Drug: 2-Chlorodeoxyadenosine

Lawrence D. Piro and Belinda Butler

OTHER NAMES: 2-CDA, CLADRABINE, LEUSTATIN

USES

- Approved by FDA for previously treated and previously untreated hairy cell leukemia (HCL)
- Commonly used for chronic lymphocytic leukemia, prolymphocytic leukemia, low-grade non-Hodgkin's lymphoma, and Langerhan's cell histiocytosis
- Also active in chronic myelogenous leukemia and cutaneous T-cell lymphomas

MECHANISM OF ACTION

- A chlorinated purine analogue resistant to the action of adenosine deaminase
- Distinguished from other purine analogues by its unique cytotoxic activity in nondividing as well as dividing lymphocytes and monocytes
- Resistance to metabolism by adenosine deaminase results in intracellular accumulation of the active triphosphate deoxynucleotide 2-chlorodeoxyadenosine triphosphate (2-CdATP)
  - in dividing cells inhibits ribonucleotide reductase and DNA polymerase alpha
  - in nondividing cells accumulation of 2-CdATP results in incorporation into DNA-inducing single- and double-strand breaks
- The broken ends of DNA activate two enzyme systems
  - calcium-magnesium dependent endonuclease produces further double-stranded DNA breaks
  - poly (ADP-ribose) polymerase consumes NAD and ATP resulting in disruption of cellular metabolism
- Consumption of NAD and ATP together with inhibition of DNA polymerase alpha prevents DNA repair
- Oligonucleosomal fragments indicative of apoptosis or programmed cell death

DOSING

- Administered IV as either a continuous infusion for 7 days or a 2 hr daily infusion for 5 consecutive days
- Oral formulation in development but not available commercially
- Schedules/doses
  - 0.09–0.1 mg/kg/d by continuous IV infusion for 7 days q4wks
  - administered as an inpatient through a peripheral IV catheter
  - as an outpatient by infusion from a Pharmacia Deltec Continuous Ambulatory Delivery Device (CADD) infusion pump through a peripherally insulated central catheter line (PICC)
  - for HCL, the 7 day continuous infusion schedule remains the most effective schedule with the longest follow-up and the highest response rate following a single course of treatment
  - for all other diseases that necessitate repetitive cycles of therapy, the 5 day brief infusion regimen appears to be equivalent to continuous infusion in terms of clinical efficacy
  - the 2 hr regimen is 0.12–0.14 mg/kg/d over 2 hrs by IV infusion on 5 consecutive days

PHARMACOKINETICS

- Believed to be cleared principally through the kidneys
- Penetrates into CSF
  - ~25% of plasma concentration
- Long terminal half-life (2–3 days)
- The intracellular half-life in leukemic cells is ~23 hrs

TOXICITY

- The principal toxicity is myelosuppression
- Nausea and vomiting unusual
- Renal, pulmonary, and neurotoxicity are infrequently reported (at standard doses)
- T-cell immunosuppression is prominent with CD4 levels often reduced to < 200 cells/μL
  - Commonly it takes 1–2 yrs for recovery to occur

RECOMMENDATIONS FOR SUPPORTIVE CARE

- When possible, steroids should not be administered to patients receiving or during the period following 2-Cda administration when T-cells are suppressed
- Pneumocystis prophylaxis with trimethoprim/sulfamethoxazole is advisable when patients are on concomitant steroids
- Steroids pose a significant danger even years after treatment if the CD4 count remains suppressed
- Prophylactic treatment for pneumocystic infection should be considered in all high-risk patients

PHARMACY ISSUES

- Most commonly used diluent is normal saline
- A 7 day infusion is prepared with bacteriostatic normal saline to a total volume of 100 ml and loaded into a Pharmacia Deltec CADD infusion pump for administration over 7 days
- With inpatient usage through a peripheral IV, 2-Cda is prepared by loading the daily dose into a 500 cc bag of normal saline and administered over 24 hrs by continuous infusion or in a 250 cc bag of normal saline and admitted as a 2 hr infusion

NURSING CONSIDERATIONS

- Monitor bone marrow, renal, and hepatic function
- Monitor for serious neurologic toxicity if patient receiving high doses with continuous infusion
- Administer cautiously in patients with renal or hepatic insufficiency
- Drug is unstable in 5% dextrose
- May precipitate when exposed to low temperature; allow to come to room temperature (do not heat or microwave)
- When peripheral counts normalize, perform bone marrow aspirate and biopsy to assess response and cellularity
- Assess
  - cardiac and pulmonary status baseline and during therapy
  - for signs and symptoms of hepatotoxicity, neurotoxicity, nephrotoxicity (for high-dose therapy), infection and fever
  - skin rash, fatigue, and alteration in nutrition
- Teach patient
  - to monitor temperature at home and report temperatures of > 101 °F
  - practice contraception
  - avoid abrasive skin products and clothing
  - expected side effects and self-care measures

KEY REFERENCE

Saven A, Piro LD: 2-chlorodeoxyadenosine: A newer purine analog active in the treatment of indolent lymphoid malignancies. Ann Intern Med 1994; 120:784–801

Drug: Suramin

Ken Kobayashi and Brenda Werner

OTHER NAMES: GERMANIN, MORANYL, BAYER 205, FOURNEAU 309, ANTRYPOL, NAGANOL, NAGANIN, NAPHURIDE SODIUM

USES

- Not approved by FDA and use in treatment of cancer is currently investigational
- Use in hormone-refractory metastatic prostate cancer has been studied most extensively

MECHANISM OF ACTION

- Multiple speculated, none proven
- Interference with glycosaminoglycan metabolism
- Inhibition of growth factor binding to receptor (e.g., TGF-alpha, TGF-beta, IGF-I, IGF-II, EGF, basic FGF)
- Inhibition of intracellular enzymes, such as DNA polymerase alpha or topoisomerase II)
- Disruption of cell motility and adhesion
- Disruption of mitochondrial energy balance
- Induction of differentiation

DOSING

- Administered IV as a 1 hr infusion
- Adaptive control (previously thought necessary) not required
- Various pharmacokinetically based dosing schemes are currently in development; only the most commonly used are cited in this chapter
- Schedules/doses
  - monotherapy: 4 days/month (University of Chicago). In order to avoid increasing peak concentrations with repetitive dosing, a scheme in which a day 1 loading dose is administered, followed by gradually decreasing doses over subsequent days in a 28 day cycle is used:

Cycle	Day	Dose, mg/m²	% of day 1 dose
1	1	1,440	
	2	720	50
	8	720	50
	9	576	40
2	1	720	50
	2	576	40
	8	576	40
	9	461	32
3	1	576	40
	2	461	32
	8	461	32
	9	374	26

Doses for cycles ≥4 are 80% of the corresponding dose from the previous cycle.

  - 2 days/month (University of Chicago):

Cycle	Day	Dose, mg/m²	% of day 1 dose
1	1	2,160	
	8	1,296	90
2	1	1,296	90
	8	1,037	72
3	1	1,037	72
	8	835	58

Doses for cycles ≥4 are 80% of the corresponding dose from the previous cycle.

  - weekly (University of Maryland):

Day	Dose, mg/m²	Infusion duration, hrs
1	200*	0.5
1	1,000	2
2	400	1
3	300	1
4	250	1
5	200	1
8	275	1
11	275	1
15	275	1
19	275	1
22	275	1
29	275	1
36	275	1
43	275	1
50	275	1
57	275	1
67	275	1
78	275	1

*Test dose.

- Commonly used combinations
  - combination therapy is investigational and cannot be recommended

PHARMACOKINETICS

- Reported elimination half-life varies from 30–60 days
- No known metabolism
- Sole route of elimination is renal
- Polyanionic compound, highly (>99%) protein bound
- Distributes to skeletal muscle, liver, kidneys, adrenal glands
- Not found in adipose tissue

TOXICITY

- Progressive demyelinating motor polyneuropathy resembling Guillain-Barre syndrome
  - usually involves peripheral and bulbar nerves
  - an axonal neuropathy has also been observed
  - some patients have required intubation and mechanical ventilation
  - some degree of reversibility in milder cases, although it is unusual for patients to recover entirely
  - a sensory neuropathy has also been observed clinically, generally characterized by a burning sensation in the lower extremities
- Malaise is frequent and consists of fatigue, general weakness, anorexia, and weight loss (described as the "suramin blues" syndrome)
- Myelosuppression (most frequently leukopenia and thrombocytopenia, but also occasionally including anemia)
- Immunosuppression, as evidenced by patients developing oral thrush, localized perioral herpetic infection, and bacterial urinary tract infections
- Dose-related asymptomatic prolongations of both the prothrombin time and partial thromboplastin time have been observed, with substantial variability in the degree of prolongation
- May complicate traumatic injuries
- Patients have undergone major surgical procedures while on suramin therapy without experiencing serious perioperative bleeding complications
- Asymptomatic hepatic transaminase and alkaline phosphatase elevations
- Transient hearing loss
- Pancreatitis
- Hyperglycemia and steroid-induced diabetes
- Pericardial effusion
- Dermatologic effects, including erythema multiforme, exfoliative dermatitis, or Stevens-Johnson syndrome, and keratoacanthomas
- A transient diffuse skin rash accompanied by fever (which occasionally reached 103°F) and rigors typically occurs around the administration of the first or second doses of suramin, but can occur with later dosing
- Chronic adrenal insufficiency and Addisonian crisis
  - possible mechanisms may include inhibition of human adrenal steroidogenesis by inhibition of key enzymes (21-hydroxylase, 17 alpha-hydroxylase, 17,20-desmolase, and 11alpha-hydroxylase) by suramin and also adrenal cortical necrosis
- A particularly unusual form of keratopathy, known as vortex keratopathy, has been described in adrenocortical carcinoma patients
  - histopathologic findings included deposits similar to those seen in lipid storage diseases and were symptomatic; the complaints were of mild pain and photophobia
- Proteinuria (up to 2 g/d) is common and declines in creatinine clearance with serum creatinine elevation have been noted
  - these generally resolve with discontinuation of therapy
- Gastrointestinal effects such as nausea, vomiting, diarrhea, colitis, and stomatitis
- Cardiac dysfunction, including instances of atrial fibrillation

■ Other metabolic abnormalities, such as hypoglycemia, hypocalcemia, and hypomagnesemia

RECOMMENDATIONS FOR SUPPORTIVE CARE

■ Patients should receive concurrent treatment with dexamethasone 0.5 mg po twice daily (or equivalent doses of another glucocorticoid) and fludrocortisone 0.1 mg po daily

■ Doses of glucocorticoid should be doubled for intercurrent illness

■ Concurrent therapy with anticoagulants, calcium channel blockers, and ketoconazole should be discouraged

■ Aspirin and NSAIDs and other drugs that may exacerbate a bleeding disorder should be used with extreme caution

PHARMACY ISSUES

■ Suramin should be administered in 0.9% normal saline in PVC containers for IV injection as an IV infusion

NURSING CONSIDERATIONS

- Suramin plasma concentration levels should remain < 300 mg/ml to avoid life-threatening toxicities
- Monitor CBC, platelet count, PT, PTT
- Monitor creatinine and LFTs
- Assess
  - signs of bleeding
  - skin integrity for rash, urticaria
  - GI toxicities
  - neurologic status for paresthesia or other neurologic toxicities
  - liver dysfunction
- Teach patient
  - avoid aspirin and NSAIDs because they are highly bound and could produce severe bleeding complications
  - salty taste in mouth

KEY REFERENCES

Eisenberger MA, Sinibaldi VJ, Reyno LM, et al.: Phase I and clinical evaluation of a pharmacologically guided regimen of suramin in patients with hormone-refractory prostate cancer. J Clin Oncol 1995; 13:2174–86

Kobayashi K, Vokes EE, Vogelzang NJ, et al.: A phase I study of suramin (NSC 34936) given by intermittent infusion without adaptive control in patients with advanced cancer. J Clin Oncol 1995; 13:2196–2207

Kobayashi K, Weiss RE, Vogelzang NJ, et al.: Mineralocorticoid insufficiency due to suramin. Cancer 1996; 78:2411–20

This section is based on work done by the author prior to his employment at the FDA and on the published literature. The opinions expressed are the author's own and may not reflect those of the Food and Drug Administration.

Drug: Homoharringtonine

Susan O'Brien and Marianne Huml

OTHER NAMES: HHT

USES

- Not yet approved by FDA
- Active in CML, AML, MDS

MECHANISM OF ACTION

- Inhibitor of protein synthesis
- Maximum activity in G_1 and G_2
- Presence of P-glycoprotein confers resistance
- Apoptosis increased in CML cells
- Induces differentiation of HL-60 cells

DOSING

- 2.5 mg/m^2 administered IV as a 24 hr continuous infusion for 5–14 days
- Bolus infusion results in hypotension and arrythmias
- Ongoing combination trials (HHT courses repeated monthly)
  - 2.5 mg/m^2/d × 5 with ara-C
  - 2.5 mg/m^2/d × 5 with IFN
  - with ara-C 10 mg/daily and IFN

PHARMACOKINETICS

- Undergoes extensive metabolism: 1 major and 2 minor products in plasma and urine
- Terminal half-life ~9 hrs
- Renal excretion minor

TOXICITY

- Hypotension was dose limiting with bolus/short infusion schedule
- Myelosuppression is only dose-limiting toxicity with continuous infusion
- Other toxicities usually mild
  - diarrhea
  - headache
  - anorexia
  - fluid retention
  - fever
  - rash
  - hyperglycemia
- Alopecia does not occur

RECOMMENDATIONS FOR SUPPORTIVE CARE

- Antiemetic prophylaxis is not required
- Loperamide may be administered for significant diarrhea

PHARMACY ISSUES

- D_5W or sodium chloride
- Not a vesicant

NURSING CONSIDERATIONS

- Continuous infusion is associated with reduced incidence of hypotension
- Stability can be an issue; drug for continuous infusions can only be mixed for 3–4 days at a time
- Diarrhea is commonly reported by patients receiving the 7 day continuous infusion; however not severe enough to require intervention
- Assess
  - baseline cardiovascular status and periodically thereafter
- Teach patient
  - expected side effects and self-care measures

KEY REFERENCES

Feldman E, Arlin Z, Ahmed T, et al.: Homoharringtonine is safe and effective for patients with acute myelogenous leukemia. Leukemia 1992; 6(11):1185–8

Feldman E, Seiter KP, Ahmed T, et al.: Homoharringtonine in patients with myelodysplastic syndrome (MDS) and MDS evolving to acute myeloid leukemia. Leukemia 1996; 10:40–2

O'Brien S, Kantarjian H, Koller C, Feldman E, Beran M, Andreeff M, Giralt S, Cheson B, Keating M, Freireich E, Rios MB, Talpaz M: Sequential homoharringtonine and interferon alpha in the treatment of early chronic phase chronic myelogenous leukemia. Blood 1999; 93(12):4149–53

O'Brien S, Kantarjian H, Keating M, Beran M, Koller C, Robertson E, Hester J, Rios MB, Andreeff M, Talpaz M: Homoharringtonine therapy induces responses in patients with chronic myelogenous leukemia in late chronic phase. Blood 1995; 86(9):3322–26

Drug: Bleomycin

Nicholas J. Vogelzang and Janine Caggiano

OTHER NAMES: BLENOXANE

USES

- Approved by FDA for treatment of testis, penile, head and neck squamous cancers, and lymphomas (Hodgkin's and non-Hodgkin's)
- Also active in esophageal cancer, squamous cell skin cancers, cervical cancer, and Kaposi's sarcoma

MECHANISM OF ACTION

- Ferrous oxidase
- Causes DNA single-strand breaks
- Drug is a large glycopeptide
- The bithiazole ring intercalates with DNA (usually at GC and GT sequences), the nitrogen-rich side chain acts as a metal coordination site to bind O_2 and Fe (required for DNA degradation)
- Actual DNA degradation occurs via active oxygen species
- Is a fermentation protein derived from the soil fungus *Streptomyces verticillus*
- Product is a mixture of bleomycin molecules: A_2 (70%), B_2 (most of remainder)

DOSING

- Has been given by multiple different routes and schedules safely
- Usual dose is 30 units (not per m^2) IV bolus weekly × 9 doses, part of combination chemotherapy for testis cancer
- Drug is usually not given on body surface area basis
- Drug can be given via direct intralesional route into skin Kaposi's sarcoma lesions. Usual dose is 2–10 U weekly
- Commonly used combinations
  - 30 U IV weekly × 9 in combination with cisplatin 20 mg/m^2 IV days 1–5 and etoposide 100 mg/m^2 IV days 1–5, (BEP) for germ cell cancers
  - 10 U/m^2 IV day 1, 15 in combination with doxorubicin (Adriamycin), 25 mg/m^2 q2wks, vinblastine 4 mg/m^2 and dacarbazine 375 mg/m^2 (ABVD for Hodgkin's disease)
  - 10 U weekly IV in combination with doxorubicin (Adriamycin) and vinblastine 3 mg/m^2 IV weekly (ABV) for AIDS-related progressive Kaposi's sarcoma
  - 15 U weekly in combination with methotrexate, doxorubicin, vincristine, cyclophosphamide 600 mg/m^2 and prednisone 60 mg/d (MACOP-B for non-Hodgkin's lymphoma)

PHARMACOKINETICS

- Terminal half-life 2–4 hrs
- Eliminated via glomerular filtration
- With decreased creatinine clearance, half-life exponentially increases as does risk of pulmonary toxicity
- Rapidly degraded by bleomycin hydroxylase
- The enzyme is found in most body tissues except skin and lung, hence lung and skin toxicity are common
- Renal dysfunction alters the excretion of bleomycin. Therefore bleomycin is given on day 2 of cisplatin in the BEP regimen in order to avoid acute renal failure, rarely caused by cisplatin

TOXICITY

- Progressive pulmonary fibrosis with increasing cumulative doses (older patients and those with prior RT are more susceptible)
- Empiric limitation of cumulative doses to 200 mg/m^2 or 360 U total dose
- Possibly caused by pulmonary vascular toxicity beginning with capillary bed inflammation and edema
- Fulminant hyperpyrexia, possibly secondary to tumor necrosis factor release. Seen anecdotally in lymphoma patients only; thus lymphoma patients receive a test dose of 1 U prior to customary dose
- Acute pulmonary insufficiency is not dose dependent
- Possibly allergic eosinophilic pneumonitis
- Usually responds to corticosteroids
- Acute and chronic skin hyperpigmentation, particularly in skin folds and creases, especially on knuckles and elbows
- Nonmyelosuppressive, although may add to myelotoxicity of cisplatin and etoposide in BEP regimen compared to EP regimen in germ cell cancers
- Allergic reactions, especially fever, common; can be abrogated with glucocorticoids
- Stomatitis, aphthous ulcers
- Raynaud's phenomenon after single agent use and particularly in 20–40% of patients treated with BEP. Does not occur when the drug is given by the continuous infusion schedule

RECOMMENDATIONS FOR SUPPORTIVE CARE

- No need for antiemetics
- IV or po dexamethasone × 1 (4–8 mg) may abrogate allergic phenomenon
- Unclear if steroids can prevent pulmonary or vascular toxicity

PHARMACY ISSUES

- Diluted in D_5W

NURSING CONSIDERATIONS

- Administer test dose and monitor for severe acute reaction including anaphylaxis and hyperpyrexia
- Question patient before each dose of bleomycin administration regarding respiratory or cutaneous symptoms. Steroids and antipyretics as needed
- Assess
  - baseline pulmonary function; obtain PFTs and CXR prior to and during therapy; earliest sign of pulmonary toxicity is fine crackles
  - risk of pulmonary toxicity is increased in elderly patients (> 70 yrs)
  - potential for skin toxicity; assess for skin eruption, hyperpigmentation, rash, and erythema; may cause irritation at injection site
- Teach patient
  - to report dyspnea, cough, or wheezing
  - avoid sun exposure
  - side effects and self-care measures

KEY REFERENCES

Comis RL: Bleomycin pulmonary toxicity: current status and future directions. Semin Oncol 1992; 19(2 suppl 5):64–70

Nichols CR, Catalano PJ, Crawford ED, et al.: Randomized comparison of cisplatin and etoposide and either bleomycin or ifosfamide in treatment of advanced disseminated germ cell tumors: an Eastern Cooperative Oncology Group, Southwest Oncology Group, and Cancer and Leukemia Group B Study. J Clin Oncol 1998; 16(4):1287–93

Yagoda A, Mukherji B, Young C, et al.: Bleomycin: An antitumor antibiotic clinical experience in 274 patients. Ann Int Med 1972; 77:861

Drug: L-Asparaginase

Richard A. Larson and Erin P. Demakos

OTHER NAMES: L-ASP, ELSPAR, ERWINIA L-ASPARAGINASE, ERWINASE (NSC-106977)

USES

- Used in combination with other agents to treat acute lymphoblastic leukemia
- Used to rescue cells after high doses of methotrexate and to increase the effectiveness of subsequent doses of methotrexate

MECHANISM OF ACTION

- The antitumor effect of L-asp is due to depletion of exogenous L-asparagine and the failure of tumor cells to generate endogenous asparagine via increased asparagine synthetase activity
- Catalyzes the hydrolysis of asparagine (a nonessential amino acid) in the plasma and extracellular fluid to aspartic acid and ammonia
- Because malignant lymphocytes may have only low concentrations of L-asparagine synthetase, these tumor cells are dependent on obtaining asparagine from the circulation
- Interrupts asparagine-dependent protein synthesis
- Most active in the G_1 phase

DOSING

- IV, IM, SubQ
- Anaphylaxis and other complications may be less common with the IM or SubQ route rather than IV
- Limit injection volume to 2 ml at a single site
- 6,000 IU/m² every other day for 3–4 wks, or daily doses of 1,000–20,000 IU/m² for 10–20 days
- 500 IU/kg IM followed 10 days later by methotrexate 100 mg/m²; repeat the cycle the following day
- Patients manifesting hypersensitivity to the *E. coli* L-asp should be switched to the Erwinia-derived formulation at the same dose

PHARMACOKINETICS

- Plasma L-asparaginase concentration is proportional to the dose administered
- The t ½ for *E. coli* L-asp is ~1.4 days and for Erwinia L-asp is ~0.65 days
- Plasma clearance is greatly accelerated in the presence of hypersensitivity, and enzyme activity may be undetectable within 4 hrs
- The enzyme distributes in the intravascular space, but asparagine levels also fall rapidly in the extracellular fluid and in CSF by an indirect effect
- There is no apparent advantage to intrathecal administration
- Blood levels of L-asparagine fall below 1 µM within minutes of L-asp injection, and remain unmeasurable for 7–10 days after the last dose

TOXICITY

- Hypersensitivity reactions to foreign protein can be severe but are uncommon (10%)
- Laryngeal edema, bronchospasm, hypotension
- Immediate reactions (common) are nausea, vomiting, fever, and chills
- Cutaneous reactions: erythema, urticaria, wheal and flare, hives, induration
- Decreased protein synthesis of albumin (edema), insulin (hyperglycemia), fibrinogen (bleeding), clotting factors V, VII, VIII, IX, antithrombin III, and protein C (thromboses)
- Cerebral dysfunction with disorientation, stupor, coma, and seizures due to low concentrations of L-asparagine or L-glutamine in the brain
- Liver dysfunction is very common due to reversible fatty metamorphosis (elevated bilirubin, AST, and alkaline phosphatase)
- Pancreatitis less common (15%)
- Thrombosis of large veins (IVC, cavernous sinus)
- Azotemia and acute renal failure are uncommon
- Minimal toxicity to the bone marrow or gastrointestinal tract

RECOMMENDATIONS FOR SUPPORTIVE CARE

- Medications to treat anaphylaxis should be available (epinephrine, diphenhydramine, hydrocortisone)
- Monitor blood pressure q15min for 1 hr after initial dose
- Patients who manifest hypersensitivity reactions to L-asp derived from *E. coli* can be safely treated with the enzyme derived from Erwinia chrysanthemi, née carotovora (obtained from the NCI's Group C Program)
- Monitor serum amylase or lipase
- Discontinue therapy if pancreatitis occurs
- Monitor fibrinogen
- Transfuse cryoprecipate to keep fibrinogen level > 100 mg/dl to reduce risk of bleeding

PHARMACY ISSUES

- Each vial of Erwinia L-asp contains 10,000 IU to be reconstituted with 2 ml NS for SubQ or IM use
- Store unreconstituted vials at 2–8°C
- They contain no preservatives

NURSING CONSIDERATIONS

- Be prepared to treat anaphylaxis with each administration of drug; epinephrine, antihistamines, corticosteroids, assure emergency measures are available
- Risk of hypersensitivity increases with repeated dosages; interdermal skin test dose should be performed prior to initiating treatment
- Potential for hepatic dysfunction or thromboembolic event; monitor LFTs and clotting factors CPT, PTT, fibrinogen
- Can enhance neurotoxicity when given with vincristine
- Potential of increased hyperglycemia when given with prednisone; monitor urine glucose before and during treatment
- Premedicate with antiemetic and continue prophylactically for 24 hrs
- Assess
  - baseline neurologic status and during treatment
  - for signs of hyperglycemia and pancreatitis
  - signs of myelosuppression; infection and bleeding
- Teach patient
  - potential for CNS toxicity
  - drug is teratogenic
  - practice contraception
  - side effects and self-care measures

KEY REFERENCE

Asselin BL, Whitin JC, Coppola DJ, Rupp IP, Sallan SE, Cohen HJ: Comparative pharmacokinetic studies of three asparaginase preparations. J Clin Oncol 1993; 11:1780–6

Drug: Valspodar

Branimir I. Sikic and Deborah T. Berg

OTHER NAMES: PSC 833, AMDRAY

USES

- Investigational agent for modulation or prevention of multidrug resistance (MDR) caused by expression of the multidrug transporter P-glycoprotein in cancer cells
- Phase III trials under way in acute myeloid leukemias, multiple myeloma, breast cancer, and ovarian carcinomas

MECHANISM OF ACTION

- Sensitizes cells to chemotherapy by binding to and inhibiting the multidrug transporter P-glycoprotein
- Specific for MDR-related drugs, including anthracyclines, vinca alkaloids, taxanes, and podophyllotoxins

DOSING

- Oral formulation: 20 mg/kg/d divided into 4 equal doses (i.e., 5 mg/kg 4 times daily) for up to 3 days, beginning 1 day prior to chemotherapy
- In multiple myeloma, the recommended oral dose is 16 mg/kg/d divided into 4 equal doses (i.e., 4 mg/kg 4 times daily)
- An increased incidence of dose-limiting cerebellar ataxia in patients on the myeloma study treated with VAD (vincristine, doxorubicin, dexamethasone) chemotherapy
- Oral valspodar drink solution should be administered at a consistent schedule with respect to meals (at least 1 hr before or 2 hrs after a meal), to avoid food-related alterations in absorption
- IV administration: 2 mg/kg loading dose over 2 hrs, followed by 10 mg/kg/d continuous infusion beginning with the administration of the first dose of chemotherapy and ending 24 hrs after the last dose of chemotherapy (up to 6 days of continuous infusion have been administered in a clinical trial)

PHARMACOKINETICS

- The bioavailability of the oral formulation of valspodar is ~50%
- The elimination half-lives are 200 hrs and 20 hrs after oral administration, and 2 hr IV infusion, respectively
- In addition to inhibition of P-glycoprotein, valspodar inhibits other membrane transporters, particularly the organic anion transporter for bilirubin, which results in hyperbilirubinemia and potential drug interactions
- Extensively metabolized by the CYP3A isoform of cytochrome P-450 via hydroxylations and demethylations
- Inhibition of CYP3A by valspodar contributes to the drug interactions caused by this drug
  - drugs that inhibit CYP3A will increase the area under the curve (AUC) exposure of valspodar
  - the drug interactions are similar to those of cyclosporine, which is a close chemical analogue of valspodar
- Extensive biliary excretion occurs, with total fecal excretion of 60% within 10 days and total urinary excretion of < 10%
- Protein binding is 98% with lipoproteins as the major binding components
- Only 10% of whole blood valspodar in distributed in red blood cells
- Valspodar increased the AUC and half-life of MDR-related anticancer drugs by 50–100%, requiring a 25–50% dose reduction of these drugs

TOXICITY

- Cerebellar ataxia is dose limiting
  - ataxia occurred 1–3 hrs after an oral dose and generally subsided within 6 hrs, before the next dose
- Other common toxicities
  - paresthesias and hypoesthesias, especially perioral numbness and tingling (20% of patients)
  - dizziness (20%)
  - headache (12%)
  - hypertension (15% after oral dosing, 13% after IV)
  - hypotension (8% after oral dosing, 15% after IV)
  - tachycardia (10%)
  - hyperbilirubinemia (30%)
  - elevated transaminases (20%)

RECOMMENDATIONS FOR SUPPORTIVE CARE

- Patients who experience grade 3 ataxia should skip the next dose of the drug and reduce subsequent doses by 1 mg/kg (e.g., a standard dose of 5 mg/kg would be reduced to 4 mg/kg)

PHARMACY ISSUES

- The oral formulation is supplied as a microemulsion drink solution in 50 ml bottles containing 100 mg/ml valspodar (5,000 mg of valspodar per bottle)
- A syringe-type dispenser is provided with a capacity of 4 ml marked in 0.1 ml increments
- The dose should be diluted at least tenfold in water, juice, cola, or other drink according to the patient's taste
- Grapefruit juice should be avoided as a diluent for the drink solution because it inhibits the metabolism of oral valspodar
- The oral solution must be used within 2 wks after opening the bottle, and within 2 hrs after dilution
- The IV concentrate is available at a concentration of 50 mg/ml in 5 ml and 10 ml ampules, which must be stored between 2–4°C
- The undiluted ampules should be warmed up to room temperature for around 20 min to redissolve the Cremophor EL component of the formulation, which may have precipitate during refrigerated storage resulting in cloudiness
- Non-PVC bags and infusion sets should be used to administer the drug, which should be diluted at least 1:20 with 5% dextrose or physiologic saline
- The diluted medication should be administered within 24 hrs if glass bottles are used
- If plastic bags or bottles are used with an infusion time of > 16 hrs, an in-line filter of pore size < 0.22 microM should be used

NURSING CONSIDERATIONS

- Monitor CBC, platelet count
- Hepatic elevations may occur
- Side effect management based on chemotherapy agents administered
- Assess
  - for signs of neurotoxicity manifested by transient ataxia or cerebral manifestations like confusion, psychosis, or seizures
  - skin for maculopapular eruption or dry desquamation
  - alterations in nutritional status
- Teach patient
  - avoid taking PSC 833 with grapefruit juice or alcohol
  - expected side effects and self-care measures
  - avoid concomitant medication use unless prescribed by the physician

KEY REFERENCES

Advani R, Saba HI, Tallman MS, et al.: Treatment of refractory and relapsed acute myelogenous leukemia with combination chemotherapy plus the multidrug resistance modulator PSC 833 (Valspodar). Blood 1999; 93(3):787–95

Fisher GA, Lum BL, Hausdorff J, et al.: Pharmacological considerations in the modulation of multidrug resistance. Eur J Cancer 1996; 32A(6):1082–8

Giaccone G, Linn SC, Welink J, et al.: A dose-finding and pharmacokinetic study of reversal of multidrug resistance with SDZ PSC 833 in combination with doxorubicin in patients with solid tumors. Clin Cancer Res 1997; 3(11):2005–15

Drug: Arsenic Trioxide

Raymond P. Warrell, Jr. and Victoria Staszak

OTHER NAMES: NONE

USES

- Investigational use: induction therapy of acute promyelocytic leukemia

MECHANISM OF ACTION

- Partial cytodifferentiation
- Caspase activation
- Induction of apoptosis

DOSING

- Administered IV over 1–4 hrs
- Schedules/Doses
  - Induction therapy of leukemia: 0.15 mg/kg infused over ~1 hr daily IV until complete remission in bone marrow has been achieved
    - □ average duration is ~25 days, but has ranged from 12–60 days
  - The drug has been successfully used in children as well as adults
  - Postremission therapy: 0.15 mg/kg IV daily for cumulative total of 25 days per course
    - □ maximum of 6 courses (including the induction course)
    - □ each course administered ~q3–6wks
    - □ weekdays-only schedule commonly used

PHARMACOKINETICS

- Primarily biliary excretion
- ~10% of daily dose recovered in urine
- Partially dialyzable
- Plasma-half life ~12 hrs
- Extensive distribution into red blood cells, which is freely exchangeable with plasma
- Binds in skin, hair, and nails

TOXICITY

- Fatigue (most common)
- Lightheadedness
  - related to infusion rate; ameliorated by slowing infusion
- Facial flushing
- Skin rash, particularly over torso
- Headache
- Cardiac
  - nonspecific ST-T wave changes on EKG
- Musculoskeletal pain
- "Retinoic acid syndrome" (in patients with acute promyelocytic leukemia only)
- Leukocytosis (~30% of leukemia patients)
- Hyperglycemia (mild, transient)
- Nausea: uncommon

RECOMMENDATIONS FOR SUPPORTIVE CARE

- Observations related to induction therapy for leukemia
  - retinoic acid syndrome
  - exacerbation of disseminated intravascular coagulopathy

PHARMACY ISSUES

- Supplied in 10 ml ampules (1 mg/ml)
- 5% dextrose is preferred diluent
- Dilutions from 100–500 ml have been used

NURSING CONSIDERATIONS

- Administer at prescribed rate using an infusion pump
- Decrease rate if patient becomes symptomatic (lightheaded)
- Monitor CBC, WBC, and platelets
- Diabetic patients may have a rise in blood glucose
- Assess
  - for clinical manifestations of leukocytosis: increase in WBC by 50% or more, vital signs, altered mental status; leukocytosis may also be associated with retinoic acid syndrome
  - for distinctive clinical characteristics of "retinoic acid syndrome": fever, respiratory distress, dyspnea, weight gain, pleural or pericardial effusion, episodic hypotension; administration of high-dose corticosteroids provides immediate response; patient may require hemodynamic and respiratory support
  - potential for ST wave changes: assess baseline cardiac status and at intervals during therapy with EKG
  - alterations in skin integrity: record description of rash and symptoms; antihistamines and corticosteroids can be administered
  - for musculoskeletal pain: implement interventions for pain control with analgesics
- Teach patient
  - stress adequate rest periods, moderate exercise, good nutritional intake
  - avoid foods that may disrupt sleep (alcohol, caffeine)
  - diabetic patients should be made aware to report a rise of their blood glucose
  - palliative measures to care for rash, control itching, protect against secondary skin infections; avoid sun exposure and hot baths; use mild soaps and warm water

KEY REFERENCES

Shen Z-X, et al.: Use of arsenic trioxide (As_2O_3) in the treatment of acute promyelocytic leukemia (APL): II. Clinical efficacy and pharmacokinetics in patients at relapse. Blood 1997; 89:3354–60

Soignet SL, Maslak P, Wang ZG, et al.: Complete remission after induction of non-terminal differentiation and apoptosis in acute promyelocytic leukemia by arsenic trioxide. N Engl J Med 1998; 339:1341–8

Drug: Pegasparaginase

Richard A. Larson and Ellen Jessop

OTHER NAMES: PEG-ASP, PEG-L-ASPARAGINASE, ONCASPAR

USES

- Used in combination with other agents to treat acute lymphoblastic leukemia

MECHANISM OF ACTION

- Polyethylene glycol (PEG) modified version of L-asparaginase *(E. coli)*
- Antitumor effect is due to depletion of exogenous L-asparagine and the failure of tumor cells to generate endogenous asparagine via increased asparagine synthetase activity
- Catalyzes the hydrolysis of asparagine (a nonessential amino acid) in the plasma and extracellular fluid to aspartic acid and ammonia
- Because malignant lymphocytes may have only low concentrations of L-asparagine synthetase, these tumor cells are dependent on obtaining asparagine from the circulation
- Interrupts asparagine-dependent protein synthesis
- Most active in the G1 phase

DOSING

- IM administration is preferred over IV
- Anaphylaxis and other complications may be less common with the IM or SC route rather than IV
- Limit injection volume to 2 ml at a single site
- Adults: 2,500 IU/m^2 IM or IV q14d
- Children with body surface area <0.6 m^2: 82.5 IU/kg IM or IV q14d
- Patients manifesting hypersensitivity to the *E. coli*–derived L-asp should be switched to the Erwinia-derived formulation and dosed appropriately

PHARMACOKINETICS

- Half-life of $\sim$5.7 days
- Plasma clearance is greatly accelerated in the presence of hypersensitivity, and enzyme activity may be undetectable within 4 hrs
- The enzyme distributes in the intravascular space, but asparagine levels also fall rapidly in the extracellular fluid and in CSF by an indirect effect

TOXICITY

- Hypersensitivity reactions to foreign protein can be severe but are uncommon (10%)
- Allergic manifestations (fever, erythematous rash, hives, bronchospasm) can be prolonged because of the long half-life
- Laryngeal edema, bronchospasm, hypotension
- Immediate reactions are mild nausea, malaise, fever, and chills in $\sim$5–10%
- Cutaneous reactions: erythema, urticaria, wheal and flare, hives, induration
- Decreased protein synthesis of albumin (edema), insulin (hyperglycemia), fibrinogen (bleeding), clotting factors V, VII, VIII, IX, antithrombin III, and protein C (thromboses)
- Cerebral dysfunction with disorientation, stupor, coma, and seizures due to low concentrations of L-asparagine or L-glutamine in the brain
- Liver dysfunction is very common due to reversible fatty metamorphosis (elevated bilirubin, AST, and alkaline phosphatase), but pancreatitis is not (15%)
- Thrombosis of large veins (IVC, cavernous sinus)
- Azotemia and acute renal failure are uncommon
- Minimal toxicity to the bone marrow or GI tract

RECOMMENDATIONS FOR SUPPORTIVE CARE

- Medications to treat anaphylaxis should be available (epinephrine, diphenhydramine, hydrocortisone)
- Monitor blood pressure q15min for 1 hr after initial dose
- Patients who manifest hypersensitivity reactions to L-asp derived from *E. coli* can be safely treated with the enzyme derived from Erwinia chrysanthemi, née carotovora (obtained from the NCI's Group C Program)
- Monitor serum amylase or lipase
- Discontinue therapy if pancreatitis occurs
- Monitor fibrinogen
- Transfuse cryoprecipate to keep fibrinogen level >100 mg/dl to reduce risk of bleeding

PHARMACY ISSUES

- Each vial of PEG-asp contains 3,750 IU in 5 ml (preservative free) for SubQ or IM use
- Store single-use vials at 2–8°C
- Stable for 48 hrs at room temperature
- Pegasparaginase terminates methotrexate action by inhibition of protein synthesis and prevention of cell entry into S phase

NURSING CONSIDERATIONS

- Hypersensitivity reactions are common and more likely to occur with IV administration versus IM or SubQ; reactions range from urticaria to true anaphylaxis; more likely to occur after several doses but can occur after first dose
- Tests doses are sometimes given prior to initiation of treatment but are not considered definitively predictive of probability of a reaction
- Drug prolongs PT, PTT, and decreases fibrinogen; monitor PT, PTT, and fibrinogen
- Monitor liver functions for increases in SGOT, Alk Phos, and decreases in albumin
- Assess
  - for signs of hypersensitivity during treatment; monitor vital signs q15min and for 1 hr after administration; emergency equipment and medications should be accessible
  - alterations in nutrition as a result of nausea and vomiting, diarrhea, and abdominal pain
  - for changes in mental status: headache, dizziness, and confusion
- Teach patient
  - potential for reaction and to report untoward signs and symptoms while receiving drug
  - expected side effects and self-care measures

KEY REFERENCE

Asselin BL, Whitin JC, Coppola DJ, Rupp IP, Sallan SE, Cohen HJ: Comparative pharmacokinetic studies of three asparaginase preparations. J Clin Oncol 1993; 11:1780–6.

Chapter 6

CYTOKINES

Introduction

Sanjiv S. Agarwala and John M. Kirkwood

DEFINITION

- Cytokines are biologic agents that in oncology are used to elicit tumor regression. Also known as biologic response modifiers, they often act by modifying the relationship between tumor and host with the goal of achieving therapeutic benefit

PROPERTIES

- Proteins of low molecular weight
- Polypeptide structure, often glycosylated
- Paracrine and autocrine function under normal circumstances (act on nearby cells)
- Interact with well-defined high-affinity receptors to alter protein synthesis
- Pleiotropic in their function with overlapping properties and intercytokine interaction

THERAPEUTIC USE

- Large quantities now available for use through recombinant DNA technology
- Used to manipulate the immune system for tumor response
- Doses vary from low dose given SubQ to high doses given IV
- Scheduling is important, especially in combination with cytotoxic agents
- Used mainly in melanoma and renal cell carcinoma

TOXICITIES

- Different from that of traditional cytotoxic agents
- Fever, chills, anorexia, flulike illness (IFN-alfa)
- Fluid retention, weight gain (IL-2)
- Leukopenia, thrombocytopenia not related to bone marrow suppression
- Toxicities resolve very quickly upon dose discontinuation

AGENTS

- Interferons (alfa, beta, gamma)
- Interleukin-2
- Other interleukins (IL-4, IL-12)
- Monoclonal antibodies
- Tumor necrosis factor

KEY REFERENCES

Rosenberg SA, Yang JC, Schwartzentruber DJ, Hwu P, Marincola FM, Topalian SL, Seipp CA, Einhorn JH, White DE, Steinberg SM: Prospective randomized trial of the treatment of patients with metastatic melanoma using chemotherapy with cisplatin, dacarbazine, and tamoxifen alone or in combination with interleukin-2 and interferon alfa-2b. J Clin Oncol 1999; 17(3):968–75

Stahl M, Wilke JH, Seeber S, Schmoll HJ: Cytokines and cytotoxic agents in renal cell carcinoma: a review. Semin Oncol 1992; 19(2 suppl 4):70–9

Drug: Interferon Alfa

Sanjiv S. Agarwala, John M. Kirkwood, and Patricia A. Sorokin

OTHER NAMES: INTRON-A (INTERFERON ALFA-2B), ROFERON (INTERFERON ALFA-2A)

USES

- Approved by FDA for the following
  - hairy cell leukemia
  - adjuvant therapy of high-risk cutaneous melanoma (resected AJCC stage IIB and III disease within 56 days of surgery)
  - follicular lymphoma
  - AIDS-related Kaposi's sarcoma
- Clinical pharmacology
  - the interferons are a family of naturally occurring proteins with antiviral activity that are secreted by cells in response to a variety of stimuli
  - binds to type I receptor
    - □ recruitment of Tyk2 and Jak1 kinases
    - □ activates Stats 1 and 2 which leads to formation of ISGF-3
    - □ ISGF-3 binds to ISRE affecting gene transcription

MECHANISM OF ACTION

- Postulated mechanisms of IFN action
  - direct antiproliferative and antitumor effects
  - immunomodulatory effects on NK cell, T-cell, macrophage/monocyte/dendritic cells
  - antiangiogenic effects

DOSING

- Can be administered by different routes including IM, SubQ, and IV
- 2 MU/m^2 SubQ tiw (hairy cell leukemia)
- 20 MU/m^2 IV every day × 5 (for 4 wks), then 10 MU/m^2 SubQ tiw × 48 wks (for melanoma)
- 5 MU SubQ tiw (with chemotherapy for follicular lymphoma)
- 8 MU SubQ every day (with antiretroviral therapy for Kaposi's sarcoma)

PHARMACOKINETICS

- Studied following administration of 5 U/m^2 in healthy male volunteers
- Following IM and SubQ administration, peak serum concentrations 3–12 hrs; elimination half-life of 2–3 hrs, serum levels undetectable in 16 hrs
- Following IV administration
- No urinary excretion (kidney primary site of metabolism)
- Serum neutralizing antibodies detected in 0–4% of patients; clinical significance unknown

TOXICITY

- Depends on dose and route of administration
- Differs for acute/early and chronic/late therapy
- Flulike illness (fever, myalgia, headache) almost universal at high doses used for melanoma (grade 3 or 4); requires dose reduction in ~ one-third of patients; also seen with low doses, and attenuates with repetitive daily or alternate-daily dosing (tachyphylaxis)
- Hematologic: (neutropenia in 25%) and less often, anemia or thrombocytopenia may require dose reduction
- Hepatic: elevated SGOT/SGPT in majority of patients at high doses; occasionally elevation of bilirubin and LDH. Elevation in triglycerides and cholesterol can occur associated with inhibition of lipoprotein lipase, but incidence and clinical significance are not well defined
- Neurotoxicity: depression common at high doses; impaired concentration, amnesia, confusion, somnolence, anxiety, nervousness, decreased libido
- Local reactions: burning, pain at injection site, inflammation, itching
- Gastrointestinal: diarrhea, anorexia, nausea, and dysgeusia in majority of patients at high doses
- Dermatologic: alopecia, skin rashes common
- Cardiovascular: angina, arrhythmias in < 5%
- Respiratory: dyspnea occasionally
- Reproductive: amenorrhea occasionally, dysmenorrhea, impotence, menorrhagia

RECOMMENDATIONS FOR SUPPORTIVE CARE

- Routine use of acetaminophen is recommended
- NSAIDs are avoided, if possible
- Liberal fluid intake
- Regular moderate aerobic exercise
- Use of antidepressants if symptoms of depression
- Use of mild antiemetics as needed

NURSING CONSIDERATIONS

- 40–60% of patients experience flulike symptoms; discuss with physician premedication and regular dosing with antipyretic
- Fatigue and malaise are cumulative and dose limiting
- Monitor CBC, WBC, differential, and platelet count, BUN, creatinine, and LFTs prior to drug initiation and periodically thereafter
- Assess
  - for hepatic dysfunction and renal impairment
  - alterations in comfort; fatigue, malaise, headache and myalgias; monitor vital signs
  - signs and symptoms of infection and bleeding related to neutropenia and thrombocytopenia
  - alterations in nutritional status related to nausea, diarrhea, and anorexia
  - sensory and perceptual alterations related to CNS effects (e.g., confusion, lack of concentration, which may interfere with self-administration of drug)
- Teach patient
  - expected side effects and self-care measures to minimize infection and bleeding
  - avoidance of aspirin-containing OTC medications
  - self-administration techniques

KEY REFERENCES

Kirkwood JM, Strawderman MH, Ernstoff MS, et al.: Interferon alfa-2b adjuvant therapy of high-risk resected cutaneous melanoma: the Eastern Cooperative Oncology Group Trial EST 1684. J Clin Oncol 1996; 14(1):7–17

Shepherd FA, Beaulieu R, Gelmon K, et al.: Prospective randomized trial of two dose levels of interferon alfa with zidovudine for the treatment of Kaposi's sarcoma associated with human immunodeficiency virus infection: a Canadian HIV Clinical Trials Network study. J Clin Oncol 1998; 16(5):1736–42

Solal-Celigny P, Lepage E, Brousse N, et al.: Doxorubicin-containing regimen with or without interferon alfa-2b for advanced follicular lymphomas: final analysis of survival and toxicity in the Group d'Etude des Lymphomes Folliculaires 86 Trial. J Clin Oncol 1998; 16(7):2332–8

Spielberger RT, Mick R, Ratain MJ, et al.: Interferon treatment for hairy cell leukemia. An update on a cohort of 69 patients treated from 1983 to 1986. Leuk Lymphoma 1994; 14(suppl 1):89–93

Wilkes GM, Ingwersen K, Burke MB: 1997–98 oncology nursing hand book. Boston: Jones and Bartlett.

Drug: Aldesleukin

Robert A. Figlin and Nancy P. Moldawer

OTHER NAMES: RECOMBINANT HUMAN INTERLEUKIN-2, IL-2, PROLEUKIN

USES

- FDA approval for metastatic renal cell carcinoma (RCCa) and metastatic melanoma
- Activity also demonstrated in leukemia and lymphoma

MECHANISM OF ACTION

- Supports growth and maturation of subpopulations of T-cells
- Stimulates activity of natural killer (NK) and cytotoxic T-cells
- Induces production of other lymphokines (gamma-interferon, TNF, IL-4, IL-6)
- Stimulates B-cell differentiation

DOSING

- 600,000 IU/kg or 720,000 IU/kg via intermittent IV bolus infusion
  - q8hrs for 5 consecutive days to a maximum of 14 doses
  - a second 5 day treatment course is given after a 10 day rest period
- Commonly used combinations
  - Figlin
    - □ rIL-2
      - ▽ 5 MIU/m^2/d × 96-h CIV q wk × 4 wks
    - □ IFN-α2b
      - ▽ 6 MIU/m^2 SubQ days 1 and 4 of each tx wk × 4
      - ▽ 4 wks of tx + 2 wks of rest = 1 treatment cycle
  - Atzpodien
    - □ rIL-2
      - ▽ 20 MIU/m^2 SubQ tiw, wks 1 and 4
      - ▽ 5 MIU/m^2 SubQ tiw, wks 2 and 3
    - □ IFN-α2b
      - ▽ 6 MIU/m^2 SubQ once per week, wk 1 and 4; tiw wks 2 and 3
      - ▽ 9 MIU/m^2, tiw, wks 5–8
    - □ 5-FU
      - ▽ 750 mg/m^2 IV bolus once per week, wks 5–8
  - Sleijfer
    - □ rIL-2
      - ▽ 18 MIU SubQ d × 5 days, wk 1
      - ▽ 9 MIU SubQ days 1 and 2 and
      - ▽ 18 MIU, days 3–5, wks 2–6
  - Legha
    - □ Interferon α2a
      - ▽ 5 × 10^6 IU/m^2/d × 5 days SubQ
    - □ Interleukin-2
      - ▽ 9 × 10^6 IU/m^2/d × 4 days CIV
    - □ Cisplatin
      - ▽ 20 mg/m^2/d × 4 days
    - □ Vinblastine
      - ▽ 1.6 mg/m^2/d × 5 days
    - □ DTIC
      - ▽ 800 mg/m^2/d × 1 day

PHARMACOKINETICS

- The kidney is the major clearance route with no biologically active IL-2 appearing in the urine

TOXICITY

- Constitutional
  - fever, chills, rigors, myalgias, arthralgias, malaise, and fatigue
- Gastrointestinal
  - nausea, vomiting, diarrhea, pancreatitis (rare), increase in gastric acid secretion, taste changes, stomatitis, anorexia, elevations of bilirubin, alkaline phosphatase, SGOT and SGPT
  - bowel hemorrhage, infarction and perforation (rare)
- Neurologic
  - somnolence, paresthesias, hallucinations, psychosis, agitation, depression, difficulty concentrating, combativeness, confusion, memory problems
- Hematologic
  - anemia, leukopenia, eosinophilia, thrombocytopenia, transient lymphopenia, rebound lymphocytosis, occasional transient granulocytopenia
- Dermatologic
  - erythematous rash, pruritus, dry desquamation, burning, redness, pain and induration at SubQ injection site, hair thinning
- Capillary leak syndrome
  - increase in vascular permeability causing intravascular fluids into the interstitium of many organs, causing hypotension, tachycardia, weight gain, oliguria with increased BUN and serum creatinine
- Pulmonary
  - shortness of breath, respiratory distress, pulmonary edema
- Cardiac
  - arrhythmias, primarily sinus or supraventricular, tachycardia, hypertension, depressed cardiac contractility
- Nephrotoxicity
  - azotemia, oliguria
- Endocrinologic
  - hypothroidism, hyperthyroidism
- IV contrast reaction
  - nausea, vomiting, diarrhea, fever, chills following the administration of IV contrast material
- Infection
  - bacterial infection secondary to staphylococcus aureus and staphylococcus epidermidis
  - risk factors are intravascular catheters, dermatologic toxicity, potentially contaminated cells (if adoptive immunotherapy [i.e., TIL] is administered)

PHARMACY ISSUES

- Reconstitute with sterile water; avoid shaking vial
- Bring to room temperature prior to infusion
- Administer proleukin within 48 hrs of reconstitution
- Do not mix proleukin for injection with other drugs

NURSING CONSIDERATIONS

- General
  - symptoms are dose, schedule, and route related. The higher the IL-2 dose, the more severe the side effects. *Do not* administer steroids including topical creams during IL-2 therapy
- Constitutional
  - fever, chills, and rigor occur 2–8 hrs after the first dose. Premedicate with acetaminophen 650 mg and continue q4hrs to reduce symptoms. NSAIDs are also used to control fevers. Rigors can be controlled with meperidine. Monitor fever patterns. Patients with continuing uncontrolled fever should be evaluated for potential infection
- Gastrointestinal
  - premedicate with antiemetics or antidiarrheal medications when symptoms occur, and continue during IL-2 treatment. Assess nutritional status. Encourage small, nonspicy meals. Recommend high-calorie dietary supplements. Assess oral cavity daily for color changes, dryness, discomfort, lesions. Administer drugs to control gastric secretions (ranitidine, cimetidine). Evaluate hydration; monitor I/O
- Central nervous system
  - obtain baseline neurologic assessment. Teach patient/caregiver reportable signs and symptoms. Assess neurologic status regularly; report changes to physician. Consider holding IL-2 dosages. Avoid medications that may potentiate CNS toxicity. Reorient patient as needed; assess concurrent meds (narcotics, antihistamines, analgesics)
- Hematologic
  - monitor blood studies: CBC, differential, platelet, and coagulation profile. Assess for signs of bleeding and/or infection. Teach patient/family measures to conserve energy
- Integument
  - assess skin daily. Patients with peripheral or central line access for IL-2 are prone to local infection, phlebitis, or sepsis. Symptoms can occur with rapid onset and are not related to degree of leukopenia. Use mild soaps. Apply water-based moisturizer bid; best applied to damp skin. Medicate with antipruritics and antihistamines: may require

around-the clock administration. Provide room humidifier; avoid hot baths. Provide bath oils, colloidal oatmeal baths

- Pulmonary
  - assess pulmonary status for shortness of breath, cough, increased respirator rate: auscultation for rales and decreased breath sounds, provide oxygen per MD order. Position patient for maximum respiratory effort. Monitor arterial blood gases. Assess oxygen saturation
- Cardiovascular
  - monitor pulse and blood pressure at each MD visit. Perform orthostatic blood pressure measurements, as clinically indicated. Administer IV fluids such as normal saline as needed. Vasopressor therapy may be required to maintain blood pressure and urine output. Assess for edema and abdominal girth daily. Report arrhythmias and chest pain. Instruct patient to rise from lying to sitting position slowly to avoid dizziness
- Renal
  - record intake and output. Weigh daily. Increase oral fluid intake. Report to physician changes in BUN and creatinine levels, significant weight gains, decreased urine output
- Hepatic
  - monitor lab work and report abnormalities
- Miscellaneous
  - monitor thyroid function while on IL-2 therapy

KEY REFERENCES

Atzpodien J, Kirchner H, Hanninen EL, et al.: Interleukin-2 in combination with interferon-alpha and 5-fluorouracil for metastatic renal cell cancer. Eur J Cancer 1993; 29A(suppl 5):S6–8

Figlin RA, Belldegrun A, Moldawer N, et al.: Concomitant administration of recombinant human interleukin-2 and recombinant interferon alfa-2A: an active outpatient regimen in metastatic renal cell carcinoma. J Clin Oncol 1992; 10(3):414–21

Heake Yarbro C, ed.: Management of patients receiving interleukin-2 therapy. Sem Oncol Nursing 1993; 9(3 suppl 1)

Legha SS, Ring S, Bedikian A, et al. Treatment of metastatic melanoma with combined chemotherapy containing cisplatin, vinblastine and dacarbaine (CVD) and biotherapy using interleukin-2 and interferon-alpha. Ann Oncol 1996; 7:827–35

Siegel JP, Puri RK: Interleukin-2 toxicity. J Clin Oncol 1991; 9(4):694–704

Sleijfer DT, Janssen RA, Buter J, et al. Phase II study of subcutaneous interleukin-2 in unselected patients with advanced renal cell cancer on an outpatient basis. J Clin Oncol 1992: 1119–23

Chapter 7

MONOCLONAL ANTIBODIES AND FUSION PROTEINS

Introduction

David G. Maloney

USES

■ Lymphomas, breast cancer, colon cancer, leukemias, others
■ Application depends on the antigen/receptor expression by tumor
■ May be synergistic or additive with chemotherapy

BIOCHEMICAL PHARMACOLOGY

■ Recognition of the antigen/receptor determines specificity of the therapy
■ Tumor expression of the target antigen/receptor determines possible use
■ Expression of target antigen/receptor by normal tissues causes potential toxicity
■ Unmodified antibodies
- serum half-life dependent on species
- immunogenicity depends on the species used (mouse > chimeric > humanized > human)
- effects depend on
  - □ interaction with human antibody-dependent cell-mediated cytotoxicity (ADCC) effector cells
  - □ interaction with human complement system
  - □ interaction with or interference with the target antigen on the tumor cell and growth inhibition or the induction of apoptosis
  - □ may increase sensitivity of tumor cells to cytotoxic chemotherapy

■ Conjugated (drug, toxins, radionucleotides) antibodies
- all have dose-limiting toxicity usually due to molecule conjugated to the mAb
- toxicity partially dependent on the expression of the antigen on normal cells
- nonspecific toxicity due to clearance of conjugated mAb and to circulation in nontumor tissues
- shorter half-life
- increased immunogenicity usually due to the conjugate
- effects depend on targeting the specific drug/toxin/radionucleotide to the tumor tissues
- less on immune (ADCC, CDC) or direct mechanisms

■ Fusion proteins
- activity dependent on the receptor targeted and on the expression of that receptor by the tumor
- all have dose-limiting toxicity
- toxicity partially dependent on the expression of the receptor on normal cells
- nonspecific toxicity due to clearance of the drug/toxin in nontumor tissues

MECHANISMS OF RESISTANCE

■ Escape of antigen/receptor negative tumors
■ Secretion of blocking antigen/receptor
■ Inefficient interaction with the human immune system effector mechanisms
■ Immunogenicity

TOXICITY

■ Due to antigen/receptor recognized
■ Due to expression of target antigen on normal tissue
■ Due to nonspecific toxicity of the targeted toxin/drug/radionucleotide on normal tissues
■ Unconjugated mAbs
- specific elimination of targeted cells (B-cell depletion for anti-CD20)
- T-cell depletion for CAMPATH mAbs
- fever, chills, rigors, hypotension

■ Radiolabeled mAbs
- myelotoxicity is dose limiting
- high dose requires stem cell transplant

REFERENCES

Bagshawe KD, Sharma SK, Springer CJ, et al.: Antibody directed enzyme prodrug therapy (ADEPT). A review of some theoretical, experimental and clinical aspects. Ann Oncol 1994; 5(10):879–91

Engert A, Sausville EA, Vitetta E: The emerging role of ricin A-chain immunotoxins in leukemia and lymphoma. Current Topics Microbiol & Immunol 1998; 234:13–33

Pietersz GA, Krauer K, McKenzie IF: The use of monoclonal antibody immunoconjugates in cancer therapy. Adv Exp Med Biol 1994; 353:169–79

Press OW: Prospects for the management of non-Hodgkin's lymphomas with monoclonal antibodies and immunoconjugates. Cancer from Scientific American 1998; 4(Suppl 2):S19–26

Saleh MN et al.: Antitumor activity of DAB389IL-2 fusion toxin in mycosis fungoides. J Am Acad Dermatol 1998; 39(1): 63–73

Sznol M, Holmlund J: Antigen-specific agents in development. Semin Oncol 1997; 24(2): 173–86

Drug: Rituximab

David G. Maloney and Janine Caggiano

OTHER NAMES: RITUXAN, IDEC-C2B8, MABTHERA

USES

- Approved by FDA for single-agent treatment of recurrent low-grade or follicular B-cell non-Hodgkin's lymphoma
- Active in other CD20 positive B-cell lymphomas: mantle cell, large cell, Waldenstrom's

MECHANISM OF ACTION

- The antibody is a mouse/human IgG1 kappa chimeric
- Lysis by antibody-dependent cell-mediated cytotoxicity
- Lysis by complement-dependent cytotoxicity
- Directly induces apoptosis in some cell lines in vitro
- May sensitize some resistant cell lines to chemotherapy

DOSING

- Administered IV by a slow infusion over 3–10 hrs as tolerated
  - start infusion at 50 mg/hr for 30 min
  - if no toxicity escalate rate by 50 mg/hr each 30 min to a maximum of 400 mg/hr
  - temporarily stop infusion for hypersensitivity or infusion-related events
  - if no toxicity, subsequent infusions can be started at 100 mg/hr and escalated by 100 mg/hr each 30 min to a maximum of 400 mg/hr
- Schedule/doses
  - 375 mg/m^2 per dose
  - weekly × 4 is the recommended dose
- Commonly used combinations
  - combinations with or following chemotherapy with CHOP

PHARMACOKINETICS

- Long terminal half-life usually exceeds 48 hrs
  - increases with subsequent dosing

TOXICITY

- Hypersensitivity and infusion-related toxicity
- Fever, chills, asthenia, or headache (50%)
- Hypotension, bronchospasm, or angioedema (10%)
- Rarely serious or life-threatening cardiac arrhythmias
- Tumor lysis syndrome
  - may occur 12–24 hrs after dosing with high levels of circulating malignant lymphocytes
  - may be serious or fatal and associated with hypotension and pulmonary toxicity
- Prolonged B-cell depletion in the peripheral blood for 6–9 mos
- Mild decreases in serum IgG and IgM levels
- No obvious increase in infections, but patients should be closely monitored
- Rare neutropenia, thrombocytopenia, or anemia

RECOMMENDATIONS FOR SUPPORTIVE CARE

- Premedication with acetaminophen and diphenhydramine and re-treatment as indicated by symptoms
- Close monitoring of vital signs during the infusion
- Epinephrine, antihistamines, and corticosteroids should be immediately available
- The infusion should be slowed or stopped until symptoms decrease
- Patients should be monitored until symptoms resolve

PHARMACY ISSUES

- Supplied as 10 mg/ml in 100 mg (10 ml) or 500 mg (50 ml) vials
- Dilute in 0.9% sodium chloride USP or D_5W USP to 1–4 mg/ml
- Stable for 24 hrs at 2–8° C. Stable an additional 12 hrs at room temperature

NURSING CONSIDERATIONS

- Nonvesicant
- Infusion reactions are related to infusion rate and are more common during the initial infusion and decrease with subsequent treatments; begin infusion slowly then increase in absence of toxicity
- Acetaminophen and diphenhydramine premedication
- Consider holding AM antihypertensive medications
- Administer premedication with Tylenol and Benadryl
- Have emergency equipment and medications accessible
- Assess
  - vital signs during administration
  - for infusional related side effects including shaking chills, hypotension, fever, respiratory symptoms, throat irritation, flushing and pain at disease site; infusion may need to be interrupted to allow symptoms to subside
  - monitor patients carefully during and after administration for toxicity
- Teach patient
  - to report untoward symptoms while receiving infusion
  - to monitor temperature
  - self-care measures

KEY REFERENCES

Coiffier B, Haioun C, Ketterer N, et al.: Rituximab (anti-CD20 monoclonal antibody) for the treatment of patients with relapsing or refractory aggressive lymphoma: a multicenter phase II study. Blood 1998; 92(6):1927–32

Czuczman MS, Grillo-Lopez AJ, White CA, et al.: Treatment of patients with low-grade B-cell lymphoma with the combination of chimeric anti-CD20 monoclonal antibody and CHOP chemotherapy. J Clin Oncol 1999; 17(1):268–76

Maloney DG, Grillo-Lopez AJ, White CA, et al.: IDEC-C2B8 (Rituximab) anti-CD20 monoclonal antibody therapy in patients with relapsed low-grade non-Hodgkin's lymphoma. Blood 1997; 90(6):2188–95

McLaughlin P, et al.: Rituximab chimeric anti-CD20 monoclonal antibody therapy for relapsed indolent lymphoma: half of patients respond to a four-dose treatment program. J Clin Oncol 1998; 16(8):2825–33

Drug: Tastuzumab

Jose Baselga and Patricia A. Sorokin

OTHER NAMES: HERCEPTIN, ANTI-P185HER2

USES

- Approved by FDA for metastatic breast cancer with HER2 protein overexpression

MECHANISM OF ACTION

- Humanized monoclonal antibody that binds with high affinity to the HER2 receptor
- Inhibits the growth of HER2 overexpressing tumor cells
- Decreases the levels of receptor expression
- Induces antibody-dependent cellular cytotoxicity (ADCC)

DOSING

- Administered IV as a 60 min infusion
- Schedules/doses
  - 4 mg/kg loading dose IV over 60 min, then 2 mg/kg weekly over 30 min
  - approved combinations
    - □ 4 mg/kg loading dose, then 2 mg/kg every week with paclitaxel 175 mg/m^2 q3wks

PHARMACOKINETICS

- Half-life is ~9 days
- Antibodies very rarely detected in patients being treated for a prolonged period of time
- Saturable immunoglobulin clearance mechanism
- Patients with high levels of serum-shed antigen may have a higher clearance

TOXICITY

- Infusion-associated symptoms, primarily with first dose
  - chills (>20%), fever (>20%), asthenia, pain, nausea, vomiting, headache
- Overall adverse events (generally mild to moderate in severity) ≥15% of patients: pain, asthenia, fever, chills, nausea, vomiting, headache, diarrhea, insomnia, catheter infections, rhinitis, dyspnea, rash
- Cardiac
  - clinical congestive heart failure or asymptomatic decrease of left ventricular ejection fraction seen in 5% of patients treated as a single agent
  - all patients had been previously treated with anthracycline or had a prior cardiac history
  - symptoms improve with standard therapy and in most cases therapy can be continued
  - cardiac toxicity does not increase when combined with paclitaxel
  - cardiac toxicity increases when combined with anthracycline
  - in the pivotal phase III study, congestive heart failure occurred in 18% of patients

RECOMMENDATIONS FOR SUPPORTIVE CARE

- During the first infusion chills and/or fever is commonly observed. Symptoms are usually mild to moderate in severity and respond to treatment with acetaminophen, diphnehydramine, and/or meperideine, without a reduction in the rate of the infusion

PHARMACY ISSUES

- The recommended diluent for the reconstituted solution is 0.9% sodium chloride injection, USP

NURSING CONSIDERATIONS

- Increased risk of cardiac dysfunction especially in patients having received previous anthracycline therapy; usually respond to medical therapy
- Fever and chills usually occur after first dose and occur less frequently thereafter
- Patients note pain at tumor sites usually within 8 hrs of therapy
- Mild increases in liver enzymes; monitor baseline LFTs and periodically thereafter
- Potential for renal insufficiency—baseline renal function and periodically
- Assess
  - skin integrity: erythema and pruritis
  - baseline neurologic status and monitor for signs of asthenia
  - alterations in nutritional status related to nausea, vomiting, and diarrhea, which can be mild to severe
- Teach patient
  - expected side effects and self-care measures
  - alterations in cardiac output (e.g., cardiomyopathy, CHF, hypotension)
  - to report alterations in their ability to concentrate, and sleep

KEY REFERENCE

Baselga J, Tripathy D, Mendelsohn J, Baughman S, Benz CC, Dantis L, Sklarin NT, Seidman AD, Hudis CA, Moore J, Rosen PP, Twaddell T, Henderson IC, Norton L: Phase II study of recombinant human anti-HER2 monoclonal antibody in stage IV breast cancer. J Clin Oncol 1996; 14:737–44

Drug: Denileukin diftitox

Timothy M. Kuzel and Ellen Samuelson

OTHER NAMES: ONTAK, DAB_{389}IL-2

USES

- FDA approved for treatment of relapsed or persistent mycosis fungoides after one previous treatment (overall response rate 30–35%)

MECHANISM OF ACTION

- Recombinant fusion protein
- Molecule consists of nucleotide sequences for the enzymatically active and membrane translocation domains of diphtheria toxin and human interleukin-2 (IL-2)
- Binds IL-2 receptor and is internalized by intermediate and high-affinity forms
- Inhibits protein synthesis by enzymatically inactivating elongation factor 2
- No known mechanism of resistance
- Unclear if detection of expression of components of IL-2 receptor by current techniques is adequately sensitive to use routinely as a screen prior to treatment with this agent

DOSING

- Administered IV as a 15–30 min infusion
- No oral formulation
- Schedules/doses
  - 9 mcg/kg/d daily for 5 days q21d (appropriate for frail patients or patients with early-stage mycosis fungoides [≤ stage IIa])
  - 18 mcg/kg/d daily for 5 days q21d (for good performance status patient or advanced stage mycosis fungoides [> stage IIa])
  - no combinations studied to date

PHARMACOKINETICS

- Metabolism to active intermediates is unclear (not definitively studied to date)
- Terminal half-life ~75 min
- No accumulation between first and fifth dose
- Peak serum concentrations (both 9 or 18 dose level) are at least 10-fold greater than required in vitro for cell cytotoxicity
- Antibody formation
  - most patients treated in clinical trials had received prior vaccination to diphtheria toxin
  - ~40% of patients with lymphoma in clinical trials had levels of anti-DAB_{389}IL-2 antibodies prior to treatment (by ELISA)
  - after 3 cycles of treatment, 97% of patients had developed significant titers of antibody
  - antibody formation is associated with several important phenomena
    - □ clearance is increased two- to threefold
    - □ dose proportionality may be lost after two to three cycles of treatment
    - □ no discernible effect on response: responders and nonresponders had similar rates and titers of antibodies to drug
    - □ tachyphylaxis to side effects (see later)

TOXICITY

- Incidence of grade III/IV events observed in phase III trials
  - fever/chills: 35%
  - fatigue: 30%
  - edema: 27%
  - rash: 21%
  - nausea/vomiting: 20%
  - dyspnea: 18%
  - hypotension: 10%
  - confusion: 9%
  - chest pain: 9%
- Several syndromes of toxicity have been observed (approximate incidences)
  - constitutional symptoms: 90%
  - acute infusion-related events: 70%
  - vascular leak syndrome: 10%
  - cardiovascular effects: 8%
- Administration in an appropriate medical setting by individuals trained in the management of side effects listed here

RECOMMENDATIONS FOR SUPPORTIVE CARE

- An anaphylaxis tray should be available containing epinephrine, diphenhydramine, and a laryngoscope with endotracheal tube
- Careful attention to fluid status is indicated to monitor for the development of the vascular leak syndrome
- Hypotension may occur in this setting, and careful fluid administration is important, with possible pressor use to minimize fluid extravasation into tissues

PHARMACY ISSUES

- Supplied in single-use vials as a sterile, clear liquid for IV administration
- A vial contains 2 ml (300 mcg) in a solution of citric acid, EDTA, polysorbate
- Store at or below −10° C
- Must be brought to room temperature before preparing dose (refrigerator for < 24 hrs or room temperature for 1–2 hrs—no artificial heating)
- Prepare and hold in containers of *soft plastic*
- Do not administer with inline filter

NURSING CONSIDERATIONS

- Nonvesicant; delayed mild reversible induration at injection site with infiltration may be seen
- Observe for immediate constitutional symptoms; antipyretic therapy prn for 24 hrs and for subsequent doses
- Premedicate with acetaminophen plus/minus diphenhydramine based on severity of side effects with the first dose(s)
- Observe for hypersensitivity-type reactions (chest tightness, back pain) with drug administration; may be ameliorated by slowing infusion rate or stopping and restarting infusion at a slower rate
- Monitor vital signs prior to each infusion and before discharge from ambulatory care center
- Monitor serum liver and renal parameters prior to and during each treatment cycle
- Assess
  - general status for fatigue, malaise, other constitutional symptoms
  - fluid status for signs and symptoms of vascular leak syndrome
  - nutritional status secondary to nausea, vomiting, and decreased appetite
  - skin for maculopapular rash
- Teach patient
  - expected side effects and related management strategies
  - report side effects in a timely manner; adherence to required follow-up

KEY REFERENCES

LeMaistre CF, Saleh MN, Kuzel TM: Phase I trial of a ligand fusion-protein (DAB389IL-2) in lymphomas expressing the receptor for interleukin-2. Blood 1998; 91(2):399–405

Saleh MN, LeMaistre CF, Kuzel TM, et al.: Antitumor activity of DAB389IL-2 fusion toxin in mycosis fungoides. J Am Acad Dermatol 1998; 39(1):63–73

Chapter 8

ANTIESTROGENS AND RELATED DRUGS

Introduction

Ruth M. O'Regan and V. Craig Jordan

EFFECTS OF ESTROGEN

- Binds to nuclear estrogen receptor (ER) resulting in dimerization of the receptor and activation of a sequence of DNA called the estrogen response element (ERE) with subsequent transcription of estrogen-regulated genes
- Association of estrogen and breast cancer well documented
  - increased incidence with early menarche, late menopause
  - decreased incidence with early surgical menopause
  - increased incidence with nulliparity, first pregnancy at age over 35
  - increased incidence with long-term birth control pills, hormone replacement therapy
- Unopposed estrogen associated with increased incidence of endometrial cancer
- Maintains bone density
- Decreases low-density lipoprotein (LDL) cholesterol and increases high-density lipoprotein (HDL) cholesterol resulting in decreased incidence of cardiovascular disease

CLASSIFICATION OF ANTIESTROGENS

- Nonsteroidal antiestrogens (tamoxifen, toremifene)
  - bind to nuclear ER in breast cancer cells but do not result in complete activation of ERE or transcription of estrogen-regulated genes
  - have paradoxical estrogenlike effects on certain target tissues
  - maintain bone density resulting in reduced hip fractures
  - decrease LDL cholesterol with no effect on HDL cholesterol
  - result in a two- to threefold increase in endometrial cancer in postmenopausal women
- Aromatase inhibitors (anastrazole, ketozole)
  - majority of circulating estrogen in postmenopausal women formed from conversion of testosterone and androstenedione to estrone and estradiol by the aromatase enzyme complex
  - nonselective aromatase inhibitors reduce circulating estrogen and result in response rates in advanced breast cancer but are associated with considerable toxicity
  - significantly reduce circulating estrogen levels

STEROIDAL ANTIESTROGENS

- Investigational agents in late clinical trials
  - ICI 182,780 (Faslode)
    - □ steroidal pure antiestrogen
    - □ inhibits transcription of estrogen-regulated genes

KEY REFERENCES

Gradishar WJ, Jordan VC: Clinical potential of new antiestrogens. J Clin Oncol 1997; 15:840–52

Jordan VC: Designer estrogens. Scientific American 1998; 279:60–7

Osborne CK: Tamoxifen in the treatment of breast cancer. N Eng J Med 1998; 339: 1609–18

Drug: Tamoxifen

William J. Gradishar and Marianne Huml

OTHER NAMES: NOLVADEX

USES

- Approved by the FDA for adjuvant therapy in axillary node-negative, premenopausal and postmenopausal women with early stage breast cancer; adjuvant therapy in axillary node-positive postmenopausal women; treatment of metastatic breast cancer in men and women with hormone-receptor positive disease

MECHANISMS OF ACTION

- Nonsteroidal triphenylethylene
- Antiestrogen activity exerted by binding to the steroid-binding domain of the estrogen receptor (ER), thereby blocking estradiol action (i.e., transcription)
- Other actions: inhibits protein kinase C and phospholipase C, stimulates phosphoinositite kinase activity, inhibits calmodulin, antioxidant activity, induction apoptosis, stimulation of transforming growth factor-beta (TGF-beta)

DOSING

- Daily dose: 20 mg
- Duration of adjuvant therapy: 5 yrs; in advanced disease: until disease progression

PHARMACOKINETICS

- Extensively metabolized after oral administration
- 65% of the administered dose excreted from the body over a period of 2 wks with fecal excretion as the primary route of elimination
- Drug excreted primarily as glucuronidated conjugates in feces
- Serum level of the main metabolite (which is active), N-desmethyltamoxifen, reaches steady state after 8 wks
- Both tamoxifen and its metabolites are highly protein bound (>95%)

TOXICITY

- Common
  - hot flashes
  - weight gain
  - nausea
  - vaginal discharge
- Less common
  - fluid retention
  - altered menses
  - vomiting
- Late complications
  - thromboembolic events
  - cataracts

RECOMMENDATIONS FOR SUPPORTIVE CARE

- Annual gynecology exam

PHARMACY ISSUES

- Oral formulation: 10, 20 mg tablets

NURSING CONSIDERATIONS

- Although hypercalcemia is uncommon, obtain serum calcium levels prior to therapy and at regular intervals during therapy
- Assess
  - skin integrity for rash
  - sensory and perceptual alterations; retinopathy has been reported with high doses
- Teach patient
  - avoid use of antacids within 2 hrs of taking enteric-coated tablets
  - of possibility of "flare" reaction, which includes bony pain and tumor pain
  - menstrual irregularity, hot flashes, small possibility of milk production in breasts
  - expected signs and symptoms and self-care measures

KEY REFERENCES

Buzdar AU, Hortobagyi GN: Tamoxifen and toremifene in breast cancer: comparison of safety and efficacy. J Clin Oncol 1998; 16:348–53

Jaiyesimi IA, Buzdar AV, Decker DA, Hortobagyi GN: Use of tamoxifen for breast cancer: twenty-eight years later. J Clin Oncol 1995; 13:513–29

Drug: Toremifene

William J. Gradishar and Janine Caggiano

OTHER NAMES: FARESTON

USES

- Approved by the FDA for the treatment of metastatic breast cancer in postmenopausal women with estrogen receptor (ER) positive and ER unknown tumors

MECHANISM OF ACTION

- Nonsteroidal triphenylethylene derivative differs from tamoxifen by the addition of a chlorine atom
- Antiestrogen activity exerted by high-affinity binding to cytoplasmic ER, thereby blocking estradiol action (i.e., transcription)
- Other actions: induces apoptosis, increases production of TGF-beta

DOSING

- Daily dose: 60 mg
- Duration of therapy: in advanced disease until disease progression

PHARMACOKINETICS

- Extensively metabolized, after oral administration, to primary metabolite N-demethyl-torememifene
- Peak plasma concentrations are obtained within 3 hrs
- Extensive binding (<99%) to serum proteins, primarily albumin
- Steady-state concentrations reached in 4–6 wks
- Elimination as metabolites in feces (90%) and urine (10%)
- Elimination half-life: 5 days

TOXICITY

- Common
  - hot flashes
  - nausea
  - vaginal discharge
- Less common
  - fluid retention
  - vomiting
  - dizziness
  - cataracts

RECOMMENDATIONS FOR SUPPORTIVE CARE

- Abnormal vaginal bleeding should be evaluated with a gynecologic examination

PHARMACY ISSUES

- Oral formulation: 60 mg tablets

NURSING CONSIDERATIONS

- Premedicate with antiemetic regimen prior to treatment
- May cause "flare" reaction with bone and tumor pain and transient increase in tumor size
- Monitor calcium and liver functions
- Assess
  - alterations in nutritional status due to epigastric pain, nausea and vomiting, and anorexia
  - for discomfort provide analgesic regimen as needed
- Teach patient
  - to take drug once daily prior to breakfast on an empty stomach
  - potential for sexual dysfunction; vaginal discharge, bleeding, and irregular menses
  - sweating and hot flashes
  - flare phenomenon

KEY REFERENCES

Buzdar AU, Hortobagyi GN: Tamoxifen and toremifene in breast cancer: comparison of safety and efficacy. J Clin Oncol 1998; 16:348–53

Hayes DF, Van Zyl JA, Hacking A, et al.: Randomized comparison of tamoxifen and two separate doses of toremifene in postmenopausal patients with metastatic breast cancer. J Clin Oncol 1995; 13:2556–66

Drug: Anastrozole

Aman U. Buzdar and Marianne Huml

OTHER NAMES: ARIMIDEX, ZD1033

USES

■ Approved by FDA for treatment of metastatic breast cancer in postmenopausal women previously refractory to tamoxifen therapy
■ Approved in most of Europe and a number of South American countries

MECHANISM OF ACTION

■ Potent selective nonsteroidal aromatase inhibitor
■ Inhibits the formation of estrogen and reduces serum estradiol concentration in postmenopausal women

DOSING

■ 1 mg daily po

PHARMACOKINETICS

■ Pharmacokinetics are linear
■ Plasma elimination half-life of 40–50 hrs
■ Drug is metabolized by N-dealkylation, hydroxylation, and glucuronidation

TOXICITY

■ Common
- nausea
- headache
- hot flashes

■ Less common
- weight gain
- slight increase in total cholesterol

DOSING

■ Changes in dose are not recommended for mild to moderate hepatic or renal impairment

PHARMACY ISSUES

■ White, biconvex, film-coated tablets containing 1 mg of anastrozole

NURSING CONSIDERATIONS

■ Well tolerated with low toxicity profile
■ Absolutely contraindicated in pregnancy
■ No dose adjustments required for mild to moderate hepatic impairment
■ Obtain baseline LFTs and periodically thereafter
■ Assess
- liver dysfunction
- sexual dysfunction related to decreased estrogen levels (e.g., hot flashes and vaginal dryness)
- potential alteration in cardiac output; identify patients at risk for thrombophlebitis
- alterations in comfort; headaches usually relieved by nonprescription analgesics

■ Teach patient
- take orally with or without food at same time daily
- expected side effects and self-care measures

KEY REFERENCES

Buzdar AU, Jonat W, Howell A, Jones SE, Blomqvist C, Vogel CL, Eiermann W, Wolter JM, Azab M, Webster A, Plourde PV: Anastrozole, a potent and selective aromatase inhibitor, versus megestrol acetate in postmenopausal women with advanced breast cancer: Results of overview analysis of two phase III trials. J Clin Oncol 1996; 14:2000–11

Buzdar AU, Jones SE, Vogel CL, Wolter J, Plourde P, Webster A: A phase III trial comparing anastrozole (1 and 10 milligrams), a potent and selective aromatase inhibitor, with megestrol acetate in postmenopausal women with advanced breast cancer. Cancer 1997; 79:730–9

Drug: Letrozole

Allan Lipton and Victoria Staszak

OTHER NAMES: FEMURA TABLETS, CGS 20267

USES

- Approved by the FDA for the treatment of advanced breast cancer in postmenopausal women with disease progression following antiestrogen therapy

MECHANISM OF ACTION

- Is a highly specific and potent nonsteroidal aromatase inhibitor
- Competitively binds to the heme of the cytochrome P-450 subunit of the aromatase enzyme
- Reduces estrogen biosynthesis in peripheral tissues
- Results in a decrease in circulating serum levels of estrone, estradiol, and estrone sulfate
- No clinically significant effect on adrenal corticosteroid synthesis, aldosterone synthesis, or synthesis of thyroid hormones

DOSING

- Dosing regimen, 2.5 mg taken orally once daily
- No dosage adjustment required
  - in the elderly
  - renally impaired patients with creatinine clearance ≥10 ml/min
  - mild to moderate hepatic impairment (patients with severe hepatic impairment have not been studied and should be dosed with caution)

DRUG INTERACTIONS

- Clinical interaction studies with cimetidine and warfarin indicate that the coadministration of letrozole with these drugs does not result in clinically significant drug interactions
- No clinical experience to date on the concomitant use of letrozole with other antineoplastic agents

PHARMACOKINETICS

- Rapid and complete absorption from the gastrointestinal tract
- Weakly bound to plasma proteins (~60%)
- The major pathway of letrozole clearance is via metabolism by the liver to an inactive carbinol metabolite
- Direct renal and fecal excretion of letrozole and formation of other metabolites play only a minor role in the overall elimination
- Elimination half-life in plasma is ~2 days
- Time to reach steady state is 2–6 wks

TOXICITY

- Most reported adverse events during clinical trials in all treatment groups were mild to moderate in severity
- Most frequently reported adverse reactions during clinical trials whether drug related or not were musculoskeletal pain, nausea, headache, arthralgia, and fatigue
- Less frequent (<5%) adverse events reported in at least 3 patients treated with letrozole included hypercalcemia, fracture, depression, anxiety, pleural effusion, alopecia, increased sweating, and vertigo

PHARMACY ISSUES

- Store at 25°C (77°F); excursions permitted to 15°–30°C (59°–86°F)
- Available in bottles of 30 tablets
- Shelf life is 2 yrs (expiration dates are on bottles)
- Can be taken without regard to meals

NURSING CONSIDERATIONS

- Suppression of aromatase may have adverse effects as is evident in postmenopausal women: increased osteoporosis, cardiovascular disease, and urogenital atrophy
- Obtain baseline BUN, creatinine, and LFTs; monitor periodically
- Assess
  - alterations in nutritional status related to anorexia, nausea, vomiting, dyspepsia, diarrhea, constipation, renal and hepatic dysfunction
  - alterations in urine elimination (e.g., urinary incontinence should be evaluated by urogynecologist)
  - baseline neurologic status
  - potential for hypertension; assess baseline blood pressure and record measurements during treatment
  - signs and symptoms of an embolic episode (e.g., pulmonary, DVT, cerebral vascular)
- Teach patients:
  - encourage weight-bearing exercise; use of calcium supplementation
  - encourage diets low in fat and high in fiber
  - avoidance of coffee, chocolate, alcohol, and spicy foods
  - urinary incontinence or painful intercourse should be reported
  - self-care measures to conserve energy
  - need for contraception

KEY REFERENCE

Dombernowsky P, et al.: Letrozole, a new oral aromatase inhibitor for advanced breast cancer: double-blind randomized trial showing a dose effect and improved efficacy and tolerability compared with megestrol acetate. J Clin Oncol 1998; 16(2):453–61

Drug: Medroxyprogesterone Acetate

John T. Carpenter, Jr. and Belinda Butler

OTHER NAMES: DEPO-PROVERA, PROVERA

USES

- Approved in the United States for palliative treatment of advanced endometrial and renal cancer, for prevention of pregnancy, and for secondary amenorrhea and abnormal uterine bleeding due to hormonal imbalance in the absence of organic pathology
- Also active in breast and prostate cancer; widely used for these indications in Europe
- Controls hot flushing

MECHANISMS OF ACTION

- Mechanism of antitumor action is unknown
- It has progestational, antiestrogenic, androgenic, and anabolic effects, as well as antiovulatory activity
- In high doses, it suppresses the production of gonadatropin hormone and cortisol
- It has a complex corticoid action and provides replacement for cortisol when used with aminoglutethimide
- Antitumor effect in breast cancer occurs in tumors that contain estrogen receptors

DOSING

- For advanced endometrial or renal cancer, 1,000 mg or more weekly have been used
- For advanced prostate or breast cancer, 400 mg or more weekly have been used
- Some evidence of a dose-response effect exists in breast cancer, suggesting that 500 mg daily may be more effective than smaller doses
- Daily IM injections produce a progressive increase in plasma concentrations for ~4 wks; this level can be maintained thereafter with twice-weekly injections
- Oral administration appears to produce comparable response rates but less dependable absorption

PHARMACOKINETICS

- Extensively metabolized
- < 3% of the drug is excreted unchanged in the urine
- Half-life is 60 hrs

TOXICITY

- Weight gain due to an increase in body mass occurs in 10–80% of patients
- 10–25% of patients gain 5% or more of their baseline body weight
- Vaginal (i.e., uterine) bleeding may occur after initiation of treatment
- Edema, muscle cramps, increase in blood pressure, and gastrointestinal effects may occur in < 5% of patients
- May increase plasma levels of coumadin
- IM injections may produce severe local irritation with sterile abcesses in a few patients

RECOMMENDATIONS FOR SUPPORTIVE CARE

- Dietary advice to avoid excessive weight gain may be helpful

PHARMACY ISSUES

- Sterile aqueous suspension available as 400 mg/ml; in 2.5 and 10 ml vials
- When multidose vials are used, special care to prevent contamination of the contents is essential

NURSING CONSIDERATIONS

- Pretreatment workup should include special reference to breasts and pelvic organs and pap smear
- Monitor liver function, coagulation tests, and thyroid function
- When submitting tissue specimens to pathology, indicate that patient is on progestin treatment
- Potential antiestrogenic properties that disturb estrogen receptor cycle; adverse effects on carbohydrate and lipid metabolism if patient is on estrogen replacement therapy
- If administered IM, give via deep IM injections; apply pressure and rotate sites systemically
- Should not be administered during first 4 mos of pregnancy
- Assess
  - for fluid retention; especially in patients with a history of epilepsy, migraines, asthma, and cardiac or renal dysfunction
  - psychic changes in patients with a history of depression
  - diabetic patients for decreased glucose tolerance
  - skin rash
- Teach patient
  - report breakthrough bleeding and skin rash
  - possibility of impaired fertility if patient is receiving high doses
  - effect on nursing infants
  - practice contraception
  - signs and symptoms of thromboembolic events
  - report sensory/perceptual changes

KEY REFERENCES

Byrne MJ, Gebski V, Forbes J, et al.: Medroxyprogesterone acetate addition or substitution for tamoxifen in advanced tamoxifen-resistant breast cancer: a phase III randomized trial. J Clin Oncol 1997; 15(9):3141–8

Carpenter JT Jr: Progestational agents in the treatment of breast cancer. Cancer Treat Res 1988; 39:147–56

Muss HB, Cruz JM: High-dose progestin therapy for metastatic breast cancer. Ann Oncol 1992; 3(suppl 3):15–20

Drug: Megestrol

John T. Carpenter, Jr. and Belinda Butler

OTHER NAMES: MEGESTROL ACETATE, MEGACE

USES

- Approved by the FDA for treatment of patients with advanced carcinoma of the breast or endometrium
- Also effective for treatment of weight loss due to malignant disease or AIDS; occasional responses have been observed in carcinomas of the prostate and kidney
- Low doses (20–40 mg daily) may suppress hot flushing

MECHANISM OF ACTION

- Unknown
- In patients with breast cancer, the presence of estrogen or progesterone receptors in tumor tissue identifies patients likely to respond

DOSING

- Administered orally in 20 mg and 40 mg tablets
- An oral suspension is also available but approved only for treatment of cachexia
- The approved dosage for breast cancer is 40 mg qid, and for endometrial cancer 40–320 mg daily in divided doses
- A once-daily schedule (i.e., 160 mg once daily) is also effective for breast cancer treatment

PHARMACOKINETICS

- Well absorbed from the GI tract
- Plasma half-life is 14 hrs

TOXICITY

- The most frequently reported toxicities are weight gain, vaginal bleeding, and fluid retention
- Dyspnea, tumor flare, and hypercalcemia may occur
- Suppression of adrenal steroid production occurs by suppression of the pituitary-adrenal axis, but usually produces no symptoms
- The frequent occurrence of weight gain, seen most frequently at doses of 400–800 mg daily, led to its use in treatment of cachexia

RECOMMENDATIONS FOR SUPPORTIVE CARE

- When the drug is used for cancer treatment, weight gain is frequently not a desired effect; dietary counseling may be helpful

NURSING CONSIDERATIONS

- Monitor for onset of new diabetes, exacerbation of preexisting diabetes, and Cushing's syndrome
- Possibility of adrenal suppression with patients receiving or being withdrawn from therapy
- Should not be administered during first 4 mos of pregnancy
- Assess
  - for thromboembolic phenomena, heart failure, edema, dyspnea, and tumor flare with or without hypercalcemia
  - need to increase insulin dosage in patients with preexisting diabetes
  - weight gain from increased appetite and fluid retention
  - mood changes and increase in pain level
- Teach patient
  - signs and symptoms of thromboembolic events
  - report breakthrough bleeding
  - practice contraception
  - effects on nursing infants
  - potential for weight gain
  - expected side effects and self-care measures

KEY REFERENCES

Lentz SS, Brady MF, Major FJ: High-dose megestrol acetate in advanced or recurrent endometrial carcinoma: A Gynecologic Oncology Group study. J Clin Oncol 1996; 14(2):357–61

Russell CA, Green SJ, O'Sullivan J, et al.: Megestrol acetate and aminoglutethimide/hydrocortisone in sequence or in combination as second-line endocrine therapy of estrogen receptor-positive metastatic breast cancer: a Southwest Oncology Group phase III trial. J Clin Oncol 1997; 15(7):2494–501

Drug: Aminoglutethimide

John T. Carpenter, Jr. and Belinda Butler

OTHER NAMES: CYTADREN

USES

- Approved by FDA for treatment of selected patients with Cushing's syndrome, particularly those with adrenal adenoma or adrenal carcinoma
- Also active in metastatic breast cancer

MECHANISMS OF ACTION

- Inhibits the enzymatic conversion of cholesterol to pregnenolone, which leads to a decrease in production of adrenal glucocorticoids and mineralocorticoids, estrogens and androgens
- Inhibits cytochrome P-450-dependent hydroxylation reactions necessary for aromatization, thus inhibiting conversion of adrogens to estrogens in extra-adrenal tissues, especially fat
- Antitumor effect in breast cancer occurs in tumors that contain estrogen receptors

DOSING

- Schedules/doses
  - 125–250 mg q6hrs with replacement hydrocortisone 40 mg daily in split doses for metastatic breast cancer
  - mineralocorticoid replacement may be needed in some patients
  - smaller doses, 125–250 mg q12hrs, inhibit aromatase and may be used in metastatic breast cancer
  - after 2 wks of treatment corticosteroids may be discontinued, since synthesis in the adrenal recovers

PHARMACOKINETICS

- Well absorbed from GI tract with 80–92% recovered in urine, 1% in feces
- Undergoes N-acetylation, thus cleared more rapidly in fast than in slow acetylators
- Half-life ~14 hrs in slow acetylators, 8 hrs in fast acetylators
- Increases clearance of tamoxifen and of progestational agents

TOXICITY

- The most frequent toxicities are lethargy, orthostatic hypotension, nausea, vomiting, hypothyroidism, reversible agranulocytosis, and rash
- The rash is usually maculopapular and pruritic
  - appears in the second week of treatment and disappears about 5 days later without discontinuation of the drugs
- Replacement of glucorticoids is needed for the first 2 wks
  - mineralocorticoid replacement is also needed occasionally

RECOMMENDATIONS FOR SUPPORTIVE CARE

- Initiating therapy with smaller doses (i.e., 125 mg every 6 or 12 hrs) may improve tolerance

PHARMACY ISSUES

- Supplied as 250 mg scored tablets

NURSING CONSIDERATIONS

- If higher doses used, consider hospitalizing patient for initiation of therapy and until regime is established
- Lower dose regimens cause fewer side effects. Individualize nursing management based on dose.
- Corticosteroids need to be administered adjuvantly
- Monitor plasma cortisol levels to point of desired suppression
- Perform baseline/periodic hematologic tests, SGOT, Alk Phos, and bilirubin
- Monitor thyroid function and serum electrolytes periodically
- Monitor for adrenalcortical hypofunction
- Patients receiving coumadin (Warfarin) should be monitored for diminished effects; may need dose increase
- Enhances dexamethasone metabolism
- Assess
  - baseline neurologic function; sensory/perceptual alterations may be severe in elderly patients
  - signs and symptoms of adrenal insufficiency: fatigue, nausea, vomiting, diarrhea, weight loss, weakness, dizziness, hyponatremia, hypoglycemia
  - blood pressure routinely for signs of postural hypotension
  - rash with fever may develop within 5–7 days and last for 8 days; if not resolved in 7–14 days, discontinue drug
- Teach patient
  - avoid alcohol
  - not to drive/operate dangerous machinery or participate in activities requiring mental alertness
  - masculinization and hirsutism may occur in females
  - practice contraception
  - expected side-effects and self-care measures (i.e., change positions slowly to avoid dizziness)

KEY REFERENCES

Cocconi G, Bisagni G, Ceci G; et al.: Low dose aminoglutethimide with and without hydrocortisone replacement as a first-line endocrine treatment in advanced breast cancer: a prospective randomized trial of the Italian Oncology Group for Clinical Research. J Clin Oncol 1992; 10(6):984–9

Gale KE, Andersen JW, Tormey DC, et al.: Hormonal treatment for metastatic breast cancer. An Eastern Cooperative Oncology Group phase III trial comparing aminoglutethimide to tamoxifen. Cancer 1994; 73(2):354–61

Garcia-Giralt E, Ayme Y, Carton M, et al.: Second and third line hormonotherapy in advanced post-menopausal breast cancer: a multicenter randomized trial comparing medroxyprogesterone acetate with aminoglutethimide in patients who have become resistant to tamoxifen. Breast Cancer Res Treat 1993; 24(2):139–45

Chapter 9

ANTIANDROGENS AND RELATED DRUGS

Introduction

Nicholas J. Vogelzang

EFFECTS OF ANDROGENS (TESTOSTERONE, DIHYDROTESTOSTERONE)

- Bind to nuclear androgen receptor (AR) resulting in dimerization of the receptor and activation of a sequence of DNA called the androgen response element (ARE) with subsequent transcription of androgen-regulated genes
- Association of androgens and male sexual function (primary and secondary)
  - loss of androgen function causes impotence and loss of libido
  - loss of muscle mass and bone mass are well documented
  - other secondary sexual characteristics also affected (hair growth, etc.)

CLASSIFICATION OF ANTIANDROGENS

- Nonsteroidal androgens (flutamide, bicalutamide, nilutamide)
  - bind to nuclear AR prostate cancer cells but result in variable activation of ARE or transcription of androgen-regulated genes
  - have paradoxical androgenlike effects on certain target tissues (maintenance of sexual libido)
  - maintain bone density
- LHRH agonists (goserelin, leuprolide)
  - two synthetic LHRH-like decapeptides
  - both associated with transient rises in testicular androgen levels and short-term "pain flares"
  - long acting (3 or 4 mo) preparations available
  - goserelin has been compared to orchiectomy in two trials and is equivalent

KEY REFERENCES

Bubley GJ, Balk SP: Treatment of metastatic prostate cancer. Lessons from the androgen receptor. Hematol Oncol Clin North Am 1996; 10(3):713–25

Small EJ, Vogelzang NJ: Second-line hormonal therapy for advanced prostate cancer: a shifting paradigm. J Clin Oncol 1997; 15(1):382–8

Drug: Leuprolide

Nicholas J. Vogelzang and Janine Caggiano

OTHER NAMES: LUPRON

USES

- FDA approved for the treatment of advanced carcinoma of the prostate, advanced metastatic breast cancer, and endometriosis

MECHANISM OF ACTION

- Drug is a decapeptide, which directly binds to the LHRH receptor on pituitary LH cells. By abolishing the tight rhythmic pulsitile secretion of LH from the hypothalamus, the pituitary LH cells cease production of LH. Preceding cessation of LH is a transient superagonist effect whereby large amounts of LH are secreted. This LH surge in turn induces a testosterone or estrogen surge, the adverse effects of which continue to be debated. The hormone surge can be blocked by premedicating the patient for 1–2 wks with a number of antiandrogens or antiestrogens. Cessation of the LHRH agonists is associated with a variable recovery period of the estrogen and testosterone levels. The LH levels recover quickly, but recovery of testosterone and estrogen levels may be protracted, especially if LHRH agonist was used for more than a year

DOSING

- 7.5 mg IM injection monthly
- 22.5 mg IM injection q3mos (84 days)
- 30 mg IM injection q4mos (16 wks)
- Also available in intermediate doses for use in pediatric and endocrinologic disorders

PHARMACOKINETICS

- Extremely short half-life, rapidly degraded by serum proteases
- Sustained-release preparations have been developed and are patent protected
- Formulated as a suspension of microspheres
- Previous work has suggested that leuprolide can be administered SubQ, IM, or via intranasal administration
- Not orally bioavailable

TOXICITY

- Toxicities are entirely due to the physiologic effects of castrate levels of testosterone or estrogen
- These castrate levels are responsible for hot flashes, weight gain, decreased libido, and mild anemia, particularly in males
- Long-term effects, such as osteoporosis and other effects of hypogonadism, are common
- Rarely allergic reactions have been reported after either IM or SubQ inoculation

RECOMMENDATIONS FOR SUPPORTIVE CARE

- Megesterol acetate 20 mg bid has been used to control hot flashes

PHARMACY ISSUES

- There are no major differences between goserelin and leuprolide; the differences are entirely due to cost (related to hospital contract issues) and drug formulation (leuprolide: suspension; goserelin: pellet). There is no evidence that monthly injections are more effective than every 3- or 4-mo injections.

NURSING CONSIDERATIONS

- Solution should be inspected for particulate matter or discoloration
- Store at room temperature
- Assess
  - for general worsening of signs and symptoms during first 2 wks of therapy
  - for peripheral edema
  - inspect injection sites
- Teach patient
  - injection schedule and proper administration techniques with rotation of sites
  - potential for weight gain
  - hot flashes will subside after 2 wks of therapy
  - decreased libido and impotence in men; amenorrhea in women after 10 wks of therapy; management of sexual dysfunction
  - possibility of temporary increase in bone pain and pain at tumor site; instruct on pain management

KEY REFERENCES

Schellhammer P, Sharifi R, Block N, et al.: A controlled trial of bicaluatamide versus flutamide, in each combination with luteinizing hormone-releasing hormone analogue therapy, in patients with advanced prostate cancer. Urology 1995; 45(5):745–52

Vogelzang NJ, Scardino P, Shipley W, Coffe D (eds): Comprehensive textbook of genitourinary oncology. 2nd ed. Baltimore: Lippincott, Williams and Wilkins, 2000

Drug: Goserelin

Nicholas J. Vogelzang and Janine Caggiano

OTHER NAMES: ZOLADEX

USES

- FDA approved for the treatment of advanced carcinoma of the prostate, advanced metastatic breast cancer, and endometriosis

MECHANISM OF ACTION

- Drug is a decapeptide, which directly binds to the LHRH receptor on pituitary LH cells. By abolishing the tight rhythmic pulsitile secretion of LH from the hypothalamus, the pituitary LH cells cease production of LH. Preceding cessation of LH is a transient superagonist effect whereby large amounts of LH are secreted. This LH surge in turn induces a testosterone or estrogen surge, the adverse effects of which continue to be debated. The hormone surge can be blocked by premedicating the patient for 1–2 wks with a number of antiandrogens or antiestrogens. Cessation of the LHRH agonists is associated with a variable recovery period of the estrogen and testosterone levels. The LH levels recover quickly, but recovery of testosterone and estrogen levels may be protracted, especially if LHRH agonist was used for more than a year

DOSING

- 3.6 mg monthly injection
- 3 mo injection of 10.8 mg

PHARMACOKINETICS

- Extremely short half-life rapidly degraded by serum proteases
- Sustained-release preparations have been developed and are patented
- Formulated as a glycolic acid copolymer in a sustained-release pellet
- Previous work has suggested that goserelin can be administered SubQ, IM, or via intranasal administration
- Not orally bioavailable

TOXICITY

- Toxicities are entirely due to the physiologic effects of castrate levels of testosterone or estrogen
- These castrate levels are responsible for hot flashes, weight gain, decreased libido, and mild anemia, particularly in males
- Long-term effects, such as osteoporosis and other effects of hypogonadism, are common
- Rarely allergic reactions have been reported after either IM or SubQ inoculation

RECOMMENDATIONS FOR SUPPORTIVE CARE

- Megesterol acetate 20 mg bid has been used to control hot flashes

PHARMACY ISSUES

- There are no major differences between goserelin and leuprolide; the differences are entirely due to cost (related to hospital contract issues) and drug formulation (leuprolide: suspension; goserelin: pellet). There is no evidence that monthly injections are more effective than every 3- or 4-mo injections.

NURSING CONSIDERATIONS

- Administer local anesthetic (lidocaine) to minimize pain at injection site
- Should be administered by a single SubQ injection q28d or q74d into skin of upper abdominal wall using sterile technique/do not aspirate with supplied needle
- Assess
  - cardiovascular function during treatment: heart rate, blood pressure, peripheral pulses
  - inspect injection sites
  - if bleeding occurs, maintain pressure on site for ~5 min
- Teach patient
  - to report palpitations, shortness of breath
  - hot flashes
  - management of sexual dysfunction
  - possibility of temporary increase in bone pain and pain at tumor site; instruct on pain management
  - potential for weight gain

KEY REFERENCES

Vogelzang NJ, Chodak GW, Soloway MS, et al.: Goserelin versus orchiectomy in the treatment of advanced prostate cancer: final results of a randomized trial. Urology 1995; 46:220–6

Vogelzang, NJ, Scardino P, Shipley W, Coffee D (eds.): Comprehensive textbook of genitourinary oncology. Baltimore: 2nd edition; Lippincott, Williams and Wilkins, 2000

Drug: Flutamide

Michael J. Morris, Howard I. Scher, and Brenda Werner

OTHER NAMES: APIMID, CHIMAX, DROGENIL, EUFLEX, EULEXIN, EULEXINE, FLUCINONE, FLUTA-GRY, FLUTACAN, FLUTAMEX, FUGEREL, GRISETIN, ONCOSAL, PROSTACUR, PROSTOGENAT, TESTAC, TESTOTARD

USES

- For the treatment of prostate cancer
- Flutamide is generally used in combination with LHRH agonists such as goserelin or leuprolide acetate

MECHANISM OF ACTION

- Competitively binds to androgen receptors, the usual binding sites of dihydrotestosterone and testosterone, and thereby inhibits androgen-induced growth of tumor cells

DOSING

- 250 mg po tid
- Treatment with goserelin or leuprolide acetate should, in most cases, continue while the patient is being treated with flutamide
- Some patients who demonstrate progression of disease while undergoing treatment with flutamide will respond to withdrawal of the drug
- Patients will generally respond to primary hormonal therapy for 12–18 mos. Flutamide should be withdrawn at relapse, to elicit a withdrawal response

PHARMACOKINETICS

- Complete and rapid absorption from GI tract
- 90% protein bound
- Time to peak concentration is 1–2 hrs
- Steady-state therapeutic levels are achieved after four doses (in geriatric patients)
- Converted to at least 10 metabolites; active metabolite is 2-hydroxyflutamide
- Half-life of biologically active metabolite is 6–9 hrs
- A diminution in tumor-related pain should be observable within 2–4 wks

TOXICITY

- Diarrhea, nausea, vomiting, elevated liver function studies, cholestasis
- Anemia
- In combination with LHRH agonists, may induce gynecomastia, breast tenderness, diminished libido, and impotence
  - flutamide alone is not associated with impotence and loss of libido

NURSING CONSIDERATIONS

- No known drug interactions
- Evaluate liver function tests prior to administration
- Assess
  - nutritional status related to diarrhea, nausea, and vomiting and abdominal distention
  - liver dysfunction
- Teach patient
  - take medication daily
  - potential for gynecomastia and hot flashes
  - effects on libido and sterility

KEY REFERENCES

Brogden RN, Clissold SP: Flutamide: a preliminary review of its pharmacodynamic and pharmacokinetic properties, and therapeutic efficacy in advanced prostatic cancer. Drugs 1989; 38:185–203

Crawford ED, Eisenberger MA, McLeod DG, et al.: A controlled trial of leuprolide with and without flutamide in prostatic carcinoma. N Engl J Med 1989; 321:419–24

Wysowski DK, Freiman JP, Tourtelot JB, et al.: Fatal and nonfatal hepatotoxicity associated with flutamide. Ann Intern Med 1993; 118:860–4

Drug: Bicalutamide

Michael J. Morris, Howard I. Scher, and Susan Noble-Kempin

OTHER NAMES: CASODEX

USES

- For the treatment of prostate cancer
- Generally used in combination with LHRH agonists such as goserelin or leuprolide acetate or surgical castration
  - the combination of an LHRH analogue and bicalutamide has a greater antitumor effect than treatment with bicalutamide alone
- At high doses (150–200 mg) bicalutamide be effective for patients previously treated with flutamide with progressive prostate cancer despite castrate levels of testosterone

MECHANISM OF ACTION

- Competitively binds to the androgen receptor, the usual binding site of dihydrotestosterone and testosterone, and inhibits androgen-induced growth of prostate cancer cells
- Prior treatment with flutamide alters the sensitivity of the tumor to subsequent treatment with other nonsteroidal antiandrogens such as bicalutamide
  - this may be related to specific mutations in the androgen receptor
- Treatment effect should be seen within 2–3 mos

DOSING

- Administered orally 50 mg daily
- In high doses it is administered as 150 mg daily
  - high-dose bicalutamide is not currently approved and is currently under investigation in the adjuvant setting and in relapsed patients
- Treatment with goserelin or leuprolide acetate should, in most cases, continue while the patient is being treated with bicalutamide
- Some patients who demonstrate progression of disease while undergoing treatment with bicalutamide will respond to withdrawal of the drug
- Therapeutic response may be seen in 1–2 wks, with a reduction in pain and biochemical markers

PHARMACOKINETICS

- Time to peak concentration is ~16 hrs after ingestiorn
- Absorption from the GI tract is slow
- Absolute bioavailability is not known
- 96% protein bound
- Undergoes stereospecific metabolism
- The active isomer is the R form and is primarily metabolized by oxidation to an active metabolite followed by glucuronidation
- The S form undergoes glucuronidation and is then rapidly cleared
- Elimination half-life is 7–10 days
  - significantly longer than that of flutamide (5 hrs) and nilutamide (2 days)

TOXICITY

- Main side effects with bicalutamide as monotherapy are gynecomastia, breast tenderness, and hot flashes
- These may occur in greater frequency in combination with LHRH agonists, as may weight gain, muscle weakness, diminished libido, impotency, diarrhea (though less so than with flutamide), and anemia

PHARMACY ISSUES

- Supplied as 50 mg tablets

NURSING CONSIDERATIONS

- When initiating bicalutamide and an LHRH agonist, careful surveillance should be maintained to prevent tumor flare. Symptoms include
  - cord compression
  - urinary obstruction
  - pain
- Patients undergoing therapy with warfarin should have coagulation profiles checked regularly. In vitro studies have shown bicalutamide displaces warfarin and therefore may induce higher than expected prothrombin times
- Use cautiously in patients with hepatic dysfunction. Monitor baseline LFTs prior to initiation of drug and periodically thereafter
- Assess
  - alterations in nutrition and elimination
- Teach Patient
  - not to stop or interrupt medication without first consulting physician
  - may be taken with food or on an empty stomach
  - advise patient to take missed doses as soon as possible but not to double up on doses
- Take measures for symptomatic relief of hot flashes and diarrhea

KEY REFERENCES

Joyce R, Fenton M, Rode P, et al.: High dose bicalutamide for androgen independent prostate cancer: effect of prior hormonal therapy. J Urol 1998; 159:149–53

Kaisary AV, Tyrrell CJ, Beacock C, et al.: A randomized comparison of monotherapy with casodex 50 mg daily and castration in the treatment of metastatic prostate carcinoma. Eur Urol 1995; 28:215–22

Schellhammer P, Sharifi R, Block N, et al.: Clinical benefits of bicalutamide compared with flutamide in combined androgen blockade for patients with advanced prostatic carcinoma: final report of a double-blind, randomized, multicenter trial. Urology 1997; 50:330–6

Drug: Ketoconazole

Frederick R. Ahmann and Ellen Jessop

OTHER NAMES: NIZORAL

USES

- FDA approved only for use as treatment for systemic fungal infections
- Secondary to ketoconazole's ability to block testicular and adrenal steroidogenesis, the drug has reported utility in prostate cancer therapy in two situations
  - when immediate testicular suppression is needed, but when an orchiectomy cannot be done (disseminated intravascular coagulation, acute epidural spinal cord compression)
  - testicular suppression can be achieved within 48 hrs
  - as second-line therapy in men failing primary testicular suppression/ablation
  - overall objective response rate is ~15% (range 10–25%) with serum PSA response rates being higher

MECHANISM OF ACTION

- Inhibits CYP3A4, thereby suppressing both testicular and adrenal androgen biosynthesis

DOSING

- 400 mg orally q8hrs (the enzyme inhibition is rapidly reversible making the q8hr dosing schedule important)
- Any agent that effects gastric acidity can block the dissolution and absorption of ketoconazole

PHARMACOKINETICS

- Peak plasma levels in 1–2 hrs
- Short half-life
- Enzyme blockage reverses rapidly as soon as drug is eliminated
- Testicular suppression is frequently overcome within 1 mo of initiating therapy secondary to rises in LH
- Drug is primarily excreted in bile

TOXICITY

- Nausea and vomiting may affect up to one-third of patients and limit the drug's utility
- Rarer toxicities include gynecomastia, dry skin, nail dystrophy, fatigue, rash, and hepatotoxicity
- Adrenal crisis has been reported, but appears to be rare
- Ketoconazole use is contraindicated in men on cisapride, terfenadine, or astemizole
- Ketoconazole will likely interfere with the metabolism of the many other drugs that are substrates for CYP3A4

RECOMMENDATIONS FOR SUPPORTIVE CARE

- None

PHARMACY ISSUES

- Comes as 200 mg tablets

NURSING CONSIDERATIONS

- Drug must be taken at 8 hr intervals
- Monitor liver functions; drug is eliminated by the liver
- Drug requires an acid environment for dissolution and absorption; drugs that decrease gastric acidity should be avoided (e.g., H2 antagonists)
- Assess
  - for alterations in nutritional status as a result of nausea and vomiting
- Teach patient
  - adherence with medication schedule, since dosing directly affects its efficacy
  - avoid OTC medications; check with physician
  - side effects and self-care measures

KEY REFERENCES

DeCoster R, et al.: P450-dependent enzymes as targets for prostate cancer therapy. J Steroid Biochem Molec Biol 1996; 56:133–43

Litt MR, et al.: Disseminated intravascular coagulation in prostatic carcinoma reversed by ketoconazole. JAMA 1987; 258:1361–2

Small EJ, et al.: Ketoconazole retains activity in advanced prostate cancer patients with progression despite flutamide withdrawal. J Urol 1997; 157:1204–7

Drug: Nilutamide

Michael J. Morris, Howard I. Scher, and Victoria Staszak

OTHER NAMES: NILANDRON, ANANDRON

USES

- Treatment of prostate cancer
- Generally used in combination with other medications such as goserelin or leuprolide acetate, or surgical castration

MECHANISM OF ACTION

- Competitively binds to the androgen receptor to block binding of dihydrotestosterone and testosterone, and thereby inhibits androgen-induced growth of prostate cancer
- Can be used for preventing disease flare during first month of initiating LHRH agonists
- Therapeutic response may be seen in 1–2 wks, with a reduction in pain and biochemical markers

DOSING

- 300 mg daily for 1 mo followed by 150 mg daily
- Nilandron is contraindicated in patients with severe hepatic impairment. Patients with mild hepatic insufficiency should receive reduced doses

PHARMACOKINETICS

- Steady state achieved in 2 wks at dosing of 150 mg twice daily
- Peak concentrations achieved in 1–4 hrs
- Drug is absorbed rapidly from the GI tract
- 80% protein bound
- Extensively metabolized in the liver to five products
- Most of the administered drug is excreted in the urine as inactive metabolites

TOXICITY

- Hot flashes, nausea, loss of libido or impotence, especially when combined with LHRH agonists or orchiectomy
- Elevated liver function studies
- Impaired visual adaptation to darkness characterized by delayed recovery of vision and/or blurry vision after exposure to bright light (13–57% of patients)
- Alcohol intolerance
- Pneumonitis (rare)

NURSING CONSIDERATIONS

- Nilutamide can delay elimination of several other drugs metabolized by the liver:
  - phenytoin: ataxia, hyperflexia, nystagmus or tremor
  - theophylline: nausea, vomiting, palpitations
  - warfarin: PT will be higher for a given dose of warfarin
- Drug should be discontinued if transaminase exceed three times normal limit
- Monitor liver functions at regular intervals during therapy
- Contraindicated in patients with severe hepatic impairment, respiratory insufficiency, or hypersensitivity to nilutamide or any component of this preparation
- Can be taken with or without food
- Store at room temperature
- Assess
  - for signs and symptoms of hepatitis: jaundice, dark urine, pruritis, abdominal pain, weight loss, fever, hepatomegaly
  - pulmonary function baseline and during therapy; note rales or rhonchi, if present, obtain chest x-ray (CXR) and note interstitial changes; if CXR is negative schedule PFT; promote adequate mucous clearance/chest physiotherapy
  - cardiovascular status baseline and during therapy; if signs of heart failure, angina, or syncope are present, CXR, EKG, and ECHO should be obtained
- Teach patient
  - altered body image; testicular atrophy, gynecomastia
  - report symptoms of cough, fever, exertional dyspnea, chest pain
  - report visual changes; patient may experience a delay in adaptation to the dark; instruct on the use of tinted glasses and caution when driving at night
  - expected side effects and self-care measures

KEY REFERENCES

Beland G, Elhilali M, Fradet Y, et al.: A controlled trial of castration with and without nilutamide in metastatic prostatic carcinoma. Cancer 1990; 66:1074–9

Bertagna C, De Gery A, Hucher M, et al.: Efficacy of the combination of nilutamide plus orchidectomy in patients with metastatic prostate cancer. A meta-analysis of seven randomized double-blind trials (1056 patients). Br J Urol 1994; 73:396–402

Harris MG, Coleman SG, Faulds D, et al.: Nilutamide: a review of its pharmacodynamic and pharmacokinetic properties, and therapeutic efficacy in prostate cancer. Drugs & Aging 1993; 3:9–25

Chapter 10

REGIONAL THERAPY

Intrathecal/Intraventricular Therapy: Introduction

Stuart A. Grossman

INDICATIONS FOR INTRATHECAL/ INTRAVENTRICULAR THERAPY

- Treatment of established neoplastic meningitis secondary to solid tumors, lymphomas, or leukemias
- CNS prophylaxis for high-risk patients with lymphoma or leukemia

AVAILABLE AGENTS

- Methotrexate
- Thiotepa
- Cytarabine

ROUTES OF ADMINISTRATION

- Intraventricular
  - via surgically implanted SubQ reservoir and ventricular catheter (SRVC)
    - □ advantages vs. lumbar administration
      - ▽ ease of drug administration
      - ▽ assurance that the administered drug has reached the spinal fluid
      - ▽ drug can be administered to thrombocytopenic patient
      - ▽ possibility that response and survival may be marginally better than via the lumbar route
    - □ disadvantages vs. lumbar administration
      - ▽ cost and adverse events associated with placement of SRVC (infection, bleeding, malfunction, improper placement)
      - ▽ adverse events associated with repeated access of SRVC (infection)
      - ▽ fluid should be withdrawn and administered slowly (<1 ml/min) to avoid rapid fluid shifts in brain
- Lumbar
  - via repeated lumbar punctures
- Systemic
  - recent study suggests that high-dose methotrexate may be advantageous

THERAPEUTIC APPROACH TO PATIENT WITH ESTABLISHED NEOPLASTIC MENINGITIS

- Early diagnosis and treatment is critical to preserving neurologic function
- Overall evaluation to assess prognostic factors and determine how aggressively the patient is to be treated
  - good prognostic factors include
    - □ natural history of systemic tumor is indolent
    - □ systemic cancer is responsive to antineoplastic therapy
    - □ no evident systemic cancer
    - □ no fixed neurologic deficits
    - □ excellent performance status
- Radiation therapy to all bulk and symptomatic sites of disease
- Intrathecal chemotherapy to treat minimal volume disease and tumor cells floating in CSF
  - this is commonly initiated by lumbar puncture
  - if it appears that the patient will benefit from long-term intrathecal therapy, an SRVC is placed
  - ^{111}Indium-DTPA CSF flow scan to document CSF flow abnormalities, which will affect the distribution of intrathecal chemotherapy
  - intrathecal therapy is begun twice weekly
  - once CSF cytology becomes negative this is given twice weekly for 1 wk/mo
  - response to intrathecal chemotherapy must be judged using CSF from the same site as the pretreatment positive cytology
    - □ ventricular CSF routinely has a higher glucose, lower protein, and lower incidence of positive cytology than lumbar CSF
    - □ doses should be in mg (rather than mg/m^2) because adults have nearly the same volume of spinal fluid regardless of their height or weight

COMMON TOXICITIES

- Myelosuppression
  - seen with thiotepa > methotrexate > cytarabine
- Potentially fatal leukoencephalopathy
  - seen with combination intrathecal chemotherapy > methothrexate > cytarabine > thiotepa
  - incidence increases >6 mos after initiating therapy
  - often first noted on MRI and followed by untreatable neurologic decline
- Staphylococcus epidermidis meningitis
  - subacute presentation in patients with SRVC

KEY REFERENCES

DeAngelis LM: Diagnosis and treatment of leptomeningeal metastases. J Neuro-Oncol 1998; 38:245–52

Grossman SA, Moynihan TJ: Neoplastic meningitis. Neurol Clin North Am 1991; 9:843–56

Drug: Methotrexate (Intraventricular)

Stuart A. Grossman and Corinne Haviley

MECHANISM OF ACTION

- Antimetabolite
- Targets dihydrofolate reductase
- Reduces carbon donor required for purine and pyrimidine synthesis
- Increases dihydrofolate polyglutamates, which further inhibits purine synthesis
- Clinical pharmacology
  - most active against rapidly dividing tissues
  - most effective when drug levels remain high for a prolonged period

DOSING

- 10 mg in 5–10 ml of Elliott's B solution twice weekly into the lumbar intrathecal space or the ventricle
- Continue until CSF cytology has cleared
- Then continue with maintenance therapy 2 treatments per week (one week per month)

PHARMACOKINETICS

- 10 mg of IT MTX provides CSF levels above 10 μM for ~48 hrs
- Intrathecal methotrexate is cleared from the CSF by the bulk flow through the arachnoid granulations and into the venous circulation
- Abnormalities of CSF flow may result in prolonged high levels of MTX entering brain parenchyma and predisposing the patient to leukoencephalopathy
- Nearly 90% of methotrexate in the systemic circulation is cleared by the kidneys
- Methotrexate may be sequestered in large fluid collections (i.e., pleural effusions or ascites), which can result in delayed release and toxicity

TOXICITY

- Primary early toxicity is to GI mucosa and bone marrow
- If these toxicities become a clinical problem, they can be prevented using oral leucovorin calcium, which "rescues" systemic tissues but does not penetrate into the CSF
- Major late toxicity is disseminated necrotizing leukoencephalopathy
- Major risk factors include
  - intrathecal methotrexate
  - cranial irradiation (especially if this precedes IT methotrexate)
  - systemic methotrexate

RECOMMENDATIONS FOR SUPPORTIVE CARE

- Antiemetics usually not required

PHARMACY ISSUES

- Only preservative-free methotrexate should be used
- Elliott's B solution (artificial CSF) is the preferred diluent

NURSING CONSIDERATIONS

- Fluid should be withdrawn and administered slowly (< 1 ml/min) to avoid rapid fluid shifts in brain
- Preservative-free methotrexate solutions of 3 mg/ml in preservative-free normal saline chloride should be used; *solutions containing preservatives should not be used*
- Avoid contamination; use strict aseptic technique
- Before administration, a volume of CSF equal to the volume of methotrexate solution to be injected should be removed (usually 5–15 ml)
- Drug should only be injected if there is an easy flow of blood-free spinal fluid
- If overdose is recognized, a lumbar puncture should be performed immediately and CSF should be allowed to drain by gravity; high-dose leucovorin calcium and corticosteroids are used for intrathecal overdose of methotrexate
- Increased toxicity has been associated with increased age and in patients with overt meningeal involvement
- Assess
  - baseline neurologic status
  - for acute arachnoiditis (most common toxic reaction): headaches, back pain, nuchal rigidity, and fever
  - subacute myelopathy: paraplegia/paraparesis of one or more nerve roots
  - chronic leukoencephalopathy: confusion, irritability, ataxia, and increased CSF pressure
  - neurotoxicity manifested by prompt burning, or numbness in lower extremities, stupor, agitation, seizures, and respiratory insufficiency
  - assessment of access site for signs of infection
- Teach patient
  - explain procedure; instruct patient to remain supine for 30 min following the procedure
  - acute complications, which could include nausea, vomiting, fever, headache, and rigidity of neck; usually they subside within 72 hrs
  - report unusual symptoms

KEY REFERENCES

Bleyer WA: Intrathecal methotrexate versus central nervous system leukemia. Cancer Drug Deliv 1984; 1(2):157–67

Drug: Thiotepa (Intrathecal/Intraventricular)

Stuart A. Grossman and Corinne Haviley

MECHANISM OF ACTION

- Polyfunctional alkylating agent
- Pharmacologically similar to nitrogen mustard
- Not a vesicant, so it can be administered into body cavities

CLINICAL PHARMACOLOGY

- Not cell cycle specific
- Primary metabolite triethylene-phosphoramide (TEPA) is responsible for most of the drug's solid tumor activity

DOSING

- 10 mg in 5–10 ml of Elliott's B solution or normal saline twice weekly into the lumbar intrathecal space or the ventricle
- Continue until CSF cytology has cleared
- Then continue with maintenance therapy 2 treatments per week (one week per month)

PHARMACOKINETICS

- Terminal half-life of intraventricular thiotepa is 8 hrs
- Ventricular clearance is ~4% of total body clearance
- Lumbar thiotepa concentrations are only 5% of ventricular levels, but still high enough to be active

TOXICITY

- Dose-limiting side effect of thiotepa is myelosuppression
- The doses administered into the CSF (10 mg biweekly) approach those one would use systemically
- Myelosuppression can be significant in this patient population
  - Often heavily pretreated with chemotherapy or radiation
  - Often have advanced cancer with bone marrow infiltration
  - Often receive concomitant radiation therapy to the spine or pelvis as part of the treatment for leptomeningeal metastases
- Major late toxicity is late acute nonlymphocytic leukemia as with many alkylating agents
- Neurotoxicity seems to be less than with intrathecal methotrexate in the one randomized study that has been conducted

RECOMMENDATIONS FOR SUPPORTIVE CARE

- Antiemetics usually not required

PHARMACY ISSUES

- Elliott's B solution (artificial CSF) or normal saline is the preferred diluent

NURSING CONSIDERATIONS

- Weekly blood counts
- Fluid should be withdrawn and administered slowly (< 1 ml/min) to avoid rapid fluid shifts in brain
- The manufacturer recommends wearing gloves when handling solutions of thiotepa because of incidence of skin rash after exposure
- Reconstituted solutions of thiotepa are hazy and must be filtered with a pore size of 0.22 mcg; if precipitate remains after filtration the solution should *not* be used
- Avoid contamination; use strict aseptic technique
- Assess
  - baseline neurologic status
  - access site for signs of infection
- Teach patient
  - to remain supine for 30 min following the procedure
  - acute complications, which could include nausea, vomiting, fever, headache, and rigidity of neck; usually they subside within 72 hrs
  - report unusual symptoms

KEY REFERENCE

Strong JM, Collins JM, Lester C, Poplack DG: Pharmacokinetics of intraventricular and intravenous N,N′, N″-thiethylenethiophosphoramide in rhesus monkeys and humans. Cancer Res 1986; 46:6101–04

Drug: Cytarabine

Robert L. Capizzi and Corinne Haviley

OTHER NAMES: ARA-C, CYTOSINE ARABINOSIDE, CYTOSAR

USES

- Approved for intrathecal use as prevention and treatment of meningeal leukemia

MECHANISM OF ACTION

- Antimetabolite
- Its intracellular metabolite, Ara-CTP, is incorporated into DNA

DOSING

- For leukemic meningitis, 30 mg/m^2 ara-C is given by direct intrathecal injection q4d
- The number of doses given is based on the severity of the leukemic meningitis
- When given intrathecally, ara-C should be dissolved in preservative-free physiologic saline solution. The product diluent containing benzyl alcohol should not be used

PHARMACOKINETICS

- The major mechanism for systemic clearance is via hepatic metabolism by cytidine deaminase forming the inactive nucleoside, ara-U

NURSING CONSIDERATIONS

- Diluent provided in the container *should not* be used (it is benzyl alcohol preserved); use sodium chloride USP (unpreserved) or Ringer's injection USP (unpreserved)
- Avoid contamination; use strict aseptic technique
- Risk of serious neurologic toxicity is less with cytarabine than with methotrexate
- Assess
  - baseline neurologic status
  - for acute arachnoiditis (most common toxic reaction): headaches, back pain, nuchal rigidity, and fever
  - access site for signs of infection
- Teach patient
  - to remain supine for 30 min following the procedure
  - acute complications, which could include nausea, vomiting, fever, headache, and rigidity of neck; usually they subside within 72 hrs
  - report unusual symptoms

KEY REFERENCES

Band PR, Holland JF, Bernard J, et al.: Treatment of central nervous system leukemia with intrathecal cytosine arabinoside. Cancer 1973; 32(4):744–8

Wang JJ, Pratt CB: Intrathecal arabinosyl cytosine in meningeal leukemia. Cancer 1970; 25(3):531–4

Intraplegural Therapy: Introduction

John C. Ruckdeschel

WHICH PATIENTS TO TREAT?

- Minimal symptoms; don't wait for significant respiratory compromise
- Reasonable prognosis; patients should have a life expectancy such that a 3–4 day hospitalization is not a significant burden
- Disease not likely to respond systematically
  - lymphoma, small cell lung cancer may only need systemic chemotherapy after a thoracentesis
  - moderately responsive tumors such as breast and ovarian cancers may respond to therapy after a thoracentesis but should be watched closely
  - most solid tumors will require intrapleural therapy

WHICH APPROACH TO DRAINAGE?

- Thoracoscopy is far and away the best procedure for assuring loculations are lysed and lung is reexpanded
  - costly and requires anesthesia/surgery
- Large-bore chest tube is the standard of care
  - maximizes lung reexpansion
  - can be inserted at bedside
- Soft catheter drainage
  - reasonable for free-flowing effusions in mildly symptomatic patients
  - can be adapted for outpatient usage
  - pleuro-peritoneal pumps work occasionally but clog frequently and are hard for the patient to use for any prolonged period

PLEURODESIS ITSELF

- The lung must be reexpanded
- Volume of drainage often said to have to be < 150–250 cc/24 hrs (or equivalent) before pleurodesis but no hard data
- Patient repositioning often done, but again little evidence that this adds anything
- When minimal loculations present, an attempt at urokinase injection may allow full lung expansion
- Systemic or intrapleural narcotic medications will relieve pain for most patients
- Intrapleural topical anesthetics also frequently used
- Drainage again needs to be < 250 cc/24 hrs when chest tube pulled

WHICH AGENT TO USE?

- Talc poudrage (blown into chest cavity at thoracoscopy) probably the most effective but enormously more costly
- Talc slurry by chest tube popular but a disturbing incidence of ARDS afterward
- May be as effective as talc poudrage
- Bleomycin
  - good efficacy but high unit cost for drug
- Doxycycline
  - mediocre efficacy but low unit cost of drug
  - need for repeat therapy often raises overall costs
- Others
  - interleukins, interferon, BCG, mitomycin, and nitrogen mustard all reported but none as frequently as above agents

KEY REFERENCE

Ruckdeschel JC: Management of malignant pleural effusions. Semin Oncol 1995; 22(2 suppl 3):58–63

Drug: Bleomycin (Intrapleural)

John C. Ruckdeschel and Heidi Downey

OTHER NAMES: BLENOXANE, BLEO, BLM

USES

- Approved by FDA for treatment of malignant pleural effusion by intrapleural route
- Also used for peritoneal or pericardial effusions

MECHANISM OF ACTION

- Purported to cause inflammatory pleurodesis but little clinical or animal evidence thereof

DOSING

- Usual dose is 60 U in 100 ml normal saline via chest or catheter with the tube held vertical for 1–2 min
- Patient empirically placed in multiple positions to provide contact with all portions of pleura
- Therapy may be repeated once, but multiple injections are not recommended

PHARMACOKINETICS

- ~45% of an intrapleural dose can reach the circulation
- Half-life in pleural space ~3 hrs
- Absorbed bleomycin is renally excreted (60–70%) and has a half-life of 2–4 hrs
- Half-life extended significantly in patients with impaired renal function

TOXICITY

- Intrapleural: common
  - fever, mild to moderate pain, nausea, local wound infection
- Intrapleural: uncommon
  - anaphylactic reactions, fluid retention, rash, diarrhea
- Systemic (45% of dose absorbed)
  - skin reactions (pruritus, hyperpigmentation, edema, erythema, thick nail beds, mucositis, alopecia)
  - anorexia
  - interstitial pneumonitis (dose related)
  - hypotension, pain at injection site, fever and chills during infusion
  - myelosuppression
  - thrombotic microangiopathy, MI, CVA (rare)
  - allergy, anaphylaxis (1%)

RECOMMENDATIONS FOR SUPPORTIVE CARE

- Lung needs to be fully reinflated in order for pleurodesis to be effective
- Acetaminophen can be given before or after procedure for fever
- Parenteral morphine (10 mg or equivalent) can be given 30 min prior to treatment
- 25 cc of 2% lidocaine can be injected into the pleural space prior to the bleomycin
- Antiemetics rarely needed
- Medications and equipment to manage an anaphylactic reaction should be readily accessible

PHARMACY ISSUES

- Intact vials stored in refrigerator; reconstituted solution stable for 1 mo if refrigerated, 2 wks at room temperature
- Normal saline is the preferred diluent
- Should not be mixed with solutions containing divalent or trivalent cations (especially copper) due to chelation problems
- Inactivated by hydrogen peroxide, compounds containing sulfhydryl groups and ascorbic acid

NURSING CONSIDERATIONS

- Emergency meds and equipment should be available
- Encourage fluids, Tylenol for fever, chills
- Patients having previous radiation treatment to the lungs or with a history of COPD are at increased risk of complications
- Instillation may be very painful; premedicate with analgesics prior to and for 24–48 hrs after procedure
- Following slurry administration (see previous section), the patient should be positioned (supine, prone, sitting, left and right lateral decutitus) to ensure uniform distribution of the sclerosing agent
- Chest tubes should remain clamped as long as the patient can tolerate or as ordered
- Amount of sclerosing agent returned following the unclamping of the chest tube should be noted on the drainage system and in the nurse's notes
- Patients having previous radiation treatment to the lungs or with a history of COPD are at increased risk for toxicities
- Assess
  - monitor for hypersensitivity reaction
  - for signs of pulmonary toxicity: shortness of breath, wheezing, rash, shaking chills, and/or new onset fever
- Teach patient
  - management of intrapleural device; dressing change
  - to report acute onset of chest pain and/or fever

KEY REFERENCES

Ruckdeschel JC, Moores D, Lee JY, et al.: Intrapleural therapy for malignant pleural effusions: a randomized comparison of bleomycin and tetracycline. Chest 1991; 100(6):1528–35

Schafers SJ, Dresler CM: Update on talc, bleomycin, and the tetracyclines in the treatment of malignant pleural effusions. Pharmacotherapy 1995; 15:228–34

Intraperitoneal Chemotherapy: Introduction

Maurie Markman

USES

■ Recognized as a rational therapeutic strategy for small-volume residual ovarian cancer (initial chemotherapy, second-line treatment, consolidation)
■ Employed in experimental trials as adjuvant therapy of gastric cancer, high-risk colon cancer
■ Examined as treatment of peritoneal mesothelioma following maximal surgical resection in the presence of minimal residual macroscopic or microscopic disease only

RATIONALE

■ Increase exposure of tumor present within the peritoneal cavity to active cytotoxic and biologic antineoplastic agents
■ Strategy most appropriate for those drugs whose antineoplastic activity against the tumor types in question (ovarian, colon, gastric cancers, mesothelioma) has been demonstrated to be enhanced by increasing either the concentration (concept of "dose intensity") or duration (cycle-specific drugs) of exposure

PHASE 1 TRIALS

■ Multiple drugs have been examined for their safety and phamacokinetic advantage following intraperitoneal delivery
■ Examples (pharmacokinetic advantage for peritoneal cavity compared to systemic exposure)
- cisplatin/carboplatin (10–20 fold)
- 5-fluorouracil (200-fold)
- methotrexate (90-fold)
- doxorubicin (300-fold)
- paclitaxel (1,000-fold)
- interferon-alfa (100-fold)

TOXICITY

■ Dose-limiting toxicity determined by drug(s) being administered into the cavity
- cisplatin/carboplatin (dose-limiting toxicity: systemic effects of agent; minimal abdominal discomfort or risk of adhesion formation)
- doxorubicin (dose-limiting toxicity: severe abdominal pain/adhesion formation)
- paclitaxel (dose-limiting toxicity: abdominal pain)

■ Risk of complications of drug administration
- infection
- bowel perforation with catheter placement

■ Risk of unique toxicities for drugs administered into the peritoneal cavity not observed with systemic delivery

METHOD OF ADMINISTRATION

■ Indwelling surgically placed semipermanent catheter or percutaneous catheter placement with each treatment
■ Generally delivered in 1–2 L treatment volume, without need to recover instilled fluid following treatment

THEORETICAL OBJECTIONS TO CONCEPT OF INTRAPERITONEAL ANTINEOPLASTIC THERAPY

■ Inability to deliver antineoplastic agents adequately throughout the peritoneal cavity
■ Decreased delivery of the drug to tumor by "capillary flow" through entry into the vascular compartment

KEY REFERENCES

Alberts D, et al.: Intraperitoneal cisplatin plus intravenous cyclophosphamide versus intravenous cisplatin plus intravenous cyclophosphamide for stage III ovarian cancer. N Engl J Med 1996; 335:1950–5

Markman M: Is there a role for intraperitoneal therapy in the management of gastrointestinal malignancies? Cancer Invest 1995; 13:625–8

Markman M: Intraperitoneal therapy of ovarian cancer. Semin Oncol 1998; 25:356–60

Drug: Cisplatin (Intraperitoneal)

Maurie Markman and Susan Budds

USES

- Initial therapy of ovarian cancer with small-volume residual disease (microscopic or largest residual tumor mass ≤0.5 cm in maximum diameter) following surgical cytoreduction
- Second-line therapy with small-volume residual disease (as above) following a documented response to initial systemic platinum-based treatment
- Consolidation therapy following attainment of a surgically documented complete response in patients with stage III–IV high-grade tumors (ultimate risk of relapse > 50%)
- Rationale
  - increase exposure to cisplatin of cancer present within the peritoneal cavity
  - maintain maximal safe delivery of cisplatin to tumor by capillary flow

DOSING

- Cisplatin administered intraperitoneally at a dose of 100 mg/m^2 in 1–2 L of normal saline
- Cisplatin has also been given intraperitoneally at a dose of 200 mg/m^2 along with systemic sodium thioulfate for nephroprotection (this "high-dose" therapeutic strategy remains experimental)
- Treatment delivery options
  - paracentesis catheter inserted at time of each course
  - indwelling Tenckhoff catheter
  - Tenckhoff catheter attached to SubQ portal delivery device
  - therapy can be repeated on a q3–4wk schedule with a maximum of 6 courses (based on prior experience with intraperitoneal cisplatin)

PHARMACOKINETICS

- Peak peritoneal concentration of free reactive cisplatin ~20-fold higher than found in the systemic compartment
- AUC for cisplatin exposure to peritoneal cavity 10-fold higher than the systemic circulation
- ~70% of cisplatin administered by the intraperitoneal route reaches the systemic compartment as reactive drug

TOXICITY

- Major side effects are from drug entering systemic compartment, producing usual cisplatin toxicities (nephrotoxicity, neurotoxicity, emesis)
- Intraperitoneal delivery of cisplatin should not be considered as a method to reduce systemic toxicities of the agent
- Local toxicity is generally limited to mild abdominal discomfort (from abdominal distention)
- Intraperitoneal adhesion formation can occur and subsequent bowel obstruction rarely encountered
- Risk of intraperitoneal infection and bowel perforation associated with catheter placement and manipulation (risk reduced with surgical placement of indwelling catheter with SubQ portal delivery system)

RECOMMENDATIONS FOR SUPPORTIVE CARE

- Use standard IV hydration regimen for cisplatin when delivered systemically at a dose of 100 mg/m^2
- Use standard antiemetic regimen for cisplatin (serotonin receptor antagonists plus dexamethasone)

PHARMACY ISSUES

- Deliver cisplatin in 1–2 L of normal saline

NURSING CONSIDERATIONS

- Pre- and postdrug hydration: monitor intake and output
- Administration of diuretics: mannitol and lasix
- Position patient in a semi-Flower's position
- Use aseptic technique to prevent catheter tunnel infection and peritonitis; infection more likely to be related to connection and disconnection (refer to earlier section for specifics of intraperitoneal therapy)
- When infusion is complete, clamp tubing for prescribed dwell time; encourage repositioning from side to side
- Clamp tubing on drainage bag after fluid has drained (usually 30 min–2 hrs) and flush catheter with nonbacteriostatic sterile saline; if using a port follow with heparinized saline
- Myelosuppression is most likely; monitor CBC, WBC, and platelet counts
- Assess
  - alterations in nutrition due to nausea and vomiting
  - catheter or port patency; assess for signs of infection
  - consider baseline audiogram; monitor for hearing loss
  - neurologic status baseline and during treatment for peripheral neuropathy
  - kidney functions, baseline and during therapy
- Teach patient
  - maintenance and care of catheter or port; patients with external catheters may require initial supervision by a home health agency
  - to report signs of infection: fever, inflammation, abdominal pain, diarrhea, and respiratory distress
  - report numbness and tingling in fingers and toes, difficulty holding a pen or buttoning clothes; reassurance that symptoms are temporary

KEY REFERENCES

Alberts D, et al.: Intraperitoneal cisplatin plus intravenous cyclophosphamide versus intravenous cisplatin plus intravenous cyclophosphamide for stage III ovarian cancer. N Engl J Med 1996; 335:1950–5

Markman M: Intraperitoneal therapy of ovarian cancer. Semin Oncol 1998; 25:356–60

Markman M, et al.: Responses to second-line cisplatin-based intraperitoneal therapy in ovarian cancer: influence of a prior response to intravenous cisplatin. J Clin Oncol 1991; 9:1801–5

Hepatic Arterial Chemotherapy (HAI): Introduction

Nancy E. Kemeny

INDICATIONS FOR HAI

- Treatment of established hepatic metastases from colorectal carcinoma
- Possible value in adjuvant therapy after liver resection

AVAILABLE AGENTS

- FUDR
- FU
- Mitomycin C

ROUTES OF ADMINISTRATION

- Via surgically implanted SubQ reservoir (port) or pump
- Advantages over systemic administration
  - ease of drug administration
  - less systemic toxicity
  - response rate higher: 50–70%
  - possibility that survival may be better
  - randomized studies so far have been flawed by being too small or allowing a crossover
  - a new study by CALGB is currently asking whether HAI increases survival over systemic therapy
- Disadvantages over systemic administration
  - cost and need for surgery
  - adverse events from catheter complications and possible biliary sclerosis

THERAPEUTIC APPROACH TO PATIENT WITH ESTABLISHED LIVER METASTASES

- Early diagnosis and surgical resection if possible
- Overall evaluation to assess prognostic factors and determine how aggressively the patient is to be treated
- If unresectable, disease-regional therapy HAI or systemic or a combination of the two modalities
  - good prognostic factors include
    - □ less than two metastases
    - □ nonsynchronous disease
    - □ no evidence of extrahepatic disease
    - □ normal LDH and normal CEA
    - □ Dukes B at the time of the primary

TOXICITY

- No myelosuppression, nausea, vomiting, and diarrhea. If diarrhea does occur, shunting to the bowel should be suspected
- Hepatobiliary toxicity
  - ischemic and inflammatory effect on the bile ducts, since bile ducts derive their blood supply from the hepatic artery and are therefore perfused
  - biliary toxicity manifests as elevations of SGOT, alk phos, and bilirubin
  - in the early stages of toxicity, hepatic enzyme elevation will return to normal when the drug is withdrawn and the patient is given a rest period; in more advanced cases it does not resolve
  - if jaundice does not resolve, an endoscopic retrograde cholangiopancreatograph (ERCP) may demonstrate lesions resembling idiopathic sclerosing cholangitis in 5–29%
  - sonograms usually do not show dilation
  - strictures may be more focal at the hepatic duct bifurcation
  - drainage procedures either by ERCP or by transhepatic cholangiogram may be helpful
  - close monitoring of liver function tests is necessary to avoid the biliary complications
  - if the serum bilirubin becomes 3 mg/dl or higher, no further treatment should be given

ULCER DISEASE

- Gastritis or ulcers may appear due to inadvertent perfusion of the stomach and duodenum drug via small collateral branches from the hepatic artery

COMPLICATIONS OF HEPATIC ARTERY INFUSION PUMP PLACEMENT AND USE

- Incomplete or extrahepatic perfusion
- The postoperative Tc^{99} macroaggregated albumin perfusion scan, when compared with the liver scan, can demonstrate incomplete or exhepation perfusion from the left gastric artery
- It may be possible to embolize an accessory vessel to get rid of extrahepatic perfusion
- A common technical error during catheter insertion is placing the catheter too far from the junction of the gastroduodenal artery and hepatic artery, which may lead to increased drug exposure

APPROACHES TO DECREASE HEPATIC TOXICITY

- Dexamethasone (Dex)
- Circadian modification
- Alternate HAI FUDR with hepatic arterial 5-FU

RECOMMENDATIONS

- Care must be taken to monitor liver function tests
- With even the slightest elevations in alkphos, SGOT, or bilirubin, doses must be adjusted
- Liver function tests should be drawn q2wks to evaluate these problems

KEY REFERENCES

Fong Y, Kemeny N, Paty P, et al.: Treatment of colorectal cancer: hepatic metastasis. Semin Surg Oncol 1996; 12(4):219–52

Kemeny NE: Regional chemotherapy of colorectal cancer. Eur J Cancer 1995; 31A(7–9):1271–6

Kemeny N, Huang Y, Cohen AM, et al.: Hepatic arterial infusion of chemotherapy after resection of hepatic metastases from colorectal cancer. N Engl J Med 1999; 341(27): 2039–48

Drug: Floxuridine (FUDR, 5-fluoro-2'-deoxyuridine)

Nancy E. Kemeny and Hollie Devine

USES

- Metastatic colorectal cancer
  - sometimes used as adjuvant treatment after curative resection
- Primary hepatobiliary cancer
- Intraperitoneal therapy

MECHANISM OF ACTION

- Pyrimidine analogue
- Thymidylate synthase indicator
- Inhibition of TS leads to a depletion of dTTP, thus interfering with DNA synthesis and repair
- Overexpression of TS results in drug resistance

PHARMACOKINETICS

- Cytotoxicity is dose and time dependent
- First-pass extraction of FUDR by the normal liver is approximately 95%; the first pass of FU, 20–50%
- Often more effective when given by prolonged infusion
- Smaller doses of FUDR need to be used when given by prolonged infusion
- Toxicity usually limited to rapidly dividing tissues (e.g., GI mucosa and bone marrow)

DOSING

- Administration is best achieved with the use of a pump to overcome pressure in large arteries and ensure a uniform rate of infusion.
  - therapeutic dose by continuous arterial infusion is 0.1–0.6 mg/kg/d
  - 0.16/kg × pump volume ÷ flow rate dose for 2 weeks if given by internal pump or 0.16 mg/kg × 14 days if given by external pump
  - dose should be combined with 20 mg dexamethasone per sterile FUDR package insert (Roche Pharmaceuticals)
- *Supplied:*
  - 500 mg sterile FUDR powder in 5-ml vial. This is to be reconstituted with 5 ml sterile water for injection (SWFI)
- *Dose and Administration:*
  - each vial must be reconstituted with 5 ml SWFI to yield solution containing approx 100 mg of FUDR/ml. The calculated daily dose is then diluted with 5% dextrose or 0.9% NaCl to a volume appropriate for the infusion apparatus to be used

NURSING CONSIDERATIONS

- Administration
  - evaluate catheter patency
    - □ after surgically placed pump, patency evaluated by intra-arterial injection of fluorescein dye
    - □ on postoperative days 4–6 and before chemotherapy, as well as every 3 months, obtain a radionuclide angiography with ^{99m}technetium macro-aggregated albumin to ensure there is no misperfusion and to assess the adequacy of whole liver perfusion
  - intrahepatic administration
    - □ withdrawing blood samples from arterial site is not recommended because of high pressure system within artery and chance for clotting
    - □ ensure free flowing infusion to assess blood return
    - □ administered by continuous intra-arterial infusion via a surgically implantable infusion pump for hepatic arterial chemotherapy
  - to alleviate or prevent epigastric distress, administer cimetidine 300 mg po qid or Zantac 150 mg po bid
  - to prevent sclerosing cholangitis, consider adding 0.3–0.5 mg/d dexamethasone concomitantly with FUDR
- Assessment/Management
  - monitor LFTs. To determine if FUDR dose modification is necessary, compare the reference value to either the value obtained on the day pump was emptied or the value obtained on day of planned pump filling. See recommended dose modifications in table below.
  - for signs of biliary sclerosis: jaundice, pruritis, right upper quadrant pain
  - diarrhea management: give IVFs, bismuth subsalicyclate, Kaolin with pectin, psyllium or loperamide hydrochloride
- Teach patient
  - procedural complications with insertion of an arterial catheter
  - FUDR side effects: nausea/vomiting, epigastric burning, abd pain/cramping, diarrhea, sudden/gradual lack of appetite, drowsiness/fatigue
  - home management: record stool character, frequency, cramping, fluid intake, antidiarrheal medications
  - pump teaching:
    - □ pamphlet or information about pump
    - □ demonstration of pump
    - □ reinforce little change in lifestyle. Resume ADLs as incision from pump placement heals. Restrict activity that may cause blunt trauma to pump pocket
    - □ avoid activity that may cause prolonged changes in body temperature, pressure, altitude changes, which could change flow rate.

KEY REFERENCES

Cozzi E, Hagle M, McGregor ML, Woodhouse D: Nursing management of patients receiving hepatic arterial chemotherapy through an implanted infusion pump. Cancer Nursing 1984; 7(3):229–34

Kemeny NE: Regional chemotherapy of colorectal cancer. Eur J Cancer 1995; 31A:1271–6

Kemeny N: The Venook article reviewed. Oncol 1997; 11(7):962, 964, 970

Lanning RM, von Roemeling R, Hrushesky W: Circadian-based infusional FUDR therapy. Oncology Nursing Forum 1990; 17(1):49–56

Venook AP: Update on hepatic-arterial chemotherapy. Oncol 1997; 11(7):947–57, 970

SGOT reference value*	≤50 μ/L	>50 μ/L	FUDR dose
SGOT at pump emptying or day of planned treatment (whichever higher)	0 – <3 × reference	0 – <2 × reference	100%
	3 – <4 × reference	2 – <3 × reference	80%
	4 – <5 × reference	3 – <4 × reference	50%
	≥5 × reference	≥4 × reference	Hold
Alk phos reference value*	**≤90 μ/L**	**>90 μ/L**	**FUDR dose**
Alk phos at pump emptying or day of planned treatment (whichever is higher)	0 – <1.5 × reference	0 – <1.2 × reference	100%
	1.5 – <2 × reference	1.2 – <1.5 × reference	50%
	≤2 × reference	≥1.5 × reference	Hold
Bilirubin reference value*	**≤1.2 mg/dL**	**>1.2 mg/dL**	**FUDR dose**
Bilirubin at pump emptying or day of planned treatment (whichever is higher)	0 – <1.5 × reference	0 – <1.2 × reference	100%
	1.5 – <2 × reference	1.2 – <1.5 × reference	50%
	≥2 × reference	≥1.5 × reference	Hold

*Reference value = value obtained on day patient received last FUDR dose.

Drug: Mitomycin C (Intrahepatic)

Nancy E. Kemeny and Deborah Berg

MECHANISM OF ACTION

- Antibiotic isolated from the broth of *Streptomyces caespitosus*

DOSING

- 10 mg/m2 IA or IV q4wks × 2 then q6wks
- Higher doses IA produced a higher biliary sclerosis rate

PHARMACOKINETICS

- Inhibits the synthesis of deoxyribonucleic acid (DNA)
- Clearance is effected primarily by metabolism in the liver, but metabolism occurs in other tissues as well

TOXICITY

- Thrombocytopenia and/or leukopenia
- May be delayed to 8 wks after therapy
- Necrosis and consequent sloughing of tissue if the drug is extravasated during injection
- Hepatic increased alkaline phosphatase and transaminases biliary sclerosis

RECOMMENDATIONS FOR SUPPORTIVE CARE

- Premedicate with dexamethasone

PHARMACY ISSUES

- Heparin 10,000 U should be placed in pump reservoir with each refill

NURSING CONSIDERATIONS

- Dose modifications are based on WBC and platelet counts, thus need to closely monitor CBC
- Monitor renal function prior to each dose. Hold dose if serum creatinine > 1.7 mg/dl
- Premedication with serotonin antagonist indicated as is post-therapy antiemetic for delayed nausea
- If extravasation occurs, stop infusion immediately and follow hospital policy
- Assess
  - renal function for signs and symptoms of renal failure/hemolytic uremic syndrome
  - pulmonary function for signs and symptoms of interstitial pneumoitis and ARDS
  - for potential for injury related to veno-occlusive disease of liver in ABMT pts
- Teach patient
  - expected side effects and self-care measures
  - importance of birth control measures

KEY REFERENCES

Atiq OT, Kemeny N, Niedzwiecki D, et al.: Treatment of unresectable primary liver cancer with intrahepatic fluorodeoxyuridine and mitomycin C through an implantable pump. Cancer 1992; 69(4):920–4

Kemeny N, Cohen A, Seiter K, et al.: Randomized trial of hepatic arterial floxuridine, mitomycin, and carmustine versus floxuridine alone in previously treated patients with liver metastases from colorectal cancer. J Clin Oncol 1993; 11(2):330–5

Schneider A, Kemeny N, Chapman D, et al.: Intrahepatic mitomycin C as a salvage treatment for patients with hepatic metastases from colorectal carcinoma. Cancer 1989; 64(11):2203–6

Intra-Arterial Chemotherapy: Introduction

Robert A. Weisman and Hollie Devine

RATIONALE

- Intra-arterial infusion achieves capillary (tumor bed) concentrations up to 2,500 times that achieved by IV infusion
- "Supradose" drug delivery may overcome drug resistance
- Selectivity can be further enhanced
  - can be combined with systemic neutralizing agents or chemoprotectants
  - can be administered by selective angiography to minimize dosing of normal tissues
  - the percentage of the tumor's blood supply from each vessel is estimated by the radiologist and used to calculate the amount of drug to be delivered through each selective or superselective arterial catheter

KEY REFERENCES

Kerber CW, Wong WH, Howell SB, Hanchett K, Robbins KT: An organ-preserving selective arterial chemotherapy strategy for head and neck cancer. Am J Neuroradiol 1998; 19(5):935–41

Thompson JF, Kam PC, Waugh RC, Harman CR: Isolated limb infusion with cytotoxic agents: a simple alternative to isolated limb perfusion. Semin Surg Oncol 1998; 14(3):238–47

Weisman RA, Christen RD, Jones VE, Kerber CW, Seagren SL, Orloff LA, Glassmeyer SL, Howell SB, Robbins KT: Observations on control of N2 and N3 neck disease in squamous cell carcinoma of the head and neck by intra-arterial chemoradiation. Laryngoscope 1998; 108(6):800–5

Drug: Cisplatin (Intra-Arterial)

Robert A. Weisman and Hollie Devine

OTHER NAMES: CIS-PLATINUM, PLATINOL, CIS-DIAMMINEDI-CHLOROPLATINUM (II)

USES

- Squamous cell carcinoma of the head and neck (highly effective when given with concurrent radiation)
- Has been used in Japan for hepatic tumors, and similar strategy has been used for ovarian cancers (intraperitoneal rather than intra-arterial)

MECHANISM OF ACTION

- Intra-arterial infusion achieves capillary (tumor bed) concentrations up to 2,500 times that achieved by IV infusion
- "Supradose" drug delivery may overcome drug resistance
- Weekly dosing at high levels yields a high "dose-intensity" treatment (150 mg/m^2/wk)
- Due to the high dose of cisplatin, must be given with the neutralizing agent sodium thiosulfate (administered IV when starting the cisplatin infusion)
- Sodium thiosulfate binds to cisplatin in serum only (not intracellularly), forming an inactive compound that is excreted in the urine

DOSING

- Prehydration and prophylactic antiemetic therapy begun 24 hrs prior to planned treatment on an inpatient basis, as for high-dose IV cisplatin
- Cisplatin 150 mg/m^2 weekly for 4 wks
- Prior to drug administration, an interventional radiologist performs transfemoral angiography and demonstrates the tumor's dominant blood supply (up to 2 vessels for well-lateralized lesions, 4 vessels for midline lesions with significant bilateral blood supply)
  - the percentage of the tumor's blood supply from each vessel is estimated by the radiologist and used to calculate the amount of cisplatin to be delivered through each selective or superselective arterial catheter
- Sodium thiosulfate 9 g dissolved in 200 ml distilled water is given by IV push over 15–20 min starting concurrent with intra-arterial infusion of cisplatin (given via a high-speed pump, 1–2 ml/sec—total infusion time 2–3 min)
- Sodium thiosulfate administration is continued at a dose of 12 g/m^2 dissolved in 1 L of distilled water infused at 167 ml/hr over the next 6 hrs
- Cisplatin can be held for up to 2 wks for grade III or IV toxicity
- Radiation commences within 24 hrs of first cisplatin dose, continues 5 days/wk, 200 cGy every day for 6–7 wks (i.e., concurrent with cisplatin)

PHARMACOKINETICS

- After initial pass through the tumor, cisplatin distributed similar to IV dosing (minus the amount neutralized by sodium thiosulfate)
- Peak intracellular concentration at 48–72 hrs

TOXICITY

- Similar to IV cisplatin
- Mucositis common with concurrent radiation (45% require long-term feeding tube)
- Nephrotoxicity, neurotoxicity, and ototoxicity uncommon, usually grade 1
- Myelosuppression uncommon; neutropenia can be supported with GCSF
- Nausea, vomiting, diarrhea usually well controlled with hydration and prophylactic antiemetics and antidiarrheals as needed

RECOMMENDATIONS FOR SUPPORTIVE CARE

- Antiemetics
- Prehydration (to limit nephrotoxicity)
- Prophylaxis with dexamethasone 4 mg IV or po started the evening before treatment and continued q6h until the morning after treatment is useful to limit tumor swelling, especially when tumor involves upper airway
- Facial edema associated with this therapy is also reduced
- PEG tube should be discussed and strongly recommended prior to treatment
- "Mucositis mix" (Benadryl, Maalox, lidocaine viscous) or other topical anesthetics helpful for anticipated mucositis

PHARMACY ISSUES

- Cisplatin dose is dissolved in normal saline to a concentration of 1mg/ml

NURSING CONSIDERATIONS

- Refer to earlier section for specifics of intra-arterial infusion therapy
- Obtain baseline CBC, platelet count, BUN, creatinine, 24 hr creatinine clearance, serum electrolytes, and audiogram
- Vigorous hydration prior to and after therapy; ensure adquate intake and output; monitor urine output to ensure a flow of 100 cc/hr, if < 100 cc/hr consider administration of Lasix
- Considerations should be given to the administration of cytoprotectants such as amifostine against nephrotoxicity, neurotoxicity, hematologic toxicity, radiation-induced toxicity
- Premedicate with corticosteroids and antihistamines to prevent anaphylaxis
- Take precaution to avoid cisplatin errors; cisplatin overdose can cause renal failure, hepatic failure, ocular toxicity, myelosuppression, severe nausea and vomiting, neuritis and death
- Drawing blood samples from arterial line is not recommended because of high-pressure system within artery and chance for clotting
- Although not a vesicant, if extravasation occurs stop infusion and remove IV tubing from Huber needle and aspirate any drug left in port reservoir; follow institutional guidelines
- Drug interactions
  - ototoxicity increased if given with loop diuretics
  - renal toxicity increased when given with aminoglycosides
  - cisplatin decreases effect of phenytoin; therefore dose of phenytoin may need to be increased; monitor phenytoin levels
- Assess
  - nausea/vomiting: administer antiemetics prior to therapy and continue for 24 hrs
  - for signs of anaphylaxis: facial edema, wheezing, tachycardia, hypotension; emergency medications should be accessible
  - monitor serum electrolytes for need to supplement
  - baseline neurologic status and during therapy; consider physical therapy for peripheral neuropathy
- Teach patient
  - demonstration and written information regarding management and care of port
  - association of transient fertility effects; consider sperm banking; a minimum of 2 yrs after treatment should elapse before considering childbearing
  - self-administration of antiemetics; encourage fluid intake by 3 L and food intake of colorless and odorless meals
  - expected side effects and self-care measures
  - report numbness and tingling or changes in hearing

KEY REFERENCES

Robbins KT, Vocario D, Murry T, Weisman R, Gold RA, Seagren SL: A novel organ preservation treatment protocol for advanced head and neck cancer. Otolaryngol Head Neck Surg 1994; 111:157–63

Weisman RA, Christen R, Los G, Kerber C, Seagren S, Glassmeyer S, Orloff LA, Wong W, Kirmani S, Howell S: Phase I trial of retinoic acid and cis-platinum for advanced squamous cell cancer of the head and neck based on experimental evidence of drug synergism. Otolaryngol Head Neck Surg 1998; 118:597–602

Intravesical Therapy: Introduction

Gary D. Steinberg

OVERVIEW

- ~70% of all newly diagnosed transitional cell carcinomas of the urinary bladder are superficial in depth of penetration, i.e., Ta (papillary), Tcis (carcinoma in situ), and T1 (lamina propria invasion)
- ~50–70% of patients will have tumor recurrences and 30–50% of patients will have progression of bladder cancer to higher stage or grade

GOALS

- Adjunctive, prophylactic, and therapeutic treatment (i.e., eliminates carcinoma in situ, superficial unresectable disease, and/or prevents recurrences)
- Decision to use intravesical therapy is based on a particular patient's bladder cancer diathesis and risks of disease progression and recurrence

CHOICE OF DRUG

- No single best drug exists; factors such as toxicity, systemic absorption, and efficacy are important
- Intravesical chemotherapy may be best for Ta grade I tumors
- The optimal treatment schedule for intravesical therapy is unknown
- Short-term courses may be equally as effective as multiple doses given over a long period of time

MECHANISM OF ACTION

- Urothelial: drug contact is necessary
- Chemotherapy requires that the agents are absorbed into cancer cells to arrest cellular division or cell growth
- Drug concentration and dwell time in the bladder is important
- Systemic absorption should be minimal to avoid systemic toxicity
- Immunotherapy (BCG) also requires direct contact and binding to the fibronectin receptors of the abnormal urothelium to create local immune or inflammatory response that may not be bladder cancer specific

KEY REFERENCE

Sarosdy, MF: Principles of intravesical chemotherapy and immunotherapy. Urol Clin North Am 1992; 19(3):509–19

Drug: Bacillus Calmette-Guerin (BCG)

Gary D. Steinberg and Patricia Tiller

USES

- Approved by FDA for transitional cell (TCC) carcinoma in situ (CIS) of the urinary bladder
- "Front-line" agent for prophylaxis of superficial papillary TCC tumor recurrence in the bladder
- Also used for treatment of unresected superficial TCC in the bladder
- Prophylaxis of upper tract superficial TCC is possible, but more difficult
- Most efficacious intravesical agent with 70% 5 yr disease-free rates in CIS
- Disease-free rate decreases to 30% at 10 yrs

MECHANISM OF ACTION

- Attenuated strain of *Mycobacterium bovis* that has stimulatory effects on immune responses
- Induces inflammatory response with production of various cytokines, including tumor necrosis factor, interferon gamma, and interleukin-2
- Possible creation of anti–bladder cancer immunity, via humoral and cellular immune systems
- BCG must adhere to bladder tumor and basal lamina via fibronectin receptors

DOSING

- Administered intravesically once weekly for 6 wks
- Retained in bladder for 2 hrs
- At least 10 million organisms in 50–75 cc of nonbacteriostatic saline are required
- Repeat 6 wk courses may be administered; however, recurrences after two 6 wk courses imply lack of BCG efficacy for particular patient

TOXICITY

- Bladder irritability, frequency, urgency, dysuria
- Hematuria, fever, malaise, nausea, chills, arthralgia, and pruritus
- BCG can cause systemic mycobacterium-like illness that can be life threatening
  - treatment is antituberculosus therapy with cycloserine and ethambutol in the acute setting and INH, pyridoxine, and rifampin for 3–6 mos afterward

NURSING CONSIDERATIONS

- Following instillation the patient should be repositioned q15min to ensure proper drug distribution
- Safe drug handling and hand washing
- Refer to earlier section for specifics of intravesical therapy
- Assess
  - for signs of systemic BCG toxicity: fever, malaise, and cough
  - for signs and symptoms of cystitis: assess urine volume, frequency, and hematuria
  - administer antispasmodics, urinary antiseptics, and NSAIDs as necessary
- Teach patient
  - strict hand washing and personal hygiene
  - drug will need to be retained in bladder for 2 hrs
  - encourage high fluid intake for 48 hrs post treatment
  - to disinfect urine for 6 hrs after drug instillation by adding undiluted bleach in equal volume to voided urine in toilet; urine should be allowed to stand in toilet for 15 min before flushing
  - to record daily temperature and to report short-term fever of 103°F or persistent fever of > 101°F for 2 days
  - report symptoms of malaise, cough, or blood in the urine

KEY REFERENCES

Giflione L: Home bacillus Calmette-Guerin therapy for the treatment of superficial bladder cancer. Home Healthcare Nurse 1991; 50–3

Lamm DL: Long term results of intravesical therapy for superficial bladder cancer. Urol Clin North Am 1992; 19:573–80

Drug: Thiotepa (Triethylenethiophosphoramide) (Intravesical)

Gary D. Steinberg and Patricia Tiller

USES

- Prophylaxis against superficial TCC bladder tumor recurrences especially grade 1
- Treatment of existing superficial tumors
- Less effective than BCG in CIS and prophylaxis
- Immediately after transurethral resection of superficial TCC tumors
- Long-term studies demonstrate minimal activity for preventing recurrence or progression of superficial TCC of the bladder

DOSING

- Intravesical instillation of either 30 mg in 30 cc of saline or 60 mg in 60 cc saline
- Should be retained in the bladder for 1–2 hrs once weekly for 6–8 wks

PHARMACOKINETICS

- Minimal systemic absorption when given intravesically; however, in patients with an extensively denuded bladder, thiotepa may be absorbed due to its small molecular size

TOXICITY

- Myelosuppression in 15–20%, typically granulocytopenia and thrombocytopenia
- Occasional cystitis

NURSING CONSIDERATIONS

- Refer to earlier section for specifics regarding administration of intravesical therapy, safe drug handling, and hand washing
- Drug has low molecular weight and propensity for vascular absorption; myelosuppression may develop; a CBC should be obtained before treatment
- Maximize contact area by repositioning patient at 15 min intervals
- Assess
  - for signs and symptoms of chemical cystitis
  - skin for bronzing, flaking, desquamation (although rare with intravesical doses)
- Teach patient
  - strict hand washing and personal hygiene
  - drug will need to be retained in bladder for 2 hrs for maximum effect
  - encourage high fluid intake after treatment
  - report urinary frequency, dysuria, or hematuria

KEY REFERENCES

Medical Research Council Working Party on Urologic Cancer, Subgroup on Superficial Bladder Cancer: The effect of intravesical thiotepa on tumor recurrence after endoscopic treatment of newly diagnosed superficial bladder cancer. A further report with long-term follow-up of the Medical Research Council's randomized trial. Br J Urol 1994; 73:632

Soloway MS, Ford KS: Thiotepa-induced myelosuppression: review of 670 bladder instillations. J Urol 1983; 130:889–91

Drug: Mitomycin C (Intravesical)

Gary D. Steinberg and Barbara Jensen

USES

- Prophylaxis against superficial TCC bladder tumor recurrences
- Treatment of existing superficial tumors
- Immediately after transurethral resection of superficial TCC tumors
- Treatment of CIS, as primary intravesical therapy or for CIS refractory to BCG
- More effective than thiotepa for high-grade superficial tumors
- Less effective for carcinoma in situ and superficial bladder cancer and much more expensive than BCG

DOSING

- 8 weekly intravesical instillations of 40 mg mitomycin C in 40 cc of saline or water followed by monthly maintenance therapy for 1 yr
- Dwell time in the bladder is 1–2 hrs

PHARMACOKINETICS

- Minimal systemic absorption from bladder surface

TOXICITY

- Chemical cystitis, mural calcification, skin rashes

NURSING CONSIDERATIONS

- Obtain urinalysis prior to treatment; note presence of bacteria, RBCs
- Dose range 20–40 mg; dilute to 1 mg/ml with sterile water; may substitute 1% lidocaine hydrochloride as diluent if chemical cystitis results from prior treatments (agent is expensive)
- Chemical cystitis/bladder irritability is the main side effect and can be treated with phenazopyridine hydrochloride, although often resolves without intervention
- Refer to earlier section for specifics regarding administration of intravesical therapy
- Oxybutynin may be prescribed for patients having difficulty holding urine for 2 hr dwell time; use cautiously in elderly patients
- Restrict fluid intake up to 8 hrs prior to treatment for less dilution of agent; increase fluid intake after treatment to flush bladder of remaining drug (up to 3–4 L in 24 hrs)
- Safe drug handling and hand washing
- Assess
  - for signs and symptoms of UTI: fever, chills
  - urine for presence of bacteria; if suspect obtain urine culture, consult physician for possible antibiotic therapy
  - for signs of allergic reactions with diffuse rash (systemic); contact dermatitis with palmar/genital rash more common
- Teach patient
  - drug will need to be retained in bladder for 2 hrs
  - importance of increasing fluid intake after treatment for 24 hrs and thereafter voiding q2–3hrs while awake
- signs and symptoms of UTI
- strict hand washing and personal hygiene
- abstinence from sexual activity or use of protective devices immediately post treatment

KEY REFERENCE

Soloway MS, Murphy WM, Defuria MD, et al.: The effect of mitomycin C on superficial bladder cancer. J Urol 1981; 125:646

Drug: Doxorubicin (Intravesical)

Gary D. Steinberg and Barbara Jensen

OTHER NAMES: ADRIAMYCIN

USES

- Prophylaxis against superficial TCC bladder tumor recurrences
- Treatment of existing superficial tumors
- Immediately after transurethral resection of superficial TCC tumors
- Treatment of CIS, as primary intravesical therapy
- Less effective than BCG in randomized trials
- More effective than thiotepa for high-grade superficial tumors
- Used infrequently in US due to inferior efficacy (compared to BCG and Mitomycin C) and local toxicity

DOSING

- Multiple intravesical instillation schedules have been used
- Most frequent is 30–90 mg weekly for 3 wks with 1–2 hr dwell times
- Another regimen is 60–90 mg in 50 cc of saline q3wks for 8 treatments, q6wks for 2, and q12wks for 2 additional treatments

PHARMACOKINETICS

- Minimal systemic absorption when given intravesically

TOXICITY

- Chemical cystitis, which may progress to permanent bladder contracture
- Leukopenia or cardiac toxicity has not been reported

NURSING CONSIDERATIONS

- Obtain urinalysis prior to treatment; note presence of bacteria, RBCs
- Dose range 40–90 mg; dilute to 1 mg/kg with normal saline; agent is expensive
- Chemical cystitis/bladder irritability is the main side effect and can be treated with phenazopyridine hydrochloride, although often resolves without intervention
- Refer to earlier section for specifics regarding administration of intravesical therapy
- Oxybutynin may be prescribed for patients having difficulty holding urine for 2 hr dwell time; use cautiously in elderly patients
- Restrict fluid intake up to 8 hrs prior to treatment for less dilution of agent; increase fluid intake after treatment to flush bladder of remaining drug (up to 3–4 L in 24 hrs)
- Safe drug handling and hand washing
- Assess
  - for signs and symptoms of UTI: fever, chills
  - urine for presence of bacteria; if suspect obtain urine culture, consult physician for possible antibiotic therapy
  - local toxicity may be severe with formation of fibrotic tissue and bladder contracture; if decreased bladder capacity is suspected drug should be discontinued
- Teach patient
  - drug will need to be retained in bladder for 2 hrs
  - importance of increasing fluid intake after treatment for 24 hrs and thereafter voiding q2–3hrs while awake
  - signs and symptoms of UTI
  - strict hand washing and personal hygiene
  - abstinence from sexual activity or use of protective devices immediately post treatment

KEY REFERENCE

Lamm DL, Blumenstein BA, Crawford ED, et al.: A randomized trial of intravesical doxorubicin and immunotherapy with bacillus Calmette-Guerin for transitional cell carcinoma of the bladder. N Engl J Med 1991; 325:1205

Chapter 11

PREVENTION AND TREATMENT OF TOXICITY

Antiemetics in Cancer Chemotherapy

R. J. Gralla, L. Hestermann, and Janan B. Geick Miller

OVERVIEW

- Nausea and vomiting continue to be rated among the greatest concerns of patients receiving chemotherapy. Emesis tends to be the more common, acute problem for patients, yet can be completely prevented in the majority of patients. The following are principles of antiemetic treatment
  - antiemetics should be given to prevent emesis, prescribed according to the chemotherapy emetic risk category (see table on page 130)
  - in risk categories in which a serotonin antagonist is the recommended agent of choice, a corticosteroid should be added unless there is a strong contraindication
  - To prevent acute emesis, a single administration of the antiemetic regimen immediately before chemotherapy is as efficacious as multiple doses
  - trials have shown that the available antiemetics (ondansetron, granisetron, dolasetron) are of equal efficacy
  - the lowest fully effective dose of a serotonin antagonist is the recommended dose, based on the threshold effect
  - oral regimens are as effective as IV dosing
  - patients receiving combination chemotherapy should be given antiemetics appropriate for the agent of the highest emetic risk
  - delayed emesis regimens should be given preventatively for patients in moderate- to high-risk categories

PATHOPHYSIOLOGY

- Emesis can be mediated by many neurotransmitters, located in the gut and in the central nervous system
  - blocking various neurotransmitter receptors, including serotonin type 3 receptors (5 HT3), dopamine type 2 receptors (D2), or neurokinin type 1 receptors (NK-1), can result in complete control of emesis, with even the chemotherapy most likely to induce emesis
  - most believe that antiemetics follow a "threshold" effect: the relevant receptors must be saturated. Antiemetic doses beyond this threshold add little efficacy, and doses below the threshold do not achieve maximal benefit

DIAGNOSIS AND PREVENTION

- Risk factors for chemotherapy-induced emesis
  - poor control with prior chemotherapy: the most effective appropriate antiemetics must be given with the first and each subsequent chemotherapy cycle to lessen this risk
  - the chemotherapeutic agent: several schemes have been devised as guides in assessing emetic risk of chemotherapy. See the table on page 130 for a listing of many commonly used agents grouped by risk category
  - gender: women are at greater risk of emesis
  - prior alcohol intake history. Patients with a low prior alcohol intake history are at greater risk. This history is important, not the current alcohol consumption
  - age: in general, it is more difficult to control emesis in younger patients
- Emetic problems: when patients receiving chemotherapy have nausea or vomiting, the emesis is typically attributed to the chemotherapy
  - acute emesis: occurs shortly after administration of chemotherapy (usually within 1.5–3 hrs in previously untreated patients)
  - delayed emesis: begins 24 hrs or more after chemotherapy. The neuropharmacology of this problem is not well understood. The greater the potential for acute emesis, the more likely it is that delayed emesis will occur. Some investigators believe that the risk for delayed emesis may begin earlier than 24 hrs after chemotherapy, specifically at 17–23 hrs
  - anticipatory emesis: conditioned by poor control of either acute or delayed emesis with previous chemotherapy
  - emesis of other causes: if emesis occurs in a pattern not common for chemotherapy (such as initiation a week after treatment), another cause should be sought. This often includes other medications (analgesics, bronchodilators, antibiotics) or tumor-related conditions (intestinal obstruction, brain metastases)

THERAPY

- Emesis prevention by chemotherapy risk category
  - very low risk (see table on page 130). For patients receiving chemotherapy of "very low risk," no preventative treatment needs to be given. It may be prudent to provide the patient with a prescription for an inexpensive oral antiemetic (for use on an as-needed basis) such as metoclopramide (10–20 mg q3–4hrs) or *prochlorperazine* (same dosage and schedule)
  - low risk (see table on page 130). Patients receiving chemotherapy of low risk generally have about a 10% risk of emesis, and should be treated prophylactically with a single antiemetic agent, usually a corticosteroid, such as *dexamethasone,* 4–10 mg, immediately prior to chemotherapy. Alternatives include the oral agents *metoclopramide* (10–20 mg), *prochlorperazine* (same dosage), *ondansetron* (8 mg), *granisetron* (1 mg), or *dolasetron* (100 mg). The latter three agents (serotonin antagonists) are markedly more expensive and are usually not necessary in this setting
  - individual patients in "low" and in the "very low risk" categories may occasionally require antiemetics more typical of moderate or higher risk groups, based on the patient's experience with chemotherapy
  - moderate and high risk (see table on page 130). Patients receiving chemotherapy of moderate (~30–60% risk of emesis) or high risk (~60–99% risk) should receive the same antiemetic regimen to prevent acute emesis. This regimen should consist of a combination of a single dose of a corticosteroid (such as *dexamethasone* 20 mg, orally or IV) plus a single dose of a serotonin antagonist (one of the following: *granisetron* 1 or 2 mg po or 10 mcg/kg IV; or *dolasetron* 100 mg orally or IV; or ondansetron 8 mg or 0.15 mg/kg IV). The combination should be given immediately before chemotherapy (dosing from 1 hr before chemotherapy to immediately before treatment)

- Delayed emesis
  - patients receiving *cisplatin* should always follow the delayed emesis prevention regimen. The key agents are corticosteroids. *Metoclopramide* and serotonin antagonists add to the efficacy; the former agent is preferred due to its equal efficacy and markedly lower cost. The following regimen is recommended: *dexamethasone,* 8 mg plus *metoclopramide,* 30–40 mg, both given orally twice a day for 3 days, beginning 16–24 hrs after the initiation of *cisplatin*
  - this same regimen, but followed for 2 days, may be useful for patients receiving chemotherapy of moderate emetic risk
- Anticipatory emesis
  - the best strategy is to use optimal antiemetics for acute and delayed emesis with each chemotherapy administration to lessen the risk of anticipatory emesis
  - if anticipatory emesis occurs, progressive desensitization, using established behavioral therapy techniques, can be helpful
  - benzodiazepines, starting a few days before chemotherapy, may be helpful (although formal trials are lacking)
- Adverse reactions with antiemetic agents
  - corticosteroids: can cause hyperglycemia, especially in diabetics and in older patients
  - serotonin antagonists: generally very well tolerated, with few allergic problems. IV ondansetron should be given over 15 min
  - dopamine antagonists (such as *metoclopramide* or *phenothiazines*): Extrapyramidal reactions and akathisia (restlessness) occur more frequently in patients < age 30, but less so in older patients (~2% risk of extrapyramidal reactions in those > 30). These reactions usually resolve spontaneously; however, *diphenhydramine* given orally or IV is appropriate for extrapyramidal reactions, and benzodiazepines are useful in lessening restlessness

KEY REFERENCES

Cleri LB: Serotonin antagonists: state of the art management of chemotherapy-induced emesis. In *Oncology Nursing: Treatment and Support* (vol. 2, pp. 1–19). Lippincott-Raven, 1995

Gralla RJ: Antiemetic therapy: a review. Semin Oncol 1998; 25:577–83

SEROTONIN ANTAGONISTS

DRUG: ONDANSETRON

- Other name: Zofran
- Uses
  - prevention of nausea and vomiting associated with initial and repeat courses of emetogenic cancer chemotherapy
  - for patients who are refractory to or have severe adverse reactions to standard antiemetic therapy
  - reserved for patients who receive chemotherapy agents with high to moderately high emetogenic potential
  - utilized on a scheduled basis, not an "as-needed" basis
    - □ data supports the use of this drug in the prevention of nausea and vomiting and not in the rescue of nausea and vomiting
    - □ data does not support any increased efficacy of ondansetron in delayed nausea and vomiting
  - ondansetron should only be used in the first 24–48 hrs of receiving chemotherapy
- Mechanism of action
  - selective 5-HT3-receptor antagonist
  - blocking serotonin, both peripherally on vagal nerve terminals and centrally in the chemoreceptor trigger zone
- Pharmacokinetics
  - absorption: is variable with oral administration
  - bioavailability of 50–60%
  - time to reach peak concentration is within 2 hrs
  - distribution: 70–76% is plasma protein-bound
  - metabolism: extensively by hydroxylation, followed by glucuronide or sulfate conjugation
  - excretion: 5% of dose is recovered in urine as parent compound
- Adverse reactions
  - central nervous system: headache, fever, dizziness, lightheadedness, seizures
  - gastrointestinal: constipation, diarrhea, abdominal cramps, xerostomia
  - neuromuscular and skeletal: weakness
  - cardiovascular: tachycardia
  - dermatologic: rash
  - endocrine and metabolic: hypokalemia
  - hepatic: transient elevations in serum levels of aminotransferases and bilirubin
  - respiratory: bronchospasm, shortness of breath, wheezing
- Dose
  - oral
    - □ children 4–11 yrs: 4 mg 30 min before chemotherapy; repeat 4 and 8 hrs after initial dose
    - □ children > 11 yrs and adults: 8 mg 30 min before chemotherapy; repeat 4 and 8 hrs after initial dose or q8hrs for a maximum of 48 hrs
  - IV
    - □ administer either three 0.15mg/kg doses or a single 24 mg dose infused over 15 min given 30 min before the start of emetogenic chemotherapy
    - □ with the 3-dose regimen, the initial dose is given 30 min prior to chemotherapy with subsequent doses administered 4 and 8 hrs after the first dose
  - dosing in hepatic impairment: maximum daily dose: 8 mg in cirrhotic patients with severe liver disease
- Pharmacy issues
  - should not be prescribed for chemotherapy agents with a low emetogenic potential
  - metabolized by the hepatic cytochrome P-450 enzymes
    - □ clearance and half-life may be changed with concomitant use of cytochrome P-450 inducers, barbiturates, carbamazepine, rifampin, phenytoin, and phenylbutazone
  - increased toxicity: inhibitors (e.g., cimetidine, allopurinol, and disulfiram)
  - may take without regard to meals
  - injectable form is stable diluted in D_5W or NS for 48 hrs at room temperature
  - does not need to be protected from light
- Nursing considerations
  - administer IV infusion over 15 min
  - administer dose 30 min before chemotherapy
  - assess baseline liver function tests and monitor during therapy

DRUG: GRANISETRON

- Other name: Kytril
- Uses
  - prevention of nausea and vomiting associated with initial and repeat courses of emetogenic cancer chemotherapy
  - may be prescribed for patients who are refractory to or have severe adverse reactions to standard antiemetic therapy
  - granisetron should be reserved for patients who receive chemotherapy agents with high to moderately high emetogenic potential
  - should be used on a scheduled basis, not as prn
    - □ data supports the use of this drug in the prevention of nausea and vomiting and not in the rescue of nausea and vomiting
    - □ data does not support any increased efficacy of granisetron in delayed nausea and vomiting
  - granisetron should only be used in the first 24–48 hrs of receiving chemotherapy
- Mechanism of action
  - selective 5-HT3-receptor antagonist
  - blocking serotonin, both peripherally on vagal nerve terminals and centrally in the chemoreceptor trigger zone
- Pharmacokinetics
  - absorption: is variable with oral administration
  - time to reach peak concentration is within 2 hrs
  - onset of action: commonly controls emesis within 1–3 min of IV administration
  - distribution: widely distributed throughout the body
  - half-life
    - □ cancer patients: 10–12 hrs
    - □ healthy volunteers: 3–4 hrs
  - metabolism: metabolized by the liver, possibly mediated by the cytochrome P-450 3A subfamily
  - excretion: primarily nonrenal, 8–15% of a dose is excreted unchanged in urine
- Adverse reactions
  - central nervous system: headache, dizziness, insomnia, anxiety, somnolence, agitation
  - cardiovascular: hyper/hypotension, arrhythmias
  - gastrointestinal: constipation, abdominal pain, diarrhea
  - neuromuscular and skeletal: weakness
  - hepatic: liver enzyme elevations
- Dose
  - oral

- □ adults: 1 mg twice daily; the first 1 mg dose should be given up to 1 hr before chemotherapy, and the second tablet, 12 hrs after the first
- IV
  - □ children and adults: 10 mcg/kg for 1–3 doses
    - ▽ doses should be administered as a single IVPB over 5 min to 1 hr or by undiluted IV push over 30 sec, given just prior to chemotherapy (15–60 min before)
  - □ no dose adjustments in renal or hepatic impairment necessary
- ■ Pharmacy issues
  - should not be prescribed for chemotherapeutic agents with a low emetogenic potential
  - metabolized by the hepatic cytochrome P-450 enzymes
  - dose should be administered as a IVBP over 5–15 min
  - undiluted over 30 sec
  - oral doses should be administered 1 hr before chemo and 12 hrs later
  - stable when mixed in D_5W or NS for 24 hrs at room temperature
  - should be protected from light
- ■ Nursing considerations
  - both IV and oral are indicated for prevention of nausea and vomiting
  - should only be administered on the days of chemotherapy
  - administer IV doses 15–60 min before chemotherapy
  - instruct patient that headache may occur but is relieved by OTC acetaminophen

DRUG: DOLASETRON

- ■ Other name: Anzemet
- ■ Uses
  - prevention of nausea and vomiting associated with initial and repeat courses of emetogenic cancer chemotherapy
  - may be prescribed for patients who are refractory to or have severe adverse reactions to standard antiemetic therapy
  - dolasetron should be reserved for patients who receive chemotherapy agents with high to moderately high emetogenic potential
  - dolasetron should be used on a scheduled basis
    - □ data supports the use of this drug in the prevention of nausea and vomiting and not in the rescue of nausea and vomiting
    - □ data does not support any increased efficacy of dolasetron in delayed nausea and vomiting
  - should only be used in the first 24–48 hrs of receiving chemotherapy
- ■ Mechanism of action
  - selective 5-HT3-receptor antagonist
  - blocking serotonin, both peripherally on vagal nerve terminals and centrally in the chemoreceptor trigger zone
- ■ Pharmacokinetics
  - absorption: is variable with oral administration
  - bioavailability of 75%
  - time to reach peak concentration is within 2 hrs
  - distribution: widely distributed throughout the body
  - metabolism: metabolized by the liver to hydrodolasetron, its primary clinically active compound
  - excretion: primarily nonrenal, 66% of a dose is excreted as hydrodolasetron in urine
- ■ Adverse Reactions
  - central nervous system: headache, fatigue, dizziness, chills/shivering, flushing, vertigo, paresthesia, tremor, agitation, sleep disorder, anxiety, abnormal dreaming
  - gastrointestinal: diarrhea, dyspepsia, abdominal pain, constipation
  - cardiovascular: bradycardia, tachycardia, hypertension, EKG interval changes, hypotension, peripheral edema
  - dermatologic: pruritus, rash
  - genitourinary: oliguria
  - respiratory: dyspnea, bronchospasm
- ■ Dose
  - oral: adults: 100 mg once daily 30–60 min prior to chemotherapy
  - IV: adults: 100 mg IVPB over 15–30 min, just prior to chemotherapy
  - no dose adjustments in renal or hepatic impairment necessary
- ■ Pharmacy issues
  - should not be prescribed for chemotherapeutic agents with a low emetogenic potential
  - metabolized by the hepatic cytochrome P-450 enzymes
  - may be diluted in D_5W or NS and infused over 15–30 min
  - undiluted over 30 sec
- ■ Nursing considerations
  - should only be administered on the days of chemotherapy
  - oral administration; give 1 hr prior to chemotherapy
  - IV preparation; give IV over 30 sec, 30 min prior to chemotherapy
  - the recommended dose of dolasetron should not be exceeded
  - administer with caution in patients who may develop cardiac conduction defects, especially prolongation of QT interval (e.g., hypokalemia, hypomagnesemia, patients receiving diuretics and antiarrhythmic drugs)
  - no dosage modifications necessary in elderly patients or in patients with hepatic or renal impairment
  - teach patient to report abdominal pain suggestive of pancreatitis with physician
- ■ Assess
  - baseline comfort; provide symptom management
  - baseline LFTs
- ■ Teach patient
  - to report abdominal pain suggestive of pancreatitis with physician

SUBSTITUTED BENZAMIDE

DRUG: METOCLOPRAMIDE

- ■ Other name: Reglan
- ■ Uses
  - symptomatic treatment of diabetic gastric stasis and gastroesophageal reflux
  - prevention of nausea and vomiting associated with emetogenic cancer chemotherapy or postsurgery
  - also useful in preventing delayed-onset nausea and vomiting
- ■ Mechanism of action
  - blocks dopamine receptors in chemoreceptor trigger zone of the CNS
  - enhances the response to acetylcholine of tissue in upper GI tract causing enhanced motility and accelerated gastric emptying
  - does not stimulate gastric, biliary, or pancreatic secretions
- ■ Pharmacokinetics
  - onset of effect
    - □ oral within 30–60 min
    - □ IV within 1–3 min
  - duration of therapeutic effect: 1–2 hrs regardless of route of administration
  - half-life, normal renal function: 4–7 hrs (may be dose dependent)
  - elimination: primarily as unchanged drug in urine and feces
- ■ Adverse reactions
  - central nervous system: restlessness, drowsiness, insomnia, depression, extrapyramidal reactions, tardive dyskinesia, fatigue, anxiety, agitation
  - gastrointestinal: diarrhea, xerostomia, constipation
  - neuromuscular and skeletal: weakness
  - dermatologic: rash
  - cardiovascular: tachycardia, hypertension, or hypotension
  - hematologic: methemoglobinemia
  - note: a recent study suggests the incidence of extrapyramidal reactions due to metoclopramide may be as high as 34% and the incidence appears more often in the elderly and patients < 30 yrs old
- ■ Dose
  - IV: 1–2 mg/kg/dose 30 min before chemotherapy and q4–6hrs (and usually given with diphenhydramine 25–50 mg IV/po)
  - oral: 10–20 mg po q4–6 hrs
  - delayed emesis: po 0.5 mg/kg qid for 4 days in combination with oral dexamethasone 8 mg bid for 2 days, then 4 mg bid for 2 days
  - dosing adjustment in renal impairment
    - □ CLcr 10–40 ml/min: administer at 50% of normal dose
    - □ CLcr < 10 ml/min: administer at 25% of normal dose
    - □ hemodialysis: not dialyzable (0–5%); do not give supplemental dose
- ■ Pharmacy issues
  - anticholinergic agents antagonize metoclopramide's action
  - opiate analgesics may increase CNS depression
  - standard dilution 10–150 mg in 50 ml of D_5W or NS
  - lower doses up to 10 mg may be given over 1–2 min
  - doses > 10 mg should be given diluted and infused over 15–30 min

- test interactions include elevated SGPT, SGOT, and amylase
- Nursing issues
  - warn patient that it may impair mental alertness or physical coordination
  - avoid alcohol, barbiturates, or other CNS depressants
  - take 30 min before meals
  - contact physician if involuntary movements occur or feelings of restlessness
  - use cautiously in patients with history of depression, Parkinson's disease, renal insufficiency, and hypertension
  - monitor vital signs if given IV; slow infusion rate if patient becomes hypotensive
- Assess
  - for signs and symptoms of extrapyramidal side effects; administer diphenhydramine as ordered
- Teach patient
  - to avoid activities requiring alertness for 2 hrs after each dose
  - report diarrhea, dry mouth, urticaria
  - self-administration of antidiarrheal medication

PHENOTHIAZINES

DRUG: CHLORPROMAZINE

- Other names: Thorazine, Ormazine
- Uses
  - antiemetic in treatment of nausea and vomiting and intractable hiccups (adults)
- Mechanism of action
  - blocks postsynaptic mesolimbic dopaminergic receptors in the brain
  - exhibits a strong alpha-adrenergic blocking effect and depresses the release of hypothalamic and hypophyseal hormones
  - believed to depress the reticular-activating system, thus affecting basal metabolism, body temperature, wakefulness, vasomotor tone, and emesis
- Dosing
  - nausea and vomiting
    - children: po 0.5–1 mg/kg/dose q4–6 hrs as needed
      - IM, IV: 0.5–1 mg/kg/dose q6–8hrs. Maximum dose for < 5 yrs (22.7 kg): 40 mg/day. Maximum for 5–12 yrs (22.7–45.5 kg): 75mg/day
      - rectal: 1 mg/kg/dose q6–8hrs as needed
    - adults: oral: 10–25mg q4–6hrs
      - IM, IV: 25–50 mg q4–6hrs
      - rectal: 50–100 mg q6–8hrs
- Pharmacokinetics
  - onset of effect: IV: within 5 min; IM: within 15–30 min; rectal: erratic
  - metabolism: extensively in the liver to active and inactive metabolites
  - half-life, biphasic: initial: 2 hrs; terminal: 30 hrs
  - elimination: < 1% excreted in urine
- Adverse reactions
  - cardiovascular: hypotension (especially with IV use), tachycardia, arrhythmias, orthostatic hypotension
  - central nervous system: pseudoparkinsonism, akathisia, dystonias, tardive dyskinesia (persistent), dizziness, blurred vision, sedation, drowsiness, restlessness, anxiety, extrapyramidal reactions, altered central temperature regulation, lowering of seizure threshold, neuroleptic malignant syndrome
  - gastrointestinal: constipation, GI upset, nausea, vomiting, stomach pain, xerostomia
  - respiratory: nasal congestion
  - dermatologic: pruritus, rash, increased sensitivity to sun
  - neuromuscular and skeletal: trembling of fingers
  - overdosage/toxicology: symptoms of overdose include deep sleep, coma, extrapyramidal symptoms, abnormal involuntary muscle movements, hypotension
- Pharmacy issues
  - cytochrome P-450 2D6 enzyme substrate
  - increased toxicity
    - additive effects with other CNS depressants
    - epinephrine (hypotension)
    - may increase valproic acid serum concentrations
- Nursing issues
  - monitor orthostatic blood pressure
  - watch for hypotension when administering IM or IV
  - avoid alcohol
  - avoid excess exposure to sun
  - may cause drowsiness; rise slowly from recumbent position

DRUG: PERPHENAZINE

- Other name: Trilafon
- Uses
  - management of nausea and vomiting in adults
- Mechanism of action
  - blocks postynaptic mesolimbic dopaminergic receptors in the brain
  - exhibits a strong alpha-adrenergic blocking effect and depresses the release of hypothalamic and hypophyseal hormones
- Dose
  - adults
    - nausea/vomiting
      - oral: 2–4 mg q4–6 hrs
      - IM: 5–10 mg q6hrs as necessary up to 15 mg/d in ambulatory patients and 30 mg/d in hospitalized patients
      - IV: (severe): 1 mg at 1–2 min intervals up to a total of 5 mg
    - dosing adjustment in hepatic impairment should be considered, although no specific guidelines are available
- Pharmacokinetics
  - absorption: well absorbed po
  - onset of effect: IV: 10 min; oral peaks within 2–4 hrs
  - duration: IV: 6–24 hrs; IM: 6 hrs
  - metabolism: in the liver
  - half-life: 9 hrs
  - elimination: in the urine
- Adverse reactions
  - cardiovascular: hypotension, orthostatic hypotension
  - central nervous system: pseudoparkinsonism, akathisia, dystonia, tardive dyskinesia (persistent), dizziness, neuroleptic malignant syndrome, impairment of temperature regulation, lowering of seizure threshold
  - gastrointestinal: constipation, dry mouth
  - dermatologic: increased sensitivity to sun, rash
  - neuromuscular and skeletal: trembling of fingers
  - overdosage/toxicology: symptoms of overdose include deep sleep, dystonia, agitation, coma, abnormal involuntary muscle movements, hypotension, arrhythmias
- Pharmacy issues
  - drug interactions: cytochrome P-450 2D6 enzyme substrate
  - decreased effect: anticholinergics, anticonvulsants; decreased effect of guanethidine, epinephrine
  - increased toxicity: CNS depressants; increased effect/toxicity of anticonvulsants
- Nursing issues
  - monitor for hypotension when administered by IM or IV
  - inform patient may cause drowsiness
  - avoid excessive sunlight
  - impairs judgment and coordination
  - notify physician of involuntary movements or feelings of restlessness

DRUG: PROCHLORPERAZINE

- Other name: Compazine
- Uses
  - most traditionally used antiemetic to control nausea and vomiting
- Mechanism of action
  - antiemetic effects are attributed to dopamine receptor blockade in the medullary chemoreceptor trigger zone
  - prochlorperazine has many other central and peripheral effects: it produces alpha and ganglionic blockade and counteracts histamine- and serotonin-mediated activity
  - exhibits a strong alpha-adrenergic and anticholinergic blocking effect and depresses the release of hypothalamic and hypophyseal hormones
  - believed to depress the reticular activating system, thus affecting basal metabolism, body temperature, wakefulness, vasomotor tone, and emesis
- Dose: antiemetic: children
  - po, rectal
    - < 10 kg: 0.4 mg/kg/24 hrs in 3–4 divided doses
    - 10–14 kg: 2.5 mg q12–24hrs as needed; maximum: 7.5 mg/day
    - 14–18 kg: 2.5 mg q8–12hrs as needed; maximum: 10 mg/day
    - 18–39 kg: 2.5 mg q8hrs or 5 mg q12hrs as needed; maximum: 15 mg/day
  - IM: 0.1–0.15 mg/kg/dose; usual: 0.13 mg/kg/dose; change to oral as soon as possible
  - IV: not recommended in children < 10 kg or < 2 yrs
- antiemetic: adults
  - po: 5–10 mg 3–4 times/day; 10–15 mg of SR preparation bid; usual maximum: 40 mg/day
  - IM: 5–10 mg q3–4hrs: usual maximum: 40 mg/day

- IV: 2.5–10 mg; maximum 10 mg/dose or 40 mg/day; may repeat dose q3–4hrs as needed
- rectal: 25 mg twice daily

■ Pharmacokinetics
- onset of effect
  - □ po: within 30–40 min
  - □ IM: within 10–20 min
  - □ rectal: within 60 min
- peak effect occurs at 2–4 hrs; steady-state serum levels are achieved within 4–7 days
- duration: persists longest with IM and po extended-release doses (12 hrs)
- shortest following rectal and immediate-release po administration (3–4 hrs)
- distribution: prochlorperazine is distributed widely into the body, including breast milk. Drug is 91–99% protein-bound
- metabolism: prochlorperazine is metabolized extensively by the liver, but no active metabolites are formed
- half-life: 23 hrs
- elimination: primarily by hepatic metabolism

■ Adverse reactions
- central nervous system: extrapyramidal symptoms (dystonia, akathisia, pseudoparkinsonism), dizziness, drowsiness, sedation, headache, neuroleptic malignant syndrome, impairment of temperature regulation, lowering of seizure threshold, blurred vision
- cardiovascular: hypotension (especially with IV use), orthostatic hypotension, tachycardia, arrhythmias
- gastrointestinal: dry mouth, constipation
- genitourinary: urinary retention
- dermatologic: increased sensitivity to sun, rash
- neuromuscular and skeletal: trembling of fingers

■ Pharmacy issues
- increased toxicity: additive effects with other CNS depressants, anticonvulsants; epinephrine may cause hypotension
- not dialyzable (0–5%)

■ Nursing issues
- inform patient may cause drowsiness
- avoid excessive sunlight
- impairs judgment and coordination
- notify physician of involuntary movements or feelings of restlessness
- administer IV 15–30 min before therapy
- monitor for orthostatic hypotension during IV infusion

■ Assess
- for signs and symptoms of extrapyramidal side effects; administer diphenhydramine as ordered

■ Teach patient
- report rash and urticaria

DRUG: PROMETHAZINE

■ Other names: Phenergan, Prometh, Phenazine, Anergan, Prorex, and others

■ Uses
- used as antiemetic similar to other phenothiazine derivatives to control nausea and vomiting
- also useful in motion sickness

■ Mechanism of action
- blocks postsynaptic mesolimbic dopaminergic receptors in the brain
- exhibits a strong alpha-adrenergic blocking effect and depresses the release of hypothalamic and hypophyseal hormones
- reduces stimuli to the brain stem reticular system

■ Dose
- nausea
  - □ adults: 12.5–25 mg po, IM, IV, or rectally q4–6hrs as needed
  - □ children: 0.25–1 mg/kg po, IM, or rectally q4–6hrs as needed
- motion sickness
  - □ adults: 25 mg po or rectally 30–60 min before departure, then q12hrs as needed
  - □ children: 0.5 mg/kg/dose po or rectally 30 min–1 hr before departure, then q12hrs as needed

■ Pharmacokinetics
- absorption: well absorbed after po administration
- onset of effect: 20 min after po, rectal, or IM administration and within 3–5 min after IV administration
- duration: 2–6 hrs
- distribution: widely throughout the body; drug crosses the placenta
- metabolism: liver
- excretion: urine and feces as metabolites

■ Adverse reactions
- central nervous system: slight to moderate drowsiness, headache, fatigue, nervousness, dizziness, sedation (pronounced), confusion, excitation, extrapyramidal reactions with high doses, dystonia, faintness with IV administration, depression, insomnia, blurred vision
- respiratory: thickening of bronchial secretions
- gastrointestinal: xerostomia, abdominal pain
- cardiovascular: tachycardia, bradycardia, palpitations, hypotension
- dermatologic: photosensitivity, rash, angioedema
- genitourinary: urinary retention
- neuromuscular and skeletal: tremor, paresthesia, myalgia

■ Pharmacy issues
- increased toxicity: epinephrine should not be used together with promethazine, since blood pressure may decrease further
- additive effects with other CNS depressants
- avoid rapid infusion as may decrease blood pressure

■ Nursing issues
- inform patient may cause drowsiness
- avoid excessive sunlight
- impairs judgment and coordination
- notify physician of involuntary movements or feelings of restlessness

DRUG: THIETHYLPERAZINE

■ Other names: Torecan, Norzine

■ Uses
- antiemetic similar to other phenothiazine derivatives to control nausea and vomiting

■ Mechanism of action
- blocks postsynaptic mesolimbic dopaminergic receptors in the brain
- exhibits a strong alpha-adrenergic blocking effect and depresses the release of hypothalamic and hypophyseal hormones
- acts directly on chemoreceptor trigger zone and vomiting center

■ Pharmacokinetics
- onset of antiemetic effect: within 30 min
- duration 3–4 hrs
- metabolism: hepatic

■ Adverse reactions
- central nervous system: drowsiness, dizziness, confusion, convulsion, extrapyramidal effects, tardive dyskinesia, fever, headache, akathisia, gait disturbances
- gastrointestinal: dry mouth
- respiratory: dry nose
- cardiovascular: tachycardia, orthostatic hypotension

■ Dose
- children > 12 yrs and adults
  - □ po, IM, rectal: 10 mg 1–3 times/day as needed
  - □ IV and SubQ: same dose as above

■ Pharmacy issues
- increased effect/toxicity with CNS depressants (e.g., anesthetics, opiates, tranquilizers, alcohol), lithium, atropine, epinephrine, MAO inhibitors, tricyclic antidepressants

■ Nursing issues
- observe for extrapyramidal symptoms
- assist with ambulation
- may cause drowsiness
- impairs judgment and coordination
- avoid excessive sunlight

BUTYROPHENONES

DRUG: HALOPERIDOL

■ Other name: Haldol

■ Uses
- antipsychotic agent and sedative with weaker antiemetic and anticholinergic effects

■ Mechanism of action
- blocks postsynaptic mesolimbic dopaminergic D1 and D2 receptors in the brain
- exhibits a strong alpha-adrenergic blocking and anticholinergic effect
- depresses the release of hypothalamic and hypophyseal hormones
- believed to depress the reticular activating system, thus affecting basal metabolism, body temperature, wakefulness, vasomotor tone, and emesis

■ Pharmacokinetics
- absorption: rate and extent of absorption vary with route of administration
  - □ oral tablet absorption yields 60–70% bioavailability
  - □ IM dose is 70% absorbed within 30 min
- peak plasma levels after oral administration occur at 2–6 hrs
  - □ after IM administration, 30–45 min
- distributed widely into the body, with high concentrations in adipose tissue
- drug is 91–99% protein-bound

- half-life: 20 hrs
- metabolism: extensively by the liver; there may be only one active metabolite that is less active than the parent compound
- excretion: ~40% of a given dose is excreted in urine within 5 days; ~15% is excreted in feces via the biliary tract

- Adverse reactions
  - central nervous system: restlessness, anxiety, extrapyramidal reactions, dystonic reactions, pseudoparkinsonian signs and symptoms, tardive dyskinesia, neuroleptic malignant syndrome seizures, altered central temperature regulation, akathisia, drowsiness
  - cardiovascular: hypotension (especially orthostatic), tachycardia, arrhythmias, abnormal T waves with prolonged ventricular repolarization
  - dermatologic: hyperpigmentation, pruritus, rash, contact dermatitis, alopecia, photosensitivity (rare)
  - genitourinary: urinary retention, overflow incontinence
  - ocular: blurred vision, decreased visual acuity
- Dose
  - adults
    - □ po or IV: 0.25–3 mg q2–6 hrs
- Pharmacy issues
  - cytochrome P-450 IID6 enzyme inhibitor
  - decreased effect: carbamazepine and phenobarbital may increase metabolism and decrease effectiveness of haloperidol
  - increased toxicity: CNS depressants may increase adverse effects
  - epinephrine may cause hypotension
  - haloperidol and anticholinergic agents may increase intraocular pressure
  - concurrent use with lithium has occasionally caused acute encephalopathy-like syndrome
  - administer IV or IVPB in D_5W solutions; avoid NS due to reports of instability
- Nursing issues
  - recommend patient avoid alcohol and other CNS depressants
  - rise slowly from recumbent position to prevent orthostatic hypotension
  - utilize haloperidol lactate injection for IV use diluted or undiluted slowly
  - decanoate injectable formulation should be administered IM only, never IV
  - monitor for orthostatic hypotension during IV infusion
  - use cautiously in elderly patients, and in those with a history of seizures, serious CV disorders, urine retention or glaucoma, and in conjunction with anticonvulsant, anticoagulant, antiparkinsonian, or lithium medications
- Assess
  - for signs and symptoms of extrapyramidal side effects; administer diphenhydramine as ordered
- Teach patient
  - avoid alcohol while taking drug
  - report rash and urticaria
  - side effects and self-care measures

DRUG: DROPERIDOL

- Other name: Inapsine
- Uses
  - sedative and antiemetic in surgical and diagnostic procedures
  - antiemetic for cancer chemotherapy
  - has good antiemetic effect as well as sedative and antianxiety effects
- Mechanism of action
  - alters the action of dopamine in the CNS, at subcortical levels, to produce sedation
  - reduces emesis by blocking dopamine stimulation of the chemoreceptor zone
- Pharmacokinetics
  - absorption: droperidol is well absorbed after IM injection
  - onset: sedation begins in 3–10 min
  - peaks at 30 min, lasts for 2–4 hrs
  - duration: lasts for 2–4 hrs, some alteration of consciousness may persist for 12 hrs
  - distribution: not well understood; drug crosses the blood-brain barrier and is distributed in the CSF
  - half-life: adults: 2.3 hrs
  - metabolism: in the liver
  - elimination: in urine (75%) and feces (22%)
- Adverse reactions
  - cardiovascular: mild to moderate hypotension with rebound tachycardia, hypertension
  - central nervous system: postoperative drowsiness, extrapyramidal reactions, dizziness, chills, postoperative hallucinations
  - respiratory: respiratory depression, laryngospasm, bronchospasm
  - miscellaneous: shivering
- Dose
  - children 2–12 yrs
    - □ nausea and vomiting: IM, IV: 0.05–0.06 mg/kg/dose q4–6hrs as needed
  - adults
    - □ nausea and vomiting: IM, IV: 0.625–5 mg/dose q3–4hrs as needed
    - □ IV doses should be given slowly over > 5 min or as IVPB
- Pharmacy issues
  - increased toxicity: CNS depressants, fentanyl, and other analgesics increase blood pressure
  - epinephrine decreases blood pressure
  - standard diluent: 2.5 mg in 50 ml of D_5W
  - administer slowly over 2–5 min
- Nursing considerations
  - monitor blood pressure, heart rate, respiratory rate
  - observe for dystonias, extrapyramidal side effects, and temperature changes

CANNABINOID

DRUG: DRONABINOL (THC)

- Other name: Marinol
- Uses
  - nausea and vomiting associated with cancer chemotherapy in patients who have failed to respond adequately to conventional antiemetics
- Mechanism of action
  - dronabinol is a synthetic cannabinoid that inhibits vomiting centers in the brain and possibly in the chemoreceptor trigger zone
- Pharmacokinetics
  - absorption: almost 90–95% of dose is absorbed
  - action begins in 30–60 min
  - peak action in 1–3 hrs
  - distribution: dronabinol is distributed rapidly into many tissue sites
  - protein-bound 97–99%
  - extensive first-pass metabolism
  - metabolized in the liver to several metabolites, some of which are active
  - half-life: 19–24 hrs
  - excretion: dronabinol is excreted primarily in feces, via the biliary tract
  - duration: drug effect may persist for several days after treatment ends; varies considerably among patients
- Adverse reactions
  - central nervous system: drowsiness, dizziness, detachment, anxiety, difficulty concentrating, mood change, ataxia, depression, headache, vertigo, hallucinations, memory lapse, nightmares, speech difficulties, tinnitus
  - cardiovascular: orthostatic hypotension, tachycardia, syncope
  - gastrointestinal: xerostomia, diarrhea
  - neuromuscular and skeletal: paresthesia, weakness, myalgia
- Dose
  - adult: 2.5 to 10 mg 1–3 hrs prior to chemotherapy, then q2hrs for 4–6 doses/d
- Pharmacy issues
  - increased toxicity (drowsiness) with alcohol, barbiturates, benzodiazepines
  - lowers FSH, LH, growth hormone, and testosterone
- Nursing considerations
  - avoid activities that require motor coordination
  - avoid alcohol and other CNS depressants
  - may impair coordination and judgment
  - assist with ambulation
  - institute safety measures
  - can produce physical and psychologic dependency
  - increased toxicity in elderly patients
- Assess
  - baseline vital signs and during therapy for tachycardia, orthostatic hypotension
  - neurologic status for signs of disorientation, drowsiness, and impaired coordination

ANTICHOLINERGIC

DRUG: SCOPOLAMINE

- Other name: Transderm Scop
- Uses
  - prevention of nausea and vomiting caused by motion sickness
- Mechanism of action
  - exact mechanism of action is unknown; probably blocks action of acetylcholine in the CNS
  - antagonizes histamine and serotonin

- may affect neural pathways affecting the vestibular input to the CNS originating in the labyrinth of the ear
- inhibiting nausea and vomiting in patients with motion sickness

■ Pharmacokinetics
- absorption: scopolamine is well absorbed percutaneously from behind the ear
- onset: antiemetic effects begin 4–5 hrs after application
- duration for 72 hrs
- distribution: widely throughout body tissues
- metabolism: probably metabolized completely in the liver; its exact metabolic fate is unknown
- excretion: in urine

■ Adverse reactions
- dermatologic: dry skin, increased sensitivity to light, rash
- gastrointestinal: constipation, xerostomia, dry throat, dysphagia
- respiratory: dry nose
- miscellaneous: diaphoresis (decreased)
- cardiovascular: orthostatic hypotension, ventricular fibrillation, tachycardia, palpitations
- central nervous system: confusion, drowsiness, headache, loss of memory, ataxia, fatigue, blurred vision

■ Dose
- children > 12 yrs and adults
  - □ apply 1 patch 0.5 mg/24 hrs (1.5 mg over 3 days) behind ear at least 4 hrs prior to exposure and q3d as needed
  - □ effective if applied as little as 2–3 hrs before anticipated need
  - □ best if 12 hrs before

■ Pharmacy issues
- increased toxicity: additive adverse effects with other anticholinergic agents
- mydriatic and cycloplegic effects persist for 3–7 days
- symptoms of overdosage include dilated pupils, flushed skin, tachycardia, hypertension, EKG abnormalities, CNS depression, respiratory failure, circulatory collapse

■ Nursing considerations
- wash hands before and after applying the disc
- avoid drug contact with the eyes
- inform patient may impair coordination and judgment
- instruct patient to contact physician with any changes of vision

CORTICOSTEROIDS

DRUG: DEXAMETHASONE

■ Other names: Decadron, Hexadrol

■ Uses
- as an adjunctive antiemetic agent for acute and delayed emesis
- usually given in combination with other antiemetic agents

■ Mechanism of action
- unknown mechanism of action for its synergy with other antiemetic agents
- probably exerts some centrally acting mechanism

■ Pharmacokinetics
- absorption: readily after oral administration
- peak effects occur in about 1–2 hrs
- distribution: removed rapidly from the blood and distributed to muscle, liver, skin, intestines, and kidneys
- half-life: normal renal function: 1.8–3.5 hrs
- biological half-life: 36–54 hrs
- time to peak serum concentration: oral within 1–2 hrs
- metabolism: in the liver to inactive glucuronide and sulfate metabolites
- excretion: the inactive metabolites and small amounts of unmetabolized drug are excreted by the kidneys
- insignificant quantities of drug are also excreted in feces

■ Adverse reactions
- central nervous system: insomnia, nervousness
- gastrointestinal: increased appetite, indigestion
- endocrine and metabolic: diabetes mellitus
- neuromuscular and skeletal: arthralgia
- dermatologic: itching, dryness, skin atrophy
- miscellaneous: secondary infection

■ Dose
- children: antiemetic (prior to chemotherapy): IV
  - □ should be given as sodium phosphate; 10 mg/m^2/dose (maximum: 20 mg) for first dose
  - □ 5 mg/m^2/dose q6hrs as needed
- adult: antiemetic (prior to chemotherapy): po/IV
  - □ should be given as sodium phosphate; 10 mg/m^2/dose (usually 20 mg) for first dose
  - □ 5 mg/m^2/dose q6hrs as needed
- due to extended half-life, single-dose therapy may be as effective as multiple doses
- delayed emesis: po 8 mg bid for 2 days, then taper to 4 mg bid for 2 days

■ Pharmacy issues
- cytochrome P-450 3A enzyme substrate
- barbiturates, phenytoin, rifampin cause decreased dexamethasone effect
- dexamethasone causes decreased effect of salicylates, vaccines, toxoids

■ Nursing considerations
- monitor serum potassium and glucose
- administer oral dose with food or milk
- give H2 antagonist to prevent gastric irritation

■ Assess
- neurologic status baseline and during therapy
- monitor weight, blood pressure, and serum electrolytes

■ Teach patient
- signs and symptoms of hyperglycemia if receiving drug for an extended period of time
- management of diarrhea, abdominal distention, and increased appetite
- not to discontinue drug abruptly or without physician's knowledge

DRUGS: METHYLPREDNISOLONE AND PREDNISONE

■ Other names: Solu-Medrol and Deltasone/Orasone/Liquid-Pred

■ Uses
- as an adjunctive antiemetic agent for acute and delayed emesis
- usually given in combination with other antiemetic agents

■ Mechanism of action
- exact mechanism of antiemetic effects are unknown
- possibly due to blockade of cerebral innervation of the emetic center via inhibition of prostaglandin synthesis

■ Pharmacokinetics
- absorption: methylprednisolone and prednisone are absorbed readily after oral administration
- after oral and IV administration, peak effects occur within 1–2 hrs
- duration 30–36 hrs IM
- peak effect within 4–8 hrs, duration 1–4 wks
- half-life: 3–3.5 hrs
- biological half-life is 18–36 hrs
- distribution: methylprednisolone and prednisone are distributed rapidly to muscle, liver, skin, intestines, and kidneys
- metabolism: in the liver to inactive glucuronide and sulfate metabolites
- prednisone is metabolized in the liver to the active metabolite prednisolone
  - □ then metabolized to inactive glucuronide and sulfate metabolites
- excretion: inactive metabolites and small amounts of unmetabolized drug are excreted by the kidneys

■ Adverse reactions
- central nervous system: insomnia, nervousness, vertigo, psychoses, headache, mood swings, delirium, hallucinations, euphoria
- gastrointestinal: increased appetite, indigestion
- endocrine and metabolic: diabetes mellitus
- neuromuscular and skeletal: arthralgia
- cardiovascular: edema, hypertension

■ Dose
- methylprednisolone: 125–250 mg IV, q4–6hrs for 4 doses
- prednisone: 2.5–20 mg po q2–4hrs

■ Pharmacy issues
- inducer of cytochrome P-450 enzymes
- cytochrome P-450 3A enzyme substrate
- decreased effect
  - □ phenytoin, phenobarbital, rifampin cause increased clearance of methylprednisolone
  - □ potassium-depleting diuretics enhance potassium depletion
- increased toxicity
  - □ skin test antigen, immunizations decrease response and increase potential infection
  - □ methylprednisolone may increase circulating glucose levels, may need adjustments of insulin or oral hypoglycemics

■ Nursing considerations
- monitor serum potassium and glucose
- administer oral form with meals to avoid GI upset
- notify physician if signs of infection occur

Chemotherapy Agents, Antiemetic Risk Categories, and Recommendations for Preventing Acute and Delayed Emesis

Emetic Category	Chemotherapy Agents	Acute Emesis Treatment	Delayed Emesis Treatment
Moderate to high risk	Cisplatin Dacarbazine Actinomycin-D Nitrogen mustard Carboplatin Cyclophosphamide Lomustine Carmustine Daunorubicin Doxorubicin Epirubicin Idarubicin Cytosine arabinoside Ifosfamide	5-HT3 antagonist plus a corticosteroid*	Metoclopramide plus a corticosteroid*
Low risk	Mitoxantrone Paclitaxel Docetaxel Mitomycin Irinotecan Topotecan Gemcitabine Etoposide Tenoposide Vinorelbine	A corticosteroid*	No routine use of antiemetics
Very low risk	Methotrexate 6-Thioguanine 6-Mercaptopurine Bleomycin l-Asparaginase Vindesine Vinblastine Vincristine Busulphan Chorambucil Alkeran Melphalan Hydroxyurea Tamoxifen	No routine use of antiemetics	No routine use of antiemetics

*See text for details, doses, and schedules.

Myelosuppression

R. G. Bociek, C. Skosey, C. Kefer, and A. Kessinger

OVERVIEW

- Myelosuppression is the dose-limiting toxicity for most chemotherapeutic agents/regimens
  - prolonged myelosuppression can result in treatment delays leading to a reduction in chemotherapeutic dose intensity
- The risk of acquiring bacterial/fungal infection is proportional to the duration and degree of neutropenia
- Chemotherapy-induced anemia can lead to symptoms of fatigue and impair quality of life
- Chemotherapy-induced thrombocytopenia can increase the risk of spontaneous bleeding
- High-dose chemotherapy/stem cell transplantation is virtually always associated with prolonged periods of marrow aplasia/peripheral pancytopenia

PATHOPHYSIOLOGY

- Endogenous hematopoietic growth factors maintain the hematopoietic organ in a steady state under basal and physiologically stressed conditions (e.g., hemorrhage, infection)
- Myelosuppression is the most common, dose-limiting side effect of combination chemotherapy regimens
- Recombinant DNA technology has made it possible to synthesize and purify a variety of hematopoietic growth factors. Given in pharmacologic quantities, they have the ability to accelerate hematopoietic recovery

DIAGNOSIS AND PREVENTION BY SYNDROME

- Anemia
  - etiology of anemia in cancer patients is multifactorial, and includes factors related to both malignancy and therapy; e.g., bone marrow metastases, depletion of nutritional stores, reticuloendothelial blockade, red cell hemolysis, blunting of erythropoietin (EPO) response to anemia, concurrent treatment with chemotherapy/irradiation
  - the decision to start therapy should be based on clinical symptomatology and the need to increase oxygen-carrying capacity rather than a particular hemoglobin level
  - level I–II evidence supports use of erythropoietin (EPO) in the prevention/treatment of anemia caused by myelosuppressive chemotherapy
- Leukopenia/neutropenia
  - leukocytes are the cell line generally most susceptible to the effects of chemotherapy
  - the probability of developing an infectious complication is proportional to the degree and duration of leukopenia/neutropenia
  - level I evidence supports use of hematopoietic growth factors such as granulocyte colony-stimulating factor (G-CSF) and granulocyte-macrophage colony-stimulating factor (GM-CSF) to reduce the incidence of neutropenic complications and optimize delivery of conventional chemotherapy regimens
    - □ primary administration should be restricted to regimens associated with a ≥40% probability of developing febrile neutropenia
- Thrombocytopenia
  - most combination chemotherapy regimens produce minimal thrombocytopenia
  - certain combinations (e.g., cytosine-arabinoside/cisplatin) and certain agents (e.g., carboplatin, gemcitabine) can produce clinically significant thrombocytopenia
  - risk of spontaneous bleeding increases significantly when platelet count $< 10 \times 10^9$/L
  - platelet transfusions are safe/effective therapy for prophylaxis of bleeding that is secondary to quantitative or qualitative platelet disorders (one unit of platelets increases platelet count by approximately 5–10 x10^9/L)

THERAPY

- Anemia
  - red cell transfusions are safe, effective, economical, and are the most effective way to rapidly increase hemoglobin levels (one unit increases hemoglobin by approximately 1 g/dl)
  - Level I–II evidence supports use of Erythropoietin (EPO) in both prevention and treatment of anemia caused by myelosuppressive chemotherapy, as well as treatment of anemia induced by malignancy
- Leukopenia/neutropenia
  - leukocyte transfusions are rarely performed because of impracticality
  - level I evidence supports use of hematopoietic growth factors to reduce duration of hematologic recovery after autologous bone marrow/peripheral blood stem cell transplantation
- Thrombocytopenia
  - platelet transfusions are safe/effective therapy for treatment of bleeding that is secondary to quantitative or qualitative platelet disorders (one unit of platelets increases platelet count by approximately 5–10 x10^9/L)
  - level II evidence supports the use of interleukin-11 (oprelvekin) to reduce the occurrence of severe thrombocytopenia in dose-intense chemotherapy regimens, or subsequent to the occurrence of severe thrombocytopenia from a prior cycle of chemotherapy

GUIDELINES FOR TRANSFUSION PRACTICE

- Red cell transfusion. Appropriate criteria may include
  - symptomatic anemia in a normovolemic patient
  - acute blood loss of > 15% estimated circulating blood volume
  - acute blood loss with symptoms/signs of compromised oxygen delivery
  - hemoglobin of ≥9 g/dl in a patient on a chronic transfusion regimen
- Platelet transfusion. Appropriate criteria may include
  - platelet count of $10–20 \times 10^9$/L in a non-bleeding patient
  - platelet count of $< 50 \times 10^9$/L in a patient requiring surgery or an invasive procedure
  - bleeding in a patient with a qualitative platelet defect (e.g., uremia) regardless of platelet count
- Evaluation of possible hemolytic transfusion reactions. Suspect acute hemolytic transfusion reaction when a rise in temperature of ≥1° C occurs in the presence of any of the following new or unexplained symptoms
  - severe chills or flushing
  - back pain
  - chest pain/dyspnea
  - nausea/vomiting
  - hypotension
  - oliguria, hemoglobinuria, anuria
- Special nursing considerations for blood component transfusions
  - nurses have a vital role in identifying reactions to transfusions; therefore they must be knowledgeable regarding the blood component being administered, the physiologic response to the product, risk factors for a reaction, adverse reactions and prevention strategies, and knowledge of institutional policies and procedures
- Workup/therapy of suspected acute hemolytic transfusion reaction
  - stop transfusion immediately
  - administer supportive care (e.g., oxygen, bronchodilators, fluids, epinephrine) as medically indicated
  - recheck unit for inadvertent clerical errors
  - return transfused unit to blood bank for repeat cross-match and culture
  - perform serum-free hemoglobin and haptoglobin levels
  - perform CBC, direct antiglobulin test
  - perform urinalysis for evidence of free hemoglobin; perform renal function studies
  - consider workup for diffuse intravascular coagulation if clinically suspected (e.g., unexplained diffuse bleeding, evidence of schistocytes on blood film; new thrombocytopenia)
- Proper sample verification/documentation is necessary. Most acute hemolytic errors occur as a result of a clerical error
  - check physician orders
  - confirm a signed witnessed patient consent form

- corroborate labeling of specimens for cross matching
  - name, product, medical record number, expiration, special issues such as CMV, filtering for each unit to be administered: compare transfusion record and physician order; compare unit tag and blood component label to verify donor number, blood type, and expiration date; compare transfusion record and unit tag to verify patient name, medical number, donor number, expiration date, donor ABO group and Rh, patient ABO group and Rh, type of component and statement regarding compatibility
- examine blood product for visual clots or discoloration, evidence of damage or leakage

■ Administration issues
- plan to initiate transfusion as soon as possible after arrival to the unit
- ensure IV line and needle size are appropriate
- prior to transfusion the patient's ID band and the blood component tag are compared to ensure patient's full name and medical record number are the same
- connect blood container, using blood administration set specific to blood components; prime filters according to manufacturer's instructions
- normal saline is the only compatible fluid that should be used to prime the blood set; IV fluids containing dextrose will cause clumping of RBCs and hemolysis
- blood transfusions should be given slowly for the first 15 min to observe for potential signs of a reaction; can increase rate as patient tolerates; the maximum time for a transfusion is 4 hrs (this decreases the risk of bacterial contamination and ensures component stability)
- platelets can be infused quickly
- flush administration set line with normal saline after completion of transfusion
- observe blood and body fluid precautions; wash hands
- *no medications* should be added to blood at any time

■ Assess patient
- patient history to determine potential risk of reaction; prior transfusions and number; history of prior reactions, type and interventions; number of pregnancies (the number of pregnancies can increase the risk of transfusion reactions)
- baseline physical exam and vital signs to detect changes during and following the transfusion; baseline, 15 min after initiation of transfusion, q30min for the first hour, then hourly (acute hemolytic and anaphylactic reactions usually occur within the first 15 min)
- observe for fluid overload

■ Teach patient
- procedure and rationale for transfusion
- risks: reactions, transmission of viruses such as HIV, hepatitis, cytomegalovirus
- benefits: lessen risk of bleeding due to low platelets; alleviation of symptoms from anemia such as shortness of breath, fatigue
- signs and symptoms of reactions to expedite intervention and minimize adverse effects
- report fever, chills, hives, difficulty breathing, pain at insertion site, low back pain, and nausea

KEY REFERENCES

Cascinu S, Fedeli A, Del-Ferro E, Luzi-Fedeli S, Catalano G: Recombinant human erythropoietin treatment in cisplatin-associated anemia: a randomized double-blind trial with placebo. J Clin Oncol 1994; 12:1058–62

Crawford J, Ozer H, Stoller R, Johnson D, Lyman G, Tabbara I, Kris M, Grous J, Picozzi V, Rausch G: Reduction by granulocyte colony-stimulating factor of fever and neutropenia induced by chemotherapy in patients with small-cell lung cancer. N Engl J Med 1991; 325:164–70

Isaacs C, Robert NJ, Bailey A, Schuster MW, Overmoyer B, Graham M, Cai B, Beach KJ, Loewy JW, Kaye JA: Randomized placebo-controlled study of recombinant human interleukin-11 to prevent chemotherapy-induced thrombocytopenia in patients with breast cancer receiving dose-intensive cyclophosphamide and doxorubicin. J Clin Oncol 1997; 15:3368–77

Nemunaitis J, Rabinowe SN, Singer JW, Bierman PJ, Vose JM, Freedman AS, Onetto N, Gillis S, Oett D, Gold M, et al.: Recombinant human granulocyte-macrophage colony-stimulating factor after autologous bone marrow transplantation for lymphoid malignancy: pooled results of a randomized, double-blind, placebo controlled trial. N Engl J Med 1991; 324:1773–8

Stehling L, Luban NLC, Anderson KC, Sayers MH, Long A, Attar S, Leitman SF, Gould SA, Kruskall MS, Goodnough LT, et al.: Committee report; guidelines for blood utilization review. Transfusion 1994; 34:438–48

G-CSF (FILGRASTIM, NEUPOGEN)

■ G-CSF is a glycoprotein synthesized by recombinant DNA technology in *E. coli* bacteria

■ Common indications
- maintenance of dose intensity in cancer patients receiving myelosuppressive chemotherapy when dose reductions/delays could compromise clinical outcome
- reduction in chemotherapy-induced neutropenic complications (e.g., febrile neutropenia)
- mobilization of peripheral blood progenitor cells (PBPC) prior to collection; promotion of hematopoietic recovery post bone marrow transplantation (BMT) or peripheral blood progenitor cell transplantation (PBPCT)
- has been used with apparent safety to augment hematopoietic recovery after chemotherapy for acute myelogenous/lymphoblastic leukemias

■ Mechanism/actions
- G-CSF binds to specific cell surface receptors and stimulates proliferation and differentiation of neutrophils from committed progenitor cells
- causes a dose-dependent increase in mature neutrophils
- mobilizes bone marrow progenitor cells into peripheral circulation

■ Dosing
- maintenance of dose intensity/reduction in probability of neutropenic complications: 4–8 mcg/kg/d SubQ beginning at least 24 hrs post chemotherapy and continued for 10–14 days or until established neutrophil recovery following expected nadir. Discontinue at least 24 hrs prior to subsequent chemotherapy cycle
- hematopoietic recovery post BMT/PBPCT: 5–10 mcg/kg/d SubQ beginning 1–7 days post stem cell infusion and continuing until ANC > 500/mm^3 on 2–3 successive days
- mobilization of PBPC prior to collection: 10 mcg/kg/d SubQ beginning at least 4 days prior to leukapheresis (e.g., G-CSF given for 7 days with leukapheresis on days 4–7). Discontinue when adequate yield of CFU-GM or CD 34$^+$ cells obtained according to institutional standards

■ Other routes of administration
- short IV infusion (15–30 min); continuous 24 hr SubQ or IV infusion

■ Possible side effects
- medullary bone pain (24%)
- reversible elevations of urate, lactate dehydrogenase, alkaline phosphatase
- rare reports of cutaneous vasculitis (< 1:7,000 patients); generally seen with chronic use

■ Other considerations
- drug interactions have not been fully evaluated; caution with drugs that may potentiate neutrophils (e.g., concurrent use of lithium or other hematopoietic growth factors)
- periodic monitoring of blood counts (e.g., three times weekly) recommended
- greater nonhematologic toxicity/thrombocytopenia may be seen as a result of higher chemotherapeutic dose intensity

  - not routinely recommended as part of primary therapy unless risk of febrile neutropenia ≥40%
  - use of G-CSF in cycles subsequent to the occurrence of a febrile neutropenic event is reasonable
- Nursing considerations
  - store in refrigerator and remove 30 min prior to injection
  - do not shake vial before use
  - discard unused portions
  - do not give within 24 hrs before and after chemotherapy
- Assess
  - for hypersensitivity to *E. coli* products
  - for signs and symptoms of side effects; skeletal pain and need for NSAIDs
- Teach patient
  - rationale for periodic blood counts
  - technique for self-injections
  - proper disposal of used syringes
  - avoid exposure to infections
  - report fever, chills, pain, or swelling at injection site

GM-CSF (SARGRAMOSTIM, LEUKINE)

- GM-CSF is a glycoprotein synthesized by recombinant DNA technology in *S. cerevisiae* yeast. It is packaged as either lyophilized powder or in liquid form and is clear and colorless in liquid form or upon reconstitution. It is suitable for SubQ administration
- Common indications
  - for promotion of myeloid recovery following induction chemotherapy for acute myelogenous leukemia (AML) in older adult patients (safety and efficacy not established in patients < 55 yrs of age)
  - mobilization of peripheral blood progenitor cells (PBPC) prior to collection
  - promotion of hematopoietic recovery post bone marrow transplantation (BMT) or peripheral blood progenitor cell transplantation (PBPCT)
  - for use in myeloid reconstitution following allogeneic bone marrow transplantation
- Mechanism/actions
  - GM-CSF binds to specific cell surface receptors
  - causes partially committed precursor cells to proliferate and differentiate principally along the granulocyte/macrophage lineage
  - can cause activation of granulocytes/macrophages
  - induces mobilization of bone marrow progenitor cells into peripheral circulation
- Dosing
  - following induction chemotherapy for AML in older adult patients: GM-CSF 250 mcg/m²/d IV over 4 hrs beginning 4 days after chemotherapy and continued until neutrophil recovery (> 1,500/mm³ for 3 days recommended)
  - mobilization of PBPC: GM-CSF 250 mcg/m²/d IV over 24 hrs or SubQ. Begin collection on day 5 or when WBC count ≥10,000/mm³. Discontinue when adequate yield of CFU-GM or CD 34⁺ cells obtained according to institutional standards
- hematopoietic recovery post BMT/PBPCT: GM-CSF 250 mcg/m²/d IV over 24 hrs or SubQ beginning immediately post stem cell infusion and continuing until absolute neutrophil recovery (e.g., > 500/mm³ on 2 successive days)
- Possible side effects
  - fever, chills, asthenia, myalgia
  - fluid retention (edema, pleural/pericardial effusions)
  - bone pain
- Other considerations
  - AML patients should have hypoplastic marrow (< 5% blasts) on day 10 (or 4 days following a second induction cycle) prior to beginning therapy with GM-CSF
  - drug interactions have not been fully evaluated; caution with drugs that may potentiate neutrophils (e.g., concurrent use of lithium or other hematopoietic growth factors)
  - periodic monitoring of blood counts (e.g., three times weekly) recommended
- Nursing considerations
  - store in refrigerator and remove 30 min prior to injection
  - do not shake vial before use
  - reconstitute per manufacturer's directions (do not use in-line membrane filter)
  - do not reenter vial; discard unused portions
  - can interfere with laboratory results by causing an increase in serum BUN, creatinine
  - do not give within 24 hrs after chemotherapy
- Assess
  - for hypersensitivity to yeast products
  - for signs and symptoms of side effects
- Teach patient
  - rationale for frequent blood counts
  - report fever, chills, pain, or swelling at injection site
  - avoid exposure to infections

ERYTHROPOIETIN (EPO, PROCRIT)

- EPO is a glycoprotein synthesized by recombinant DNA technology. It stimulates division and differentiation of erythroid progenitors in the bone marrow. It is packaged as a sterile clear colorless liquid suitable for SubQ or IV administration
- Indications
  - anemia associated with chronic renal failure
  - anemia associated with zidovudine
  - anemia caused by chemotherapeutic treatment of nonmyeloid malignancies
- Mechanism/Actions
  - synthetic EPO binds to specific cell surface receptors
  - same biologic activity/actions as endogenous EPO
- Dosing
  - for chemotherapy-induced anemia, recommended starting dose is 150 U/kg three times weekly SubQ or 40,000 U SubQ once weekly
  - patients who fail to respond after 8 wks, increase to 300 U/kg three times weekly SubQ
  - patients who fail to respond to 300 U/kg SubQ three times weekly are unlikely to benefit from further increased dosage
- Possible side effects
  - rare increases in blood pressure noted in patients with cancer; monitor appropriately
  - association with seizures unclear; weigh risks/benefits and monitor appropriately in patients with history of seizures
  - association of EPO with thrombotic events in cancer patients is uncertain
- Treatment considerations
  - patients must be replete in iron (serum ferritin at least 100 mcg/ml, transferrin 20%), folate, and B12
  - patients may require ongoing iron supplementation during therapy
  - anemias due to other mechanisms (e.g., reticuloendothelial blockade, red cell hemolysis) unlikely to respond to EPO
  - patients with baseline endogenous levels of EPO > 200 m U/ml unlikely to benefit
  - increase in hemoglobin not usually seen until 1 mo after beginning therapy
  - if hematocrit exceeds 0.40, discontinue EPO until hematocrit falls to 0.36, then restart EPO at 75% of previous dose
  - if rapid rise in hematocrit seen (e.g., > 4% over 2 wks) reduce dose of EPO
- Nursing considerations
  - gently mix; *do not shake vial*, as it may denature the glycoprotein
  - vials must be refrigerated
  - discard unused portion
  - do not give with any other drug solution
  - monitor access line for signs of clotting
  - contraindicated in patients with uncontrolled hypertension
- Assess
  - for hypersensitivity to mammalian cell-derived products
  - urinary output, renal function, blood pressure, and reflexes
- Teach patient
  - rationale for frequent blood counts to determine effects of drug
  - report difficulty breathing, numbness or tingling, chest pain, seizures

IL-11 (OPRELVEKIN, NEUMEGA)

- Oprelvekin is a polypeptide synthesized by recombinant DNA technology in *E. coli* bacteria and administered by SubQ injection

Myelosuppression *(Continued)*

- Common indications
  - prevention of severe thrombocytopenia/ reduction in need for platelet transfusions in patients with nonmyeloid malignancies undergoing myelosuppressive chemotherapy associated with a high probability of severe thrombocytopenia
  - patients at high risk for severe thrombocytopenia: patients with extensive prior chemotherapy; patients with severe thrombocytopenia on previous treatment cycles; patients receiving dose-intense chemotherapy regimens associated with a high risk for thrombocytopenia
- Mechanism/actions
  - oprelvekin is a hematopoietic growth factor that stimulates the proliferation of hematopoietic stem cells/megakaryocyte precursors, resulting in increased platelet production
  - in nonmyelosuppressed cancer patients, causes a dose-dependent increase in platelets after 5–9 days of a 14 day dosing schedule
  - platelet counts continue to rise for up to 7 days after beginning therapy, returning toward baseline by day 14 of therapy
  - platelet function (in vitro studies of reactivity, aggregation) appears to be unaffected by oprelvekin
- Dosing
  - safety/efficacy not established when given prior to/concurrently with chemotherapy; therefore dosing should begin 6–24 hrs post completion of chemotherapy
  - recommended adult dose is 50 mcg/kg/d SubQ given for 10–21 days or until established platelet recovery (e.g., platelets ≥50,000/mcL) following expected nadir
  - discontinue at least 48 hrs prior to subsequent chemotherapy cycle
- Possible adverse effects
  - fluid retention/edema (up to 59% of patients)
  - amblyopia, blurred vision, papilledema
  - paresthesiae, dehydration, skin discoloration, exfoliative dermatitis
  - asthenia, chills
  - abdominal pain, anorexia, dyspepsia, constipation
  - myalgias, bone pain
- Other considerations
  - safety/efficacy not established in regimens/agents associated with delayed myelosuppression (e.g., nitrosoureas, mitomycin-C)
  - caution in patients with history of atrial arrhythmias; oprelvekin may be associated with increased incidence of transient atrial fibrillation/flutter; not known to be directly related; arrhythmogenic and arrhythmias observed may have been related to increases in plasma volume
  - caution in patients with fluid retention states (e.g., congestive heart failure)
  - CBC at baseline and at periodic intervals recommended
  - safety/efficacy of chronic administration not established (e.g., beyond 6 cycles of therapy)
  - safety/efficacy following myeloablative chemotherapy not established
- Nursing considerations
  - drug should be used within 3 hrs after reconstitution; if not used immediately store in refrigerator or at room temperature. *Do not* freeze or shake
- Assess
  - baseline fluid/electrolyte balance
  - baseline heart rate and monitor during therapy
- Teach patient
  - dizziness may occur; change positions slowly
  - report palpitations, dizziness, lightheadedness, or dyspnea

Chemotherapy-Induced Mucositis/Stomatitis

S. H. Okuno, D. Watts, and C. L. Loprinzi

OVERVIEW

- Mucositis can be a dose-limiting toxicity for antimetabolite cytotoxic agents such as 5-FU, methotrexate, and other purine antagonists
- Antitumor antibiotics, such as doxorubicin, and other cytotoxic agents, such as hydroxyurea and procarbazine, can also occasionally cause mucositis when used in nonablative doses

PATHOPHYSIOLOGY

- The precise mechanism by which cytotoxic drugs cause mucositis has not been clearly delineated
- Presumably, causative agents damage rapidly reproducing mucosal epithelial cells leading to mucosal inflammation and ulceration
- In some situations secondary infection may play a role

DIAGNOSIS AND PREVENTION

- Prevention of 5-fluorouracil–induced mucositis
  - the only definitive studies conducted regarding prevention of chemotherapy-induced mucositis have evaluated the prevention of 5-fluorouracil–induced oral mucositis
  - two clinical trials have demonstrated that oral cryotherapy decreases 5-FU–induced mucositis by ~50%. These trials utilized 30 min of oral cryotherapy
  - the oral cryotherapy program had patients place ice chips in their mouths 5 min prior to being given a bolus injection of 5-fluorouracil. Patients continuously swished the ice around in the oral cavity for 30 min, replenishing the chips so that the ice was continuously in contact with the oral mucosa during this 30 min time period
  - a third randomized trial compared 30 vs. 60 min of oral cryotherapy, finding no additional benefit from the longer treatment period
  - since the mechanism of action from oral cryotherapy is thought to be vasoconstriction of the oral mucosa during times of peak serum 5-FU concentrations (noting that bolus dose 5-FU has a half-life of ~10 min), it would not be expected that this therapy would be efficacious for continuous infusion 5-FU therapy
  - this therapy would not be expected to be beneficial for patients receiving methotrexate, given the prolonged serum half-life of this drug
  - while a number of other potentially promising agents have been evaluated by randomized trials to test whether they might prevent 5-FU–induced mucositis, these trials failed to demonstrate any benefit for such things as camomile tea, glutamine, or an allopurinol mouthwash

THERAPY

- The treatment of established mucositis from 5-fluorouracil or other chemotherapeutic agents has not been well studied
  - a time-honored standard has been to have the patient gargle with a salt and baking soda solution (a teaspoon of each in a cup of water)
  - a topical anesthetic such as viscous lidocaine has commonly been utilized (again, not well studied). A number of cocktails (containing such drugs as magnesium hydroxide, diphenhydramine, lidocaine, and/or sucralfate) have also been established at many institutions. These cocktails have not been well studied
  - of note, however, a randomized trial of sucralfate for treatment of established 5-FU–induced mucositis failed to demonstrate any benefit from such
  - other antidotes that are undergoing testing include vitamin E and a variety of cytokines, such as colony-stimulating factors
  - a more comprehensive review of the prevention and treatment of mucositosis related to chemotherapy (and radiation therapy) can be found in the final key references
- Special nursing considerations
  - considerable controversy exists within the oncology community regarding the best treatment of oral mucositis. The need for comprehensive and consistent oral hygiene to modify the severity and incidence of mucositis in patients who are receiving chemotherapy has been well documented in the literature
  - currently, there is no standardized oral care protocol. However, research has shown that regardless of agents used, a protocol that emphasizes adequate teaching, consistent assessment and documentation of changes, and reinforcement of oral care (cleaning, lubricating, adequate pain control, and mechanisms to avoid further injury) can decrease the severity of mucositis. A comprehensive and systematic method to describe and rate the severity of mucositis was developed at the University of Nebraska Medical Center. This Oral Assessment Guide (OAG) consists of eight categories, each with three levels of grading on a 1-2-3 scale. The eight categories encompass quality of the voice, swallowing, saliva, and integrity of the lips, tongue, mucous membranes, gingiva, and teeth. The three descriptive levels rate each category from most normal (1) to most abnormal (3). The total scores are the sums of the eight categories ranging from 8 (normal in all categories) to 24 (breakdown or loss of function in all categories)
- General principles of care
  - avoid foods that are rough, hot, spicy, or acidic to minimize irritation and pain to the oral mucosa
  - avoid commercial mouthwashes
  - eat foods high in protein to promote cellular repair and healing
  - drink plenty of fluids to maintain adequate hydration
  - perform oral hygiene after meals and especially at bedtime to minimize bacteria formation during sleep
  - assess the oral cavity carefully for signs and symptoms of infection
  - use a soft sponge-tipped swab for cleaning oral cavity

KEY REFERENCES

Cascinu S, Fedeli A, Fedeli SL, Catalano G: Oral cooling (cryotherapy), an effective treatment for the prevention of 5-fluorouracil-induced stomatitis. Eur J Cancer 1994; 30:324–6

Loprinzi CL, Gatineau D, Foote RL: Oral complications. In *Clinical Oncology* (pp. 741–53). MD Abeloff, JO Armitage, AS Lichter, JE Niederhuber (eds.). New York, Edinburg, London, Melbourne, Tokyo: Churchill Livingstone, 1995

Loprinzi CL, Ghosh C, Camoriano J, Sloan JA, Steen PD, Michalak JC, Stevens B, Novotony PJ, Vukov AM, White DF, Hatfield AK, Quella SK: Phase III controlled evaluation of sucralfate for alleviating stomatitis in patients receiving 5FU based chemotherapy. J Clin Oncol 1997; 15(3):1235–8

Mahood DJ, Dose AM, Loprinzi CL, Veeder MH, Athmann LM, Therneau TM, Sorensen JM, Gainey DK, Mailliard JA, Gusa NL, et al.: Inhibition of fluorouracil-induced somatitis by oral cryotherapy. J Clin Oncol 1991; 9:449–52

Rocke LK, Loprinzi CL, Lee JK, Junselman SJ, Iverson RK, Finck G, Lifsey D, Glaw KC, Stevens BA, Hatfield AK, et al.: A randomized clinical trial of two different durations of oral cryotherapy for prevention of 5-fluorouracil-related stomatitis. Cancer 1993; 72:2234–8

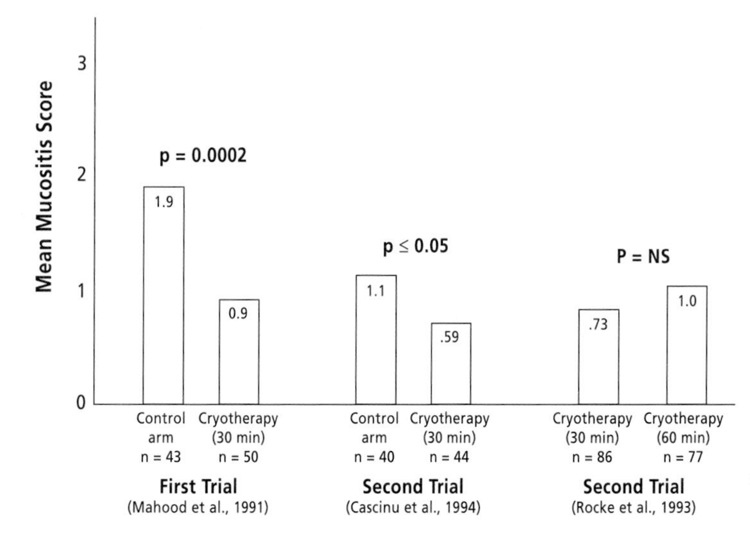

Mean comparative mucositis scores (higher is worse) on patients entered on two randomized clinical trials.

Agents used to Treat Mucositis

Agents	Action	Dose/Administration	Pros and Cons
Cleansing Agent			
Saline solution	Aids granulation, promotes healing. Increased rinsing frequency decreases bacterial load by removing loose debris	½ tsp. salt in 8 oz H_2O or 1 tsp. in 1L H_2O. If pt has ulcers or neutropenia, sterile saline is recommended	– Economical, readily available, least damaging – Does not effectively remove hardened mucous, debris, or crust
Sodium bicarbonate solution	Mucosolvent; loosens debris and crust. Decreases odor. Reduces oral acidity	1 tsp. baking soda in 8 oz H_2O. Swish, gargle, spit. Rinse mouth with water or normal saline afterward	– Particularly effective for thick saliva – May cause irritation and burning sensation if too concentrated – Unpleasant taste; flavoring with non-alcoholic mouthwash may improve taste – Risk of potential absorption in pts with sodium restrictions
Perox-A-Mist	Loosens degenerated tissue, debris and mucous	Rinse up to 4 times/day. If foaming action occurs, rinse with saline or water	– Alcohol free – Ready-to-use formula
Lip Lubricant			
K-Y Jelly	Lubricates; prevents cracking and bleeding	Apply as often as needed. Periodic removal of dried film to prevent excessive buildup may be required	– Nonirritating, water soluble, inexpensive – Can be used for long periods – Can be used on pts receiving oxygen – Can be applied to oral mucosa
Petrolatum	Lubricates. Prevents evaporation of moisture by forming an occlusive film on lips	Apply as needed. Clean lips periodically with normal saline to prevent excessive buildup if mucositis is present	– Cannot be used w/pts receiving oxygen – May cause aspiration in pts with an altered state of consciousness
Coating Agents/Topical Anesthetics			
Oratect-gel	Topical anesthetic. Contains 20% benzocaine	Apply small amount to dry lesion up to 4 times /day	– Gel dries within 1 min to form a protective film for up to 2 hrs – Mild, transient stinging immediately after application – Mainly indicated for Grade I–II (mild to moderate) mucositis
Orahesive	A thin dressing that forms a protective coat, which leads to pain relief	Hold dressing against oral site for 1–2 mins. Lesions should be dry before application to facilitate a seal	– Not harmful if swallowed – Can adhere to oral surfaces up to 30 hrs. Duration of adhesive depends on location of lesion and application technique
Xylocaine-Viscous 2% solution	Numbs oral cavity	5 ml swish and swallow prior to meals. 15 ml swish, gargle, and expectorate q3hrs as needed. Do not exceed 120 ml in a 24 hr period	– Simple to use, readily accessible and inexpensive – Quick onset of action (5 min) – Duration of relief is short term, 20 mins – Pts may dislike taste and feeling of numbness – May mask sensitivity to hot or irritating foods if swallowed – May interfere with the pharyngeal phase of swallowing – May have systemic effects (cardiovascular and CNS)
Diclone hydrochloride	Topical anesthetics for generalized areas of pain	15 ml swish and spit as needed q3–4hrs	– Minimal absorption and decreased likelihood of any systemic effects – Longer duration than viscous xylocaine; numbing effect lasts up to 1 hr – Contains no alcohol but may cause local discomfort upon contact w/oral tissues
Infection Control and Treatment			
Nystatin Swish and Troches	Treats or prevents candida by altering cell wall permeability, thereby inhibiting fungal growth	Swish and swallow 15–30 ml 4 times/day (400,000–600,000 units) to treat oral or esophageal infection. When used prophylactically solution may be expectorated. Swish in mouth at least 5 mins. Cleanse mouth prior to administration to maximize drug contact w/mucosal surfaces. Do not eat or drink for at least 30 mins afterward. Let troche dissolve completely in mouth	– Topical effects may be diminished, since pt may have difficulty complying with minimal time for swish – Troche may take longer to dissolve in pts w/xerostomia – Long-term use of troches may result in dental caries due to large quantities of sugar – May exacerbate nausea
Fluconozole	System oral antifungal agent	100 mg tablet daily	– Once a day dosing leads to increased compliance – Potentially toxic to liver

Diarrhea

Thomas J. Garrett, Patricia Ferrill, and Marianne Huml

OVERVIEW

■ Diarrhea commonly occurs in cancer patients and can significantly degrade the patient's quality of life, as well as be life threatening through dehydration and electrolyte depletion

■ Diarrhea can have many causes but in most oncology patients, it is a complication of therapy

■ Patients with diarrhea must be evaluated to determine both the likely etiology and the severity of the illness

■ Those with volume depletion and serum electrolyte abnormalities will require appropriate repletion. The IV route may be necessary, especially in patients with nausea or oropharyngeal mucositis, which limits oral intake

■ Patients treated with diarrhea-associated medication also must be instructed about the significance of this condition and the indications for contacting the health care provider

■ With some anticancer treatments, such as irinotecan, where the likelihood of diarrhea is high, it may be appropriate to outline preliminary steps the patients should take before calling

PATHOPHYSIOLOGY

■ Mechanism of action
  - osmotic: ingestion of a nonabsorbable molecule that retains fluid in the gastrointestinal tract
  - secretory: the net elaboration of water and electrolytes from the intestinal epithelial cells exceeds reabsorption. Result: watery diarrheal fluid that is isosmotic to plasma
  - exudative: inflammatory injury to the epithelial cells of the intestinal tract
  - hypermotile: the rapid transit of fluid through the gastrointestinal tract prevents the normal degree of absorption of water and electrolytes
  - *secretory* or *exudative* mechanisms explain the diarrhea seen in most cancer patients

DIAGNOSIS AND PREVENTION

■ Unfortunately, pharmacological agents are not available to prevent the diarrhea that may develop as a complication of antineoplastic medications

■ Chemotherapy induced
  - diarrhea can be a complication of many of the antineoplastic drugs and is seen with some of the DNA-binding agents, with antimetabolites and the topoisomerase inhibitors. The incidence with the antimetabolite 5-fluorouracil varies from $<10\%$ to $\sim 30\%$, depending on the regimen used
  - diarrhea may be a dose-limiting toxicity with the topoisomerase inhibitor irinotecan with grade 3 or 4 morbidity reported in $\sim 40\%$ of patients. Two patterns of diarrhea have been described
    □ early onset (within 24 hrs of administration) is cholinergically mediated and associated with diaphoresis and cramping
    □ late onset (more than 24 hrs following administration) can be severe and result in life-threatening dehydration and electrolyte depletion
  - few studies have explored the pathophysiology of chemotherapy-induced diarrhea in detail. However, it is likely that most cases fall into the *secretory* category. Chemotherapy drugs may cause changes in the normal maturation process of the epithelial cells, resulting in a shift in the balance between fluid secretion and absorption with the former exceeding the latter
  - some cases of diarrhea may be *exudative* if the degree of mucosal damage from chemotherapy drugs results in necrosis and inflammation
  - diarrhea is a common and often severe complication of many of the high-dose chemotherapy regimens used in stem cell transplant protocols

■ Radiation therapy induced
  - patients receiving radiation therapy to a field that includes the small intestine and/or colon may develop diarrhea, which occurs within several weeks of initiating the therapy
  - the diarrhea may have a *secretory* component as a result of impaired epithelial cell function, as well as an *exudative* component due to the inflammatory responses to radiation damage to the mucosa

■ Diarrhea due to comorbid conditions
  - with leukopenia caused by chemotherapy, antineoplastic drugs may cause *C. difficile* colitis if broad-spectrum antibiotics are administered when fever develops
  - patients undergoing allogeneic stem cell transplantation almost always develop diarrhea
  - the high-dose chemotherapy and/or radiation therapy conditioning regimens may cause diarrhea, as noted above. In addition, diarrhea is a manifestation of graft-versus-host disease, which often complicates allogeneic transplantation

THERAPY

■ Loperamide or diphenoxylate
  - the mainstay of therapy for patients with antineoplastic-related diarrhea are these synthetic opioids, which interact with receptors on enteric neurons, as well as on intestinal epithelial and smooth muscle cells
  - effects on smooth muscle cells reduce gastrointestinal tract peristalsis, causing longer intestinal time while allowing more opportunity for fluid absorption. The effect on epithelial cell function is a reduction in water secretion and electrolytes
  - these synthetic opioids have largely supplanted the naturally occurring opiates because of their lower penetration of the central nervous system, resulting in greater antidiarrheal action relative to side effects. This is especially the case with loperamide, which may be the preferred agent for initial therapy

■ Atropine
  - anticholinergic drugs, such as atropine, can reduce intestinal peristalsis. However, side effects, such as dry mouth, blurred vision, and urinary retention, limit their usefulness. Atropine may be especially useful in treating the early type of diarrhea that occurs with irinotecan

■ Octreotide
  - this somatostatin analogue has been approved for treating secretory diarrhea seen with functional endocrine tumors. It currently is being evaluated for the management of diarrhea due to chemotherapy and graft-versus-host disease

KEY REFERENCES

Abigerges D, Armand JP, Chabot GG, Da Costa L, Fadel E, Cote C, Herait P, Gandia D: Irinotecan (CPT-11) high-dose escalation using intensive high-dose loperamide to control diarrhea. J Natl Cancer Inst 1994; 86:446–9

Cascinu S: Drug therapy in diarrheal diseases in oncology/hematology patients. Crit Rev Oncol Hematol 1995; 18:37–50

Machover D: A comprehensive review of 5-fluorouracil and leucovorin in patients with metastatic colorectal carcinoma. Cancer 1997; 80: 1179–87

Pitot HC, Wender DB, O'Connell MJ, Schroeder G, Goldberg RM, Rubin J, Mailliard JA, Knost JA, Ghosh C, Kirschling RJ, Levitt R, Windschitl HE: Phase II trial of irinotecan in patients with metastatic colorectal carcinoma. J Clin Oncol 1997; 15:2910–19

Wadler S, Benson AB, Engelking C, Catalano R, Field M, Kornblau SM, Mitchell E, Rubin J, Trotta P, Vokes E: Recommended guidelines for the treatment of chemotherapy-induced diarrhea. J Clin Oncol 1998; 16:3169–78

Wright PS, Thomas SL: Constipation and diarrhea: the neglected symptoms. Semin Oncol Nurs 1995; 11:289–97

DRUG: DIPHENOXYLATE

■ Other name: Lomotil

■ Uses: approved by FDA for relief of acute nonspecific diarrhea

■ Mechanism of action
  - synthetic opiate with little uptake into central nervous system

- effects receptors on neurons within the gut as well as receptors on intestinal smooth muscle and epithelial cells
- reduction in peristalsis with prolonged transit time allowing more fluid reabsorption
- reduction in net fluid secretion by effects on epithelial cell function

- Dosing
  - tablet containing 2.5 mg diphenoxylate and 0.025 mg atropine sulfate and liquid with 5 ml containing 2.5 mg diphenoxylate and 0.025 mg atropine sulfate
  - recommended dose is 2 tablets or 10 ml four times daily (total dose 20 mg diphenoxylate per 24 hrs)
- Pharmacokinetics
  - readily absorbed
  - rapid deesterification with metabolite active with a half-life of 12 hrs
- Side effects
  - hypersensitivity reactions including cutaneous
  - constipation
  - sedation
  - atropine effects—tachycardia, dry mouth, flushing, urinary retention
- Other considerations
  - caution advised in patients with liver disease, although specific guidelines not readily available
  - atropine added to formulation to reduce addiction potential through anticholinergic side effects
  - patients must be monitored for indications of dehydration and/or colitis
- Nursing considerations
  - assess for history of medication allergies
  - evaluate change in frequency and water content of stools with medication
  - advise patients that continued use after diarrhea stops may cause constipation
  - may be habit forming when used in high doses
  - use cautiously in patients with hepatic cirrhosis; may precipitate hepatic coma
  - use cautiously in patients with acute ulcerative colitis
  - not recommended for use in patients with fevers and bloody or profuse diarrhea suggestive of an infectious or inflammatory process
- Assess
  - baseline neurologic status and during treatment for signs of sedation, lethargy, restlessness, or insomnia; drug crosses blood-brain barrier
  - baseline nutritional status; monitor during therapy
  - skin integrity
- Teach patient
  - self-care of rectal mucosa and surrounding skin; use of skin barriers, warm soaks, good personal hygiene to keep area clean and dry
  - drug should only be used for 2 days; if diarrhea persists notify physician
  - importance of drinking 3 L a day, avoiding caffeine drinks, and intake of a low-residue diet
  - may cause constipation and abdominal cramping; notify physician
  - monitor temperature; report a temperature of 100.5° F (38° C)

DRUG: LOPERAMIDE

- Other name: Imodium
- Uses
  - approved by FDA for relief of acute nonspecific diarrhea
- Mechanism of action
  - synthetic opioid with little uptake into central nervous system
  - effects receptors within the gut as well as receptors on intestinal smooth muscle and epithelial cells
  - reduction in peristalsis with prolonged transit time allowing more fluid retention
  - reduction in net fluid secretion by effects on epithelial cell function
- Dosing
  - oral preparation of 2 mg/capsule; liquid 1 mg/5 ml
  - initial dose of 4 mg with 2 mg after each loose stool to a maximum of 16 mg in 24 hrs
  - irinotecan dosing in clinical trials exceeds the above standard recommendation
  - one regimen used when diarrhea occurs following irinotecan is 4 mg at the start of diarrhea with 2 mg q2hrs during the day and 4 mg q4hrs at night until the patient has no diarrhea for 12 hrs
- Pharmacokinetics
  - readily absorbed
  - hepatic metabolism with biliary excretion main route of clearance
  - most excreted in feces, little in urine
- Side effects
  - hypersensitivity reactions including cutaneous
  - constipation
- Other considerations
  - caution advised in patients with liver disease, although specific guidelines are not readily available
  - antidiarrheal action relative to CNS effects greater than diphenoxylate
  - patients must be monitored for indications of dehydration and/or colitis
- Nursing considerations
  - assess for history of medication allergies
  - evaluate change in frequency and water content of stools with medication
  - advise patients that continued use after diarrhea stops may cause constipation
  - discontinue if abdominal distention occurs
  - record frequency and volume of diarrhea
  - not recommended for use in patients with fevers and bloody or profuse diarrhea suggestive of an infectious or inflammatory process
- Assess
  - baseline nutrition and elimination status
  - for side effects related to drug: constipation, abdominal cramps, gastric upset, dry mouth, headache, and rash
  - skin integrity
- Teach patient
  - self-care of rectal mucosa and surrounding skin; use of skin barriers, warm soaks, good personal hygiene to keep area clean and dry
  - maintenance of care log to record date and time of diarrheal event and time of dosing
  - drug should only be used for 2 days; if diarrhea persists notify physician
  - importance of drinking 3 L a day, avoiding caffeine drinks, and intake of a low-residue diet
  - monitor temperature; report a temperature of 100.5° F (38° C)

DRUG: OCTREOTIDE ACETATE

- Other name: Sandostatin
- Uses
  - approved by the FDA for the treatment of diarrhea due to metastatic carcinoid tumor or vasoactive intestinal peptide (VIP) secreting tumor
  - evaluated in the treatment of diarrhea due to graft-versus-host disease following allogeneic transplantation
  - evaluated in the treatment of diarrhea due to chemotherapy, especially 5-fluorouracil–based regimens
- Mechanism of action
  - inhibits secretion of serotonin, vasoactive intestinal peptide, and secretin as well as other hormonally active molecules
  - suppression of release of active molecules from tumor cells is the primary mechanism for antidiarrheal effect
- Dosing
  - metastatic carcinoid tumor: doses during the first 2 wks range from 100–600 mcg/d administered SubQ in 2–4 divided doses with a median maintenance dose of 450 mcg/d
  - VIP secreting tumor: doses during the first 2 wks range from 200–300 mcg/d administered SubQ in 2–4 divided doses with maintenance doses usually not exceeding 450 mcg/d

Diahrrea *(Continued)*

- graft-versus-host–related diarrhea: doses range from 50–250 mcg administered 2–3 times daily
- chemotherapy-related diarrhea: doses range from 100 mcg twice a day to 500 mcg 3 times a day

■ Pharmacokinetics
- rapidly absorbed from SubQ injection site with peak level reached within 30 min
- plasma half-life ~2 hrs but longer in older individuals, which may require dose adjustment
- biologic action variable and may extend up to 12 hrs

■ Side effects
- pain at injection site
- hypoglycemia and hyperglycemia

■ Nursing considerations
- for outpatient management, caregiver and/or patient needs instruction in technique of SubQ injection
- instruct patient/caregiver to report symptoms that could be related to changes in blood glucose including drowsiness, polyuria, polydipsia, dry mouth, increased thirst
- rotate injection site if administered SubQ
- if given IV, it is not compatible with total parenteral nutrition solutions
- not recommended for use in patients with fevers and bloody or profuse diarrhea suggestive of an infectious or inflammatory process

■ Assess
- baseline nutritional status; monitor during therapy
- skin integrity

■ Teach patient
- side effects: nausea, abdominal cramps; notify physician
- self-care of rectal mucosa and surrounding skin; use of skin barriers, warm soaks, good personal hygiene to keep area clean and dry
- monitor temperature; report a temperature of 100.5° F (38° C)

Cardiotoxicity

J. Doroshow and P. Tiller

OVERVIEW

- Cardiac toxicity related to antineoplastic agents occurs principally after therapy with an anthracycline antibiotic, such as doxorubicin, daunorubicin, or idarubicin
- It also occurs when related quinone-containing anticancer agents, including *mitoxantrone* or *mitomycin C*, are utilized following a full course of anthracycline therapy
- The incidence of clinically significant cardiac injury is related to the total cumulative dose of drug administered; however, each dose produces subclinical myocyte damage
- Abundant recent evidence demonstrates that children have a heightened sensitivity to the cardiotoxicity of the anthracycline antibiotics

PATHOPHYSIOLOGY

- Anthracycline antibiotics produce a wide variety of biochemical alterations in the heart that include
  - loss of high-affinity calcium binding sites on the sarcoplasmic reticulum
  - diminished mitochondrial ATP generation
  - down-regulation of cardiac actin and troponin mRNAs
- All of these effects contribute to a loss of efficient excitation-contraction coupling
  - anthracycline antibiotics are also effective substrates for mitochondrial and sarcoplasmic flavin dehydrogenases, which reduce the quinone moiety of these drugs to semiquinone free radical intermediates
  - the free radical metabolism of the anthracyclines produces reactive oxygen species in each of the cardiac compartments damaged by anthracycline exposure
  - because the heart has limited enzymatic defenses against free radical attack, drug-induced oxygen radical formation leads to compromised mitochondrial energy production, altered calcium sequestration, and release of protein-bound iron that enhances free radical injury

DIAGNOSIS AND PREVENTION

- Acute cardiac toxicity. Two manifestations (syndromes) of acute, anthracycline-related cardiac injury
  - more commonly, doxorubicin and daunorubicin have been associated with both supraventricular and ventricular arrhythmias, as well as heart block
  - a less well-characterized myopericarditis syndrome has been associated with bolus administration of relatively large doses of daunorubicin during induction therapy for acute leukemia
- Chronic cardiac toxicity
  - when anthracycline-related congestive heart failure is diagnosed early, it is fully treatable with standard measures; however, it is possible that a continuing, subtle deterioration of cardiac function may present as heart failure several months after anthracycline therapy has been discontinued
  - the risk of congestive heart failure after anthracycline administration is increased in patients with poorly controlled hypertension or those individuals who have received ~2,000 cGy of radiation to the heart
  - progressive injury to the heart is produced with each dose of doxorubicin when it is administered as a bolus or short infusion
  - major pathologic changes observed: disintegration of myofibrils and dilatation of the sarcoplasmic reticulum
  - the clinical picture of anthracycline cardiac toxicity: a congestive cardiomyopathy, which recent studies have demonstrated increases significantly in risk above a cumulative doxorubicin dose of 350–400 mg/m^2
  - measurement of cardiac ejection fraction by gated radioisotopic blood pool scanning has been demonstrated to correlate significantly with anthracycline-related damage to the heart; thus, evidence of significant cardiac toxicity can now be detected earlier
  - cardiac injury in anthracycline-treated patients may also be exacerbated by subsequent exposure to modest total doses of either mitoxantrone or mitomycin C

THERAPY

- Infusional administration
  - the risk of anthracycline cardiac toxicity is a function of peak drug concentration rather than systemic exposure
  - identical cumulative drug doses administered by 96 hr continuous IV infusion produce significantly less cardiac toxicity than does bolus drug administration
  - the use of an infusion pump and central venous line is necessary
- Co-administration of the cardioprotective agent dexrazoxane (Zinecard)
  - the iron-chelating agent dexrazoxane, when delivered together with doxorubicin, increases by at least a factor of two the cumulative drug dose that produces definite cardiac injury
  - the cost of dexrazoxane approximates that involved in the use of an anthracycline infusion to lessen the risk of heart damage
- Cardiac toxicities from other therapeutic agents: cardiac arrhythmias
  - 5-fluorouracil (5-FU)
    - □ administration of 5-FU by either bolus or infusional schedules has been associated in < 10% of treated patients with the development of cardiac arrythmias (usually supraventricular tachyarrythmias) with or without chest pain and associated ischemic electrocardiographic abnormalities
    - □ these episodes occur most commonly in patients with prior ischemic heart disease or a prior history of chest irradiation
    - □ numerous reports of coronary arteriography performed in this circumstance have failed to document clear evidence of atherosclerotic coronary artery disease. Hence, this syndrome has been ascribed to drug or drug-metabolite–related vasospasm
    - □ the mechanism of 5-FU–related cardiac toxicity remains unclear; however, the drug may increase the vasoreactivity of vascular smooth muscle. In vitro, nitroglycerin has been shown to diminish drug-related vasoconstriction. Both the arrythmias and chest discomfort associated with 5-FU therapy resolve following withdrawal of treatment
  - paclitaxel
    - □ treatment with paclitaxel produces asymptomatic bradyarrythmias in 15–30% of patients. In general, this effect is transient and without hemodynamic consequences; asymptomatic bradycardia is not an indication for discontinuation of therapy. A much smaller number of patients experience higher grades of heart block, which in general are also asymptomatic
    - □ continuous cardiac monitoring of patients receiving paclitaxel is not required. In vitro studies have demonstrated a direct effect of paclitaxel on the beating frequency of cultured myocytes similar to the conduction abnormalities observed in humans; the mechanism of the toxic effect of paclitaxel on cardiac automaticity is unknown. Recent pharmacokinetic trials have also demonstrated an effect of the Cremophor vehicle in which paclitaxel is solubilized on the metabolism of doxorubicin
    - □ simultaneous administration of paclitaxel by 3 hr infusion with concomitant doxorubicin can decrease the clearance of doxorubicin and potentiate the cardiotoxicity of the anthracycline
- Miscellaneous forms of cardiac injury
  - high-dose cyclophosphamide
    - □ when cyclophosphamide is used in the high-dose chemotherapy setting with bone marrow or peripheral blood progenitor cell support, its dose-limiting toxicity is cardiac necrosis
    - □ heart damage from cyclophosphamide therapy occurs most commonly at doses over 150 mg/kg delivered over 24–48 hrs. It is characterized clinically by the rapid onset of congestive heart failure that may be fatal. Pathological-

ly, myocardial necrosis, edema, and interstitial hemorrhage are present, with alterations also seen in the coronary arteriolar endothelium
  - □ recent evidence suggests that the etiology of cyclophosphamide cardiac toxicity is related to severe depletion of cardiac-reduced thiol pools, which occurs when hepatic detoxification pathways are saturated following high-dose administration
  - □ damage to the heart has not been observed, either acutely or after chronic administration, following repeated treatment with the standard doses of cyclophosphamide usually employed in the outpatient setting
- Herceptin (recombinant humanized anti-p185^{HER2} monoclonal antibody; rhuMAB HER2)
  - □ recent studies have demonstrated that rhuMAB HER2 when administered to women with advanced breast cancer whose disease had progressed after one or two prior chemotherapy regimens produces an ~7% incidence of significant cardiac toxicity
  - □ most of the patients who develop cardiac toxicity after treatment with rhuMAB HER2 had received doxorubicin or left chest wall radiation previously
  - □ the cardiac toxicity of the antibody in patients previously treated with doxorubicin is equivalent to the level of heart damage produced by doxorubicin itself when the anthracycline is used as first-line therapy for metastatic breast cancer. Furthermore, the addition of rhuMAB HER2 to the combination of doxorubicin and cyclophosphamide administered as initial treatment for advanced breast cancer significantly increased the incidence of anthracycline cardiac toxicity in a recent study (from 7 to 28%)
  - □ there is no currently accepted mechanism that explains the cardiac injury produced by rhuMAB HER2 alone or in combination with doxorubicin

KEY REFERENCES

Gianni L, Munzone E, Capri G, et al.: Paclitaxel by 3-hour infusion in combination with bolus doxorubicin in women with untreated breast cancer: high antitumor efficacy and cardiac effects in a dose-finding and sequence-finding study. J Clin Oncol 1995; 13:2688–99

Gianni L, Vigano L, Locatelli A, et al.: Human pharmacokinetic characterization and in vitro study of the interaction between doxorubicin and paclitaxel in patients with breast cancer. J Clin Oncol 1997; 15:1906–15

Slamon D, Leyland-Jones B, Shak S, et al.: Addition of Herceptin (humanized anti-HER2 antibody) to first line chemotherapy for HER2 overexpressing metastatic breast cancer (HER2 +/MBC) markedly increase anticancer activity: a randomized multinational controlled phase III trial. Proc Amer Soc Clin Oncol 1998; 17:98a

Speyer JL, Green MD, Kramer E, et al.: Protective effect of the bispiperazinedione ICRF-187 against doxorubicin-induced cardiac toxicity in women with advanced breast cancer. N Engl J Med 1988; 319: 745–52

Swain SM: Adult multicenter trials using dexrazoxane to protect against cardiac toxicity. Semin Oncol 1998; 25:43–7

DRUG: DEXRAZOXANE

- Other names: Zinecard, ICRF-187
- Use: approved by the FDA for use in combination with doxorubicin for women with metastatic breast cancer who have received a cumulative doxorubicin dose of 300 mg/m^2 and who would benefit from continued doxorubicin therapy
- Mechanism of action
  - dexrazoxane is a lipophilic derivative of EDTA that enters cardiac myocytes by passive diffusion. Intracellularly it is rapidly hydrolyzed nonenzymatically to a ring-opened derivative (ICRF-198) that actively chelates iron; the iron-ICRF-chelate can be effluxed efficiently from the cell, removing toxic-free iron species that may be released from cardiac iron-binding proteins by a flux of anthracycline-induced reactive oxygen
  - in cultured tumor cells, dexrazoxane also directly inhibits the enzymatic activity of topoisomerase II without producing protein-associated single-strand cleavage in DNA
- Dosing
  - supplied as a lyophilized powder in 250 or 500 mg vials for parenteral use; dexrazoxane is stable for no more than 6 hrs at room temperature or under refrigerated conditions
  - the approved dosage is a 10:1 ratio of dexrazoxane:doxorubicin (e.g., 600 mg/m^2 dexrazoxane: 60 mg/m^2 doxorubicin) administered as a slow IV bolus or short infusion. Doxorubicin must be delivered within 30 min after the initiation of the dexrazoxane infusion. Dexrazoxane should not be mixed with other drugs
- Pharmacokinetics
  - following IV administration, dexrazoxane is cleared from plasma following a biexponential decay with an initial $T_{1/2}\alpha$ of 8–10 min and a $T_{1/2}\beta$ of 2–3 hrs
  - the volume of distribution is equivalent to total body water (25 L/m^2)
  - no binding to plasma proteins has been observed
  - ~40% of an administered dose is excreted in the urine; both unchanged drug and ring-opened hydrolysis products have been detected in the urine, including species bound to iron
  - guidelines for usage in the presence of renal or hepatic dysfunction are not available
  - dexrazoxane does not alter the pharmacokinetics or metabolism of doxorubicin
- Side effects
  - the major side effects of treatment with dexrazoxane and doxorubicin are related to the use of the anthracycline antibiotic; however, the incidence of granulocytopenia and thrombocytopenia when dexrazoxane is combined with doxorubicin appears to be higher than that observed without the cardioprotective agent
- Other considerations
  - dexrazoxane is reconstituted with either 0.9% sodium chloride for injection or 5% dextrose for injection up to a concentration of 1.3–5.0 mg/ml
- Nursing considerations
  - dose-dependent elevations in SGOT, SGPT, and bilirubin occur infrequently
  - initiate therapy after patient has received a cumulative dose of 300 mg/m^2
  - give by slow IV push or rapid IV infusion, starting 30 min before doxorubicin is administered
- Assess
  - for alterations in nutritional status; most common toxicities are nausea and vomiting, malaise, fatigue, and anorexia

Cytotoxic Pulmonary Injury

R. N. Aurora, C. Skosey, and D. E. Stover

OVERVIEW

■ Cytotoxic pulmonary injury can result from several categories of chemotherapeutic agents. Patterns of presentation (syndromes) include:
- chronic pneumonitis/fibrosis
  - □ drugs associated
    - ▽ all categories
    - ▽ atypical for antimetabolites and procarbazine
  - □ risk factors
    - ▽ dose dependent: bleomycin (especially with doses > 350 total units but also with much lower doses; and BCNU (especially with dose > 1,000 mg)
    - ▽ increasing age (especially > 60 yrs)
    - ▽ concurrent radiation therapy—or chemotherapy with other agent(s)
    - ▽ oxygen use
- hypersensitivity pneumonitis
  - □ drugs associated
    - ▽ methotrexate (most commonly)
    - ▽ procarbazine
    - ▽ bleomycin
    - ▽ taxol
  - □ risk factors: none known
- noncardiogenic pulmonary edema
  - □ drugs associated
    - ▽ cytosine arabinoside
    - ▽ teniposide (VM-26)
    - ▽ methotrexate
    - ▽ cyclophosphamide
    - ▽ all trans-retinoic acid
    - ▽ vinca alkaloid
    - ▽ mitomycin
    - ▽ gemcitabine
  - □ risk factors: none known

PATHOPHYSIOLOGY

■ Mechanisms of injury
- matrix repair system: alteration of fibroblast activity, imbalance between collagenesis and collagenolysis
- immunologic mechanisms: alteration of normal effector/suppressor balance and influx of PMNs, eosinophils, lymphocytes, macrophages
- generation of reactive oxygen metabolites and alterations of the normal balance between oxidants and antioxidants

■ Histopathology
- chronic pneumonitis/fibrosis
  - □ early endothelial cell damage
  - □ extensive type I pneumocyte destruction
  - □ neutrophil and lymphocyte influx
  - □ fibroblast proliferation and subsequent pulmonary fibrosis
- hypersensitivity pneumonitis
  - □ mononuclear cell interstitial infiltration
  - □ eosinophilic cell infiltration
  - □ atypical type II pneumocytes
  - □ granuloma formation seen with methotrexate pulmonary toxicity
- noncardiogenic pulmonary edema
  - □ acute inflammation with influx of neutrophils in the lung parenchyma
  - □ subsequent release of proteolytic enzymes and toxic oxygen metabolites
  - □ increased pulmonary microcirculation "leakiness"
  - □ high levels of protein in edema fluid

DIAGNOSIS AND PREVENTION

■ Presenting signs and symptoms
- chronic pneumonitis/fibrosis
  - □ dyspnea, initially with exertion over weeks to months to years (especially with nitrosoureas)
  - □ nonproductive cough
  - □ fatigue and/or malaise
  - □ end expiratory crackles ("velcro rales")
- hypersensitivity pneumonitis
  - □ symptoms may occur over hours or days
  - □ fever
  - □ nonproductive cough
  - □ dyspnea
  - □ fatigue and/or malaise
  - □ skin rash (rarely seen)
- noncardiogenic pulmonary edema
  - □ dyspnea over hours or days
  - □ cough

■ Diagnostic tests
- chronic pneumonitis/fibrosis
  - □ radiographic tests: chest radiographs/CT may show a reticulonodular pattern, pulmonary fibrosis, or nodular infiltrate; chest x-radiograph may be normal but HRCT scan usually shows one of these patterns
  - □ pulmonary function tests: most common manifestation is a restrictive ventilatory defect; earliest defect is a reduced diffusing capacity
  - □ desaturation with exercise
  - □ tissue biopsy is not definitive but may be necessary to rule out infection and malignancy; VATS or open-lung biopsy is usually required for adequate tissue sample
- hypersensitivity pneumonitis
  - □ radiographic test: chest radiograph/CT scan usually shows bilateral, patchy infiltrates and, less commonly, pleural effusions. Methotrexate toxicity may be associated with hilar adenopathy; chest radiograph may be normal
  - □ laboratory data may show a 10–20% peripheral eosinophilia (especially with methotrexate and procarbazine)
- noncardiogenic pulmonary edema
  - □ radiographic tests: chest radiograph/CT show diffuse bilateral acinar and/or reticulonodular infiltrates (commonly resembles pulmonary edema)
  - □ tissue biopsy may be needed to rule out other causes of respiratory failure, i.e., infection and/or malignancy

THERAPY

■ Chronic pneumonitis/fibrosis
- discontinue offending agent(s)
- corticosteroids (1 mg/kg/d) may be helpful; treatment course is usually prolonged

■ Hypersensitivity pneumonitis
- discontinue offending agent(s)
- corticosteroids (1 mg/kg/d): prognosis is especially favorable with corticosteroids

■ Noncardiogenic pulmonary edema
- discontinue offending agent(s)
- supportive care (may require positive-pressure ventilation and pressors)
- possibly corticosteroids (1 mg/kg/d): exact role unclear

■ Nursing considerations for administration of corticosteroids (also see corticosteroid profile in cachexia and anorexia section)
- adverse effects depend on the specific corticosteroid used, dose, route, and duration of therapy
- use cautiously in patients at risk for peptic ulcers
- taper corticosteroid doses when discontinuing high-dose or long-term therapy

■ Assess
- baseline physical exam and body weight
- monitor for signs of hypertension and observe for fluid retention (weight gain, edema)

■ Teach patient
- corticosteroids may be associated with GI toxicities, mood swings, and insomnia
- undesirable effects such as myopathy, hyperglycemia, weight gain, dysphoria, accelerates osteoporosis and cataract formation.

KEY REFERENCES

Cooper JA, White DA, Matthay RA: Drug induced pulmonary toxicity. Am Rev Respir Dis 1986; 133:321–40

Stover DE, Daner RJ: Pulmonary toxicity. In *Cancer* (pp. 2729–39), VT DeVita, S Hellman, SA Rosenberg (eds). Philadelphia: JB Lippincott, 1997

Agents Associated with Pulmonary Toxicity

Nitrosureas	Alkylating agents	Antimetabolites
Carmustine (BCNU)	Busulfan	Methotrexate
Lomustine (CCNU)	Cyclophosphamide	Azathioprine
Semustine (methyl-CCNU)	Chlorambucil	Mercaptopurine
Chlorozotocin (DCNU)	Melphalan	Cytosine arabinoside
	Thiotepa	Gemcitabine
Vinca alkaloids	**Antibiotics**	**Miscellaneous**
Vinblastine	Bleomycin	VM-26
Vindesine	Mitomycin	Retinoic acid
	Neocarzinostatin	Procarbazine
		Taxol
		Etoposide

Nephrotoxicity

R. L. Capizzi and C. Skosey

OVERVIEW

- The kidney is an important metabolic and excretory organ for many drugs and toxins
- Impaired renal function, either directly or indirectly related to chemotherapy effects, could have serious consequences
  - direct drug toxic effects to one or more portions of the nephron or intra-renal obstruction is not as common in cancer medicine as is marrow suppression and mucosal toxicity
- Impaired renal function, with a subsequent delay in the renal elimination of a cancer drug—or its metabolite—can significantly amplify its toxicity profile, affecting multiple organ systems

PATHOPHYSIOLOGY

- Direct renal toxicity
  - cisplatin
    - □ acute toxicity can be determined within 1–3 hrs of administration by measurement of sensitive indicators of proximal tubular injury, i.e., urinary beta-2 microglobulin
    - □ chronic, cumulative toxicity is noted as a progressive, typically irreversible decline in the glomerular filtration rate
    - □ heavy metal toxicity to renal tubules initially affects the proximal tubule, but also the distal tubule and collecting ducts
    - □ proximal tubular damage is evident as magnesium wasting, which at times can be symptomatic requiring appropriate replacement therapy
  - ifosfamide
    - □ proximal tubule defect causing a Fanconi-like syndrome
  - mitomycin-C
    - □ hemolytic-uremia syndrome related to cumulative dose of drug
  - nitrosoureas (primarily streptozocin and to a lesser degree, carmustine (BCNU) and lomustine (CCNU)
    - □ tubulo-interstitial nephritis and tubular atrophy
- Indirect renal toxicity
  - high-dose methotrexate (MTX)
    - □ 90% of the administered dose is excreted unchanged in the urine
    - □ MTX is filtered at the glomerulus, reabsorbed and secreted by the tubular epithelium
    - □ concentration of MTX in the urine following administration of gram doses that exceed the solubility of MTX in the acid urine (pH 5.0) precipitates in the renal tubules, causing crystal-induced intrarenal obstruction and azotemia
  - tumor lysis syndrome
    - □ primarily associated with therapy of high, bulky chemosensitive tumors, such as the acute leukemias, lymphomas, and testicular cancer
    - □ rapid lysis of tumor tissues frees intracellular constituents and metabolites into the bloodstream, and may cause a potentially life-threatening situation, due to sudden hyperkalemia and hypocalcemia with consequent cardiac arrhythmias
    - □ other manifestations include hyperphosphatemia and hyperuricemia (acute hyperuricemia, the end product of purine catabolism, causes uric acid nephropathy, due to the poor solubility of uric acid in the acid urine—pH 5.0)
    - □ precipitation of uric acid crystals in the renal tubules causes intrarenal obstruction and azotemia

DIAGNOSIS AND PREVENTION

- Cisplatin
  - careful assessment of renal function prior to each dose; avoid concurrent use of other nephrotoxic agents, i.e., aminoglycosides, nephrotoxic contrast agents, etc.
  - saline hydration is the mainstay prevention of acute cisplatin nephropathy: 1–3 L of saline hydration to induce a brisk diuresis—urine flow of 100–125 cc/hr—is indicated prior to cisplatin, depending on dose of drug (20–100 mg/m^2)
  - pretreatment with amifostine has been approved for prevention of nephrotoxicity associated with cumulative doses of cisplatin (see section on amifostine)
  - because of the hyperbolic relationship between serum creatinine and creatinine clearance, the serum creatinine is a poor measure of renal impairment associated with cisplatin—a modest rise in serum creatinine within the clinically acceptable range, i.e., 0.7–1.4 mg/dl, represents a substantial decline in the glomerular filtration rate (GFR)
- Mitomycin-C
  - no available preventive agents
  - careful monitoring of hematologic and renal function
- Ifosfamide
  - mesna not useful as a preventive agent
  - careful monitoring of hematologic and renal function
- Nitrosoureas
  - no available preventive agents
  - careful monitoring of hematologic and renal function
- High-dose methotrexate (MTX)
  - MTX is not dialyzable (see Therapy)
- Tumor lysis syndrome and urate nephropathy
  - IV hydration to ensure brisk diuresis and allopurinol—600 mg/d, started 24 hrs prior to chemotherapy
  - alkalinize the urine with bicarbonate and acetazolamide
- Special nursing considerations for IV saline hydration
  - institute preventive measures early
  - administer IV hydration to maintain urinary output
  - urinary alkalinization to keep urine pH > 7.0
  - monitor for symptoms of fluid overload: shortness of breath, anxiety, pedal edema, and lung sounds
  - monitor I/O and weight
  - monitor electrolytes

THERAPY

- Cisplatin
  - an osmotic diuretic, such as mannitol, may be used with higher doses of drug
  - magnesium supplements may be indicated
- High-dose methotrexate (MTX)
  - IV and/or oral sodium bicarbonate sufficient to increase urine pH to 7.0 (generally, 100 mEq/m^2/d); acetazolamide also may be useful
  - IV and/or oral hydration is necessary to ensure a brisk diuresis

KEY REFERENCES

Capizzi RL: Amifostine reduces the incidence of cumulative nephrotoxicity from cisplatin: laboratory and clinical aspects. Semin Oncol 1999; 26:72–81

Capizzi RL: Clinical status and optimal use of amifostine. Oncology 1999; 13:47–59

Cohen LF, Balow JE, Magrath IT, Poplack DG, Ziegler JL: Acute tumor lysis syndrome. Am J Med 1980; 68:486–91

Goren MP, Wright RK, Horowitz ME, Pratt CB: Ifosfamide-induced sub-clinical tubular nephrotoxicity despite mesna. Cancer Treat Rep 1987; 71:127–30

Kemp G, Rose P, Lurain J, Berman M, Manetta A, Roullet B, Homesley H, Belpomme D, Glick J: Amifostine pretreatment for protection against cyclophosphamide- and cisplatin-induced toxicities: results of a randomized control trial in patients with advanced ovarian cancer. J Clin Oncol 1996; 14:2101–12

List AF, Brasfield F, Heaton R, Glinsmann-Gibson B, Crook L, Taetle R, Capizzi R: Stimulation of hematopoiesis by amifostine in patients with myelodysplastic syndrome. Blood 1997; 90:3364–9

Viele CS, Carlile Holmes B: Amifostine: drug profile and nursing implications of the first pancytoprotectant. Oncol Nurs Forum 1998; 25(3):515–23

DRUG: AMIFOSTINE

- Other names: Ethyol, WR-2721
- Uses
  - approved by FDA as a cytoprotector to prevent cumulative nephrotoxicity from cisplatin in patients with advanced ovarian cancer and non–small cell lung cancer

- also useful as a cytoprotector from cisplatin-induced neuropathy, acute and cumulative bone marrow toxicities associated with cisplatin, cyclophosphamide, and carboplatin
- also useful as a cytoprotector from radiation-induced stomatitis and xerostomia in patients with head and neck cancer
- also useful in patients with myelodysplastic syndromes

■ Mechanism of action
- amifostine is a prodrug anabolized by dephosphorylation at the tissue site by membrane-bound alkaline phosphatase to form the free thiol, WR-1065
- the free thiol is rapidly taken up by normal tissues by a carrier-mediated facilitated diffusion process
- the free thiol binds to and thereby detoxifies reactive nucleophiles generated by alkylating agents and organoplatinums. The free thiol also acts as a scavenger of oxygen-free radicals

■ Dosing
- available as a parental agent for IV infusion
- no oral bioavailability
- patient should be in supine position during IV infusion
- baseline blood pressure should be taken and repeated at 5 min intervals during the infusion and 5 min after the infusion
- used with intermittent chemotherapy regimens at a dose of 740–910 mg/m^2 given as a 10–15 min infusion IV, 15–30 min before chemotherapy. Dose reduction based on degree of amifostine-induced hypotension (see package insert)
- used with daily standard fraction radiation at a dose of 200–340 mg/m^2 as a 5–10 min IV infusion
- used as a marrow stimulant in patients with myelodysplastic syndromes at a dose of 100 mg/m^2–200 mg/m^2 as a 5 min IV infusion 3 times a week (typically on Monday, Wednesday, and Friday)

■ Pharmacokinetics
- distribution half-life is < 1 min
- elimination half-life is ~ 8 min
- 90% of the parent drug is cleared from the systemic circulation in 6 min
- systemic clearance is via dephosphorylation to the thiol, WR-1065, with rapid uptake into normal tissues with little to no uptake into tumor tissues
- < 5% of the parent drug and its metabolites is excreted in the urine

■ Side effects
- no tissue irritation with extravasation
- asymptomatic hypotension usually occurs toward the end of a 15 min infusion and lasts 5–15 min (average 6 min); hypotension has rarely been associated with dizziness or fatigue
- nausea and vomiting
- flushing, sensation of warmth
- hiccups

■ Other considerations
- hypotension and nausea and vomiting are related to dose and duration of infusion. Both side effects are lesser in frequency with the dose of 740 mg/m^2 given as a 10 min infusion than with 910 mg/m^2 given as a 15 min infusion
- side effects are minimal with three weekly or daily doses of 200 mg/m^2

■ Nursing considerations
- contraindicated in patients who are dehydrated, hypotensive, or receiving concomitant antihypertensive medications or other drugs that can contribute to hypotension and cannot be stopped within 24 hrs of treatment
- in most settings the antiemetic regimen used includes 5HT$_3$ antagonist, dexamethasone 20 mg IV, and diphenhydramine 25–50 mg IV or lorazepam 1–2 mg IV given at least 1 hr prior to chemotherapy
- allergic reactions are rare
- dosing and management
  - □ 740 mg/m^2
    - ▽ infusion should not be prolonged beyond 10–15 min
    - ▽ do not administer with other agents
  - □ administration
    - ▽ premedicate with antiemetics 45–60 min before infusion
    - ▽ have patient empty bladder prior to infusion
    - ▽ adequate prehydration with 1 L of normal saline 1 hr prior to amifostine
    - ▽ administer amifostine 30 min before chemotherapy
    - ▽ administer in 50 cc normal saline over 10–15 min (rapid infusion reduces risk of hypotension)
    - ▽ patient should be in reclining/supine position during infusion and for 15 min after infusion to minimize hypotension
    - ▽ a pump regulates infusion

■ Assess
- for transient hypotension symptomatic or asymptomatic; monitor blood pressure baseline and during infusion; if systolic blood pressure decreases below threshold, stop infusion; give normal saline and monitor pressure; if pressure returns to baseline within 5 min restart infusion; if pressure does not return to baseline within 5 min discontinue amifostine infusion for that cycle
- common side effects: nausea, vomiting, somnolence, hypocalcemia, sneezing, and a warm flushed feeling are manageable with appropriate medical and nursing interventions
- assess neurologic status baseline and during therapy; monitor blood calcium levels and provide OTC calcium supplement if symptoms of hypocalcemia develop

■ Teach patient
- potential to experience a flushed sensation with the infusion but will subside within 30–60 min postinfusion
- report feelings of numbness, twitching, muscle weakness, or stiffness
- potential for drug-induced sneezing and/or hiccups

Bladder Toxicity

J. D. Shepherd, D. I. Warkentin, and L. Haser

OVERVIEW

■ Many chemotherapeutic agents have been reported to cause hemorrhagic cystitis; the most common are the oxazaphosphorine derivatives, cyclophosphamide and ifosfamide
■ Incidence depends on dose and schedule; most common with higher cyclophosphamide doses, such as used for stem cell transplantation (≥2 g/m^2)
■ Prevention is more effective than therapy in most cases
■ Chronic use of these drugs may lead to bladder fibrosis and predispose patient to bladder neoplasms

PATHOPHYSIOLOGY

■ Oxazaphosphorines are metabolized in the liver to both active and inactive metabolites, including acrolein
- acrolein is excreted by the kidneys and is probably responsible for most cases of hemorrhagic cystitis
- ifosamide is broken down more slowly than cyclophosphamide and into more metabolites. This drug is often used in higher doses, representing a potentially greater risk for hemorrhagic cystitis
- the urinary system is low in natural thiols (e.g., glutathione) that bind acrolein and other metabolites; thus the mucosa is exposed to higher concentrations for longer periods of time

■ Chemical hemorrhagic cystitis may predispose patients to late viral infections
- implicated viruses are adenovirus and polyomaviruses (especially BK virus)

■ Radiation-induced cystitis may result from obliterative endarteritis and cellular hypoxia
- in addition, radiation also may break down the normal protective mechanisms of the bladder and cause direct interstitial inflammation
- it may also facilitate secondary infection

■ The combined effects of radiation and chemotherapy may be cumulative
■ A number of other agents have also been implicated, including busulfan, L-asparaginase, mitomycin-C, DTIC, and others
- these are uncommon enough that no firm prophylactic or therapeutic guidelines exist. In many cases, the etiology may be multifactoral, such as coagulopathy superimposed on epithelial damage from drugs

PREVENTION AND DIAGNOSIS

■ Effective prophylaxis against radiation cystitis is not well documented
- alkalinization may be of benefit but this is not proven

■ Mainstays of prophylaxis are hyperhydration with diuresis, bladder irrigation, and sulfhydryl compounds such as 2-mercaptoethane sulfonate (mesna)
- since the risk of hemorrhagic cystitis is higher with ifosfamide, data support the prophylactic use of mesna
- a recent retrospective analysis from one stem cell transplant center using combined hyperhydration, diuresis, and bladder irrigation for high-dose cyclophosphamide showed an incidence of microscopic hematuria of 19% with virtually no symptomatic hemorrhagic cystitis
- randomized trials of mesna versus hyperhydration and bladder irrigation in stem cell transplant patients receiving high-dose cyclophosphamide showed equivalence, and it is hard to make firm recommendations

■ Although many patients may have microscopic hematuria, the clinical diagnosis of hemorrhagic cystitis is usually based on macroscopic hematuria, urinary frequency, and/or symptomatic dysuria
- clots may form in the bladder and cause spasm or pain on urination; they may also obstruct the urethra

■ Bacterial cultures are appropriate to rule out infectious etiology
- viral studies should be considered if onset is delayed after administration of chemotherapy drugs

THERAPY

■ Patients with asymptomatic hematuria and/or minimal symptoms can be managed with fluid diuresis
■ More pronounced symptoms, presence of clots or obstruction, mandates more aggressive therapy. Most would use indwelling 3-way catheter for irrigation, hydration, and, possibly, alum irrigation
■ Direct interventions include prostaglandin administration, interventional cystoscopy, bladder fibrosing with formalin or phenol, and cystectomy
- the use of fibrosing agents or cystectomy should only be undertaken in desperate situations

■ The role of cystoscopy is controversial
- large amounts of clot will delay healing, and clot removal is essential before administration of prostaglandin
- local lesions may be seen that are amenable to fulguration. More often, the entire bladder mucosa will be hyperemic and cautery will be of little benefit

■ It is important to maximize hemostasis by ensuring adequate platelet count, reversing any coagulopathies, and avoiding drugs that can affect coagulation
■ Reports exist of radiation-induced hemorrhagic cystitis responding to hyperbaric oxygen; data in chemical hemorrhagic cystitis are scant, although some animal models support possible role
■ Symptomatic relief can sometimes be obtained with phenazopyridine (Pyridium)
- bladder spasm may respond to anticholinergics (oxybutynin or belladonna and opium suppositories)
- some patients with severe pain may require narcotic analgesics

■ Specific drugs
- hyperhydration/diuresis and bladder irrigation
- mercaptoethane sulfonate (mesna)
- aluminum sulfate (alum)
- prostaglandin F_2a (carboprost tromethamine, carboprost)

KEY REFERENCES

deVries CR, Freiha FS: Hemorrhagic cystitis: a review. J Urol 1990; 143:1–9

Ippoliti C, Przepiorka D, Mehra R, Neumann J, Wood J, Claxton D, Gajewski J, Khouri I, Van Besien K, Andersson B, Deisseroth AB, Dinney CP: Intravesicular carboprost for the treatment of hemorrhagic cystitis after marrow transplantation. Urology 1995; 46:811–15

Meisenberg B, Lassiter M, Hussein A, Ross M, Vredenburgh JJ, Peters WP: Prevention of hemorrhagic cystitis after high-dose alkylating agent chemotherapy and autologous bone marrow support. Bone Marrow Transplant 1994; 14:287–91

Murphy CP, Cox RL, Harden EA, Stevens DA, Heye MM, Herzig RH: Encephalopathy and seizures induced by intravesical alum irrigations. Bone Marrow Transplant 1992; 10:383–5

Shepherd JD, Pringle LE, Barnett MJ, Klingemann HG, Reece DE, Phillips GL: Mesna versus hyperhydration for the prevention of cyclophosphamide-induced hemorrhagic cystitis in bone marrow transplantation. J Clin Oncol 1991; 9:2016–2020.

Trigg ME, O'Reilly J, Rumelhart S, Morgan D, Holida M, de Alarcon P: Prostaglandin E1 bladder instillations to control severe hemorrhagic cystitis. J Urology 1990; 143:92–4

Vose JM, Reed EC, Pippert GC, Anderson JR, Bierman PJ, Kessinger A, Spinolo J, Armitage JO: Mesna compared with continuous bladder irrigation as uroprotection during high-dose chemotherapy and transplantation: a randomized trial. J Clin Oncol 1993; 11:1306–10

West NJ: Prevention and treatment of hemorrhagic cystitis. Pharmacotherapy 1997; 17:696–706

PREVENTION OF HEMORRHAGIC CYSTITIS

DRUG: HYPERHYDRATION AND DIURESIS; BLADDER CATHETERIZATION AND IRRIGATION

■ Mechanism of action
- reduces the time in which toxins such as acrolein are in contact with the genitourinary mucosa

- Dosing
  - hyperhydration
    - □ hydrate patient prior to starting cyclophosphamide (CY) or ifosfamide (IF) (minimum of 1 L)
    - □ infuse normal saline at 3 L/m^2 per 24 hr period; may also include KCl; and $MgSO_4$ in hydration fluid
    - □ continue hyperhydration until 24–48 hrs after completion of CY or IF infusion
    - □ maintain urine output of 150–200 ml/hr; furosemide may be needed to sustain appropriate rate
  - continuous bladder irrigation
    - □ normal saline infused through indwelling double or triple lumen catheter at 250–1,000 ml/hr
    - □ many centers attempt to maintain measured fluid balance, but this may be difficult
    - □ continue irrigation until 12–24 hrs after completion of chemotherapy dosing
- Side effects
  - hyperhydration
    - □ volume overload may occur; electrolytes need to be monitored regularly
    - □ careful attention to fluid balance and patient weight important
    - □ because CY may induce inappropriate secretion of antidiuretic hormone, be aware of increasing positive fluid balance
  - bladder irrigation
    - □ carries risk of infection and local trauma, especially if platelets are low
    - □ may cause patient discomfort
- Nursing considerations
  - hyperhydration and diuresis
    - □ monitor I/O closely; have patient void q2–4hrs
    - □ diligent nursing supervision is required for bladder irrigation
    - □ monitor patient for symptoms of fluid overload: shortness of breath, anxiety, pedal edema, lung sounds
    - □ monitor I/O accurately; report positive fluid balance to MD
    - □ daily weights
    - □ monitor electrolytes
  - bladder catheterization and irrigation
    - □ maintain patency of urinary drainage
    - □ solution should run rapidly enough to maintain urinary drainage of light pink-red color
    - □ manually irrigate clots as prescribed
    - □ encourage patient to drink 2–3 L of fluid per day unless contraindicated
    - □ instruct patient on bladder spasms and constant urge to void initially after catheter is inserted, and indicate the sensation will decrease within 24–48 hrs. Administer antispasmodics and analgesics as prescribed
    - □ avoid use of enemas or rectal thermometers or tubes
    - □ maintain scrupulous catheter care every shift and prn; alert MD to any signs of infection
    - □ assess adequacy of bladder emptying once catheter is removed
  - teach patient
    - □ instruct patient not to try to void around the catheter
    - □ teach patient perineal exercises to promote bladder control after catheter is discontinued

PREVENTION OF HEMORRHAGIC CYSTITIS (HC)

DRUG: MESNA (2-MERCAPTOETHANE SULFONATE, MESNEX, UROMITEXAN)

- Designated orphan drug by the FDA for prophylactic use as a uroprotective agent to decrease the incidence of HC in patients receiving ifosfamide and other oxazaphosphorine compounds
- Mechanism of action
  - rapidly excreted in the urinary tract and contributes a sulfhydryl group, which binds acrolein and other metabolites in a stable thioether bond, thus detoxifying them. Also enhances the urinary excretion of cysteine, which may also contribute to the uroprotective activity
- Dosing
  - suggested dose based on dose of oxazaphosphorine administered; various methods and doses have been used and the optimum has not been determined. Total IV dose of mesna in most references is 60–160% of the daily dose of the oxazaphosphorine
  - IF: the manufacturer recommends a dose of 60% of the IF dose given in 3 divided doses 15 min before and 4 and 8 hrs after the IF. Alternatively, the mesna has been given in 4 doses just prior to IF and at 4, 8, and 12 hrs. It has also been administered as a continuous infusion at 100% of the IF dose
  - CY: mesna has been given at a total daily dose of 60–160% of the CY dose by both bolus dosing and continuous infusion. In BMT patients a loading dose of 10 mg/kg followed by 60 mg/kg over 24 hrs has been used in patients receiving 60 mg/kg of CY
  - since mesna has a shorter half-life than IF and CY, it should be continued for 8–24 hrs after IF infusion is completed. Mesna dose must be repeated each day IF or CY is given
- Pharmacokinetics
  - oxidized in the body to the inert and stable dimesna; reduced in the kidney to the active thiol
  - volume of distribution 0.64 L/kg; 10% protein-bound; does not cross the blood-brain barrier
  - plasma concentrations decline linearly; eliminated in the urine (no hepatic metabolism)
  - most of a single dose is eliminated within 4 hrs
- Side effects
  - mesna is well tolerated and side effects are reported to be rare
- Nursing considerations
  - obtain early morning void to evaluate for hemorrhagic cystitis
  - administer for at least one half-life longer than the drug that can cause the hemorrhagic cystitis (e.g., give at least 4 hrs after the completion of Ifex)
  - assess
    - □ alteration in nutritional status and comfort; most common side effects are diarrhea, headache, fatigue, nausea, and vomiting
  - teach patient
    - □ if given orally, dilute in carbonated cola drinks or in chilled juices to mask odor and taste; recommend candy or chewing gum to mask taste

TREATMENT OF HEMORRHAGIC CYSTITIS

DRUG: ALUM (ALUMINUM POTASSIUM SULFATE; ALUMINUM AMMONIUM SULFATE)

- Mechanism of action
  - astringent
  - induces protein precipitation on cell surfaces and interstitial spaces
  - causes contraction of bladder surface and tamponade of bleeding vessels; also hardens capillary endothelium and inhibits transcapillary movement of plasma proteins
- Dosing
  - administered as a 1% solution via continuous bladder irrigation using 3-way catheter
  - rate of 300–1,000 ml/hr; rate adjusted to maintain light pink to clear drainage
  - best response obtained when bladder evacuated of clots prior to therapy
  - duration of therapy unclear; most centers use until urine clear for 24–48 hrs
- Pharmacokinetics
  - minimal absorption by bladder mucosa; absorption more likely when bladder mucosa denuded
  - absorbed aluminum is normally rapidly excreted by the kidneys; accumulation may occur in renal dysfunction
- Side effects
  - suprapubic pain, fever, bladder spasm, and urinary retention or frequency
  - rarely, aluminum toxicity can occur and is manifested by CNS disturbances, metabolic acidosis, or coagulopathy; more likely to occur in patients with renal dysfunction and with prolonged therapy. In such cases, monitoring of serum aluminum levels may be appropriate
  - rare patients may have an allergic reaction to topical application; if so irrigation should be discontinued immediately

■ Nursing considerations
  - aluminum may precipitate out of solution and clog catheter
  - evacuate clots prior to instillation
  - observe solution for precipitate prior to instillation
  - maintain catheter patency
  - assess
    □ observe for allergic reaction
    □ patient for signs of aluminum toxicity/encephalopathy: fever, headaches, vomiting, nuccal rigidity, drowsiness, behavioral changes, seizures
    □ renal function: impaired function may be associated with aluminum toxicity
    □ for vesicle pain and/or irritability

TREATMENT OF HEMORRHAGIC CYSTITIS

DRUG: PROSTAGLANDIN F_2A (CARBOPROST TROMETHAMINE, HEMABATE)

■ Other prostaglandin preparations also used (PGE_1, PGE_2)

■ Mechanism of action
  - several mechanisms postulated including strengthening of cell membranes, stimulation of platelet aggregation, local vasoconstriction, and direct cytoprotection of mucosa

■ Dosing
  - doses used range from 0.2–1.0 mg/dl; most effective dose appears to be 0.8–1.0 mg/dl
  - diluted in 50 ml saline and instilled into bladder; catheter clamped and solution allowed to dwell for 60 min; repeat 6×/hr
  - evacuation of clots from bladder by hand irrigation necessary before each dose for best effect
  - after emptying of solution, continue bladder irrigation between doses
  - median time to response 3 days; most patients who respond will do so by 5–7 days
  - relapses occur in up to 50% of patients who respond initially; re-treatment indicated but may not be successful

■ Pharmacokinetics
  - no data on absorption after intravesical administration
  - when given systemically, most drug is eliminated via the urinary tract within 5–10 hrs
  - half-life following discontinuation of continuous IV infusion 30–45 min

■ Side effects
  - bladder spasm is common; symptomatic treatment with oxybutynin chloride or belladonna and opium suppositories

■ Nursing considerations
  - have patient change positions q15min while carboprost in bladder
  - requires intensive nursing care for instillation, drainage, and management of spasm
  - medicate with oxybutynin chloride or belladonna and opium suppositories prior to procedure
  - assess
    □ provide emotional support and reassurance during procedure
  - teach patient
    □ to change position q15min to ensure adequate drug contact of entire bladder lining
    □ high incidence of bladder spasms and relaxation techniques to help minimize the incidence

Neurotoxicity

D. Glover

OVERVIEW

- Neurotoxicity is a dose-limiting complication of several chemotherapeutic agents
- Neurotoxicity is seen most commonly among patients treated with vincristine, and to a lesser extent with other vinca alkaloids, cisplatin, taxanes, ifosfamide, and IL-2

PATHOPHYSIOLOGY BY CERTAIN DRUG TYPE

- Vinca alkaloids: vincristine, vinblastine, and vinorelbine
  - pathophysiology is due to disruption of microtubule function in the neuronal axons. There is a reduced amplitude of the action potentials and, histologically, axonal degeneration
    - □ electrophysiologic studies showed distal axonal dysfunction
    - □ nerve conduction studies showed that sensory nerves are most affected
- Cisplatinum
  - the peripheral neuropathy is usually related to the accumulation of inorganic platinum within the neurons, which may be irreversible
    - □ pathologic postmortem studies indicated changes in the ganglia in platinum-treated patients
  - the tissue levels of platinum correlates with the neuronal histologic changes and clinical neurotoxicity

DIAGNOSIS AND PREVENTION BY DRUG TYPE

- Preliminary studies have demonstrated that amifostine (Ethyol) may prevent cisplatin's neurotoxicity, allowing physician to administer a higher dose of certain chemotherapy agents without an increase in neuropathy, ototoxicity, hematologic toxicity, and nephrotoxicity
- Vinca alkaloids
  - these drugs can cause neurologic injury in both the peripheral and central nervous systems, related to both individual and cumulative doses
  - with vincristine, neurotoxicity is dose limiting, whereas with vinblastine and navelbine (Vinorelbine), the most common dose-limiting toxicity is myelosuppression
  - neurotoxicity symptoms of vincristine
    - □ the most common, initial manifestations are a decrease in the deep tendon reflexes (usually asymptomatic) and parathesias of the distal extremities, usually beginning with the Achilles tendon reflexes
    - □ the fingertips are the first site to develop numbness and loss of sensation
    - □ motor dysfunction due to vincristine, and rarely with other agents, is usually first seen as leg weakness. Foot drop will occur if agents are continued
    - □ vincristine can also affect cranial nerves, causing facial palsy and disorders of eye movement. Parasympathetic neurotoxicity is manifested by constipation and problems starting urination, and can lead to paralytic ileus and bladder atony if the drug is continued
    - □ autonomic neuropathy can produce orthostatic hypotension, problems with penile erection, and ejaculatory dysfunction
    - □ rarely, vocal cord paralysis and cortical blindness can occur following high doses of vincristine
    - □ the parathesias commonly progress as the therapy continues
    - □ peripheral neurotoxicity progresses in a glove stocking distribution in both upper and lower extremities
- Cisplatinum
  - cisplatinum's neurotoxicity can be dose limiting, with neuropathy seen with higher individual and cumulative doses
  - the majority of patients who continue on cisplatinum will eventually develop peripheral neuropathy (a cumulative dose of 300–500 mg/m^2)
  - neurotoxicity symptoms
    - □ initial signs are loss of deep tendon reflexes, vibratory sense, and position sense, which occurs more commonly in the feet than the hands
    - □ Lhermitte's sign and autonomic neuropathy
    - □ seizures, which may be related to hypomagnesemia due to renal tubular injury
    - □ encephalopathy, transient cortical blindness, retrobulbar neuritis, and retinal injury are very rare
  - amifostine (Ethyol) has been shown to be beneficial in decreasing the risk of neuropathy in cisplatinum treatments used for melanoma and advanced ovarian cancer
- Taxanes: paclitaxel (Taxol) and docetaxel USP (Taxotere)
  - these drugs cause neurotoxicity similar to that seen with cisplatinum and vincristine, with onset of neuropathy directly related to high cumulative doses
  - peripheral neuropathy can be a dose-limiting toxicity
  - depending on drug dose used, the onset of symptoms can occur within the days after the first dose
  - a cumulative dose of Taxotere (400 mg/m^2) can cause severe symptoms with documented electrical changes in nerves
  - preliminary studies suggest that amifostine may protect against the neurologic toxicity of taxanes
- Cytarabine (Ara-C)
  - cytarabine given both IV or intrathecally for lymphomatous or carcinomatous meningitis can result in neurotoxicity. Intrathecal cytarabine rarely can produce an ascending myelopathy
  - between 17–37% of patients receiving high doses of cytarabine therapy develop neurotoxicity
  - the most common form of neurotoxicity is cerebellar dysfunction, which can occur within the first few days of treatment. These effects can be accompanied by headache, altered mentation, memory loss, and somnolence
  - peripheral neuropathy is rare, but can range from a purely sensory neuropathy to a sensory motor polyneuropathy in a glove stocking distribution
- Ifosfamide
  - neurotoxicity is seen in 10% of patients
  - some believe that toxicity is most commonly caused from a dechloroethylated metabolite, which is produced in high quantities with this therapy
  - neurotoxicity symptoms
    - □ this drug can cause acute visual and auditory hallucinations, vivid dreams, personality changes, anxiety, and restlessness
    - □ cerebellar and cranial nerve dysfunction.
    - □ hemiparesis, seizures, coma, and, occasionally, death
    - □ myoclonus, muscular spasticity, and peripheral neuropathy have been reported
  - risk factors
    - □ low albumin
    - □ renal dysfunction
    - □ prior use of neurotoxic drugs
    - □ presence of a CNS tumor
    - □ age, since children are more susceptible
- 5 Fluorouracil (5-FU)
  - neurotoxicity is seen in 10% of patients, and can be acute at onset. Cerebellar dysfunction is the most commonly seen, although occasionally confusion has been observed
  - patients who develop neurotoxicity tend to have a genetic enzyme deficiency for metabolizing 5-FU
  - those with complete or partial deficiency of dihydropyrimidine dehydrogenase are particularly subject to neurotoxicity
  - 5-FU and levamisole have been shown to produce a multifocal leukoencephalopathy with agitation, confusion, short-term memory loss, diplopia, cerebellar dysfunction, and expressive aphasia
  - MRI scans of the brain may show multiple, enhancing, white matter lesions (sometimes ring enhancement) in the cerebellum and focal demyelination
- Methotrexate

- when given intrathecally, methotrexate can cause meningeal irritation, transient paraphrases or encephalopathy, along with headache, nausea, vomiting, lethargy, nuchal rigidity
  - □ with repeated intrathecal doses, this drug can rarely cause a progressive, necrotizing leukoencephalopathy, accompanied by memory loss, dementia, and seizures
  - – increased risk factors with intrathecal doses
    - □ cranial radiation
    - □ presence of neoplastic cells in the spinal fluid
    - □ cumulative drug doses
  - – IV methotrexate can produce leukoencephalopathy, especially if cranial radiation is used concurrently with high doses
    - □ these neurotoxic effects may be acute and transient—or delayed in onset
    - □ preventative treatment consists of active hydration to facilitate methotrexate clearance and leucovorin, an adenosine receptor antagonist that has been used to successfully reverse the toxic effect of the drug
- Procarbazine
  - – this drug can cause central and peripheral neurotoxicity
  - – the most common symptoms
    - □ lethargy, depression, confusion, hallucinations, and, rarely, psychosis
    - □ parathesias and decreased tendon reflexes are signs of peripheral neuropathy
- Fludarabine
  - – central nervous toxicity is dose limiting. Patients receiving recommended doses usually do not develop more than mild toxicity, although rarely fatal neurotoxicity has been seen even at lower doses
  - – neurotoxicity symptoms
    - □ altered mental status and/or dementia
    - □ photophobia
    - □ amaurosis
    - □ seizures
    - □ spastic or flaccid paralysis or quadriparesis
    - □ coma
- Azacytidine
  - – neural-muscular effects, such as weakness, lethargy, and muscle pain, have rarely occurred. Confusion and coma are possible
- Carboplatinum
  - – neurotoxicity is much less common than with cisplatinum, although symptoms can occur with higher dose regimens
  - – neurotoxicity appears to be cumulative in patients with a higher risk of underlying neuropathies. These patients should be carefully observed
- Oxaliplatinum
  - – a platinum derivative
    - □ the dose-limiting side effect of this drug is a sensory neuropathy, presenting as dysthesias or involving the area around the mouth
    - □ neuropathy is similar to that seen with cisplatinum
    - □ after 6 cycles, 10% will develop grade II or III neuropathy, which will resolve over 3–4 mos
    - □ onset occurs shortly after the infusion and resolves within a few days
    - □ with repeated doses, the symptoms can last longer between cycles
- Suramin
  - – this drug has had a profound neuropathy, which mimics Guillian-Barre syndrome, that can occur within weeks of therapy. Symptoms can progress over 3–6 mos after the drug is discontinued
    - □ Guillian-Barre syndrome has occurred in 11% of patients receiving doses of 350/mg/m^2 per day by continuous infusion; 40% had these symptoms when dose exceeded 350 mg/m^2
  - – neuropathy can range from mild glove stocking parathesias to paralysis requiring mechanical ventilation
  - – suramin can lead to progressive, reversible myelopathy, hyperesthesias of the palms and soles, headache, and altered taste. These symptoms could also be due to metabolic problems, including hyponatremia, hypokalemia, hypocalcemia, hypomagnesemia, hypophosphatemia, hypouricemia, and renal dysfunction
- Retinoids
  - – these drugs can cause headaches within hours after treatment, most commonly after oral trans-retinoic acid. These headaches usually resolve after discontinuation
  - – disorientation and coma have been reported, usually with higher dose regimens
  - – pseudotumor cerebri and hypocalcemia also have been reported with this drug
- Hexamethylmelamine (Altretamine)
  - – this drug works as an alkalating agent after conversion in the liver and can cause peripheral neuropathy and CNS side effects
  - – the incidence of neuropathy can be up to 40% of patients
  - – neurotoxicity symptoms
    - □ confusion, dysphagia, personality changes
    - □ ataxia, fatigue, somnolence
    - □ seizures
    - □ respiratory problems and parkinsonian tremors
  - – neuropathy can have an early onset if patient has preexisting neuropathy or if other agents, such as cisplatinum, are used concurrently
- Pyrazoloacridine (PZA)
  - – the primary dose-limiting toxicity of this drug is neurotoxicity, which can be seen during infusion, and myelosuppression
  - – neurotoxicity has only been seen with doses of over 600 mg/m^2 and seen more commonly with high, repeated plasma concentrations, prolonged infusions
  - – neurotoxicity symptoms
    - □ anxiety or paranoid-like behavior, agitation and fright
    - □ neuromotor symptoms, such as leg twitching, with an inability to walk
- L-Asparaginase
  - – this drug can occasionally cause confusion, aphasia, stupor, or coma in 25–35% of patients
  - – CSF levels of this drug disappear rapidly
- Interferon
  - – with high doses, interferon can cause neurologic complaints, such as fatigue, changes in personality, and depression, all of which resolve within weeks after discontinuation of treatment

THERAPY

- Treatment for most therapies that cause neurotoxicity is discontinuation of the therapy. Neurologic recovery can take place within hours, days, weeks, or months, depending on chemotherapy agent used
- Amifostine (Ethyol) may be beneficial in decreasing the risk of neuropathy in some drugs
  - – cisplatinum
  - – paclitaxel and docetaxel
- To prevent complications, continuous infusions of ifosfamide with concurrent administration with methylene blue should be considered
- Treatment of complications from retinoids involve lumbar puncture and high doses of cortical steroids

KEY REFERENCES

Bleyer WA: The clinical pharmacology of methotrexate: new applications for an old drug. Cancer 1995; 41:36–51

Glick J, Kemp G, Rose P, et al.: A randomized trial of cyclophosphamide and cisplatin plus amifostine in treatment of advanced epithelial ovarian cancer. Proc ASCO 1994; 13:437

McMahon SB, Priestley JV: Peripheral neuropathies and neurotrophic factors: animal models and clinical perspectives. Curr Opin Neurobiol 1995; 5:616–24

Graft-versus-Host Disease (GVHD)

K. R. Terrill, H. Devine, and P. G. Beatty

OVERVIEW

- GVHD remains a common complication from bone marrow/stem cell transplants, most frequently and more severe in patients receiving mismatched donations from family members or unrelated donors
  - GVHD occurs in roughly half of all transplant patients, although mild in most cases
- GVHD occurs when the new donor marrow develops lymphocytes reactive against the host (patient) and tries to destroy the host as if it were a disease or foreign material
- GVHD appears to increase the probability of engraftment, although the mechanism remains unclear, by decreasing or eliminating patient immune cells that are capable of rejecting the graft, and/or providing factors that facilitate engraftment. Further, GVHD may destroy residual malignant cells (the so-called graft-versus-leukemia effect)
  - it is also unclear whether the dangerous GVHD effect and the beneficial graft-versus-leukemia effect can be separated

PATHOPHYSIOLOGY

- In GVHD, the effector cells in the donor's bone marrow attacks the patient's organs and tissues, most often those of the patient's skin, liver, and gastrointestinal tract, and also increases the risk for infections
  - early experiments demonstrated that removing the T cells from the donated marrow prior to transplant can significantly reduce severe GVHD. However, the chance of disease relapse, graft rejection, and stimulation of endogenous viral infections is markedly increased

DIAGNOSIS AND PREVENTION

- Acute symptoms begin 2 wks after transplant
  - rashes, diarrhea, fever, blisters, toxic state
  - erythroderma, hyperbilirubinemia, lymphocytosis, edema
- Chronic symptoms usually occur after 3 mos, and resemble autoimmune diseases
  - malaise, fatigue, dry mouth, muscle aches, skin changes, weakness, increased infections
  - multisystem autoimmune symptoms: lupus erythematosus, scleroderma, Sjogren's syndrome, fasciitis, infection
- Prophylaxis of GVHD attempts to prevent the development of a significant allogeneic response of the bone marrow/stem cell donor's immune system toward tissue antigens expressed on vital organs in the patient's body
  - early animal experiments demonstrated that antimetabolic agents, such as methotrexate, were relatively effective, presumably by destroying proliferating T-lymphocytes directed against patient antigens
  - more recently, cyclosporin has been shown to also be effective in preventing GVHD, and a combination of the two is superior to either alone
  - another method for preventing GVHD is to deplete from the hematopoietic stem cell inoculum mature T-lymphocytes, which appear to be the inciting agent for GVHD
- All current maneuvers for preventing GVHD have potentially severe or even fatal side effects, particularly by increasing the risk for infection, but also by increasing risk of graft rejection, and by increasing the risk of leukemic or lymphomatous relapse
- Having many similarities to autoimmune diseases, such as scleroderma and primary biliary cirrhosis, CGVHD can involve virtually any mucous membrane, the liver, and, most profoundly, the immune system
  - staging of disease is key to determining the most appropriate treatment
  - screening tests include skin biopsy, lower lip biopsy, Schirmer's test, pulmonary function tests, liver function tests, CBCs, nutritional assessment, and careful physical exam, with particular attention to mucous membranes, hair distribution, and skin and fascia
  - patients with disease limited to skin tend to have a favorable course, compared to patients with multiorgan involvement

THERAPY

- Once GVHD is established, the first-line treatment is normally corticosteroids
  - other agents, such as antithymocyte globulin, tacrolimus, and mycophenolate mofetil, have activity, but are not clearly superior to steroids
- If first-time treatment fails, second-line treatment includes potent immunosuppressive agents, such as antithymocyte globulin and anti-CD3 monoclonal antibodies
- There is clearly a need for more effective agents, as mortality approaches 75% for first-line failures
  - the major organ toxicities leading to major morbidity and death are normally gut or liver
  - the final common pathway of death is usually infection, probably of a multifactorial origin, including the breaching of natural barriers to infection in the gut and liver, the impact of immunosuppressive agents being delivered to suppress the GVHD, and the immune disregulation intrinsic to GVHD
- Late after transplant, it is possible for a separate entity to develop: chronic graft-versus-host disease (CGVHD)
  - in general, CGVHD is seen in ~33% of HLA-matched sibling transplants and 64% of matched unrelated donors
  - risk factors include increasing patient age, previous serious acute GVHD, previous use of corticosteroids, and perhaps use of allogeneic peripheral blood stem cells rather than marrow stem cells
  - early-stage CGVHD can usually be treated with single-agent therapy: cyclosporin, imuran, or corticosteroids
  - extensive CGVHD requires combination therapy, usually cyclosporin and corticosteroids
    - □ steroid failures can be treated with imuran or thalidomide. If disease is limited to the skin, responses can be seen with the use of PUVA
- Attention to supportive care is crucial for CGVHD
  - physical therapy to prevent joint contractures, local skin care, and attention to dry eyes
  - most important, patients under treatment for CGVHD are profoundly immunodeficient and require antimicrobial prophylaxis
  - when free of GVHD, most patients require reimmunization to childhood diseases
  - treatment is often successful and involves chronic immunosuppression and careful taper of immunosuppressive agents

KEY REFERENCES

Jacobson P, Uberti J, Davis W, Ratanatharathorn V: Tacrolimus: a new agent for the prevention of graft-versus-host disease in hematopoietic stem cell transplantation. Bone Marrow Trans 1998; 22:217–25

Martin PJ, Schoch G, Fisher L, Byers V, Anasetti C, Appelbaum F, Beatty PG, Doney K, McDonald GB, Sanders JE, et al.: A retrospective analysis of therapy for acute graft-versus-host disease: initial treatment. Blood 1990; 76:1464–72

Martin PJ, Schoch G, Fisher L, Byers V, Appelbaum FR, McDonald GB, Storb R, Hansen JA: A retrospective analysis of therapy for acute graft-versus-host disease: secondary treatment. Blood 1991; 77:1821–8.

Storb R, Deeg HJ, Whitehead J, Appelbaum F, Beatty P, Bensinger W, Buckner CD, Clift R, Doney K, Farewell V, et al.: Methotrexate and cyclosporin compared with cyclosporin alone for prophylaxis of acute graft-versus-host disease after marrow transplantation for leukemia. N England J Med 1986; 314:729–35

Sullivan KM, Agura E, Anasetti C, Appelbaum F, Badger C, Bearman S, Erickson K, Flowers M, Hansen J, Loughran T, et al.: Chronic graft-versus-host disease and other late complications of bone marrow transplantation. Semin Hematol 1991; 28:250–9

Sullivan KM, Witherspoon RP, Storb R, Deeg HJ, Dahlberg S, Sanders JE, Appelbaum FR, Doney KC, Weiden P, Anasetti C, et al.: Alternating-day cyclosporin and prednisone for treatment of high-risk chronic graft-v-host disease. Blood 1988; 72:555–61

Vogelsang GB, Farmer ER, Hess AD, Altamonte V, Beschorner WE, Jabs DA, Corio RL, Levin LS, Colvin OM, Wingard JR, et al.: Thalidomide for the treatment of chronic graft-versus-host disease. New Engl J Med 1992; 326:1055, 1058

CYCLOSPORIN

- Other names: Sandimmune, Neoral, SangCya, Gengraf
- FDA-approved use
  - prevention and treatment of rejection following solid organ transplant
  - rheumatoid arthritis (Neoral only)
  - psoriasis (Neoral only)
- Unlabeled uses
  - prevention and treatment of acute and chronic GVHD following bone marrow transplant
  - aplastic anemia
- Mechanism of action
  - cyclosporin binds to a cytosolic protein: cyclophylin
  - the cyclosporin-cyclophylin complex inhibits calcineurin phosphatase
  - inhibition of calcineurin phosphatase may prevent transcription of genes encoding interleukin-2 and other cytokines involved in the immune response
- Pharmacokinetics
  - assay method and biologic fluid influences pharmacokinetic parameters
  - one-third of an oral dose is bioavailable (Sandimmune). One-half of an oral dose is bioavailable with new formulations – Neoral, SangCya, Gengraf
  - bile flow, liver function, diarrhea, and administration with food may affect absorption
  - peak plasma concentrations (C_{max}) are achieved between 2 and 6 hrs
  - cyclosporin is highly tissue-bound
  - volume of distribution ranges from 4–8 L/kg
  - cyclosporin may be measured in tissues for at least 2 wks after discontinuation of cyclosporin therapy
  - cyclosporin binds to erythrocytes; erythrocyte-binding increases with decreased temperature and increased hematocrit
  - plasma protein binding is associated with high-density lipoproteins (HDL) and low-density lipoproteins (LDL)
  - protein binding is higher at 20° C (90–95%) than at 4° C (70%)
  - cyclosporin is extensively metabolized through cytochrome P-450 3A family of enzymes in the gut wall and liver
  - cyclosporin is a substrate for P-glycoprotein, which may prevent systemic absorption
  - clearance is higher in children and lower in individuals with reduced LDL and hepatic impairment
  - elimination half-life may range from 6 to > 24 hrs
  - 90% of cyclosporin is excreted in the bile with < 1% as unchanged drug
  - 6% of cyclosporin is excreted in the urine with 0.1% as parent drug
- Dosing
  - available in oral and parenteral dosage forms
    - □ oral capsules 100 mg and 25 mg
    - □ oral solution at 100 mg/ml
    - □ injectable 250 mg/5 ml ampules
  - for acute GVHD
    - □ IV cyclosporin (Sandimmune). Initiate at 1.5 mg/kg q12hrs and adjust according to clinical status
    - □ oral cyclosporin (Sandimmune) if tolerated. Initiate at 12.5 mg/kg/day in two divided doses and adjust according to clinical status (lower doses may be needed with newer oral formulations)
- Adverse effects
  - most common adverse reactions are renal dysfunction, tremor, hirsutism, hypertension, and gum hyperplasia
- Monitoring
  - measure cyclosporin trough concentrations at approximately the same time of day, due to clearance of cyclosporin varying diurnally. Draw cyclosporin sample from an IV port not used for cyclosporin administration. Cyclosporin concentrations may vary depending on the assay and sample (blood vs. plasma). Therapeutic range varies from institution to institution

Drugs Reported to Influence Cyclosporin Concentrations

Drugs that decrease cyclosporin concentration	Drugs that increase cyclosporin concentration
Anticonvulsants	Acetazolamide
Carbamazepine	
Phenobarbital	Azole antifungal drugs
Phenytoin	Fluconazole
	Itraconazole
Nafcillin	Ketoconazole
Octreotide	
Rifampin	Calcium antagonists
Sulfonamides and Trimethoprim	Diltiazem
	Nicardipine
	Verapamil
	Cimetidine
	Colchicine
	Ethanol
	Imipenem/Cilastin
	Macrolide antibiotics
	Erythromycin
	Josamycin
	Metoclopramide
	Norfloxacin
	Steroid hormones
	Methylprednisolone
	Methyltestosterone
	Oral contraceptives/danazol
	Sulindac
	Other
	Grapefruit juice

- Nursing considerations
  - hypersensitivity reaction can occur with IV formulation secondary to Cremophor diluent; close monitoring during first 30 min is strongly recommended
  - mix IV solution well; unmixed solutions may be associated with increased incidence of anaphylactic reactions caused by delivery of uneven concentrations of Cremophor in bottle
  - when converting IV to po, use a 1:3 ratio; divide into two doses and schedule 12 hrs apart
  - oral solution may be mixed with milk, chocolate milk, orange or apple juice at room temperature

- because absorption is erratic and elimination variable, monitor cyclosporin blood levels; adjust dose requirements to avoid toxicity
- cyclosporin levels are not useful in protecting patients from renal toxicity and cannot be advocated as a 100% protective measure in prevention of GVHD
- nephrotoxicity is dose limiting; avoid administration of nephrotoxic medications (aminoglycosides, amphotericin, etc.)
- may induce lymphoma when given in conjunction with other immunosuppressive agents
- monitor following parameters: cyclosporin trough levels, electrolytes, renal function, hepatic function, cholesterol, blood pressure

■ Assess
- hypertension
- for signs of infection
- neurologic status, baseline and during therapy

■ Teach patient
- possibility of a second malignancy
- signs of neurotoxicity: fine sustension tremors, seizure activity, headaches; tremors decrease when dose is tapered
- not to stop therapy abruptly
- importance of regular dental hygiene
- avoid immunizations unless approved by physician

TACROLIMUS

■ Other names: Prograf, FK506

■ FDA-approved uses: organ rejection prophylaxis in liver transplantation

■ Unlabeled uses
- autoimmune disorders
- severe recalcitrant psoriasis
- GVHD

■ Mechanism of action
- tacrolimus is a macrolide immunosuppressant produced by *Streptomyces tsukubaensis.* Tacrolimus inhibits activation of T-lymphocyte cells by binding to an intracellular protein, FKBP-12. Bound tacrolimus to FKBP-12 forms a complex with calcium, calmodulin, and calcineurin, which inhibits calcineurin phosphatase activity. Calcineurin phosphatase inhibition prevents transcription of genes responsible for the formation of cytokines involved in the immune response

■ Pharmacokinetics
- absorption of tacrolimus varies between individuals and food reduces bioavailability
- oral bioavailability ranges from 14.4–17.4%
- peak plasma concentrations (C_{max}) are achieved at 1.5–3.5 hrs
- volume of distribution is 0.85 L/kg
- tacrolimus is bound to plasma proteins, albumin, and alpha-1-acid glycoprotein
- protein binding ranges from 75–99% depending on concentration, 0.1 to 100 ng/ml, respectively
- distribution of tacrolimus between whole blood and plasma depends on factors such as hematocrit, temperature of separation of plasma, drug concentration, and plasma protein concentration
- tacrolimus is highly bound to erythrocytes
- half-life was measured at 11.7 hrs
- metabolism occurs extensively through cytochrome P-450 3A subfamily of enzymes
- < 1% of tacrolimus is excreted unchanged in the urine

■ Dosing
- available in oral and parenteral dosage forms
  - □ oral capsules of 0.5 mg, 1 mg, and 5 mg
  - □ injectable 5 mg/ml ampules
- for immunosuppression
  - □ IV tacrolimus. Initiate at 0.03–0.05 mg/kg/day as a continuous infusion and adjust according to clinical status. IV doses should be based on lean body weight
  - □ oral tacrolimus. Initiate at 0.15–0.3 mg/kg/day in 2 divided doses q12hrs and adjust according to clinical status

■ Adverse effects
- most common adverse reactions include tremor, headache, diarrhea, hypertension, nausea, and renal dysfunction. Hyperglycemia (glucose intolerance) has occurred in multiple patients with liver transplantation and may require insulin therapy

■ Monitoring
- blood concentrations may aid in evaluating rejection and toxicity, dose adjustment, and compliance. Trough concentrations depend on the assay employed. Therapeutic trough whole blood concentrations range from 5–20 ng/ml. Therapeutic range may vary from institution to institution. Dose modifications should be individualized

■ Drug interactions
- vaccinations may be less effective when administered while a patient is on an immunosuppressant such as tacrolimus. Concomitant administration of aminoglycosides or amphotericin B may increase the potential for renal dysfunction. Antifungals, such as ketoconazole and itraconazole, calcium channel blockers, cimetidine, clarithromycin, erythromycin, methylprednisolone, and metoclopramide, are examples of drugs that inhibit the cytochrome P-450 3A enzyme system and may increase the concentration of tacrolimus. Carbamazepine, phenobarbital, phenytoin, and rifampin are examples of drugs that induce cytochrome P-450 3A enzymes and may decrease concentrations of tacrolimus. Grapefruit juice may increase tacrolimus concentrations

■ Nursing considerations
- polyvinyl-containing sets absorb significant amounts of drug leading to a lower dose being delivered to patient
- when converting IV to po use a 1:3–4 ratio; divide into two doses and schedule 12 hrs apart
- tacrolimus levels are initially evaluated 3 times/wk starting on day +1 until engraftment then weekly until day 100, then q2–3wks until off immunosuppression; target dose levels are 5–20 ng
- monitor tacrolimus blood levels and adjust dose requirements to avoid toxicity; levels are useful in protecting patients from renal toxicity
- the following dose adjustments are necessary in patients with renal dysfunction:

serum creatinine	1.0–1.5 × BL	1.6–1.9 × BL	>1.9 × BL
tacrolimus dose	75–100% of current dose	25–50% of current dose	Hold and resume at 50% of current dose if renal dysfunction is stable

- dose adjustments may be necessary depending on Tacrolimus level

tacrolimus level (ng/ml)	<5	5–9	10–15	16–20	21–25	>25
% dose adjustment	increase 25–50%	↑ by 0–25%	No change	decrease 0–25%	HOLD for 6 hrs; then resume at 50% dose	Hold and resume at 25% dose when level < 20

- nephrotoxicity is dose limiting; use caution with potentially nephrotoxic medications (aminoglycosides, amphotericin, etc.)
- presence of moderate-to-severe hepatic dysfunction (serum bilirubin > 2 mg/dl) appears to effect metabolism of tacrolimus
- monitor following parameters: tacrolimus trough levels, BUN, creatinine, magnesium, potassium, glucose, and liver functions

■ Assess
- for signs of infection
- neurologic status, baseline and during therapy

- Teach patient
  - signs of neurotoxicity: fine sustension tremors, seizure activity, headaches; tremors decrease when dose is tapered
  - not to stop therapy abruptly
  - do not take pills 3 hrs before having tacrolimus levels drawn
  - drink 2 L of fluid a day
  - no immunizations while on therapy w/o MD approval

CORTICOSTEROIDS (PREDNISONE AND METHYLPREDNISOLONE)

- Other names
  - prednisone: Deltasone, Meticorten, Orasone
  - Methylprednisolone: Solu-Medrol, A-Methapred, Medrol (oral)
- Mechanism of action
  - adrenal cortical steroids possess anti-inflammatory (glucocorticoid) and salt-retaining (mineralocorticoid) activity. Corticosteroids may inhibit T-cell proliferation, T-cell dependent immunity, and expression of genes encoding for cytokines such as IL-1, IL-2, IL-6, tumor necrosis factor (TNF), and interferon. Suppression of these cytokines modifies the body's immune response
- Pharmacokinetics
  - corticosteroids are readily absorbed from the gastrointestinal tract
  - plasma protein binding is variable, but distribution to liver, muscle, kidney, intestine, and skin occurs rapidly
  - half-life of prednisone is 1 hr, and methylprednisolone ranges from 1–3 hrs
  - prednisone is extensively metabolized by the liver
  - prednisone is inactive and metabolized to its active metabolite prednisolone by the liver
- Dosing
  - prednisone is available as an oral dosage form
    - □ oral tablets at 1 mg, 2.5 mg, 5 mg, 10 mg, 20 mg, and 50 mg
  - methylprednisolone is available in oral and parenteral dosage forms
    - □ oral tablets of 2 mg, 4 mg, 8 mg, 16 mg, 24 mg, and 32 mg
    - □ powder for injection 40 mg, 125 mg, 250 mg, 500 mg, 1 g and 2 g per vial
  - for immunosuppression (prednisone): treatment of AGVHD
    - □ in adults: oral dose 2 mg/kg/day in 2 divided doses (usually start with 2 mg/kg/day, then taper accordingly)
    - □ in children: oral dose 2 mg/kg/day in 2 divided doses
  - for immunosuppression (methylprednisolone): treatment of AGVHD
    - □ in adults: high-dose therapy (IV): 2 mg/kg/day over at least 30 min
    - □ oral, IV in children: methylprednisolone 2 mg/kg/day divided bid
- Adverse Effects
  - short-term administration of corticosteroids is well tolerated, but long-term therapy may produce harmful effects. Adverse reactions include adrenal suppression (avoided with a gradual taper), muscle weakness, osteoporosis, increased susceptibility to infection, fluid and electrolyte disturbances, cataracts, exophthalmos, glaucoma, hyperglycemia, development or delayed healing of peptic ulcers, mental status changes, impaired wound healing, facial erythema, edema, acne, hirsutism, and easy bruising
- Monitoring
  - signs and symptoms of progression of disease state
- Drug interactions
  - inducers of metabolism (i.e., carbamazepine, phenytoin, and rifampin) may increase the metabolism of corticosteroids
  - diuretics or other potassium-depleting drugs (i.e., amphotericin B) may enhance potassium wasting
  - decreases the effectiveness of vaccinations
  - increased potential for gastrointestinal irritation when given in combination with NSAIDs
  - anticoagulant requirements may decrease or, conversely, corticosteroids may oppose anticoagulation
  - corticosteroids may increase potential for digitalis toxicity
  - may increase cyclosporin concentrations
- Nursing considerations
  - antacids or histamine H2-antagonist should be considered prophylactically to lessen risk of ulceration
  - patients receiving high-dose steroids should receive prophylactic bacterial and fungal antibiotics to decrease risk of infection
  - high doses must be tapered slowly; abrupt withdrawal produces symptoms of adrenal insufficiency
  - monitor glucose, particularly with diabetic patients, because steroids will cause hyperglycemia
  - obtain routine surveillance blood cultures
- Assess
  - for signs of infection; large doses increase susceptibility of infection and can mask signs and symptoms of infection
  - neurologic status, baseline and during therapy; observe for signs of depression with steroid tapering
  - monitor vital signs, weight, blood glucose, and stools for occult blood
- Teach patient
  - oral doses should be taken with meals or snacks to decrease gastric irritation
  - if weight is excessive, counsel on reduction diets (decrease sodium and increase potassium)
  - diabetic patients should monitor blood glucose closely; may require a change in diet or insulin
  - report tarry stools or coffee ground emesis; signs of infection and injuries that do not heal
  - if skin is fragile, avoid rough activity to prevent bruising
  - avoid immunizations unless approved by physician
  - keep health care professionals informed of medications being taken
  - avoid contact with individuals with infection

METHOTREXATE

- Other names: Folex, Mexate
- FDA-approved uses
  - treatment of gestational choriocarcinoma, chorioadenoma destruens, and hydatidiform mole. Treatment and prophylaxis of meningial leukemia. Treatment of breast cancer, epidermoid cancer of the head and neck, mycosis fungoids, squamous cell and small cell lung cancer, advanced-stage nonHodgkin's lymphoma, acute lymphocytic leukemia, non-metastatic osteosarcoma, psoriasis, and rheumatoid arthritis
- Unlabeled uses
  - testicular carcinoma, bladder carcinomas, soft tissue sarcomas, prevention of acute GVHD
- Mechanism of action
  - methotrexate is an antimetabolite and competitively inhibits dihydrofolic acid reductase (DHFR). Inhibition of dihydrofolic acid reductase prevents the formation of tetrahydrofolic acid (FH_4). Methotrexate in its inhibiting action of DHFR interrupts the synthesis of DNA and RNA necessary for cell replication. Methotrexate inhibits the proliferation and differentiation of T cells and B cells
- Pharmacokinetics
  - oral absorption is dose dependent
  - oral doses ≤30 mg/m² are well absorbed with bioavailability measured at 60%
  - absorption of oral doses > 80 mg/m² is decreased significantly
  - food delays absorption and reduces peak plasma concentrations
  - initial volume of distribution is 0.18 L/kg and increases at steady state to 0.4–0.8 L/kg
  - methotrexate competes with reduced folates for active transport across cell membranes, except at higher concentrations (> 100 micromolar) where methotrexate transport across membranes relies on passive diffusion
  - serum protein binding is 50%

- 80–90% of a single dose is excreted unchanged in the urine
- < 10% of methotrexate dose relies on biliary excretion
- half-life of doses < 30 mg/m² ranges from 3–10 hrs. Half-life of higher doses ranges from 8–15 hrs

■ Dosing
- available in oral and parenteral dosage forms
  - □ oral tablets, 2.5 mg
  - □ parenteral, preservative-free injection: 2.5 mg/ml; 2 ml, 4 ml, 8 ml, and 10 ml vials
  - □ parenteral injection: 2.5 mg/ml; 2 ml vials
  - □ parenteral injection: 2.5 mg/ml; 2 ml, 4 ml, 8 ml, 10 ml vials
  - □ parenteral powder for injection; 20 mg, 50 mg, 100 mg, 250 mg, and 1 g vials
- for prevention of acute GVHD
  - □ IV methotrexate
    - • dose at 15 mg/m² IV on the first day after bone marrow transplant (day 1), followed by 10 mg/m² on days 3, 6, and 11; often in combination with cyclosporin. Methotrexate is administered weekly at 10 mg/m² following day 11 in some protocols. Methotrexate may be used as a single agent for prophylaxis

■ Adverse effects
- side effects are related to dose and frequency of administration
- most common side effects are ulcerative stomatitis, nausea, leukopenia, abdominal distress, malaise, fatigue, chills, fever, dizziness, and decreased resistance to infection

■ Monitoring
- monitor methotrexate concentrations at 0 hr, 24 hrs, and q24hrs until concentration < 0.05 micromolar

■ Drug interactions
- increased concentrations of methotrexate have been caused by NSAIDs, probenecid, salicylates, sulfonamides, amiodarone, procarbazine (may increase the potential of nephrotoxity), Ethanol and etritinate (may increase the potential for hepatotoxicity), phenylbutazone, and high-dose penicillins. Decreased methotrexate concentrations have been associated with administration of oral antibiotics (tetracyclines, chloramphenicol, oral aminoglycosides, and nonabsorbable broad-spectrum antibiotics), activated charcoal, and cholestyramine. Increased bone marrow suppression with trimethoprim/sulfamethoxazole, and other sulfonamides. Phenytoin concentrations may decrease and theophylline concentrations may increase with administration of methotrexate
- may lower efficacy of G-CSF (Neupogen) and other growth factors

■ Nursing considerations
- methotrexate 15 mg/m² or mini-dose methotrexate 5 mg/m² is commonly administered on day + 1, + 3, + 6, and + 11 (day 11 may not be included in all regimens)
- dose should be held or reduced if patient has severe mucositis and an impairment in renal or hepatic function
- monitor liver functions tests; if bilirubin is 3.1–5 mg/dl or AST > 180, administer 75% of usual dose; if bilirubin is > 5, do not administer dose and notify physician
- monitor renal function and dose adjust as follows

Creatinine clearance	Dose
creatinine clearance 60–80 ml/min	give 75% of total dose
creatinine clearance 51–60 ml/min	give 70% of total dose
creatinine clearance 10–50 ml/min	give 30–50% of total dose
creatinine clearance <10 ml/min	HOLD

- in renal dysfunction (creatinine clearance < 60 ml/min) monitor methotrexate levels at 24 hrs and 48 hrs after dose; leucovorin rescue may be initiated

■ Assess
- obtain comprehensive oral exam to evaluate for mucositis/ulcerative stomatitis; lubrication of lips, topical analgesics formulations and systemic analgesics provide pain relief
- for infection: examine catheter sites, lungs, integument, oral mucosa, and rectal area; if neutropenic, institute infection control practices
- monitor for diarrhea: hemorrhagic enteritis and death may occur from intestinal perforation; initiate antidiarrheals

■ Teach patient
- meticulous oral and perineal hygiene
- report stomatitis, diarrhea, tarry stools, abd discomfort
- report signs of infection: fever, chills, sore throat, cough, shortness of breath
- report yellow color to skin and eyes and unusual bleeding

AZATHIOPRINE

■ Other name: Imuran

■ FDA-approved uses
- renal transplantation, rheumatoid arthritis

■ Unlabeled uses
- chronic ulcerative colitis, generalized myasthenia gravis, controlling the progression of Behçet's syndrome, treatment of Crohn's disease, and treatment of chronic GVHD

■ Mechanism of action
- azathioprine is cleaved to 6-mercaptopurine. Azathioprine is an antagonist of purine metabolism and may inhibit DNA and RNA synthesis. Azathioprine suppresses cell-mediated immunity and causes alterations in antibody production. Azathioprine affects proliferation and differentiation of T cells and B cells. Azathioprine's effect on T cells is related to the temporal relationship between antigenic stimulus and engraftment. Azathioprine has little effect on established organ rejections or secondary responses

■ Pharmacokinetics
- azathioprine is readily absorbed after oral administration
- azathioprine is rapidly cleared from the blood, and normal doses produce blood concentrations of < 1 mcg/mL
- 30% bound to plasma proteins
- azathioprine is rapidly eliminated from the blood and oxidized or methylated in erythrocytes and liver
- very small amounts of azathioprine are excreted unchanged
- renal clearance may not be important when predicting effectiveness or toxicity
- dose reduction is practiced with poor renal function

■ Dosing
- available in oral and parenteral dosage forms
  - □ oral tablets, 50 mg
  - □ parenteral, powder for injection: 100 mg; 20 ml vials
- for immunosuppression in adults and children
  - □ initiate oral or IV dose at 3–5 mg/kg/d followed by a maintenance dose of 1–3 mg/kg/d

■ Adverse effects
- principal and potentially serious toxic effects are hematologic and gastrointestinal. These include severe bone marrow depression, severe leukopenia or thrombocytopenia, macrocytic anemia, and severe nausea and vomiting. Secondary infections, neoplasia, and hepatotoxicity are noted

■ Monitoring
- monitor hematologic indices (i.e., WBC, CBC) and liver function tests

■ Drug interactions
- ACE inhibitors may increase risk of severe leukopenia. Allopurinol may increase potential for toxic effects of azathioprine. Methotrexate may increase plasma concentrations of metabolite 6-mercaptopurine. Azathioprine may decrease activity of anticoagulants. Cyclosporin concentrations may be decreased. Activity of neuromuscular blockers may be reduced or reversed

■ Nursing considerations
- hematologic suppression is the usual dose-limiting toxic effect (leukopenia, thrombocytopenia, anemia)
- patients are at risk for serious infections (bacterial, fungal, protozoal) and should receive appropriate prophylactic antibiotics

- Assess
  - pulmonary status, baseline and during therapy; severe pulmonary edema has occurred in patients with fluid overload; monitor I/O and weight
  - vomiting and diarrhea are common at higher doses
  - skin integrity
- Teach patient
  - take drug in divided doses with food
  - may develop serum sickness (rash, fever, arthralgias, and/or pleuritis) 10–14 days after dose
  - avoid immunizations unless approved by physician
  - report signs and symptoms of infection and avoid contact with individuals with infections
  - report unusual bleeding, bruising, mouth sores, abdominal pain, diarrhea, dark urine or pale stools, and nausea and vomiting
  - keep health care professionals informed of medications being taken

MYCOPHENYLATE MOFETIL

- Other name: Cellcept
- FDA-approved uses
  - prophylaxis of organ rejection in patients receiving allogeneic renal transplant
  - used in combination with cyclosporin and corticosteroids
- Mechanism of action
  - mycophenylate is hydrolyzed to form the active metabolite, mycophenolic acid (MPA). MPA inhibits inosine monophosphate dehydrogenase and, therefore, interrupts the de novo pathway of guanosine nucleotide synthesis without incorporation into DNA. T- and B-lymphocytes are dependent on de novo synthesis of purines for proliferation. Therefore, MPA inhibits the proliferative response of T- and B-lymphocytes. MPA may also inhibit antibody formation from B cells
- Pharmacokinetics
  - bioavailability of mycophenylate mofetil is 94% and absorption is rapid
  - mcophenylate mofetil is metabolized to active metabolite, MPA
  - volume of distribution is 4 L/kg
  - MPA is 97% bound to plasma proteins
  - MPA is metabolized to a MPA glucuronide
  - < 1% of mycophenylate mofetil is excreted as MPA
  - 90% of MPA glucuronide is excreted in the urine and 6% is recovered in feces
  - half-life of oral dose is 17.9 hrs, and half-life of IV dose is 16.6 hrs
- Dosing
  - available in oral dosage forms
    - □ oral capsule, 250 mg
    - □ oral tablets, 500 mg
  - for immunosuppression in adults
    - □ initiate oral mycophenylate mofetil at 1 g twice daily. May increase to 1.5 g twice daily. Patient toleration was greater with 2 g/day dose. In patients with severe chronic renal impairment (GFR < 25 ml/min/1.73 m^2), avoid doses > 1 g twice daily
  - for immunosuppression in children
    - □ initial dose is 600 mg/m^2 twice daily
- Adverse effects
  - most common adverse effects include diarrhea, leukopenia, sepsis and vomiting, and increased potential for infection
- Monitoring
  - perform CBCs weekly during the first month, twice monthly for the second month, then monthly for the first year. If neutropenia develops (ANC < 1,300 mcL) stop mycophenylate mofetil or reduce the dose
- Drug interactions
  - MPA glucuronide, acyclovir, and ganciclovir may compete for tubular secretion, and concentrations of these drugs may increase
  - antacids may decrease the absorption. Cholestyramine may interfere with hepatic recirculation
  - probenecid may increase MPA glucuronide concentrations due to inhibition of tubular secretion
  - salicylates increased the free fraction of MPA. MPA decreases binding of phenytoin and theophylline
- Nursing considerations
  - monitor CBC, differential, platelets, renal function tests
- Assess
  - alterations in nutritional status due to diarrhea, nausea, and vomiting
- Teach patient
  - capsules should be taken on an empty stomach and should not be opened, chewed, or crushed
  - report signs and symptoms of infection
  - report unusual bleeding, bruising, mouth sores, abdominal pain, diarrhea, dark urine or pale stools, and nausea and vomiting

LYMPHOCYTE IMMUNE GLOBULIN, ANTI-THYMOCYTE GLOBULIN (EQUINE)

- Other name: Atgam
- FDA-approved uses
  - management of allograft rejection in renal transplantation
  - aplastic anemia
- Unlabeled uses

  immunosuppressant in the course of liver, bone marrow, heart, and other solid organ transplants. Multiple sclerosis, myasthenia gravis, pure red-cell aplasia, and scleroderma. Treatment and prevention of acute and chronic GVHD
- Mechanism of action
  - lymphocyte immune globulin, antithymocyte globulin (ATG) is a lymphocyte-selective immunosuppressant. ATG binds to the surface of T-lymphocytes reducing the number of circulating T cells. ATG impairs the T cell immune response
- Pharmacokinetics
  - rapid onset of action
  - distribution of ATG into body fluids and tissues has not been fully described
  - ATG has poor penetration into lymphoid tissues
  - ATG likely crosses the placenta, since other immune globulins cross the placenta
  - < 1% of ATG is excreted in the urine as unchanged equine IgG
  - half-life ranges between 3–9 days
- Dosing
  - available in a parenteral dosage form
    - □ parenteral injection: 50 mg/ml; 5 ml ampules
  - test dose should be administered prior to first infusion
    - □ *test dose:* intradermal injection 0.1 ml of a 1:1000 dilution (5 mcg of horse IgG)
  - Premedications
    - □ diphenhydramine: 0.5–1 mg/kg po or IV (max 50 mg)
    - □ acetaminophen: 10–15 mg/kg po (max 1000 mg)
    - □ hydrocortisone: 1–5 mg/kg IV (max 100 mg)
  - for treatment
    - □ 15 mg/kg dose qd 7–14 days
- Adverse effects
  - fever (51%), thrombocytopenia (30%), rashes (27%), chills (16%), leukopenia (14%), systemic infection (13%). Adverse reactions that had 5–10% occurrence: abnormal renal function tests, serum sickness–like symptoms, dyspnea or apnea, arthralgia, chest/back/flank pain, diarrhea, nausea, and vomiting. Adverse reactions that had < 5% occurrence: hypertension, herpes simplex infection, pain, swelling or anaphylaxis, tachycardia, edema, localized infection, malaise, seizures, GI bleeding/perforation, deep-vein thrombosis, sour mouth/throat, hyperglycemia, acute renal failure, abnormal liver function tests, confusion, disorientation, cough, neutropenia, granulocytopenia, anemia, thrombophlebitis, dizziness, epigastric/stomach pain, lymphadenopathy, pulmonary edema, CHF, abdominal pain, nosebleed, vasculitis, aplasia, pancytopenia, abnormal involuntary movement, tremor, rigidity, sweating, laryngospasm, hemolysis/hemolytic anemia, viral hepatitis, faintness, enlarged/ruptured kidney, paresthesias, renal artery thrombosis

- Monitoring
  - patients should be observed for possible allergic reactions during initial and subsequent infusions of ATG
- Drug interactions
  - ATG administered with other immunosuppressants (i.e., cyclosporin, azathioprine, corticosteroids) may increase the potential for infection, including cytomegalovirus (CMV)
- Nursing considerations
  - test dose is strongly recommended
  - premedicate with Benedryl 25 mg IV, Solumedrol 1 mg/kg, Tylenol 650 mg po
  - using a pump, administer infusion through a central line with an inline filter preferred due to chemical phlebitis
  - if patient develops chills, Demerol 25 mg IV every hour prn, can be given for comfort measures
  - epinephrine and resuscitative equipment should be readily available
- Assess
  - observe patient for possible anaphylactic reaction during initial and subsequent infusions; be aware of development of a wheal at injection site, erythema or swelling
  - for hypotension, respiratory distress, serum sickness, and viral infection, which may indicate anaphylaxis
  - notify physician if patient develops shortness of breath, wheezing, fevers, chills, severe myalgias, rash, or chest pain
- Teach patient
  - may develop serum sickness (rash, fever, arthralgias, and/or pleuritis) 10–14 days after dose
  - diabetic patients should monitor blood glucose closely; may require a change in diet or insulin

MUROMONAB-CD3

- Other name: Orthoclone, OKT3
- FDA-approved uses
  - reversal of heart and liver transplant rejection in adults
- Unlabeled uses
  - treatment of acute GVHD, lung, kidney, and pancreas transplant rejection. Psoriasis vulgaris
- Mechanism of action
  - Muromonad-CD3 (OKT3) is a monoclonal antibody that binds to CD3 glycoprotein found on the surface of T-lymphocytes. OKT3 inhibits antigen recognition by T-lymphocytes. OKT3 also binds to T-lymphocytes resulting in early activation of the T cell and increased cytokine release, followed by blocking T-cell function
- Pharmacokinetics
  - rapid decrease in T-lymphocytes is observed within minutes following OKT3 administration
    - □ time to reversal of rejection averages 3–4 days
    - □ volume of distribution is $\sim$6.5 L
    - □ elimination occurs through the reticuloendothelial system
    - □ half-life of OKT3 is 18 hrs
- Dosing
  - Premedications
    - □ methylprednisolone: 1 mg/kg, 2 hrs prior to OKT3 infusion
    - □ hydrocortisone: 1–5 mg/kg (max 100 mg) given 30 mins after the administration of OKT3 to reduce reactions to the first dose. Reactions to subsequent doses seem to be less severe, but premedications are still used
    - □ diphenhydramine 0.5–1 mg/kg IV or po (max: 50 mg)
    - □ acetaminophen 10–15 mg/kg po (max: 1000 mg)
  - available as a parenteral dosage form
    - □ parenteral injection: 1 mg/ml; 5 ml ampules
  - usual dose in adults
    - □ OKT3 5 mg IV daily for 10–14 days
  - usual dose in children <12 yrs old
    - □ OKT3 0.1 mg/kg/day IV daily for 10–14 days; in patients >30 kg: 5 mg IV daily for 10–14 days
- Adverse reactions
  - fever, chills/rigors, flulike syndrome, fatigue/malaise, generalized weakness, anorexia, tachycardia, hypertension, hypotension, perioral and peripheral cyanosis, aseptic meningitis, seizures, headache, confusion, pruritus, rash, diarrhea, nausea, vomiting, arthralgia, myalgia, tremor, photophobia, elevated serum creatinine/BUN, dyspnea, chest pain/tightness, wheezing, pulmonary edema, anaphylactic-type reactions
- Monitoring
  - chest x-ray, weight gain, CBC with differential. Immunologic monitoring of T cells and OKT3 concentrations. OKT3 concentrations maintained at 1 mcg/ml should yield low CD3 counts
- Drug interactions
  - encephalopathy and other CNS effects have been reported with OKT3 in combination with indomethacin
  - the risk of psychosis and infection may increase with OKT3 and corticosteroids
  - increased risk of infection or malignancies when OKT3 is given with other immunosuppressant such as cyclosporin or azathioprine
- Nursing considerations
  - contraindicated in patient with a recent exposure to chicken pox or herpes zoster; fluid overload or pulmonary edema; fever >37.8 C; and pregnancy
  - effects of first dose (flulike symptoms, anaphylactic-type reaction) may occur within 30 min up to 24 hrs; effect can be minimized by premedicating with methylprednisolone 15 mg/kg po, hydrocortisone 100 mg IV, Tylenol 1,000 mg po, and Benedryl 50 mg po
  - emergency medications for intubation and respiratory support should be readily available
  - Assess
    - □ remain with patient and monitor vital signs during the first 30 min of the first infusion; chest pain may occur with first dose, but rare thereafter
    - □ pulmonary status, baseline and during therapy; severe pulmonary edema has occurred in patients with fluid overload; monitor I/O and weight
  - Teach patient
    - □ difficulty breathing, chest congestion, fever and chills, trembling and shaking of the hands can occur following first dose; reassure patient will be monitored closely
    - □ report chest pain, difficulty breathing, nausea and chills
    - □ effects of medication may last a week
    - □ report signs and symptoms of infection

KEY REFERENCES

Basara N, Blau WI, Römer E, Rudolphi M, Bischoff M, Kirsten D, Sanchez H, Gunzelmann S, Fauser AA: Mycophenolate mofetil for the treatment of acute and chronic GVHD in bone marrow transplant patients. Bone Marrow Trans 1998; 22:61–5

Clark JB, Queener SF, Burke Karb: *Pharmacological Basis of Nursing Practice* (3rd ed.). St. Louis: CV Mosby Company, 1990

Forman SJ, Blume KG, Thomas ED: *Bone Marrow Transplantation.* Boston: Blackwell Scientific Publications, 1994

Karch A, Boyd E: *Handbook of Drugs and the Nursing Process.* Pittsburgh: Lippincott, 1989

PDR: Oncology Prescribing Guide (2nd ed). Pharmacia and Upjohn, 1998

Przepiorka D, Devine SM, Fay JW, Uberti JP, Wingard JR: Practical considerations in the use of tacrolimus for allogeneic marrow transplantation. Bone Marrow Transplantation 1999; 24(10):1053–56

Tierney LM, McPhee SJ, Papadakis MA: *Current Medical Diagnosis and Treatment* (36th ed.) Norwalk, Conn: Appleton and Lange, 1997

Extravasation of Vesicant Anticancer Agents

R. T. Dorr

OVERVIEW

■ Vesicant (locally ulcerogenic) anticancer agents include three main categories of compounds
- DNA-binding agents: mechlorethamine, mitomycin C, and rarely, cisplatin
- DNA-intercalating agents: dactinomycin, daunorubicin, doxorubicin, idarubicin, and rarely, mitoxantrone
- tubulin-binding agents: vincristine, vinblastine, vinorelbine, and rarely, paclitaxel

■ Only a few antidotes to vesicant extravasations have been adequately tested
- 1/6 molar (isotonic) sodium thiosulfate for mechlorethamine, and cisplatin
- topical cooling and dimethylsulfoxide (DMSO) for DNA intercalators
- hyaluronidase (spreading factor enzyme) for tubulin-binding agents

■ Locally elevated levels of vesicant drugs can cause severe tissue destruction if untreated, but most vesicant extravasations will not lead to ulceration if conservatively treated

■ approximately one-third of vesicant extravasations will result in local necrosis

PATHOPHYSIOLOGY

■ Tissue damage is a direct extension of the drug's pharmacologic (cytotoxic) activity

■ Time course and pathology of symptom/lesions varies by class of vesicant
- rapid onset of symptoms of pain and swelling are typical for most vesicant extravasations (DNA intercalators, mechlorethamine, most vinca alkaloid extravasations)
- a defined subset of some agents have delayed symptoms
  - □ 1–24 hrs for ~20% of vinca alkaloids (vincristine, vinblastine, vinorelbine) extravasations
  - □ up to 4 wks for ~10% of mitomycin extravasations
  - □ visible tissue damage is prolonged for all agents (weeks to months), which is especially problematic on dorsum of the hand, where nerves and tendons are superficial

■ Some agents are relatively weak vesicants and require large extravasations to produce toxicity
- rare cases of paclitaxel-induced necrosis involve large-volume extravasations: >60% of intended dose
- rare cisplatin-induced necrosis involve extravasations of highly concentrated solutions: >1 mg/ml

■ Doxorubicin, the most common vesicant, slowly involves a widening and deepening lesion due to months-long drug entrapment at the site
- early surgical excision can remove significant amounts of drug
- hallmark for surgical referral is moderate/severe pain (with or without significant swelling) 2 wks after extravasations
- histopathology of lesions shows extensive coagulative necrosis with little or no inflammatory reaction (no rationale for corticosteroids)

DIAGNOSIS AND PREVENTION

■ Prevention is imperative by exercising great caution during vesicant administration
- adequate training (ONS certification) of personnel administrating vesicants
- use central access for repeated or long-term vesicant infusions
- challenge/test vein patency with isotonic saline or D_5W
- stop infusions at first sign of difficulty
- withdraw any material possible from line if extravasations confirmed
- refer to surgery immediately for severe (expanding) ulcers

■ At the first sign of difficulty, stop infusion and evaluate site
- significant resistance to continued infusion flow or inability to withdraw blood or fluid (use isotonic test solution for challenge)
- immediate pain, with or without localized swelling
- swelling, which can be distal to infusion site (especially seen with mitomycin C extravasations). Swelling may not occur at the exact catheter tip, and may even be retrograde to expected venous flow path
- for indwelling port or catheter extravasations
  - □ pain can be referred through the back or up the neck
  - □ swelling can occur into the chest wall and dependent tissue, i.e., breast
  - □ document catheter tip placement and device patency status by radiologic dye study

■ Pain and swelling can be delayed days to weeks for some agents
- vinca alkaloids
- mitomycin C

THERAPY

■ No universal antidote exists for vesicant agents
- specific antidotes are available for each category of vesicant
- there is no role for corticosteroids as local antidotes

■ Only true vesicant agents should be treated. Other irritating anticancer drug extravasations should be conservatively managed

■ Rapid use of specific local antidotes may substantially reduce subsequent ulceration; these vary by vesicant drug class
- mechlorethamine (nitrogen mustard) and large cisplatin extravasations
  - □ 1/6 M sodium thiosulate (4 ml of 10% solution combined with 6 ml sterile water) and inject 3–5 ml into extravasations site to bind and inactivate drug
- DNA intercalators, especially doxorubicin
  - □ apply topical cool packs to site for 15 min every half hour for 6–8 hrs. If suspected large extravasations, apply ~1 ml of 99% (w/v) dimethylsulfoxide (DMSO) solution to site, allow to dry (no occlusive cover), and repeat 3–4 times daily for 1–2 wks
- vinca alkaloids and large paclitaxel extravasations
  - □ prepare hyaluronidase solution in 0.9% sodium chloride to 150 U/ml concentration; inject 1–2 ml into extravasations site to facilitate systemic uptake of entrapped drug

■ Documentation of extravasations, close follow-up, and early surgical referral for evolving lesions (especially doxorubicin) is important to mitigate damage

KEY REFERENCES

Bertelli G, Dini D, Forno GB, Silvestro S, Venturini M, Rosso R, Prozato P: Hyaluronidase as an antidote to extravasations of vinca alkaloids: clinical results. J Cancer Res Clin Oncol 1994; 120:505–6

Bertelli G, Gozza A, Forno GB, Vidilli MG, Silvestro S, Venturini M, Del Mastro L, Garrone O, Rosso R, Dinni D: Topical dimethylsulfoxide for the prevention of soft tissue injury after extravasations of vesicant cytotoxic drugs: a prospective clinical study. J Clin Oncol 1995; 13(11):2851–5

Dorr RT: Antidotes to vesicant chemotherapy extravasations. Blood Rev 1990; 4:41–60

Rudolph R, Larson DL: Etiology and treatment of chemotherapeutic agent extravasation injuries: a review. J Clin Oncol 1987; 5(7):1116–26

Allergic Toxicity

N. Kalil, H. Streicher, Erin P. Demakos, and S.G. Arbuck

OVERVIEW

■ Allergic or hypersensitivity reactions (HSR) reflect immunologic mechanisms rather than pharmacologic actions of a drug. HSRs typically occur in individuals sensitized by previous exposure to an allergen, when antibodies or lymphocytes react against the drug or its metabolites

■ A careful patient history that includes prior exposures and reactions is vital before any drug is given. However, reactions may occur at any time, including with an initial exposure

■ HSRs are more frequently associated with some compounds than others, most notably taxanes and l-asparaginase. However, all administrated drugs and their components should be considered when evaluating the cause of an allergic reaction. The rate and route of exposure to drug can also influence the frequency and severity of reactions

■ Types of HSRs
- immediate hypersensitive reaction (type I or IgE-mediated). These HSRs are the most prevalent and also may produce life-threatening, anaphylactic reactions. Airway obstruction and hypotension are the main causes of death. Type I reactions include anaphylaxis, angioedema, bronchospasm, and uticaria
- cytotoxic reaction (type II)
- immune-complex-mediated reaction (type III)
- delayed hypersensitivity reaction (type IV)

PATHOPHYSIOLOGY

■ Immediate hypersensitivity reaction (type I)
- sensitization and production of drug-specific IgE is dependent on T helper cells, which produce cytokines including IL-4 and IL-5
- IgE binds to a high-affinity receptor on mast cells (Fc-epsilonR1). Within minutes, mast cells degranulate and release preformed mediators, histamine, heparin, tryptase, and chymotryptase from cytoplasmic granules
- lipid mediators, prostaglandins D2, leukotriene C4 are synthesized for later release and are associated with inflammation and late-phase reactions that may occur for up to 24 hrs

■ Cytotoxic reaction (type II)
- IgG or IgM may bind to antigens on cell membranes, thereby activating the complement cascade and causing Coombs-positive hemolytic anemia, thrombocytopenia, and neutropenia

■ Immune-complex-mediated reaction (type III)
- immune complexes composed of antigen and antibody occur in the circulation or are deposited in target organs, such as kidneys, joints, and skin
- they may cause serum sickness–like illness, manifested as hypersensitivity vasculitis, glomerulonephritis, nephrotic syndrome, arthritis, and urticarial skin rashes
- clearance of immune complexes often requires a week or more. During this time, serum complement levels are usually decreased

■ Delayed hypersensitivity reaction (type IV)
- type IV HSR results from the expansion of activated antigen-specific T cells that produce cytokines, such as IL-2, IL-4, TNF-alpha, and IFN-gamma
- macrophages may form giant cells, resulting in granulomatous inflammation
- these cellular events frequently occur in the skin, lungs, and kidneys
- classic examples of type IV HSR are intradermal skin tests and contact sensitivity to poison ivy
- delayed-type hypersensitivity (DTH) is the probable mechanism for immunologically mediated pulmonary reactions to methotrexate, a drug that can also cause type I and type III HSRs

DIAGNOSIS AND PREVENTION

■ Presenting signs and symptoms of type I reactions
- minor symptoms
  - □ flushing
  - □ anxiety
  - □ gastrointestinal cramping
  - □ pruritus
  - □ local or generalized urticaria
  - □ minor symptoms that progress rapidly may precede cardiovascular collapse and respiratory failure
- anaphylactoid reactions, mediated by complement activation or possibly by direct release of mediators from mast cells, are indistinguishable from HSRs. Anaphylactoid reactions may occur with the first exposure to a drug
- symptoms of severe systemic HSRs
  - □ hypotension
  - □ tachycardia
  - □ laryngeal edema with hoarseness and stridor
  - □ bronchospasm with wheezing

■ Differential diagnosis
- myocardial infarction
- arrhythmia
- hypovolemic shock; septic shock
- vasovagal syncope
- pulmonary embolism
- airway obstruction due to foreign body
- anxiety or panic disorder

■ Prophylaxis
- prophylactic regimens include corticosteroids in association with H1 and H2 antihistamines as premedication and slowing the infusion rate, which may ameliorate HSRs but will not always be effective
- history, monitoring of patients by personnel skilled in recognizing the signs and symptoms of HSR, and the availability of emergency treatment is essential
- for patients who have had a HSR, when the risk/benefit ratio and general medical status justifies retreating, additional premedication and desensitization or slowing the infusion rate may ameliorate subsequent reactions
  - □ these approaches must be used cautiously by those trained to manage anaphylactic reactions
  - □ patients should understand the potential risks. Severe, life-threatening reactions may recur
  - □ patients with HSRs to *E. coli* l-asparaginase: *Erwinia* l-asparaginase or the polyethylene glycol-modified (PEG) formulation may have lower risk

■ Standard premedication regimen for paclitaxel
- dexamethasone, 20 mg po 12 and 6 hrs before treatment. Manufacturer recommends that HIV patients receive 10 mg of the oral dose of dexamethasone
- diphenhydramine hydrochloride, 50 mg IV 30–60 min before drug infusion
- ranitidine, 50 mg (or Cimetidine—300 mg) IV 30–60 min before drug infusion
- monitor and observe patient during and after treatment
- this standard regimen is associated with an incidence of severe HSRs in $<2\%$. The efficacy of abbreviated regimens remains unproven

■ Standard premedication regimen for docetaxel
- dexamethasone, 8 mg po twice a day for 3 days starting 1 day prior to docetaxel administration. Other side effects, such as effusions and edema, are also ameliorated or delayed with this premedication regimen
- H1 and H2 antihistamines may be helpful, on an individual basis

THERAPY

■ Treatment of reactions requires a diagnostic evaluation
- first priority is to maintain an open airway
- obtain vital signs and quickly assess patient, even if only minor symptoms are present
- hypotension and shock due to vasodilation, capillary leak, and hypoxemia, if present, must be treated without delay
- when administrating anticancer therapy, one must always be prepared to treat allergic reactions. HSR, especially IgE-mediated, may recur with a small amount of drug, even years after initial sensitization

- Anaphylaxis treatment
  - discontinue the drug immediately. Expertise and equipment should be immediately available for airway management
  - administer 100% oxygen by mask or cannula
    - □ endotracheal intubation and ventilation with 100% oxygen for upper airway obstruction or laryngeal edema with respiratory failure that does not respond to epinephrine
  - surgical airway management is rarely needed but should not be delayed when required
  - epinephrine is the primary therapy for anaphylaxis. Administer SubQ dose of 0.3–0.5 mg initially, then repeat q15–20min until reaction subsides (to a maximum total dose of 2 mg)
    - □ for severe unresponsive hypotension or airways compromise: epinephrine 0.1–0.25 mg IV may be given slowly over 5–10 min, with further cardiovascular support as needed
    - □ epinephrine can precipitate acute cardiovascular events in elderly patients and those with underlying coronary artery disease
  - patients taking beta-adrenergic antagonists may have a poor response to treatment
  - volume expanders (crystalloid or colloid), as needed, to support cardiac output
  - bronchodilators: inhaled nebulized solution of beta 2-selective adrenergic agonists. Metaproterenol, 10–20 mg/dose or albuterol, 2.5–5.0 mg/dose q20min for up to 3 doses; then q4hrs for persistent bronchospasm
  - corticosteroids: methylprednisolone, 125 mg, or hydrocortisone, 500 mg, IV q6hrs. These agents are not helpful during an acute event, but may be very useful for persistent bronchospasm and delayed effects that may occur following severe allergic reactions
  - diphenhydramine 50 mg IM or IV over 5 min particularly for urticaria and angioedema without airways compromise
  - observation for 6–8 hrs, even for rapidly responsive patients. Late-phase reactions may occur for up to 24 hrs
  - patients should be fully informed about the nature of the reaction and given instructions for prevention and response to further events
  - treatment of other allergic reactions, such as rash and fever, is symptomatic; H1 antihistamines and corticosteroids for more severe reactions
- Special nursing considerations
  - nursing expertise in the administration and management of side effects of chemotherapy is critical
  - must have knowledge of the chemotherapy drug's potential to cause a hypersensitivity reaction
  - knowledge of the drugs used to treat anaphylaxis and method of administration
  - knowledge and skill to perform cardiopulmonary resuscitation
  - baseline assessment of patient prior to drug administration; monitor vital signs during infusion
  - administer chemotherapy drug slowly and with caution; emergency medications and equipment must be available and accessible
  - close observation of the patient during administration for local or systemic reaction; usually occur within 15 min of start of infusion
- Specific drugs
  - epinephrine hydrochloride (adrenaline)
    - □ monitor for signs of tachycardia, hypertension, anginal pain, dizziness, disorientation
    - □ use cautiously in elderly patients with hyperthyroidism, history of respiratory ailments, and cardiac disease
    - □ assess
      - ▽ vital signs; monitor for hypotension
      - ▽ baseline neurologic status and during therapy
      - ▽ avoid extravasation
  - diphenhydramine (Benadryl)
    - □ use cautiously in patients with history of hypertension, hyperthyroidism, cardiovascular disease, respiratory ailments
    - □ may be given IV push by registered nurse; not to exceed 25 mg/min
    - □ Assess
      - ▽ vital signs; monitor for hypotension
      - ▽ baseline neurologic status and during therapy
    - □ teach patient
      - ▽ avoid alcohol ingestion; operation of equipment or driving a car while drowsy
      - ▽ take medication with food
  - methylprednisolone
    - □ use caution when given to patients with history of GI ulceration, renal disease, hypertension, diabetes mellitus, hypothyroidism, GI disturbances, emotional instability
    - □ diabetic patients may require insulin altered during treatment; monitor glucose levels
    - □ drug may mask or exacerbate infections, including latent amebiasis
    - □ gradually titrate off medication for those patients receiving prolonged therapy
    - □ assess
      - ▽ patient weight, blood pressure, electrolytes, and sleep patterns
    - □ teach patient
      - ▽ take medication with milk or food
      - ▽ not to stop taking drug abruptly
  - hydrocortisone
    - □ use caution when administering to patients with history of GI ulcerations, renal disease, hypertension, diabetes mellitus, hypothyroidism, GI disturbances, emotional instability
    - □ drug may mask or exacerbate infections, including latent amebiasis
    - □ gradually titrate off medication for those patients receiving prolonged therapy
    - □ assess
      - ▽ baseline neurologic status and during therapy; watch for depression or psychotic episodes, especially in those patients receiving high doses
    - □ teach patient
      - ▽ not to stop taking drug abruptly

KEY REFERENCES

Baker JR, Zylke JW (eds): *Primer on Allergic and Immunologic Diseases* (4th. ed.). JAMA 1997; (Dec. 10):1799–2034

Golden BD, Schwartz HJ, Graft DF, et al.: Position statement: the use of epinephrine in the treatment of anaphylaxis. J Allergy Clin Immunol 1994; 94:666–8

Fisher DS, Knobf MT, Durivage HJ (eds): *The Cancer Chemotherapy Handbook* (5th ed.). St. Louis: Mosby, 1997

Lichtenstein LM: Anaphylaxis. N Engl J Med 1991; 324:1785–90

Markman M, Kennedy A, Webster K, Webster K, Elson P, Peterson G, Kulp B, Belinson J: Features of hypersensitivity reactions to carboplatin. J Clin Oncol 1999; 17:1141–5

Nursing 98 Drug Handbook. Springhouse, PA: Springhouse Corporation, 1998

Weiss RB: Hypersensitivity reactions. Semin Oncol 1992; 19:458–77

Wilkes GM, Ingwersen K, Barton-Burke MB (eds): *Oncology Nursing Handbook.* Sudbury: Jones and Bartlett, 1997–8

Table1: Estimated Incidence of Hypersensitivity Reactions Associated with Anticancer Agents

HSR type	Agents	Grade 1, 2	Grade 3, 4	Clinical examples
I** Immediate type or IgE mediated	*E.coli* l-asparaginase*	12%–25%	2.4%–8%	Anaphylaxis, angioedema, bronchospasm, urticaria
	Erwinia l-asparaginase	17%–22%	2.4%–14%[a]	
	PEG l-asparaginase	8%–24%	1%–8%[b]	
	Paclitaxel*[e]	8%–44%	2%[c]	
	Docetaxel[d]	4%–40%	2.2%[c]	
	Teniposide	2.4%	2.1% (mostly grade 3)	
	Etoposide IV*	4%	—	
	Cisplatin IV*	—	< 1%	
	Carboplatin	1.4%	0.2%	
	Melphalan IV	0.9%	1.4%	
	Procarbazine	6–18%	—	
II Cytotoxic reaction	Fludarabine*	Case reports		Coombs' positive hemolytic anemia/thrombocytopenia
	Interferon-alpha			
	Teniposide			
	Cisplatin IV*			
III Immune complex mediated	Procarbazine	Case reports		Serum sickness
	Mitomycin			
	Monoclonal antibodies			
	Levamisole			
IV Delayed	Topical mechloretamine	Case reports		Contact dermatitis
	Intravesical mitomycin			
	Methotrexate			
	Mesna			

*Agent-related deaths have been reported.

**Case reports have also been published for amifostine, aminoglutethimide, amsacrine, bleomycin, chlorambucil, intraperitoneal cisplatin, cyclophosphamide, cytosine arabinoside, dacarbazine, 5-fluorouracil, GM-CSF and G-CSF (no cross-reactivity), gonadotropin-releasing hormone, 5-HT3-receptor antagonists (possible cross-reactivity), ifosfamide, interleukin-2, mechlorethamine IV, oral melphalan, mesna, methotrexate, mitoxantrone, monoclonal antibodies, pamidronate, pentostatin, progesterone, tamoxifen, trimetrexate, vinblatine, vincristine.

[a]Pts with previous HSR to *E.coli* l-asparaginase.

[b]Pts with previous HSR to *E.coli* l-asp and/or *Erwinia* l-asparaginase.

[c]Pts with premedication.

[d]Pts without premedication: up to 28% grade 3 or 4 HSRs have been reported.

[e]Pts without premedication 7.8% grade 3 or 4 HSRs.

Table 2: National Cancer Institute/Common Toxicity Criteria (NCI/CTC)

	Grade*				
Toxicity	**0**	**1**	**2**	**3**	**4**
Allergic reaction/ hypersensitivity (including drug fever)	none	transient rash, drug fever < 38°C (<100.4°F)	urticaria, drug fever ≥38°C (≥ 100.4°F), and/or asymptomatic bronchospasm	symptomatic bronchospasm, requiring parenteral medication(s), with or w/o urticaria; allergy-related edema/angioedema	anaphylaxis
Note: Isolated urticaria, in the absence of other manifestations of an allergic reaction, is graded in the dermatology/skin category					
Allergic rhinitis (including sneezing, nasal stuffiness, postnasal drip)	none	mild, not requiring treatment	moderate; requiring treatment	—	—
Autoimmune reaction	none	serologic or other evidence of autoimmune reaction but patient is asymptomatic (e.g., vitiligo); all organ function is normal and no treatment is required	evidence of autoimmune reaction involving a nonessential organ or function (e.g., hypothyroidism), requiring treatment other than immunosuppressive drugs	reversible autoimmune reaction involving function of a major organ or other toxicity (e.g., transient colitis or anemia), requiring short-term immunosuppressive treatment	autoimmune reaction causing major grade 4 organ dysfunction; progressive and irreversible reaction; long-term administration of high-dose immunosuppressive therapy required
Note: Also consider hypothyroidism, colitis, hemoglobin, hemolysis					
Serum sickness	none	—	—	present	—
Vasculitis	none	mild, not requiring treatment	symptomatic; requiring medication	requiring steroids	ischemic changes or requiring amputation
Allergy—other (specify)	none	mild	moderate	severe	life-threatening or disabling

*Grade 5: Death related to toxicity

Chapter 12

PREVENTION AND TREATMENT OF COMPLICATIONS OF DISEASE

Cancer Pain Management

Beth Popp, C. Skosey, Nancy Velez-Piñeiro, and Joey Vitanza

OVERVIEW

■ 30% of patients have pain at the time of cancer diagnosis

■ 65–85% of patients with advanced disease have pain

■ A majority of cancer patients (85–95%) can achieve adequate analgesia without unacceptable side effects from a systematic application of analgesic therapy that is integrated with appropriate oncologic management

■ The patient's experience of pain may not directly correlate with the magnitude of abnormalities seen on imaging studies
- the human nervous system is more sensitive than our best scans
- don't fall into the trap of discounting the patient's complaints when imaging studies are nondiagnostic

PATHOPHYSIOLOGY

■ Disease related
- bone metastases, neuropathic pain, visceral pain, etc.

■ Therapy related
- myalgias due to taxanes or interferon, vincristine neuropathy, etc.

■ Unrelated to cancer
- osteoarthritis, low back pain, headache, etc.

DIAGNOSIS AND PREVENTION

■ Diagnostic evaluation
- a careful history is most important, followed by a thorough physical exam, with attention to the neurologic aspects of the exam
- choice of imaging studies should be guided by information from the history and physical exam
- remember to treat the pain as necessary (in an empiric fashion) to facilitate diagnostic evaluation

■ General principles of pain management based on the WHO three-step analgesic ladder (Figure 1) and AHCPR guidelines

Table 1: Opioids used in cancer pain management

	Approximate equianalgesic dose			
Opioid analgesic	**PARENTERAL**	**ORAL**	**Duration of analgesic effect**	**Comments**
Morphine	10 mg	30 mg	2–4 hrs	• sustained-release products (MS Contin, Oramorph, Kadian) are not dosed prn • MSContin reaches peak effect in 3–4 hrs
Hydromorphone	1.5 mg	7.5 mg	2–4 hrs	
Oxycodone	Not available in the US	30 mg	3–6 hrs	• OxyContin is sustained-release oxycodone, dosed q12hrs ATC (*not prn*) • OxyContin reaches peak effect in 1–2 hrs • combination products available with 5 mg oxycodone and varying amounts of acetaminophen
Fentanyl transdermal	TTS 50 patch (50 mcg/hr) equivalent to MSO4 1 mg/hr infusion		48–72 hrs	• requires 12–24 hrs to reach peak effect with first application or new dose • should not be used in patients with acute pain or rapidly changing analgesic needs
Codeine	130 mg	200 mg	2–4 hrs	• combination products containing 15, 30, or 60 mg of codeine with acetaminophen are available • combination products are DEA schedule III narcotics; single-agent codeine is DEA schedule II
Hydrocodone	not available	30 mg	3–6 hrs	• Combination products with 2.5, 7.5, or 10 mg of hydrocodone with acetaminophen are available
Levorphanol	2 mg	4 mg	3–6 hrs	
Oxymorphone	1 mg	not available	3–6 hrs	• suppositories of 5 mg oxymorphone available • 10 mg oxymorphone PR = 1 mg oxymorphone IV
Methadone	10 mg	20 mg	4–8 hrs	• half-life changes with chronic use • because of long half-life, give 25% of calculated equianalgesic dose initially; titrate dose to effect q3–7d
Meperidine	75 mg	300 mg	2–4 hrs	• *not recommended, due to accumulation of metabolite normeperidine* • use should be limited to 600 mg/d for 48 hrs

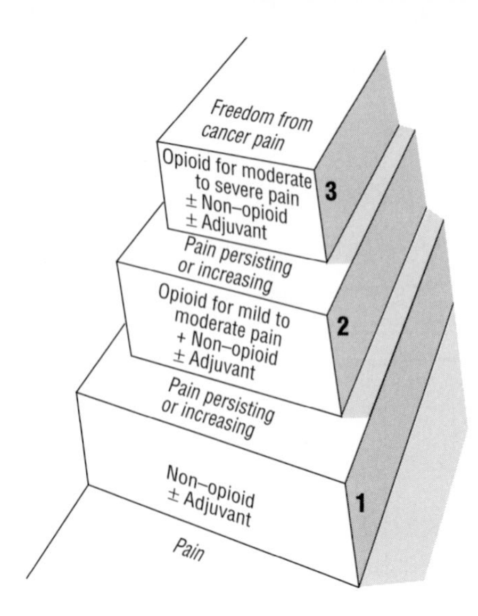

Figure 1: WHO analgesic ladder. (Reproduced by permission of WHO, from: *Cancer pain relief,* 2nd ed. Geneva, World Health Organization, 1996)

- patients should receive scheduled dose medication (around the clock, ATC) unless there is a contraindication
- patients should also have available supplemental doses to take if needed (prn) for episodes of breakthrough pain
- the optimal dose of an opioid is determined by the balance between analgesic and toxic effects; it is different in each patient
- there is no absolute maximum dose for the pure opioid agonists
- the distinction between "low-potency" opioids, used for moderate pain (step 2 of the WHO analgesic algorithm) and "high-potency" opioids, used for severe pain (step 3), has much to do with their availability in combination with nonopioids, which limit dose escalation (the acetaminophen content) or, as single agents, where dose escalation is limited only by opioid toxicity

THERAPY

- Choice of analgesic based on patient-reported pain intensity
  - mild pain: start with a nonopioid (acetaminophen or an NSAID) and adjust, based on clinical response (see Table 2)
  - moderate pain: an opioid in a dose equianalgesic to 10 mg *oral* morphine (MSO_4) po q4hrs and adjust, based on clinical response
  - severe pain: an opioid in a dose equianalgesic to 10 mg MSO_4 SubQ q4hrs and adjust, based on clinical response
  - when changing from one opioid to another, consider the relative analgesic potencies of the drugs (Table 1)
    - □ these figures were derived from single-dose studies, so in clinical use with chronic pain bear in mind that there is *incomplete cross-tolerance* between opioids. This means a patient will be less tolerant to a new opioid, and therefore more sensitive to its analgesic effects, when compared with the previously used opioid (see section on dose titration)
  - meperidine should be avoided in chronic cancer pain due to its short half-life and toxic metabolite, normeperidine
- Routes of administration
  - use the oral route when possible
    - □ sustained-release preparations usually cannot be crushed without loss of their sustained-release characteristics
  - sublingual, buccal, and rectal routes can be used for rescue dosing in patients unable to swallow
  - transdermal route is useful for patients with stable pain and chronically impaired swallowing or enteral absorption
  - SubQ, IV, and IM routes are therapeutically equivalent for opioid analgesics when a parenteral route is needed
    - □ avoid the IM route, since it is painful for the patient and offers no safety or therapeutic advantage over SubQ or IV (and absorption of drugs from the muscle may be less predictable in cachectic patients)
    - □ methadone should not be given SubQ, since it causes irritation at the injection site
    - □ codeine can cause more hypotension when administered IV than other opioids
    - □ repeated SubQ injections for scheduled or rescue doses of opioid can be given via an indwelling SubQ butterfly needle to minimize the number of needle sticks the patient requires
- Dose intervals
  - the goal is to prevent pain recurrence with the minimal number of daily doses
  - short-acting opioids (morphine, hydromorphone, oxycodone, codeine, hydrocodone) usually should be dosed q4hrs (the half-life of the drug), whether oral or parenteral, with the interval adjusted, based on clinical response
  - sustained-release morphine preparations should generally be dosed q8, q12, or q24hrs depending on clinical effect and the preparation used
  - sustained-release oxycodone preparations should generally be dosed q12hrs
  - there is some increased risk of opioid toxicity, due to the accumulation of active metabolites, when morphine is used in patients with renal or hepatic insufficiency
    - □ consider starting with a slightly lower dose or a slightly longer dosing interval, or using hydromorphone or oxycodone in these patients
- Rescue dosing
  - use the same opioid and route of administration for rescue dosing and scheduled dosing when possible
  - use a short-acting, rapid-onset formulation for rescue doses

Table 2: Nonopioid analgesics

Analgesic	Dose range	Duration of analgesic effect	Pharmacologic $t_{1/2}$
aspirin	650 mg po q6hrs	4–6 hrs	varies with dose
acetaminophen	650–1,000 mg po q4–6hrs maximum 4,000–6,000 mg/d	4–6 hrs	1–4 hrs
ibuprofen	200–400 mg po q6hrs maximum 2,400 mg/d	4–6 hrs	2 hrs
naproxen	250–500 mg po q6hrs	8–12 hrs	14 hrs
choline magnesium trisalicylate	500–750 mg po q8–12hrs	8–12 hrs	9–17 hrs
diflunisal	500–1,000 mg po q12hrs	8–12 hrs	8–12 hrs
ketorolac (parenteral)	30–60 mg IM or IV loading dose then 15–30 mg q6hrs maximum daily dose 120 mg/d (150 mg/d on first day) Should not be used for more than 5 consecutive days	6–8 hrs	4–6 hrs

- sustained-release products or the transdermal route of administration is not appropriate for rescue dosing
- rescue doses should be 5–15% of the total daily dose of the ATC opioid
  - *oral* rescue doses should be available q1–2hrs, as needed, for breakthrough pain. When the drug has reached peak effect, persistent pain should be treated with an additional dose if no toxicity is present
  - parenteral rescue doses should be available q30–60min, as needed, for breakthrough pain. When the drug reaches peak effect, persistent pain should be treated with an additional dose if no toxicity is present
- an analgesic regimen is considered well titrated if the patient requires no more than 4–5 rescues/d

■ Dose titration
- when making a dose adjustment or changing from one opioid to another, consider the quality of analgesia and the presence or absence of toxicity
- if the patient has *adequate analgesia* and *no dose-limiting toxicity,* continue regular reassessments of pain, but there is no need to change the analgesic regimen
- if the patient has *inadequate analgesia* and *no dose-limiting toxicity,* increase the scheduled dose by the total amount of the rescue doses taken in the previous 24 hrs, or by 50% if the amount of medication taken as rescue doses is not known
- if the patient has *adequate analgesia* and *dose-limiting toxicity is present,*
- treat the toxicity, if this can be done without adding multiple additional drugs
- consider a small dose decrement, with or without the addition of an adjuvant analgesic, in an attempt to maintain analgesia at a dose which is below the threshold for toxicity
- consider changing to an alternate opioid. Start the new opioid at 50–75% of the calculated equianalgesic dose, due to incomplete cross-tolerance
- if the patient has *inadequate analgesia* and *dose-limiting toxicity is present*
  - change to an alternate opioid
  - start the new opioid at 75–100% of the calculated equianalgesic dose, due to incomplete cross-tolerance
  - alternatively, consider treating the side effects and adding an adjuvant analgesic, although this is likely to result in excessive polypharmacy

■ Tapering opioids
- patients become tolerant to opioids with regular administration as soon as 7 days
  - opioids must be tapered to prevent withdrawal in situations where the pain resolves, due to successful anticancer therapy or invasive pain treatment, i.e., neurolytic blocks
- taper by 25–50% q48hrs until the patient is taking the equivalent of 30 mg/d of morphine; then the drug can usually be discontinued without precipitating withdrawal

■ Adjuvant analgesics
- adjuvant analgesics are drugs whose primary indication is something other than analgesia, but may act to improve the therapeutic window of the opioids or alter the pain stimulus in the nervous system
  - see Table 3 for a list of examples of adjuvant analgesics and Table 4 for pain syndromes in which adjuvant analgesics are commonly useful

■ Management of opioid side effects
- tolerance to each of the opioid effects develops at a different rate
  - many side effects need only short-term treatment after initiation of opioid therapy, until tolerance develops and the side effect resolves
  - adverse effects may briefly recur with each upward dose titration
- the threshold for toxicity at a given analgesic potency is different for each opioid and for each patient
  - this is a major rationale behind "opioid rotation" in patients who experience adverse effects with or without adequate analgesia

Table 3: Adjuvant analgesics

Drug	Analgesic indication	Usual dose	Therapeutic blood level	Primary indication
Dexamethasone	bone pain, deafferentation pain	4–8 mg po or IV q6hrs	N/A	various
	epidural spinal cord compression, brain metastases	100 mg IV loading dose then 24 mg q6hrs, tapered over several weeks as tolerated		
Methotrimeprazine	terminal agitation	5–10 mg parenterally q6 hrs or by infusion up to 80 mg/d	N/A	major tranquilizer
Clonazepam	lancinating neuropathic pain	0.5 mg po q8–12hrs initially up to 2 mg po q6hrs	N/A	anticonvulsant anxiolytic
Amitriptyline	neuropathic pain	10–25 mg po every bedtime initially titrated up to 100–150 mg/d	50–150 mcg/ml	antidepressant
Mexiletine	neuropathic pain	50–100 mg po q8hrs initially titrated up to 450–600 mg/d	N/A	cardiac arrhythmias
Carbemazepine	neuropathic pain	200 mg–1600 mg/d	4–12 mcg/ml	anticonvulsant
Phenytoin	neuropathic pain	300–500 mg/d	10–20 mcg/ml	anticonvulsant
Baclofen	neuropathic pain	5 mg po q8–12hrs titrated up to 30–90 mg/d	N/A	spasticity

Table 4: Pain syndromes in which adjuvant analgesics are used

Continuous neuropathic pain	Lancinating neuropathic pain	Bone pain	Visceral pain
Antidepressants	Anticonvulsants	Corticosteroids	Glycopyrrolate
Corticosteroids	Baclofen	Calcitonin	Atropine
Local anesthetics	Clonazepam	Strontium-89	Scopolamine
Clonidine	Local anesthetics	Pamidronate	
Capsaicin	Antidepressants	NSAIDs	

- be alert to other causes of adverse effects, especially sedation and confusion, rather than falling into the trap of "blaming" the opioid first
  - □ this may result in a missed opportunity for early intervention in cases of infection, metabolic abnormalities, etc.
- respiratory depression does not occur without concomitant CNS depression and mental status changes
  - □ tolerance to respiratory depressant effects of opioids develops more rapidly than to other opioid effects
  - □ with careful dose titration, respiratory depression is a rare phenomenon, even in patients with minimal pulmonary reserve due to underlying pulmonary disease
  - □ when it does occur, it should be treated conservatively by stimulating the patient to remain awake and talking if possible, while withholding subsequent opioid doses until enough drug has been cleared to relieve the problem
- constipation is almost universal in patients on scheduled doses of opioids
  - □ a prophylactic regimen should be prescribed at the initiation of opioid therapy and titrated based on effect
  - □ most patients do well with a combination of a stool softener and a stimulant such as senna. The doses required may be higher than conventionally used in patients who are not on opioid therapy
  - □ additional laxatives should be given if the patient evacuates less often than every other day
- nausea may occur to a specific opioid or to all the drugs as a class
  - □ centrally acting antiemetics are usually effective, such as prochlorperazine, haloperidol, or metoclopramide
  - □ some patients have nausea triggered by movement or an upright posture and may respond well to transdermal scopalamine, as used for treatment of motion sickness
- sedation may be improved by use of adjuvant analgesics that facilitate the use of a lower opioid dose. Stimulants, such as caffeine, methylphenidate, or pemoline, have been effective in relieving persistent opioid-induced sedation
- confusion or delirium may also be improved by the use of opioid-sparing, adjuvant drugs
  - □ haloperidol is useful in the treatment of persistent delirium when opioid rotation is not desirable
  - □ parenteral administration of haloperidol results in fewer extrapyramidal reactions and is preferred in patients requiring higher doses
  - □ benzodiazepines may exacerbate delirium in patients on opioid therapy, especially in the elderly
- myoclonic jerks usually respond to clonazepam
- naloxone should be given only for life-threatening opioid toxicity, such as hypoxemia and hypoventilation, not merely for a decreased respiratory rate when adequate oxygenation and ventilation are maintained
  - □ when used, it should be given in small aliquots (40 mcg every minute) only until the opioid toxicity has been reversed, and not with the intent of fully reversing the analgesic effect of the opioid
  - □ naloxone has a shorter half-life than most opioids. As a result, repeated dosing of naloxone or administration of a naloxone infusion may be required

■ Special considerations
- *tolerance:* a pharmacologic effect whereby a stable dose of drug results in a gradually diminished effect over time
  - □ conversely, it can be viewed as the need for an increasing dose of drug to achieve a constant effect
  - □ tolerance develops to the analgesic and nonanalgesic (respiratory depression, sedation, etc.) effects of opioids at different rates
- *physical dependence:* a pharmacologic effect whereby abrupt discontinuation of a drug results in a withdrawal syndrome
  - □ this is not unique to opioids and is not an indication of addiction (consider the result of the abrupt discontinuation of corticosteroids, beta blockers, or clonidine)
- *opioid withdrawal:* a constellation of signs and symptoms that result from the abrupt cessation of a drug
  - □ opioid withdrawal is extremely unpleasant, but not life threatening. In general, it is characterized by lacrimation, yawning, rhinorrhea, piloerection, abdominal cramping, and diarrhea. In patient taking opioids for pain, severe pain is also a characteristic of withdrawal
- *opioid addiction:* a syndrome of inappropriate and uncontrolled use of opioids
  - □ it is a difficult diagnosis to make in the patient with cancer-related pain, since some of the psychiatric criteria for the diagnosis are those of physical dependence
  - □ it can most succinctly be characterized as opioid use despite harm, or use that results in a deterioration in, rather than a restoration of, function

■ Special nursing considerations for administration of nonopioids (NSAIDs)
- each patient should be given an adequate trial of a nonopioid on a regular basis before switching to another drug
- doses should be given regularly to maintain plasma level
- monitor lab values routinely: CBC, WBC, platelets
- some NSAIDs are contraindicated in patients with existing renal disease, CHF, vascular disease; monitor renal and hepatic function
- consider administration of misoprostol for patients with significant risk factors for GI complications

■ Assess
- baseline neurologic and mental status; changes in perception/sensation of pain
- for signs and symptoms of salicylism
- for bleeding
- for hepatic dysfunction
- for gastric ulceration; may potentiate peptic ulcer disease, especially in the elderly
- alterations in nutritional status

■ Teach patient
- to report signs of bleeding: black stools, epistaxis, menorrhagia
- avoid aspirin or aspirin-containing drugs; may increase risk of bleeding
- take drug with food or milk
- monitor temperature and report temperature over 38.3° C (101° F); fever could be disguised by self-dosing with acetaminophen

■ Special nursing considerations for administration of opioids
- respiratory depression most serious of adverse effects; occurs most commonly after short-term administration and is associated with other signs of CNS depression, including sedation and drowsiness
- use cautiously in patients with bronchial asthma and COPD
- use cautiously in patients with renal or hepatic dysfunction
- increased opioid requirements are most commonly associated with disease progression rather than tolerance alone
- nausea and vomiting increase in ambulatory patients; nausea occurring with one drug does not indicate that all drugs will produce it; consider an alternative opioid
- use antiemetics that stimulate the chemoreceptor trigger zone (CTZ)
- long-term administration is associated with development of physical dependence; taper drug slowly

■ Assess
- alterations in elimination: need for cathartics and stool softeners; urinary retention
- baseline cardiovascular status: hypotension, bradycardia
- baseline pulmonary status and routinely during therapy
- baseline neurologic status: monitor for CNS depression or hyperirritability

■ Teach patient
- self-administration of laxative preparations
- avoid driving and operating machinery
- avoid alcohol
- potential for sexual dysfunction: impotence and decreased libido
- maintain a pain diary and record pain intensity, time of drug administration, and factors that alleviate or accelerate pain
- self-administration for relief of chronic pain around the clock, not prn

KEY REFERENCES

Brogden RN, Heel RC, Pakes GE, Speight TM, Avery GS: Diflunisal: A review of its pharmacological properties and therapeutic use in pain and musculoskeletal strains and sprains and pain in osteoarthritis. Drugs 1980; 19(2):84–106

Calis KA, Kohler DR, Corso DM: Transdermally administrated fentanyl for pain management. Clin Pharm 1992; 11(1):22–36. PMID: 1730176; UI: 92111097

Cancer pain relief and palliative care: Report of a WHO expert committee. WHO Tech Rep Ser 1990; 804:1–73

Clissold SP: Aspirin and related derivatives of salicylic acid. Drugs 1986 (Suppl 32); 4:8–26. PMID: 3552588; UI: 87189880

Clissold, SP: Paracetamol and phenacetin. Drugs 1986 (Suppl 32); 4:46–59 PMID: 3552585; UI: 87189877

Foley KM, Inturrisi CE: Analgesic drug therapy in cancer pain; principles and practice. Med Clin North Am 1987; 71:207–32. PMID: 2881032; UI: 87143233

Food and Drug Administration, HHS. 21, Code of Federal Regulations, Washington, DC: Office of Federal Register National Archives and Records Administration. 1993; Ch 1 (8320.22):74–5

Gillis JC, Brogden RN. Ketorolac: A reappraisal of its pharmacodynamic and pharmacokinetic properties and therapeutic use in pain management. Drugs 1997; 53(1):139–88. PMID: 9010653; UI: 97163898

Goetting MG, Thirman MJ: Neurotoxicity of meperidine. Ann Emerg Med 1985; 14(10): 1007–9. PMID: 4037466; UI: 85305042

Jacox A, Carr DB, Payne R, et al.: Management of cancer pain: clinical practice guideline. No. 9. Rockville, MD: Agency for Health Care Policy and Research, 1994 (AHCPR publication no. 94–0592)

Lacey C, Armstrong L, Ingrim N, Lance L: *Drug information handbook.* 6th Edition. (pp. 783–5; 937–8). Hudson, OH: Lexi-Comp Inc., 1998

Levy MH: Pharmacologic treatment of cancer pain (drug therapy). N Engl J Med 1996; 335(15): 1124–32. PMID: 8813044; UI: 96434829

Levy MH: Pharmacologic management of cancer pain. Semin Oncol 1994; 21(6):718–39, 1994. PMID: 7527595; UI: 95084201

Portenoy, RK: *Contemporary diagnosis and management of pain in oncologic and AIDS patients* (pp. 74, 78–80) Newton, PA: Handbooks in Healthcare, 1997

Todd PA, Clissold S: Naproxen: a reappraisal of its pharmacology and therapeutic use in rheumatic diseases and pain states. Drugs 1990; 40(1):91–137. PMID: 2202585; UI: 90360915

OPIOID ANALGESICS

DRUG: MORPHINE

- Other names: MS Contin, Roxanol, Kadian, MSIR, OramorphSR
- Uses
  - for the relief of moderate to severe acute and chronic pain; for pain due to acute myocardial infarction
  - relief of dyspnea due to acute left ventricular failure and pulmonary edema
- Mechanism of action
  - binds to opiate receptors in the CNS, causing inhibition of ascending pain pathways, altering the perception of and response to pain; produces generalized CNS depression
- Dosing
  - oral formulations
    - □ immediate-release tablets: 15 mg, 30 mg
    - □ oral solution (immediate release): 10 mg/5 ml, 20 mg/5 ml, 20 mg/ml, 100 mg/5 ml, and 10 mg/2.5 ml
    - □ controlled-released tablets: 15 mg, 30 mg, 60 mg, 100 mg, and 200 mg
  - rectal suppositories: 5 mg, 10 mg, 20 mg, and 30 mg
  - injectable formulations: 0.5 mg/ml, 1 mg/ml, 4 mg/ml (prefilled syringe), 5 mg/ml, 10 mg/ml, 15 mg/ml (prefilled syringe), and 25 mg/ml
  - dose depends on balance of analgesic effect and adverse side effects (see text)
  - immediate-release tablets and oral solution are dosed q4hrs around the clock or as needed (see text)
  - controlled-release tablets dosed q8–12hrs around the clock (*not* for "as needed" or prn administration)
  - rectal suppositories are dosed q4hrs around the clock or as needed
  - intermittent parenteral dosing (IM, IV, or SubQ) is q4hrs around the clock or as needed. Dose must be adjusted in each patient depending on balance between analgesia and adverse effects. Typical starting dose is 10 mg q4hrs
  - continuous infusion dosing (IV or SubQ) must be adjusted in each patient depending on balance between analgesia and adverse effects. The usual dose range is 1–80 mg/hr
- Pharmacokinetics
  - absorption: oral; variable
  - metabolism: liver via glucuronide conjugation
  - half-life: 2–4 hrs elimination; unchanged in urine

Morphine sulfate

Dosage, form/route	Peak analgesic effect	Duration of analgesic
Tablets	1 hr	4–5 hrs
Oral solution	1 hr	4–5 hrs
Extended-released tablets	3 hrs	8–12 hrs
Rectal suppository	20–60 min	3–7 hrs
SubQ injection	50–90 min	4–5 hrs
IM injection	30–60 min	4–5 hrs
IV injection	20 min	4–5 hrs

- Side effects
  - > 10%: palpitations, bradycardia, hypotension, dizziness, nausea, vomiting, constipation, and xerostomia
  - 1–10%: urinary retention, headache, confusion
- Other considerations
  - morphine is the prototype opioid agonist for treatment of moderate to severe pain
  - patients with impaired renal or hepatic function are at increased risk for toxicity. These patients should be monitored more closely for signs of adverse effects. Dose may need to be decreased or dosing interval may need to be increased as clinically indicated
  - dosage adjustment for renal impairment: CrCl 10–50 ml/min decrease dose by 25%; CrCl < 10 ml/min decrease dose by 50%
  - controlled-released dosage forms *should not be crushed*

DRUG: METHADONE

- Other name: Dolophine
- Uses: for management of severe pain
- Mechanism of action
  - binds to opiate receptors in the CNS, causing inhibition of ascending pain pathways, altering the perception of and response to pain; produces generalized CNS depression
- Dosing
  - available in oral and injectable forms
  - oral formulations
    - □ tablets: 5 mg and 10 mg
    - □ solution: 5 mg/5 ml (also available as an oral concentrate—10 mg/ml—but use of this form restricted to methadone maintenance and is subject to special regulations)
  - formulations for parenteral injection: 10 mg/ml
  - dose depends on balance of analgesic effect and adverse side effects (see text)
  - typical starting doses for treatment of pain in adults: 2.5–10 mg q3–8hrs
- Pharmacokinetics
  - oral: onset of action is 0.5–1 hr
  - duration: 4–8 hrs, increases to 22–48 hrs with repeated doses
  - parenteral: onset of action is 10–20 min
  - peak effect: 1–2 hrs

- protein binding: 80–85%
- metabolism: in the liver
- half-life: 15–29 hrs (may be prolonged with alkaline pH)
- elimination: in the urine, increased renal excretion with urine pH of <6

■ Side effects
- >10%: palpitations, vomiting and constipation, hypotension, bradycardia, peripheral vasodilation, drowsiness, dizziness, nausea
- 1–10%: headache, confusion, urinary retention, anorexia

■ Other considerations
- dose must be titrated slowly because of the long and variable half-life of methadone and resultant risk of accumulation
- does not cross-react with other opioids, so it can be used in cases of true morphine allergy

DRUG: FENTANYL TRANSDERMAL

■ Other name: Duragesic

■ Uses: management of chronic pain

■ Mechanism of action
- binds to opiate receptors in the CNS, causing inhibition of ascending pain pathways, altering the perception of and response to pain; produces generalized CNS depression

■ Dosing
- available as a transdermal system, or "patch," containing a membrane that limits the rate of absorption of drug from the patch
- transdermal systems are available in doses of 25 mcg/hr, 50 mcg/hr, 75 mcg/hr, and 100 mcg/hr
- in most patients these doses will reliably be absorbed from the transdermal system for 72 hrs (occasional patients require dosing q48hrs)
- fentanyl is also available for parenteral injection and for oral transmucosal administration in the form of an "Oralet"
- for pain control in adults who have not previously been on an opioid, the initial dose is a 25 mcg/hr system
- for patients currently receiving opioid analgesics, dosing is based on the response to the current opioid and the relative potency of fentanyl compared to the current opioid (see text and Table 1)

■ Pharmacokinetics
- transdermal system onset of analgesia: 12–24 hrs
- duration: 72 hrs
- bioavailability: 92%
- half-life: 17 hrs
- metabolism: in the liver
- elimination: hepatic biotransformation and urinary excretion
- distribution: like other highly lipid soluble drugs, fentanyl is widely distributed throughout organs and tissues

■ Side effects
- 10%: drowsiness, sedation, nausea, hypotension, bradycardia, vomiting, constipation
- 1–10%: erythema, pruritus, urticaria, itching, confusion, CNS depression, orthostatic hypotension, urinary retention

■ Other considerations
- fentanyl should not be used in patients with acute pain or rapidly changing analgesic needs
- supplementary doses of short-acting, immediate-release analgesics should be administered until the transdermal system is providing fentanyl absorption at full effect. They should also be available as needed for breakthrough pain
- absorption of fentanyl from the transdermal system can be increased by nearly 35% when the body temperature exceeds 40° C
- transdermal fentanyl should be avoided in patients with head injuries because it may obscure their clinical course
- fentanyl may also cause bradycardia and therefore should be used cautiously in patients with bradyarrhythmias

DRUG: OXYMORPHONE

■ Other name: Numorphan

■ Uses: relief of moderate to severe pain

■ Mechanism of action
- oxymorphone is a potent opioid analgesic with uses similar to those of morphine. The drug is a semisynthetic (phenanthrene) derivative of morphine and is closely related to hydromorphone chemically. Binds to opiate receptors in the CNS, causing inhibition of ascending pain pathways, altering the perception of and response to pain; produces generalized CNS depression

■ Dosing
- available in parenteral and suppository formulations
  - □ parenteral injection: 1 mg/ml, 1.5 mg/ml (ampules)
  - □ rectal suppositories: 5 mg
- dose depends on balance of analgesic effect and adverse side effects (see text)
- typical initial adult dosing regimens
  - □ IM, SubQ: 0.5 mg initially, 1–1.5 mg q4–6 hrs as needed
  - □ IV: 0.5 mg initially
  - □ rectal dose: 5 mg q4–6hrs

■ Pharmacokinetics
- onset of analgesia: IV, IM, SubQ: within 5–15 min; rectal: 15–30 min
- duration of analgesia: 3–4 hrs
- metabolism: conjugated with glucuronic acid
- elimination: in urine

■ Side effects
- >10%: hypotension, drowsiness, dizziness, nausea, vomiting, constipation
- 1–10%: anorexia, headache, urinary retention, confusion

DRUG: OXYCODONE

■ Other names: Percocet, Percodan, OxyContin, OxyIR, Roxicodone, others

■ Uses: management of moderate to severe pain, often used in combination with nonnarcotic analgesics (aspirin, acetaminophen)

■ Mechanism of action
- binds to opiate receptors in the CNS, causing inhibition of ascending pain pathways, altering the perception of and response to pain; produces generalized CNS depression

■ Dosing
- available oral formulations
  - □ immediate-release tablets: 5 mg
  - □ combination products available with 2.5–10 mg oxycodone and varying amounts of acetaminophen or aspirin
  - □ oral solution: 5 mg/5 ml and 20 mg/ml
  - □ controlled-release tablets: 10 mg, 20 mg, 40 mg, and 80 mg
- immediate-release tablets and oral solution are dosed q4hrs or as needed
- controlled-release tablets are dosed q12hrs
- dosing of combination oxycodone/acetaminophen products is limited by acetaminophen content, which should not exceed 4–6 g/d

■ Pharmacokinetics
- OxyContin reaches peak effect in 1–2 hrs

■ Side effects
- 10%: drowsiness, dizziness, nausea, vomiting
- 1–10%: stomach cramps, constipation, headaches, confusion

■ Other considerations
- controlled-release products cannot be crushed or chewed
- controlled-release products are not appropriate for "as needed" or prn dosing
- patients with hepatic impairment are at increased risk for toxicity and should be monitored more closely for adverse effects. These patients may require dosage reduction or lengthening of dosing interval based on clinical effect

DRUG: HYDROCODONE

■ Other names: Vicodin, Lortab (in combination with acetaminophen), Vicoprofen (in combination with ibuprofen)

■ Mechanism of action
- binds to opiate receptors in the CNS, causing inhibition of ascending pain pathways, altering the perception of and response to pain; produces generalized CNS depression

■ Dosing
- available oral formulations
  - □ 5 mg hydrocodone and 500 mg acetaminophen tablet
  - □ 7.5 mg hydrocodone and 650 mg acetaminophen tablet
  - □ 7.5 mg hydrocodone and 200 mg ibuprofen tablet

- tablets are dosed 1–2 tablets q4–6hrs. Dose is limited by coanalgesic (nonopioid) content, which should not exceed 4–6 g/d of acetaminophen or 3.2 g/d of ibuprofen
- ■ Pharmacokinetics
  - onset of analgesia: within 10–20 min
  - duration: 3–6 hrs
  - metabolism: hepatic
  - half-life: 3.8 hrs
  - elimination: in urine
- ■ Side effects
  - > 10%: hypotension, dizziness, drowsiness, sedation, nausea
  - 1–10%: vomiting, confusion, urinary retention, hemolytic anemia, rash

DRUG: HYDROMORPHONE

- ■ Other names: Dilaudid, Dilaudid-HP
- ■ Uses: relief of moderate to severe pain
- ■ Mechanism of action
  - hydromorphone is a semisynthetic (phenanthrene) opioid derivative. It is a pure opioid agonist. It binds to opioid receptors in the CNS, causing inhibition of ascending pain pathways, altering the perception of and response to pain
- ■ Dosing
  - available in oral, parenteral, and rectal suppository formulations
    - □ tablets: 1 mg, 2 mg, 3 mg, 4 mg, and 8 mg
    - □ oral solutions: 1 mg/ml and 5 mg/5 ml
    - □ for parenteral injection: 1 mg/ml, 2 mg/ml, 3 mg/ml, 4 mg/ml, and 10 mg/ml
    - □ powder for injection: 250 mg
    - □ rectal suppositories: 3 mg
  - hydromorphone is dosed q4hrs. Dose magnitude depends on balance of analgesia and adverse effects (see text). Typical starting dose for adults is 2–4 mg by mouth. Suppositories may have a slightly longer duration of action
- ■ Pharmacokinetics
  - hydromorphone is well absorbed following oral, rectal,or parenteral administration
  - onset of analgesic effect: 15–30 min
  - peak of effect: within 0.5–1.5 hrs
  - duration: 3–4 hrs (depending on route of administration)
  - metabolism: primarily in the liver, where it undergoes conjugation with glucuronic acid
  - bioavailability: 62%
  - half-life: 1–3 hrs
  - elimination: in urine, principally as glucuronide conjugates
- ■ Side effects
  - > 10%: hypotension, dizziness, drowsiness, anorexia
  - 1–10%: headache, nausea, vomiting, stomach cramps, urinary retention
- ■ Other considerations
  - the highly concentrated injection should only be used in patients who are tolerant to opioid agonists
  - the primary advantage of hydromorphone over morphine is its higher potency and solubility, which allow it to be administered in a smaller injection volume than equianalgesic doses of morphine

DRUG: MEPERIDINE

- ■ Other names: Demerol, (Pethidine in Europe)
- ■ Uses: for relief of moderate to severe pain
- ■ Mechanism of action
  - binds to opioid receptors in the CNS causing inhibition of ascending pain pathways, altering the perception of and response to pain; produces generalized CNS depression
- ■ Dosing
  - available in oral and parenteral formulations
    - □ tablets: 50 mg, 100 mg
    - □ oral liquid: 50 ml/5 ml (glucose, saccharin, and alcohol-free banana-flavored syrup)
    - □ injectable forms: 10 mg/ml, 25 mg/ml, 50 mg/ml, 75 mg/ml, and 100 mg/ml
    - □ multidose vials are available for the 50 mg/ml and 100 mg/ml concentrations
  - typical adult dosing regimens for postoperative pain: 50–150 mg IM or IV q3–4hrs
- ■ Pharmacokinetics
  - onset of analgesic effect: within 5–15 min of parenteral administration depending on route used
  - peak effect: within 1 hr
  - duration: 2–4 hrs
  - protein binding: 65–75%
  - metabolism: in the liver
  - bioavailability ~50–60%; increased with liver disease
  - half-life: 2.5–4 hrs; half life prolonged to 7–11 hrs in adults with liver disease
  - normeperidine (active metabolite) has a half-life of 15–30 hrs. Normeperidine is cleared by the kidneys and can accumulate with prolonged use, high doses, or renal dysfunction
- ■ Side effects
  - < 10%: drowsiness, dizziness
  - 1–10%: nausea, vomiting, headaches, constipation, insomnia, nightmares, confusion, urinary retention
- ■ Other considerations
  - not recommended for treatment of chronic pain, pain in the elderly, or in patients with renal insufficiency, due to the accumulation of the active metabolite normeperidine. Normeperidine is a weaker analgesic, but has twice the convulsant activity of the parent compound
  - for acute pain, meperidine use should be limited to 600 mg/d for no more than 48 hrs
  - meperidine should not be administered to patients who have received MAO inhibitors within 14 days
  - meperidine does not cross-react with other opioids, so it can be used in patients with a true allergy to morphine

DRUG: LEVORPHANOL TARTRATE

- ■ Other name: Levo-Dromoran
- ■ Uses: management of moderate to severe pain
- ■ Mechanisms of action
  - levorphanol is a synthetic (morphinan) opioid derivative. It is a pure agonist. It binds to opioid receptors in the CNS causing inhibition of ascending pain pathways, altering the perception of and response to pain; produces generalized CNS depression
- ■ Dosing
  - available in oral or parenteral formulations
    - □ tablets: 2 mg
    - □ for parenteral injection: 2 mg/ml (1 ml and 10 ml vials)
  - levorphanol has a longer duration of analgesic effect than the other immediate-release opioids and is typically dosed q6hrs. In clinical practice, some patients have a longer duration of effect and can be dosed at a longer interval
  - dose magnitude depends on the balance between analgesia and adverse effects (see text)
- ■ Pharmacokinetics
  - onset of action: with oral administration ~1 hr; with parenteral injections 10–30 min
    - □ metabolism: liver
    - □ duration: 6–8 hrs
    - □ elimination: primarily in urine as the glucuronide conjugate
- ■ Side effects
  - < 10%: hypotension, drowsiness, dizziness, pruritus, nausea, vomiting
  - 1–10%: headache, constipation, anorexia, confusion, urinary retention
- ■ Other considerations
  - levorphanol has a long plasma half-life (8–12 hrs), which makes it a useful alternative to sustained-release preparations of morphine, oxycodone, or fentanyl
  - patients with hepatic impairment are at increased risk for toxicity and should be monitored more closely for adverse effects. These patients may require dosage reduction or lengthening of dosing interval based on clinical effect

DRUG: CODEINE SULFATE

■ Uses: for relief of mild to moderate pain. Antitussive in lower doses for patients with a nonproductive cough

- ■ Mechanism of action
  - codeine is metabolized to morphine in the liver. Morphine binds to opioid receptors in the CNS, causing inhibition of ascending pain pathway, altering the perception of and response to pain; produces generalized CNS depression. Opioids produce cough suppression by direct central action in the medulla
- ■ Dosing
  - available in oral formulations
    - □ oral solution: 15 mg/5 ml
    - □ oral tablets: 15 mg, 30 mg, and 60 mg
    - □ also available in various fixed-dose combinations with acetaminophen

- dose magnitude depends on the balance between analgesia and adverse effects
- codeine is dosed q4–6hrs when used to treat pain or as a cough suppressant

■ Pharmacokinetics
- see morphine

■ Side effects
- see morphine

■ Other considerations
- patient taking inhibitors of the hepatic microsomal enzyme CYP2D6 such as quinidine, cimetidine, or fluoxetine may not be able to convert codeine into morphine and as a result may get little or no analgesic or antitussive effect from codeine
- use caution in patients with severe liver or renal insufficiency
- patients with hepatic impairment are at increased risk for toxicity and should be monitored more closely for adverse effects. These patients may require dosage reduction or lengthening of dosing interval based on clinical effect

NONOPIOID ANALGESICS

DRUG: IBUPROFEN

■ Other names: Motrin, Nuprin, Advil

■ Uses: inflammatory diseases and rheumatoid disorders, mild to moderate pain, fever, dysmenorrhea, gout, ankylosing spondylitis, acute migraine headache

■ Mechanism of action
- ibuprofen is a nonsteroidal anti-inflammatory (NSAID) agent with analgesic and antipyretic properties. It is an effective inhibitor of cyclo-oxygenase. It reversibly alters platelet function

■ Dosing
- available oral preparations
  - □ tablets: 100 mg, 200 mg, 300 mg, 400 mg, 600 mg, 800 mg
  - □ suspension: 100 mg/5 ml
- for mild to moderate pain: 200–400 mg q4–6hrs
- for rheumatoid arthritis and osteoarthritis: 400–800 mg 4 times per day
- maximum dose: 3.2 g/d

■ Pharmacokinetics
- onset of analgesia: 30–60 min
- duration: 4–6 hrs
- onset of anti-inflammatory effect: up to 7 days
- peak action: 1–2 wks
- absorption: oral: rapid 85%
- time to peak serum concentration: within 1–2 hrs
- protein binding: 90–99%
- metabolism: in the liver by oxidation
- half-life: 2–4 hrs
- end-stage renal disease: unchanged
- elimination: in urine (1% as free drug): some biliary excretion occurs

■ Side effects
- > 10%: dizziness, fatigue, rash, urticaria, abdominal cramps, dyspepsia, nausea, UGI bleeding
- 1–10%: headache, nervousness, itching, fluid retention, tinnitus
- < 1%: edema, congestive heart failure, arrhythmias, confusion, hallucinations, depression, drowsiness, insomnia

■ Other considerations
- avoid use in severe hepatic problems
- contraindicated in patients allergic to aspirin or other NSAIDs

DRUG: DIFLUNISAL

■ Other name: Dolobid

■ Uses
- for the management of inflammatory disorders including rheumatoid arthritis and osteoarthritis; can also be used as an analgesic for the treatment of mild to moderate pain

■ Mechanism of action
- diflunisal is a salicylic acid derivative with analgesic and anti-inflammatory activity, related to its inhibition of prostaglandin synthesis. Diflunisal inhibits the enzyme cyclo-oxygenase, which results in decreased formation of prostaglandin precursors. The analgesic effect of diflunisal is longer than that of aspirin, lasting for at least 8 hrs and up to 12 hrs

■ Dosing
- available oral preparations: 250 mg and 500 mg tablets
- for pain: 500–1,000 mg initially followed by 250–500 mg q8–12 hrs
- for inflammatory conditions: 500–1,000 mg/d in 2 divided doses
- maximum daily dose: 1.5 g

■ Pharmacokinetics
- onset of analgesia: within 1 hr
- duration of action: 8–12 hrs
- absorption: well absorbed from the GI tract
- metabolism: extensively in the liver
- half-life: 8–12 hrs, prolonged with renal impairment
- time to peak concentration: oral within 2–3 hrs

■ Side effects
- > 10%: gastric ulcers, upper GI bleeding, fluid retention
- 1–10%: rash, itching, tinnitus, dizziness, headaches

■ Other considerations
- dosage adjustment in renal impairment: Cl or < 50 ml/min; give 50% of normal dose
- tablets must be swallowed whole and may not be crushed or chewed

DRUG: ASPIRIN

■ Other names: Empirin, Ecotrin, Genprin

■ Uses: mild to moderate pain; fever; various inflammatory conditions such as rheumatic fever, rheumatoid arthritis, and osteoarthritis; to reduce the risk of death or nonfatal myocardial infarction in patients with previous infarction or unstable angina pectoris; to reduce the risk of recurrent transient ischemic attacks or stroke in men

■ Mechanism of action
- inhibits prostaglandin synthesis, acts on the hypothalamus heat-regulating center to reduce fever, blocks prostaglandin synthetase action that prevents formation of the platelet-aggregating substance thromboxane A2

■ Dosing

Oral formulations	Rectal suppository formulations
81 mg (chewable) ("baby aspirin")	120 mg
165 mg (enteric coated)	200 mg
325 mg tablets and enteric-coated tablets	300 mg
500 mg tablets and enteric-coated tablets	600 mg
650 mg enteric-coated tablets	
975 mg enteric-coated tablets	

- as an analgesic or antipyretic: 650 mg q6hrs (up to 4 g per day)

■ Pharmacokinetics
- absorption: from the stomach and small intestine
- distribution: readily distributes into most body fluids and tissues
- metabolism: hydrolyzed to salicylate (active) to esterases in the GI mucosa, red blood cells, synovial fluid, and blood; metabolism of salicylate occurs primarily by hepatic microsomal enzymes; metabolic pathways are saturable
- half-life of parent drug: 15–20 min
- half-life of salicylate metabolites is dose dependent, ranging from 3 hrs (at doses of 300–600 mg) to 5–6 hrs (at doses of 1 g) to 10 hrs with higher doses
- time to peak serum concentrations: 1–2 hrs

■ Side effects
- > 10%: nausea, vomiting, dyspepsia, epigastric discomfort, heartburn, stomach pains, gastric ulceration, UGI bleeding
- 1–10%: fatigue, rash, urticaria, hemolytic anemia, muscle weakness, dyspnea, anaphylaxis

■ Other considerations
- patients allergic to tartrazine dye should avoid aspirin
- use with caution in patients with G-6-PD deficiency

DRUG: NAPROXEN

■ Other names: Aleve, Naprosyn, Anaprox, Naprelan

■ Uses: management of inflammatory disease and rheumatoid disorders (including juvenile rheumatoid arthritis); acute gout; mild to moderate pain, dysmenorrhea; fever, migraine headache

■ Mechanism of action
- naproxen exhibits dose-related anti-inflammatory, analgesic, and antipyretic effects. These effects are generally

thought to be related to its inhibition of cyclo-oxygenase and consequent decrease in prostaglandin concentrations in various fluids and tissues. Naproxen, like other NSAIDS, is a potent inhibitor of the secondary phase of platelet aggregation

- Dosing
  - available oral preparations
    - oral suspension: 125 mg/5 ml
    - naproxen sodium tablets (Anaprox): 220 mg (200 mg base), 275 mg (250 mg base), and 550 mg (500 mg base)
    - naproxen tablets: 200 mg (Aleve), 250 mg, 375 mg, and 500 mg
    - controlled-release tablets (Naprelan): 375 mg, 500 mg
  - for fever in children > age 2: 2.5–10 mg/kg/dose (to a maximum of 10 mg/kg/d)
  - for pain and inflammation of juvenile arthritis: 10 mg/kg/d in 2 divided doses
  - for pain and inflammation of rheumatoid arthritis, osteoarthritis, and ankylosing spondylitis in adults: 500–1,000 mg/d in 2 divided doses
  - dose may be increased to 1.5 g/d for a limited time period
  - for treatment of mild to moderate pain or dysmenorrhea: 500 mg initially, then 250 mg q6–8hrs
  - maximum dose: 1,250 mg/d naproxen base
- Pharmacokinetics
  - absorption: oral: almost 100%
  - time to peak serum concentration: 1–2 hrs with levels persisting for up to 12 hrs
  - protein binding: > 90% (increased free fraction in the elderly)
  - half-life: normal renal function: 12–15 hrs
  - end-stage renal disease: unchanged
- Side effects
  - > 10%: dizziness, pruritus, rash, abdominal discomfort, nausea, heartburn, constipation, GI bleeding, ulcers, perforation, indigestion
  - 1–10%: headache, nervousness, fluid retention
  - < 10%: edema, congestive heart failure, hypertension
- Other considerations
  - administer with food, milk, or antacids to decrease GI adverse effects

DRUG: KETOROLAC

- Other names: Toradol, Acular
- Uses: short-term management of pain (< 5 d)
- Mechanism of action
  - ketorolac is an NSAID that has strong analgesic activity. Its primary mechanism of action is to inhibit the enzyme cyclo-oxygenase, the enzyme responsible for the biosynthesis of prostaglandins, prostacyclin, and thromboxane. NSAIDS produce analgesia by attenuating the hyperalgesic state caused by the sensitization of afferent nerve fibers by prostaglandins
- Dosing
  - available formulations
    - for parenteral injection: 15 mg/ml (1 ml), 30 mg/ml (2 ml)
    - for oral use: 10 mg tablets
  - IV: initially 30 mg, then 15–30 mg q6hrs as needed for up to 5 days total
  - IM: initially 30–60 mg, then 15–30 mg q6hrs as needed for up to 5 days
  - oral dosing: 10 mg q4–6hrs as needed for a maximum of 40 mg/d
  - dosing for patients > 65 yrs of age, with renal insufficiency or < 50 kg
    - IM or IV: 15 mg q6hrs
  - maximum parenteral dose 120 mg/24 hrs for up to 5 days total (150 mg/d during the first 24 hrs)
  - maximum dose on the day of transition from parenteral route to oral administration is 120 mg by all routes and 40 mg by the oral route
  - maximum oral dose 40 mg/d
- Pharmacokinetics
  - analgesic effect: onset of action: IM within 10 min
  - peak effect: within 75–150 min
  - duration of action: 6–8 hrs
  - absorption: oral: well absorbed
  - time to peak serum concentration: IM: 30–60 min
  - protein binding: 99%
  - metabolism: liver
  - half-life: 2–8 hrs; increased 30–50% in the elderly
  - elimination: renal excretion; 61% appearing in urine as unchanged
- Side effects
  - > 10%: renal impairment; wound bleeding, postoperative hematomas
  - 1–10%: edema, drowsiness, dizziness, headache pain, nausea, dyspepsia, diarrhea, gastric ulcers, indigestion, diaphoresis
  - < 1%: depression, dyspnea, purpura, oliguria, rectal bleeding, change in vision
- Other considerations
  - see alternate dosing regimen in the elderly due to decreased clearance and increased sensitivity to the renal effects of NSAIDs
  - use with caution in patients with congestive heart failure, hypertension, decreased renal or hepatic function, history of GI bleeding, or taking anticoagulants

DRUG: CHOLINE MAGNESIUM TRISALICYLATE

- Other name: Trilisate
- Uses: for the treatment of osteoarthritis, rheumatoid arthritis, and other inflammatory conditions. Choline magnesium trisalicylate does not inhibit platelet aggregation and should not be substituted for aspirin in the prophylaxis of thrombosis
- Mechanism of action
  - inhibits prostaglandin synthesis; acts on the hypothalamus heat-regulating center to reduce fever; blocks the generation of pain impulses
- Dosing
  - available oral formulations
    - liquid: 500 mg/5 ml
    - tablets: 500 mg, 750 mg, and 1,000 mg
  - for the treatment of pain or inflammation in adults: 500–1,500 mg in divided doses 2–3 times daily
- Pharmacokinetics
  - absorption: from the stomach and small intestine
  - distribution: readily distributes into most body tissues and fluids
  - half-life: dose dependent ranging from 2–3 hrs at low doses to 30 hrs at higher doses
  - time to peak serum concentration ~ 2 hrs
- Side effects
  - > 10%: nausea, heartburn, stomach pains, dyspepsia, epigastric discomfort
  - 1–10%: fatigue, rash, gastrointestinal ulceration, hemolytic anemia, weakness, dyspnea, anaphylactic shock
- Other considerations: avoid use in severe renal impairment

DRUG: ACETAMINOPHEN

- Other names: Tylenol, Panadol, Abenol
- Uses: as an analgesic and antipyretic
- Mechanism of action
  - acetaminophen has both analgesic and antipyretic properties that do not significantly differ from those of aspirin. However, acetaminophen lacks the potent anti-inflammatory actions of aspirin. It appears that acetaminophen is a potent inhibitor of prostaglandin production within the CNS. This mechanism accounts for its analgesic and antipyretic properties
- Dosing

Oral formulations	Rectal suppository formulations
80 mg chewable tablets	80 mg
160 mg tablets	120 mg
325 mg tablets	300 mg
500 mg tablets	325 mg
650 mg tablets	650 mg

  - suspension: 160 mg/5 ml
  - for pain or fever in adults: 325–650 mg po q4–6hrs, *or* 1 g po 3–4 times daily, *or* 650 mg PR q4–6hrs
  - maximum daily dose in patients with normal hepatic function: 4–6 g/d (less in patients with hepatic insufficiency)

Cancer Pain Management *(Continued)*

- Pharmacokinetics
  - protein binding: 20–50%
  - metabolism
    - □ *at therapeutic dosages,* the majority of the parent compound is metabolized in the liver to sulfate and glucuronide metabolites; a small amount is metabolized by microsomal mixed function oxidases to a highly reactive intermediate (acetylimidoquinone), which is conjugated with glutathione and inactivated
    - □ *at toxic doses,* glutathione conjugation becomes insufficient to meet the metabolic demand, causing an increase in acetylimidoquinone concentration, which is thought to cause hepatic cell necrosis
  - half life
    - □ neonates: 2–5 hrs
    - □ in adults with normal renal function: 1–3 hrs
    - □ in end-stage renal disease: 1–3 hrs
  - time to peak serum concentration (with oral administration): 10–60 min (may be longer in acute overdoses)
- Side effects
  - < 1%: rash, nausea, vomiting, blood dyscrasias (neutropenia, pancytopenia, leukopenia, anemia), analgesic nephropathy, nephrotoxicity (with chronic overdose)
- Other considerations
  - dosing interval in renal impairment: CrCl 10–50 ml/min: dose q6hrs; CrCl < 10 ml/min: dose q8hrs
  - excessive intake of alcohol may increase the risk of hepatotoxicity: avoid or limit alcohol intake
  - antidote in acute overdose: N-acetylcysteine: 140 mg/kg orally loading followed by 70 mg/kg q4hrs for 17 doses

Neutropenic Fever

L. Hestermann, B. Werner, and E. Reed

OVERVIEW

- Neutropenic fever is most often defined as a single temperature of 38.5° or 38° for an hour or more, and the patient's absolute neutrophil count is < 1,000/mcl
- A causative agent is identified in < 50% of patients
- The goal of therapy is to cover gram-negative and gram-positive organisms broadly with agents that are bactericidal, well tolerated, and cost effective
  - particularly important is to choose antibiotics that are active against resistant bacteria, which occur in the institution or unit

PATHOPHYSIOLOGY

- Gram-positive bacteria, especially coagulase-negative *Staphylococci,* are the most commonly found causative agents
  - coagulase-negative *Staphylococci* most often identified in patients with vascular access devices
  - *Staphylococcus aureus, Streptococci, Enterococci,* and *Corynebacterium* are other causative agents
  - alpha hemolytic *Streptococci* may have a particularly virulent course in neutropenic patients, presenting as septic shock
  - vancomycin-resistant *Enterococci* are bacteremias; uncommon but serious
- Gram-negative organisms are less common than gram-positive organisms, but more likely to cause septic shock
  - most common among these are *E. coli, Klebsiella,* and *Pseudomonas*

DIAGNOSIS AND PREVENTION

- The potential neutropenic patient should be evaluated with a complete history, a mental status assessment, and physical, with attention directed toward the periodontium and pharynx, and lungs and skin, including the axillae and perineum
  - careful examination of all vascular access devices
- Diagnostic studies should include a CBC, with differential, platelet count, measurement of renal and hepatic function, as well as electrolytes
  - at least 20 cc of blood needs to be obtained for culture
  - the blood volume sampled is more important than timing of samples or site (peripheral vein vs. venous access device)
  - any suspicious skin or mucosal lesions should be scraped and/or biopsied for bacterial and/or viral culture
  - if the patient presents with any upper respiratory symptoms, nasal washings for respiratory virus cultures should be obtained
    - □ two-view plain films of the chest and oximetry should be part of the routine evaluation
  - neutropenic fever does not necessitate removal of right atrial catheters
    - □ catheter should be removed if infection involves tissues where catheter is tunneled under the skin, there is persistent bacteremia, infections with *Corynebacterium* or *Diphtheroids,* fungemia, or evidence of septic emboli is present

THERAPY

- Single-agent antibiotics or a combination can be given IV or po in selected, low-risk patients
  - single-agent antibiotics include ceftazidime, cefipime, imipenem, trovofloxacin, and aztreonam
  - an aminoglycoside and a third-generation cephalosporin, such as ceftazidime, or an antipseudomonas penicillin, such as piperacillin, are often used for combined therapy
- To avoid resistant organisms, such as vancomycin-resistant *Enterococci,* vancomycin should not be used routinely
  - it also requires IV administration and is irritating to peripheral veins
  - vancomycin should be used if a high incidence of methicillin-resistant *S. aureus* or alpha hemolytic *Streptococci* is present
    - □ drug should be discontinued after 72 hrs if cultures are negative for such organisms
- Patients with neutropenic fever, who have well-controlled tumor and no serious medical conditions, can be treated as outpatients, as long as the patient is compliant and can be evaluated frequently
- Patients with progressing cancer, other serious medical conditions, or have had a stem cell or bone marrow transplant are at higher risk and should be treated in an acute-care setting
- Antifungal therapy
  - antifungal therapy should be started for patients with new or persistent fever after 5 days of broad-spectrum antibiotics; can be stopped if patients are afebrile; have an absolute neutrophil count of at least 200 cells/mcl and rising; and have had therapy for 4 days with no documented infection
  - the choices for antifungal therapy are amphotericin or a liposomal preparation of amphotericin or an azole, usually fluconazole or itraconazole
    - □ amphotericin has several side effects but is broad spectrum and has been widely experimented
    - □ the liposomal preparations are not more effective than amphotericin but may be better tolerated
    - □ fluconazole is well tolerated, highly water soluble, available in IV formulation, but does not cover *Aspergillus* species, *C. Kruseii,* or *Torulopsis*
    - □ itraconazole has a broader spectrum. It is available in oral preparations and IV formulation may not be well absorbed

KEY REFERENCES

Koc Y, Snydman DR, Schenkein DS, Miller KB: Vancomycin-resistant enterococcal infections in bone marrow transplant recipients. Bone Marrow Transpl 1998; 22:207–9

Malik IA, Khan WA, Karim M, Aziz Z, Khan MA: Feasibility of outpatient management of fever in cancer patients with low-risk neutropenia: results of a prospective randomized trial. Am J Med 1995; 98:224–31

Talcott JA, Finberg R, Mayer RJ, Goldman L: The medical course of cancer patients with fever and neutropenia: clinical identification of a low-risk subgroup at presentation. Arch Intern Med 1988; 148:2561–8

Walsh TJ, Finberg RW, Arndt C, Hiemenz J, Schwartz C, Bodensteiner D, Pappas D, Seibel N, Greenberg RN, Dummer S, Schuster M, Holcenberg JS: Liposomal amphotericin B for empirical therapy in patients with persistent fever and neutropenia. N Engl J Med 1999; 340:764–71

Whimbey E, Champlin RE, Englund JA, Mirza NQ, Piedra PA, Goodrich JM, Przepiorka D, Luna MA, Morice RC, Neumann JL, Elting LS, Bodey GP: Combination therapy with aerosolized ribavirin and intravenous immunoglobulin for respiratory syncytial virus disease in adult bone marrow transplant recipients. Bone Marrow Transpl 1995; 16:393–9

DRUG: VANCOMYCIN HYDROCHLORIDE

- Other names: Vancocin, Lyphocin, Vancoled
- Uses
  - infections due to documented or suspected methicillin-resistant *S. aureus* or beta-lactam–resistant coagulase-negative *Staphylococcus*
  - serious or life-threatening infections (e.g., endocarditis, meningitis) due to documented or suspected staphylococcal or streptococcal infections in patients who are allergic to penicillins and/or cephalosporins
  - empiric therapy of infections associated with gram-positive organisms; used orally for staphylococcal enterocolitis or for antibiotic-associated pseudomembranous colitis produced by *C. difficile*
- Mechanism of action
  - vancomyin is bactericidal
    - □ hinders bacterial cell wall synthesis by blocking glycopeptide polymerization
    - □ binds tightly to D-alanyl-D-alanine portion of cell wall precursor

- Dosing
  - initial dosage recommendation: IV
    - □ infants > 1 mo and children: 10 mg/kg/dose q6hrs
    - □ adults (select dosage based on weight)
      - ▽ < 60 kg: 750 mg
      - ▽ 60–100 kg: 1 g
      - ▽ 100–120 kg: 1.25 g
      - ▽ > 120 kg: 1.5 g
  - dosing interval in renal impairment
    - □ CrCl > 90 ml/min: administer q12hrs
    - □ CrCl 40–90 ml/min: administer q24hrs
    - □ CrCl 30–40 ml/min: administer q48hrs
    - □ CrCl 20–30 ml/min: administer q72hrs
    - □ CrCl 10–20 ml/min: administer q96hrs
    - □ CrCl < 10 ml/min: administer q5–7d
  - hemodialysis: not dialyzable (0–5%); generally not removed; exception minimal to moderate removal by some of the newer high-flux filters
  - continuous ambulatory peritoneal dialysis (CAPD): not significantly removed
  - continuous arteriovenous hemofiltration: dose similar to Clcr of ~ 10–15 ml/min
  - dosing adjustments in hepatic impairment: reduce dose by 60%
  - antibiotic lock technique (for catheter infections): 2 mg/ml in SWI/NS or D_5W; instill 3–5 ml into catheter port as a flush solution instead of heparin lock (note: do not mix with any other solutions)
  - oral: pseudomembranous colitis produced by *C. difficile*
    - □ children: 40 mg/kg/d in divided doses q6–8hrs, added to fluids
    - □ adults: 125 mg 4 times/d
- Pharmacokinetics
  - absorption
    - □ oral: poor
    - □ IM: erratic
    - □ intraperitoneal: can result in 38% absorption systemically
  - distribution
    - □ widely distributed in body tissues and fluids except for CSF
    - □ relative diffusion of antimicrobial agents from blood into CSF
    - □ good only with inflammation (exceeds usual MICs)
    - □ normal meninges: nil
    - □ inflamed meninges: 20–30% of blood levels
  - protein binding: 10–50%
  - half-life (biphasic): terminal
    - □ children > 3 yrs: 2.2–3 hrs
    - □ adults: 5–11 hrs; prolonged significantly with reduced renal function
    - □ end-stage renal disease: 200–250 hrs
  - time to peak serum concentration: IV: within 45–65 min
  - elimination: as unchanged drug in the urine via glomerular filtration (80–90%); oral doses are excreted primarily in the feces
- Adverse reactions
  - oral
    - □ gastrointestinal: bitter taste, nausea, vomiting
    - □ CNS: chills, drug fever
    - □ hematologic: eosinophilia, thrombocytopenia
    - □ cardiovascular: vasculitis
    - □ otic: ototoxicity
    - □ renal: renal failure, interstitial nephritis
- Parenteral
  - □ cardiovascular: hypotension accompanied by flushing, vasculitis
  - □ dermatologic: erythematous rash on face and upper body (red-neck or red-man syndrome)
  - □ hematologic: eosinophilia, thrombocytopenia
  - □ otic: ototoxicity
  - □ renal: renal failure
- Pharmacy issues
  - symptoms of overdose include ototoxicity, nephrotoxicity
  - increased toxicity with anesthetic agents
  - vancomycin reconstituted IV solutions are stable for 14 days at room temperature or refrigeration
  - standard diluent: 500 mg/150 ml D_5W; 1 g/250 ml D_5W
- Nursing considerations
  - use cautiously in patients receiving other drugs for neurotoxicity, nephrotoxicity, or ototoxicity
  - use cautiously in patients > 60 yrs of age and in those with hepatic dysfunction, preexisting hearing deficit, or allergies to other antibiotics
  - do not infuse drug rapidly; red-neck syndrome can occur; if this happens stop infusion
  - assess renal function during therapy
  - patient information
    - □ report pain at infusion site, dizziness, fullness or ringing in ears with IV use; nausea or vomiting with oral use
    - □ complete full course of therapy

DRUG: AZITHROMYCIN

- Other name: Zithromax
- Uses
  - children
    - □ acute otitis media due to *H. influenzae, M. catarrhalis*, or *S. pneumoniae*
    - □ pharyngitis/tonsillitis due to *S. pyogenes*
  - adults
    - □ mild to moderate upper and lower respiratory tract infections
    - □ infections of the skin and skin structure
    - □ susceptible strains of *C. trachomatis, M. catarrhalis, H. influenzae, S. aureus, S. pneumoniae, Mycoplasma pneumoniae*, and *C. psittaci*
    - □ also for prevention of disseminated *Mycobacterium avium* complex in patients with advanced HIV infection
- Mechanism of action
  - inhibits RNA-dependent protein synthesis at the chain elongation step; binds to the 50S ribosomal subunit resulting in blockage of transpeptidation
- Dosing
  - oral
    - □ children > 6 mos: otitis media: 10 mg/kg on day 1 (maximum: 500 mg/d) followed by 5 mg/kg/d once daily on days 2–5 (maximum: 250 mg/d)
    - □ children > 2 yrs: pharyngitis, tonsillitis: 12 mg/kg/d once daily for 5 days (maximum: 500 mg/d)
    - □ children: *M. avium*–infected patients with acquired immunodeficiency syndrome: not currently FDA approved for use; 10–20 mg/kg/d once daily (maximum: 40 mg/kg/d) has been used in clinical trials; prophylaxis for first episode of MAC: 5–12 mg/kg/d once daily (maximum: 500 mg/d)
    - □ adolescents > 16 yrs and adults
      - ▽ respiratory tract, skin and soft tissue infections: 500 mg on day 1 followed by 250 mg/d on days 2–5 (maximum: 500 mg/d)
      - ▽ uncomplicated chlamydial urethritis or cervicitis: single 1 g dose
      - ▽ prophylaxis of disseminated *M. avium* complex disease in patient with advanced HIV infection: 1,200 mg once weekly
- Pharmacokinetics
  - absorption: rapid from the GI tract
  - distribution: extensive tissue distribution
  - protein binding: 7–50% (concentration dependent)
  - metabolism: in the liver
  - bioavailability: 37%; decreased by food
  - half-life, terminal: 68 hrs
  - peak serum concentration: 2.3–4 hrs
  - elimination: 4.5–12% of dose is excreted in urine; 50% of dose is excreted unchanged in bile
- Adverse reactions
  - gastrointestinal: diarrhea, nausea, abdominal pain, cramping, vomiting
  - cardiovascular: ventricular arrhythmias
  - CNS: fever, headache, dizziness
  - dermatologic: rash, angioedema
  - genitourinary: vaginitis
  - hematologic: eosinophilia
  - hepatic: elevated LFTs, cholestatic jaundice
  - local: thrombophlebitis
  - otic: ototoxicity
  - renal: nephritis
  - miscellaneous: allergic reactions
- Pharmacy issues
  - symptoms of overdose include nausea, vomiting, diarrhea, prostration; treatment is supportive and symptomatic
  - decreased peak serum levels: aluminum- and magnesium-containing antacids by 24% but not total absorption
  - increased effect/toxicity: azithromycin increases levels of tacrolimus, alfentanil, astemizole, terfenadine, loratadine, bromocriptine, carbamazepine,

cyclosporine, digoxin, disopyramide, and triazolam; azithromycin did not affect the response to warfarin or theophylline, although caution is advised when administered together
- take capsule on an empty stomach; 1 hr prior to a meal or 2 hrs after
- do not take with aluminum- or magnesium-containing antacids
- tablet form may be taken with food to decrease GI effects

■ Nursing considerations
- assess history of sensitivity to erythromycins and note previous experience with macrolide antibiotics
- teach patient to avoid exposure to sun, use sunscreens

QUINOLONE ANTIBIOTICS

DRUG: CIPROFLOXACIN

■ Other name: Cipro

■ Uses
- documented or suspected infections of the lower respiratory tract, skin and skin structure, bone/joints, and urinary tract due to susceptible bacterial strains
- pseudomonal infections (e.g., home care patients)
- multidrug resistant gram-negative organisms
- chronic bacterial prostatitis
- infectious diarrhea
- complicated gram-negative and anaerobic intra-abdominal infections (with metronidazole)
- *E. coli* (enteropathic strains), *B. fragilis, P. mirabilis, K. pneumoniae, P. aeruginosa, Campylobacter jejuni* or *Shigella*
- osteomyelitis when parenteral therapy is not feasible

■ Mechanism of action
- inhibits DNA-gyrase in susceptible organisms; inhibits relaxation of supercoiled DNA and promotes breakage of double-stranded DNA

■ Dosing
- adults: oral
  - □ administer 2 hrs after a meal; may administer with food to minimize GI upset; administer 2 hrs before or 2 hrs after antacids, dairy products, sucralfate, iron products, didanosine, enteral feedings, oral multivitamins, and mineral supplements
  - □ urinary tract infection: 250–500 mg q12hrs for 7–10 days, depending on severity of infection and susceptibility
  - □ lower respiratory tract, skin/skin structure infections: 500–750 mg twice daily for 7–14 days depending on severity and susceptibility
  - □ bone/joint infections: 500–750 mg twice daily for 4–6 wks, depending on severity and susceptibility
  - □ infectious diarrhea: 500 mg q12hrs for 5–7 days
- adults: IV
  - □ urinary tract infection: 200–400 mg q12hrs for 7–10 days
  - □ lower respiratory tract, skin/skin structure infection (mild–moderate): 400 mg q12hrs for 7–14 days
  - □ dosing adjustment in renal impairment
    - ▽ Clcr < 30 ml/min: administer q18hrs (oral) and q18–24hrs (IV)
    - ▽ dialysis: only small amounts of ciprofloxacin are removed by hemo- or peritoneal dialysis (< 10%); usual dose: 250–500 mg q24hrs following dialysis

■ Pharmacokinetics
- absorption: oral: rapid from GI tract (~ 50–85%)
- distribution: crosses the placenta; appears in breast milk; distributes widely throughout body; tissue concentrations often exceed serum concentrations, especially in the kidneys, gallbladder, liver, lungs, gynecologic tissue, and prostatic tissue; CSF concentrations reach 10% with noninflamed meninges and 14–37% with inflamed meninges
- protein binding: 16–43%
- metabolism: partially metabolized in the liver
- bioavailability: oral: Tmax: 0.5–2 hrs
- half-life
  - □ children: 2.5 hrs
  - □ adults with normal renal function: 3–5 hrs
- elimination: 30–50% excreted as unchanged drug in urine; 20–40% of dose excreted in feces primarily from biliary excretion

■ Adverse reactions
- CNS: headache, restlessness, dizziness, confusion, seizures
- gastrointestinal: nausea, diarrhea, vomiting, abdominal pain
- dermatologic: rash
- hematologic: anemia
- hepatic: increased liver enzymes *(acute liver failure with trovafloxacin)*
- neuromuscular and skeletal: tremor, arthralgia, ruptured tendons
- renal: acute renal failure

■ Pharmacy issues
- symptoms of overdose include acute renal failure, seizures; GI decontamination and supportive care; not removed by peritoneal or hemodialysis
- not recommended in children < 18 yrs of age
  - □ has caused transient arthropathy in children
  - □ CNS stimulation may occur (tremor, restlessness, confusion, and very rarely hallucinations or seizures)
  - □ use with caution in patients with known or suspected CNS disorder
  - □ green discoloration of teeth in infants has been reported
  - □ prolonged use may result in superinfection
  - □ may rarely cause inflamed or ruptured tendons (discontinue use immediately with signs of inflammation or tendon pain)
- drug interactions: inhibitor of cytochrome P-450 1A2 enzymes
- increased toxicity: caffeine and theophylline: CNS stimulation when concurrent with cipro
- cyclosporine may increase serum creatinine levels
- administer by slow IV infusion over 60 min to reduce the risk of venous irritation (burning, pain, erythema, and swelling); final concentration for administration should not exceed 2 mg/ml

■ Patient teaching
- medication may cause dizziness; avoid activity requiring alertness or coordination
- report persistant diarrhea, vomiting, or abdominal pain
- avoid caffeine because of potential for cumulative caffeine effects
- if skin rash or other allergic reaction occurs, stop taking medication and notify physician
- oral: administer 2 hrs after a meal; may administer with food to minimize GI upset; avoid antacid use; drink plenty of fluids to maintain proper hydration and urine output

DRUG: CINOXACIN, ENOXACIN, LEVOFLOXACIN, LOMEFLOXACIN, NALIDIXIC ACID, NORFLOXACIN, OFLOXACIN, PEFLOXACIN, AND TROVAFLOXACIN

■ Other names: Cinobac, Penetrex, Levaquin, Maxaquin, NegGram, Noroxin, Floxin, Trovan

■ Uses
- levofloxacin oral and IV
  - □ acute maxillary sinusitis due to *S. pneumoniae, H. influenzae,* or *M. catarrhalis*
  - □ acute bacterial exacerbation of chronic bronchitis and community-acquired pneumonia due to *S. aureus, S. pneumoniae, H. influenzae, H. parainfluenza* or *M. catarrhalis, C. pneumoniae, L. pneumophilia* or *M. pneumoniae*
  - □ may be used for uncomplicated skin and skin structure infection (due to *S. aureus* or *S. pyogenes*)

■ Dosing
- adults: oral, IV (infuse IV solution over 60 min)
  - □ acute bacterial exacerbation of chronic bronchitis: 500 mg q24hrs for at least 7 days
  - □ community-acquired pneumonia: 500 mg q24hrs for 7–14 days
  - □ acute maxillary sinusitis: 500 mg q24hrs for 10–14 days
  - □ uncomplicated skin infections: 500 mg q24hrs for 7–10 days

- □ complicated urinary tract infections including acute pyelonephritis: 250 mg q24hrs for 10 days
- dosing adjustment in renal impairment
  - □ Clcr 20–49 ml/min: administer 250 mg q24hrs (initial: 500 mg)
  - □ Clcr 10–19 ml/min: administer 250 mg q48hrs (initial: 500 mg for most infections; 250 mg for renal infections)
  - □ hemodialysis/CAPD: 250 mg q48hrs (initial: 500 mg)

■ Pharmacy issues
- may be taken with or without food; drink plenty of fluids; do not take antacids within 4 hrs before or 2 hrs after dosing
- contact your physician immediately if signs of allergy occur
- do not discontinue therapy until your course has been completed
- take a missed dose as soon as possible, unless it is almost time for your next dose

■ Uses
- trovafloxacin: oral and IV (alatrofloxacin mesylate), a prodrug of trovafloxacin
  - □ nosocomial pneumonia caused by *E. coli, P. aeruginosa, H. influenzae,* or *S. aureus*
  - □ when *P. aeruginosa* is a documented or presumptive pathogen, combination therapy with either an aminoglycoside or aztreonam may be clinically indicated
  - □ community-acquired pneumonia caused by *S. pneumoniae, H. influenzae, K. pneumoniae, S. aureus, M. pneumoniae, M. catarrhalis, Legionella pneumophilia,* or *Chlamydia pneumoniae*
  - □ complicated intra-abdominal infections, including post-surgical infections caused by *E. coli, B. fragilis,* viridans group streptococci, *P. aeruginosa, Klebsiella pneumoniae, Peptostreptococcus* species, or *Prevotella* species
  - □ skin and skin structure infections caused by *S. aureus, S. pyogenes,* or *S. agalactiae*

■ Dosing
- adult: oral, IV (infuse IV solutions over 60 min); no adjustment necessary when switching from IV to oral dosing
  - □ nosocomial pneumonia: 300 mg IV followed by 200 mg oral daily for 10–14 days
  - □ community-acquired pneumonia: 200 mg oral or IV followed by 200 mg oral daily for 7–14 days
  - □ skin and skin structure, uncomplicated: 100 mg oral daily for 7–10 days
  - □ complicated intra-abdominal infections, including post-surgical infections: 300 mg IV followed by 200 mg orally for 7–14 days
  - □ no adjustment necessary in renal impairment; may need to adjust dose with mild or moderate cirrhosis

■ Pharmacy issues
- oral doses should be administered at least 2 hrs before or 2 hrs after antacids containing magnesium or aluminum, as well as sucralfate, citric acid buffered with sodium citrate (e.g., Bicitra), and metal cations (e.g., ferrous sulfate)
- may be taken without regard to meals
- dizziness/lightheadedness was the most common adverse reaction reported; may decrease incidence of dizziness if taken at bedtime or with food

■ Nursing considerations
- absorption is reduced with administration of antacids; if necessary administer antacids 2 hrs before
- monitor liver functions
- baseline neurologic status
- inform patient to report GI disturbances
- report skin rash or itching; female patients should report vaginal itching or discharge
- limit caffeine-containing fluids, since trovafloxacin delays caffeine excretion and could exacerbate sensory/perceptual patterns
- exposure to sun can cause sunburn; use sunscreen

DRUG: CEFTAZIDIME

■ Other names: Ceptaz, Fortaz, Tazicef, Tazidime

■ Uses
- third-generation cephalosporin; generally reserved for the treatment of serious infections caused by susceptible gram-negative organisms
- *Pseudomonas aeruginosa*
- Enterobacter
- *Hemophilus influenzae*
- *E. coli*
- nonmethicillin-resistant streptococcus and staphylococcus
- may have enhanced synergistic activity when used in combination with other antibiotics

■ Mechanism of action
- inhibits bacterial cell wall synthesis by binding to one or more of the penicillin-binding proteins (PBPs)

■ Dosing
- IM, IV
  - □ infants and children 1 mo–12 yrs: 30–50 mg/kg/dose q8hrs; maximum dose 6 g/d
  - □ adults: 1–2 g q8–12hrs
  - □ urinary tract infections: 250–500 mg q12hrs
- dosing interval in renal impairment
  - □ Clcr 30–50 ml/min: administer q12hrs
  - □ Clcr 10–30 ml/min: administer q24hrs
  - □ Clcr < 10 ml/min: administer q48–72hrs
  - □ hemodialysis: dialyzable (50–100%)

■ Pharmacokinetics
- distribution: widely distributes throughout the body including bone, bile, skin, CSF (diffuses into CSF with higher concentrations when the meninges are inflamed), endometrium, heart, pleural and lymphatic fluids
- protein binding: 17%
- half-life: 1–2 hrs (prolonged with renal impairment)
- time to peak serum concentration: IM: within 1 hr
- elimination: glomerular filtration with 80–90% of the dose excreted as unchanged drug within 24 hrs

■ Adverse reactions
- gastrointestinal: diarrhea, nausea, vomiting, pseudomembranous colitis
- local: pain at injection site, phlebitis
- CNS: fever, headache, dizziness
- dermatologic: rash, angioedema
- hematologic: eosinophilia, thrombocytosis, transient leukopenia, hemolytic anemias
- hepatic: transient elevation in liver enzymes
- neuromuscular and skeletal: paresthesia
- renal: transient elevation of BUN/creatinine
- miscellaneous: candidiasis

■ Pharmacy considerations
- observe for signs and symptoms of anaphylaxis during first dose
- modify dosage in patients with severe renal impairment
- prolonged use may result in superinfection
- low incidence of cross-sensitivity to penicillins exists
- symptoms of overdose include neuromuscular hypersensitivity, convulsions
- aminoglycosides: in vitro studies indicate additive or synergistic effect against some strains of Enterobacteriaceae and *Pseudomonas aeruginosa*
- increased toxicity: furosemide, aminoglycosides may be a possible additive to nephrotoxicity

■ Nursing considerations
- note patient allergies to penicillin
- drug results in a false-positive Coombs' test

DRUG: CEFEPIME

■ Other name: Maxipime

■ Uses
- cefepime is a fourth-generation cephalosporin
- used in treatment of respiratory tract infections (including bronchitis and pneumonia)
- cellulitis and other skin and soft tissue infections, and urinary tract infections
- good gram-negative coverage similar to third-generation cephalosporins, but better gram-positive coverage

- Mechanism of action
  - inhibits bacterial cell wall synthesis by binding to one or more of the penicillin-binding proteins (PBPs)
  - inhibits the final transpeptidation step of peptidoglycan synthesis in bacterial cell walls
  - inhibiting cell wall biosynthesis. Bacteria eventually lyse due to ongoing activity of cell wall autolytic enzymes (autolysis and murein hydrolases) while cell wall assembly is arrested
- Dosing
  - IV
    - □ children: unlabeled: 50 mg/kg q8hrs, maximum 2 g per dose
    - □ adults: most infections: 1–2 g q12hrs for 5–10 days; higher doses or more frequent administration may be required in pseudomonal infections
    - □ manufacturer recommends a dose of 2 g q8hrs in febrile neutropenia
  - dosing adjustment in renal impairment
    - □ Clcr 10–30 ml/min: administer 500 mg q24hrs (500 mg q12hrs in febrile neutropenia)
    - □ Clcr < 10 ml/min: administer 250 mg q24hrs
    - □ hemodialysis: removed by dialysis; administer supplemental dose of 250 mg after each dialysis session
    - □ peritoneal dialysis: removed to a lesser extent than hemodialysis; administer 250 mg q48hrs
- Pharmacokinetics
  - absorption: IM: rapid and complete; Tmax: 0.5–1.5 hrs
  - Vd: adults: 14–20 L
  - distribution: penetrates into inflammatory fluid at concentrations ~80% of serum levels and into bronchial mucosa at levels ~60% of those reached in the plasma
  - protein binding, plasma: 16–19%
  - metabolism: very little
  - half-life: 2 hrs
  - elimination: nearly completely eliminated as unchanged drug in urine
- Adverse reactions
  - CNS: headache, lightheadedness
  - gastrointestinal: dyspepsia, antibiotic-associated diarrhea
  - hepatic: transient elevations in LFTs
  - local: phlebitis
  - ocular: blurred vision
- Pharmacy issues
  - symptoms of overdose include neuromuscular hypersensitivity, convulsions
  - hemodialysis may be helpful to aid in the removal of the drug from the blood
  - increased effect: high-dose probenecid decreases clearance
  - increased toxicity: aminoglycosides increase nephrotoxic potential
  - test interactions: false-positive Coombs' test
  - may falsely elevate creatinine values when Jaff reaction is used
  - may cause false-positive results in urine glucose tests when using cupric sulfate (Benedict's solution, Clinitest), false-positive urinary proteins and steroids
- Nursing considerations
  - anticipate dose reductions in patients with renal dysfunction
  - document other medications being taken by patient; aminoglycosides and furosemide may increase risk of nephrotoxicity or ototoxicity
  - drug may cause a positive Coombs' test result
  - educate patient to report pain, inflammation, and rash at injection site

DRUG: AMIKACIN

- Other name: Amikin
- Uses
  - documented gram-negative enteric infection resistant to gentamicin and tobramycin
  - bone infections, respiratory tract infections, endocarditis, and septicemia
  - documented infection of mycobacterial organisms susceptible to amikacin including Pseudomonas, *Proteus, Serratia*, and gram-positive *Staphylococcus*
- Mechanism of action
  - inhibits protein synthesis in susceptible bacteria by binding to ribosomal subunits
- Dosing
  - individualization is critical because of the low therapeutic index
  - use of ideal body weight (IBW) for determining the mg/kg/dose appears to be more accurate than dosing on the basis of total body weight (TBW)
  - adults (18 yrs and older)
    - □ IBW in kg (male) = 50 + (2.3 × height in inches over 5 feet)
    - □ IBW in kg (female) = 45.5 + (2.3 × height in inches over 5 feet)
    - □ in morbid obesity, dosage requirement may best be estimated using an adjusted dosing weight of IBW + 0.4 (TBW – IBW)
  - infants, children, and adults: IM, IV: 5–7.5 mg/kg/dose q8hrs
  - dosing interval in renal impairment: some patients may require larger or more frequent doses if serum levels document the need (e.g., cystic fibrosis or febrile granulocytopenic patients)
    - □ Clcr > 60 ml/min: administer q8hrs
    - □ Clcr 40–60 ml/min: administer q12hrs
    - □ Clcr 20–40 ml/min: administer q24hrs
    - □ Clcr 10–20 ml/min: administer q48hrs
    - □ Clcr < 10 ml/min: administer q72hrs
  - hemodialysis: dialyzable (50–100%); administer dose postdialysis or administer two-thirds normal dose as a supplemental dose postdialysis and follow levels
  - peritoneal dialysis: dose as Clcr < 10 ml/min and follow levels
  - continuous arteriovenous or venovenous hemodiafiltration (CAVH) effects: dose as Clcr < 10 ml/min and follow levels
- Therapeutic levels
  - peak
    - □ life-threatening infections: 25–30 mcg/ml
    - □ serious infections: 20–25 mcg/ml
    - □ urinary tract infections: 15–20 mcg/ml
    - □ synergy against gram-positive organisms: 15–20 mcg/ml
  - trough
    - □ life-threatening infections: 4–8 mcg/ml
    - □ serious infections: 1–4 mcg/ml
    - □ toxic concentration: Peak: > 35 mcg/ml; trough: > 10 mcg/ml
  - timing of serum samples: draw peak 30 min after completion of 30 min infusion or at 1 hr following initiation of infusion or IM injection; draw trough immediately before next dose
- Pharmacokinetics
  - absorption: may be delayed in the bedridden patient
  - distribution: crosses the placenta; primarily distributes into extracellular fluid (highly hydrophilic)
  - relative diffusion of antimicrobial agents from blood into CSF: good only with inflammation (exceeds usual MICs); ratio of CSF to blood level (%)
    - □ normal meninges: 10–20
    - □ inflamed meninges: 15–24
  - half-life (dependent on renal function)
    - □ infants
      - ▽ low birth weight (1–3 days): 7–9 hrs
      - ▽ full term > 7 days: 4–5 hrs
      - ▽ children: 1.6–2.5 hrs
    - □ adults
      - ▽ normal renal function: 1.4–2.3 hrs
      - ▽ anuria: end-stage renal disease: 28–86 hrs
  - time to peak serum concentration
    - □ IM: within 45–120 min
    - □ IV: within 30 min following 30 min infusion
  - elimination: 94–98% excreted unchanged in urine via glomerular filtration within 24 hrs; clearance dependent on renal function and patient age
- Adverse reactions
  - CNS: neurotoxicity, headache, drowsiness, drug fever
  - otic: ototoxicity (auditory), ototoxicity (vestibular)
  - renal: nephrotoxicity
  - cardiovascular: hypotension
  - dermatologic: rash
  - gastrointestinal: nausea, vomiting
  - hematologic: eosinophilia
  - neuromuscular and skeletal: paresthesia, tremor, arthralgia, weakness
  - respiratory: dyspnea

- Pharmacy issues
  - initial and periodic peak and trough plasma drug levels should be determined, particularly in critically ill patients with serious infections
  - once daily dosing
    - □ higher peak serum drug concentration to MIC ratios
    - □ demonstrated aminoglycoside postantibiotic effect
    - □ decreased renal cortex drug uptake
    - □ improved cost-time efficiency
    - □ effective for non-life-threatening infections, with no higher incidence of nephrotoxicity than those requiring multiple daily doses
    - □ doses are determined by calculating the entire day's dose via usual multiple dose calculation techniques and administering this quantity as a single dose
    - □ doses are then adjusted to maintain mean serum concentrations above the MIC(s) of the causative organism(s)
    - □ example: 14–35 mg/kg as a single dose/24 hrs; peak (maximum) serum concentration may approximate 40–55 mcg/ml and trough (minimum) serum concentration < 3 mcg/ml
    - □ further research is needed for universal recommendation in all patient populations
  - monitoring parameters
    - □ urinalysis, BUN, serum creatinine, appropriately timed peak and trough concentrations
    - □ vital signs, temperature, weight, I/O, hearing parameters (audiology testing warranted in extended treatment courses > 10 days)
    - □ the presence of fever may decrease peak levels
    - □ in vitro data indicate the presence of high concentrations of penicillins concurrent with sampling of aminoglycoside levels may result in inactivation (decreased values)
    - □ increased toxicity of aminoglycoside: indomethacin IV, amphotericin, loop diuretics, vancomycin, enflurane, methoxyflurane
    - □ increased toxicity of depolarizing and nondepolarizing neuromuscular blocking agents and polypeptide antibiotics with administration of aminoglycosides
    - □ cross-sensitivity may exist with other aminoglycosides
- Nursing considerations
  - obtain baseline weight and renal function prior to initiation of therapy and monitor during therapy
  - baseline audiogram should be obtained prior to and during therapy
  - aminoglycoside levels measured from blood taken from Silastic central catheters can sometimes give falsely high reading (draw levels from alternate lumen or peripheral stick, if possible)
  - reference range: sample size: 0.5–2 ml blood (red-top tube) or 0.1–1 ml serum (separated)
  - if no response after 3–5 days of therapy, discontinue and obtain another set of specimens
  - report loss of hearing, ringing or roaring in the ears, or feeling of fullness in head

OTHER AMINOGLYCOSIDE ANTIBIOTICS

DRUG: GENTAMICIN, KANAMYCIN, NEOMYCIN, NETILMICIN, STREPTOMYCIN, TOBRAMYCIN

- Other names: Garamycin, Kantrex, Neo-Tabs, Netromycin, Nebcin
- Uses: Gentamicin and Tobramycin: IM and IV
  - treatment of susceptible bacterial infections, normally gram-negative organisms
  - Pseudomonas, Proteus, Serratia, and gram-positive Staphylococcus
  - bone infections, respiratory tract infections, skin and soft tissue infections, as well as abdominal and urinary tract infections, endocarditis, and septicemia
- Dosing
  - adults: IM, IV
    - □ severe life-threatening infections: 2–2.5 mg/kg/dose
    - □ urinary tract infections: 1.5 mg/kg/dose
    - □ synergy (for gram-positive infections): 1 mg/kg/dose. Dosing interval in renal impairment
      - ▽ Clcr > 60 ml/min: administer q8hrs
      - ▽ Clcr 40–60 ml/min: administer q12hrs
      - ▽ Clcr 20–40 ml/min: administer q24hrs
      - ▽ Clcr 10–20 ml/min: administer q48hrs
      - ▽ Clcr < 10 ml/min: administer q72hrs
    - □ hemodialysis: dialyzable
      - ▽ removal by hemodialysis
      - ▽ 30% removal of aminoglycosides occurs during 4 hrs of HD
      - ▽ administer dose after dialysis and follow levels
      - ▽ removal by continuous ambulatory peritoneal dialysis (CAPD)
- Pharmacy issues
  - therapeutic levels
    - □ peak
      - ▽ serious infections: 6–8 mcg/ml
      - ▽ life-threatening infections: 8–10 mcg/ml
      - ▽ urinary tract infections: 4–6 mcg/ml
      - ▽ synergy against gram-positive organisms: 3–5 mcg/ml
    - □ trough
      - ▽ serious infections: 0.5–1 mcg/ml
      - ▽ life-threatening infections: 1–2 mcg/ml
    - □ monitor serum creatinine and urine output
    - □ obtain drug levels after cultures identified and decision made to continue therapy
- Nursing considerations
  - do not mix with other drugs
  - monitor CBC, electrolytes, liver functions, and kidney functions
  - potential for neuromuscular blockade when given concurrently with general anesthetics
  - increased risk of toxicity with other ototoxic drugs
  - assess
    - □ respiratory depression
    - □ baseline neurologic status
    - □ baseline hearing during therapy with an audiogram
    - □ renal function: keep patient well hydrated
  - teach patient
    - □ to report difficulties in hearing/perceptual problems
    - □ importance of hydration and to report symptoms of fatigue, bleeding, or infection

DRUG: IMIPENEM AND CILASTATIN

- Other name: Primaxin
- Uses
  - treatment of documented multidrug resistant gram-negative infection
  - organisms proven or suspected to be susceptible to imipenem/cilastatin
  - treatment of multiple organism infection in which other agents have an insufficient spectrum of activity or are contraindicated due to toxic potential
  - antibacterial activity includes resistant gram-negative bacilli (*P. aeruginosa* and *Enterococcus* sp)
  - gram-positive bacteria (methicillin-sensitive *Staphylococcus aureus* and *Enterococcus* sp)
  - anaerobes
- Mechanism of action
  - imipenem is a broad-spectrum antibiotic chemically related to the penicillins and cephalosporins
  - inhibits cell wall synthesis by binding to penicillin-binding proteins on the bacterial outer membrane
  - cilastatin prevents renal metabolism of imipenem by competitive inhibition of dehydropeptidase along the brush border of the proximal renal tubules
- Dosing
  - IM and IV (dosing based on imipenem component)
    - □ children: IV: 60–100 mg/kg/24 hrs divided q6hrs (maximum: 4 g/d)
    - □ adults: IV: 500 mg q6–8hrs (1 g q6–8hrs for severe *Pseudomonas* infection)

- □ infuse each 250–500 mg dose over 20–30 min; infuse each 1 g dose over 40–60 min
- – dosing adjustment recommended in renal impairment

■ Pharmacokinetics
- – imipenem
  - □ distribution: appears in breast milk; crosses the placenta
  - □ metabolism: in the kidney by dehydropeptidase
  - □ half-life: 1 hr, extended with renal insufficiency
  - □ elimination: when given with cilastatin, urinary excretion of unchanged imipenem increases to 70%
- – cilastatin
  - □ metabolism: partially in the kidneys
  - □ half-life: 1 hr, extended with renal insufficiency
  - □ elimination: 70–80% of dose excreted in urine as unchanged cilastatin

■ Adverse reactions
- – gastrointestinal: nausea, diarrhea, vomiting, pseudomembranous colitis
- – local: phlebitis, pain at injection site
- – cardiovascular: hypotension, palpitations
- – CNS: lowers seizure threshold, especially in renal failure
- – dermatologic: rash
- – hematologic: neutropenia, eosinophilia
- – miscellaneous: emergence of resistant strains of *P. aeruginosa*

■ Pharmacy issues
- – symptoms of overdose include neuromuscular hypersensitivity, seizures
- – drug interactions: increased toxicity: beta-lactam antibiotics, probenecid may increase toxicity
- – use with caution in patients with a history of seizures or hypersensitivity to beta-lactams
- – elderly patients often require lower doses
- – standard diluent: 500 mg/100 ml NS; 1 g/250 ml NS prepared fresh due to limited stability

■ Nursing considerations
- – obtain urine specimen for culture and sensitivity before the first dose
- – use cautiously in patients allergic to penicillins or cephalosporins
- – patients with renal dysfunction may need a lower dose or longer dose intervals
- – should nausea occur during infusion, decrease infusion rate

AMPHOTERICIN B

■ Other name: Fungizone

■ Uses
- – treatment of severe systemic infections and meningitis caused by susceptible fungi
- – candida species, *Histoplasma capsulatum, Cryptococcus neoformans, Aspergillus* species, *Blastomyces dermatitidis, Torulopsis glabrata,* and *Coccidioides immitis*
- – fungal peritonitis; irrigant for bladder fungal infections; and topically for cutaneous and mucocutaneous candidal infections

■ Mechanism of action
- – binds to ergosterol, altering cell membrane permeability in susceptible fungi and causing leakage of cell components with subsequent cell death

■ Dosing
- – IV
  - □ adults and children
    - ▽ test dose (not required): 1 mg infused over 20–30 min
    - ▽ initial dose: 0.25 mg/kg administered over 2–6 hrs, gradually increased on subsequent days to the desired level by 0.25 mg/kg increments per day
    - ▽ critically ill patients, may initiate with 1–1.5 mg/kg/d with close observation
    - ▽ maintenance dose: 0.25–1 mg/kg/d or 1.5 mg/kg over 4–6 hrs every other day
    - ▽ do not exceed 1.5 mg/kg/d; cumulative dose: 1–4 g over 4–10 wks
    - ▽ duration of therapy varies with nature of infection: histoplasmosis, cryptococcus, or blastomycosis may be treated with total dose of 2–4 g
- – IT
  - □ adults: 25–300 mcg q48–72hrs; increase to 500 mcg to 1 mg as tolerated
- – oral: 1 ml (100 mg) 4 times daily

■ Pharmacokinetics
- – distribution: minimal amounts enter the aqueous humor, bile, CSF (inflamed or noninflamed meninges), amniotic fluid, pericardial fluid, pleural fluid, and synovial fluid
- – protein binding: 90%
- – half-life, biphasic
  - □ initial: 15–48 hrs
  - □ terminal: 15 days
  - □ time to peak: within 1 hr following a 4–6 hr infusion

■ Adverse reactions
- – CNS: fever, chills, headache, malaise, generalized pain, delirium, arachnoiditis, convulsions, vision changes, hearing loss
- – endocrine and metabolic: hypokalemia, hypomagnesemia
- – gastrointestinal: anorexia, nausea, vomiting
- – hematologic: anemia, leukocytosis, bone marrow suppression, coagulation defects, leukopenia
- – renal: nephrotoxicity, tubular acidosis, renal failure, anuria
- – cardiovascular: hypotension, hypertension, flushing, cardiac arrest
- – genitourinary: urinary retention
- – local: thrombophlebitis
- – neuromuscular and skeletal: paresthesia (especially with IT therapy)
- – hepatic: acute liver failure
- – respiratory: dyspnea

■ Pharmacy issues
- – may premedicate patients with acetaminophen and diphenhydramine 30 min prior
- – meperidine (Demerol) may help reduce rigors
- – avoid rapid injection
- – increased toxicity: cyclosporine and aminoglycosides (nephrotoxicity), corticosteroids (hypokalemia)
- – reconstitute only with sterile water without preservatives
- – standard diluent: dose/500 ml D_5W
- – minimum volume: 250 ml D_5W (concentrations should not exceed 0.1 mg/ml for peripheral administration or 1.4 mg/ml for central administration)
- – avoid additive toxicity with other nephrotoxic drugs
- – monitor BUN and serum creatinine levels frequently while therapy is increased and at least weekly thereafter
- – IV amphotericin is used primarily for the treatment of patients with progressive and potentially fatal fungal infections

■ Nursing considerations
- – infuse slowly and monitor vital signs frequently
- – monitor I/O; report changes in urine appearance or volume
- – instruct patient to report neurologic symptoms such as tinitus, blurred vision, or vertigo

DRUG: AMPHOTERICIN B LIPID COMPLEX, ABLC

■ Other name: Abelcet

■ Uses
- – treatment of aspergillosis or any type of progressive fungal infection in patients who are refractory to or intolerant of conventional amphotericin B therapy
- – orphan drug status for cryptococcal meningitis

■ Mechanism of action
- – as a modification of dimyristoyl phosphatidylcholine: dimyristoyl phosphatidylglycerol 7:3(DMPC:DMPG) liposome, amphotericin B lipid-complex has a higher drug to lipid ratio and the concentration of amphotericin B is 33 M
- – ABLC is a ribbonlike structure, not a liposome
- – mechanism is like amphotericin—includes binding to ergosterol, altering cell membrane permeability in susceptible fungi and causing leakage of cell components with subsequent cell death

■ Dosing
- – children and adults: IV: 2.5–5 mg/kg/d as a single infusion
  - □ significantly higher doses of ABLC are tolerated

- it appears that attaining higher doses with ABLC produces more rapid fungicidal activity in vivo than standard amphotericin B preparations
- dosing adjustment in renal impairment not necessary
- effects of renal impairment are not currently known
- hemodialysis/peritoneal dialysis/continuous arteriovenous or venovenous hemofiltration (CAVH/CAVHD): no supplemental dosage necessary

- Adverse reactions
  - reduced nephrotoxicity as well as frequent infusion related side effects have been reported with this formulation
  - CNS: chills, fever, headache
  - renal: increased serum creatinine
  - cardiovascular: hypotension, cardiac arrest
  - dermatologic: rash
  - endocrine and metabolic: bilirubinemia, hypokalemia, acidosis
  - gastrointestinal: nausea, vomiting, diarrhea, gastrointestinal hemorrhage, abdominal pain
  - renal: renal failure
  - respiratory: respiratory failure, dyspnea, pneumonia
  - miscellaneous: multiple organ failure
- Pharmacy issues
  - anaphylaxis has been reported with amphotericin B desoxycholate and other amphotericin B–containing drugs
  - facilities for cardiopulmonary resuscitation should be available during administration
  - if severe respiratory distress occurs, the infusion should be immediately discontinued and the patient should not receive further infusions
  - during the initial dosing, the drug should be administered IV and under close clinical observation by medically trained personnel
  - acute reactions (including fever and chills) may occur 1–2 hrs after starting an IV infusion. These reactions are usually more common with the first few doses and generally diminish with subsequent doses
  - increased toxicity: toxic effect of nephrotoxic drugs may be additive; corticosteroids may increase potassium depletion caused by amphotericin; may predispose patients receiving cardiac glycosides or skeletal muscle relaxants to toxicity secondary to hypokalemia
  - BUN and serum creatinine levels should be determined every other day while therapy is increased and at least weekly thereafter; monitor I/O
  - serum potassium and magnesium should be monitored closely; monitor for signs of hypokalemia (muscle weakness, cramping, drowsiness, EKG changes, etc.)
  - monitor electrolytes, liver function, hematocrit, CBC, blood pressure, and temperature regularly

DRUG: FLUCONAZOLE

- Other name: Diflucan
- Uses
  - oral or vaginal candidiasis unresponsive to nystatin or clotrimazole
  - nonlife-threatening candida infections (e.g., cystitis, esophagitis)
  - treatment of hepatosplenic candidiasis
  - treatment of other candida infections in persons unable to tolerate amphotericin B
  - treatment of cryptococcal infections
  - secondary prophylaxis for cryptococcal meningitis in persons with AIDS
  - antifungal prophylaxis in allogeneic bone marrow transplant recipients
- Mechanism of action
  - interferes with cytochrome P-450 activity, decreasing ergosterol synthesis (principal sterol in fungal cell membrane) and inhibiting cell membrane formation
- Dosing
  - the daily dose of fluconazole is the same for oral and IV administration
  - oral fluconazole should be used in persons able to tolerate oral medications
  - parenteral fluconazole should be reserved for patients who are both unable to take oral medications and unable to tolerate amphotericin B
  - a small number of patients from 3–13 yrs of age have been treated with fluconazole using doses of 3–6 mg/kg/d once daily
    - doses as high as 12 mg/kg/d once daily have been used to treat candidiasis in immunocompromised children
    - prophylactic doses of 10–12 mg/kg/d have been used against fungal infections in pediatric bone marrow transplant patients
  - adults: oral, IV
    - oropharyngeal candidiasis: 200 mg once, then 100 mg daily for a minimum of 14 days
    - esophageal candidiasis: 200 mg once, then 100 mg daily for a minimum of 21 days
    - systemic candidiasis: 400 mg once, then 200 mg daily for a minimum of 28 days
    - cryptococcal meningitis
      - (acute): 400 mg once, then 200 mg daily for a minimum 10–12 wks after CSF culture becomes negative
      - (relapse): 200 mg daily for 10–12 wks after CSF culture becomes negative
  - dosing adjustment/interval in renal impairment
    - Clcr 21–50 ml/min: administer 50% of recommended dose or administer q48hrs
    - Clcr <20 ml/min: administer 25% of recommended dose or administer q72hrs
    - hemodialysis: 50% removed by hemodialysis
- Pharmacokinetics
  - distribution: relative diffusion of antimicrobial agents from blood into CSF
  - adequate with or without inflammation (exceeds usual MICs)
  - ratio of CSF to blood level (%)
    - normal meninges: 70–80
    - inflamed meninges: >70–80
  - protein binding, plasma: 11–12%
  - bioavailability: oral: >90%
  - half-life: 25–30 hrs with normal renal function
  - time to peak serum concentration: oral: within 2–4 hrs
  - elimination: 80% of a dose excreted unchanged in the urine
- Adverse reactions
  - CNS: headache, dizziness
  - dermatologic: rash
  - gastrointestinal: nausea, vomiting, abdominal pain, diarrhea
  - cardiovascular: pallor
  - endocrine and metabolic: hypokalemia
  - hepatic: elevated AST, ALT, or alkaline phosphatase
- Pharmacy issues
  - should be used with caution in patients with renal and hepatic dysfunction or previous hepatotoxicity from other azole derivatives
  - patients who develop abnormal liver function tests during fluconazole therapy should be monitored closely and discontinued if symptoms consistent with liver disease develop
  - drug interactions: cytochrome P-450 3A4 enzyme inhibitor and cytochrome P-450 2C enzyme inhibitor
  - decreased effect: rifampin decreases concentrations of fluconazole; fluconazole may decrease the effect of oral contraceptives
  - increased toxicity: may increase cyclosporine levels when high doses used
  - may increase phenytoin serum concentration
  - fluconazole may also inhibit warfarin metabolism
  - infuse over 1–2 hrs; do not exceed 200 mg/hr
  - may take with food; consider an alternative method of contraception if taking concurrently with birth control pills
- Nursing considerations
  - incidence of adverse reactions appears to be greater in HIV-infected patients
  - liver functions should be monitored during therapy

- if rash develops monitor closely, and if lesions progress notify physician

DRUG: ITRACONAZOLE

- Other name: Sporanox
- Uses
  - treatment of susceptible fungal infections in immunocompromised and immunocompetent patients including blastomycosis and histoplasmosis
  - indicated for aspergillosis and onychomycosis of the toenail
  - activity against *Aspergillus, Candida, Coccidioides, Cryptococcus, Sporoathrix, Tinea unguium*
  - oral solution is marketed for oral and esophageal candidiasis
  - unlabeled uses
    - □ superficial mycoses including dermatophytoses (e.g., *Tinea capitis*), pityriasis versicolor, sebopsoriasis
    - □ vaginal and chronic mucocutaneous candidiasis
    - □ systemic mycoses including candidiasis, meningeal and disseminated crptococcal infections, paracoccidioidomycosis, coccidioidomycoses
    - □ miscellaneous mycoses such as sporotrichosis, chromomycosis, leishmaniasis, fungal keratitis, alternariosis, zygomycosis
- Dosing
  - oral (absorption) requires an acid medium
    - □ best to administer itraconazole after meals
    - □ children: efficacy and safety have not been established
    - □ small number of patients 3–16 yrs of age have been treated with 100 mg/d for systemic fungal infections with no serious adverse effects
  - adults: 200 mg once daily
  - if no obvious improvement or there is evidence of progressive fungal disease
    - □ increase the dose in 100 mg increments to a maximum of 400 mg/d
    - □ doses > 200 mg/d are given in 2 divided doses
    - □ length of therapy varies from 1 day to > 6 mos depending on the condition and mycologic response
  - life-threatening infections: loading dose: 200 mg 3 times/d (600 mg/d) for the first 3 days of therapy
  - dosing adjustment in renal impairment: not necessary
  - hemodialysis: not dialyzable
  - dosing adjustment in hepatic impairment: may be necessary, but specific guidelines are not available
  - administration doses > 200 mg/d are given in 2 divided doses; do not administer with antacids
- Pharmacokinetics
  - absorption: enhanced by food and requires gastric acidity
  - distribution: apparent volume averaged 796 + 185 L or 10 L/kg
  - highly lipophilic and tissue concentrations are higher than plasma concentrations
  - the highest itraconazole concentrations are achieved in adipose
    - □ omentum
    - □ endometrium
    - □ cervical and vaginal mucus
    - □ skin/nails
  - aqueous fluids, such as cerebrospinal fluid and urine, contain negligible amounts
  - steady-state concentrations are achieved in 13 days with multiple administrations 100–400 mg/d
  - protein binding: 99.9% bound to plasma proteins
    - □ metabolite hydroxy-itraconazole is 99.5% bound to plasma protein
  - metabolism: extensive by the liver into > 30 metabolites
    - □ hydroxy-itraconazole the major metabolite has in vitro antifungal activity
    - □ the main metabolic pathway is oxidation
    - □ may undergo saturation metabolism with multiple dosing
  - bioavailability: increased from 40% fasting to 100% postprandial
  - absolute oral bioavailability: 55%
  - hypochlorhydria has been reported in HIV-infected patients
    - □ oral absorption in these patients may be decreased
  - half-life: after single 200 mg dose: 21 ± 5 hrs
  - elimination: ~ 3–18% excreted in feces; ~ 0.03% of parent drug excreted renally, and 40% of dose excreted as inactive metabolites in urine
- Adverse reactions
  - gastrointestinal: nausea, abdominal pain, vomiting, diarrhea, anorexia
  - CNS: headache, fatigue, fever, malaise, dizziness, somnolence
  - dermatologic: rash, pruritus
  - cardiovascular: edema, hypertension
  - endocrine and metabolic: hypokalemia, decreased libido
  - hepatic: abnormal hepatic function
  - renal: albuminuria
- Drug interactions
  - inhibitor of cytochrome P-450 2C and cytochrome P-450 3A enzymes
  - decreased effect
    - □ decreased serum levels with isoniazid and phenytoin
    - □ may cause a decreased effect of oral contraceptives; alternative birth control is recommended
    - □ decreased/undetectable serum levels with rifampin—should not be administered concomitantly with rifampin
  - absorption requires gastric acidity
    - □ antacids, H2 antagonists (cimetidine, ranitidine, and famotidine), omeprazole and lansoprazole, and sucralfate significantly reduce bioavailability resulting in treatment failures and should not be administered concomitantly
    - □ amphotericin B or fluconazole should be used instead
  - increased effect
    - □ may increase cyclosporine levels (by 50%) when high doses are used
    - □ itraconazole increases lovastatin levels (possibly 20-fold) due to inhibition of CYP3A4
    - □ may increase phenytoin serum concentration
    - □ may inhibit warfarin metabolism
    - □ may increase digoxin serum levels
    - □ may increase terfenadine levels—concomitant administration is not recommended
- Pharmacy issues
  - doses > 200 mg/d are given in 2 divided doses; do not administer with antacids
  - manufacturer states the solution is 60% more bioavailable than the capsule
- Nursing considerations
  - take with food
  - report any signs and symptoms that may suggest liver dysfunction so the appropriate laboratory testing can be done
  - signs and symptoms may include unusual fatigue, anorexia, nausea and/or vomiting, jaundice, dark urine, or pale stool
  - liver functions baseline and during therapy should be obtained
  - assess patient for symptoms that may indicate reactivation of histoplasmosis

DRUG: AZTREONAM

- Other name: Azactam
- Uses
  - treatment of patients with documented aerobic gram-negative bacillary infection in which beta-lactam therapy is contraindicated (e.g., penicillin or cephalosporin allergy)
  - urinary tract infections
  - lower respiratory tract infections
  - septicemia
  - skin/skin structure infections
  - intra-abdominal infections
  - multiple-drug regimen for the empiric treatment of neutropenic fever in persons with a history of beta-lactam allergy or with known multidrug-resistant organisms
- Mechanism of action
  - monobactam, which is active only against gram-negative bacilli (unlikely cross-allergenicity with other beta-lactams)

- inhibits bacterial cell wall synthesis during active multiplication, causing cell wall destruction

- ■ Dosing
  - children > 1 month: IM, IV: 90–120 mg/kg/d divided q6–8hrs
    - □ maximum: 6–8 g/d
  - adults
    - □ urinary tract infection: IM, IV: 500 mg–1 g q8–12hrs
    - □ moderately severe systemic infections: 1 g IV or IM or 2 g IV q8–12hrs
    - □ severe systemic or life-threatening infections (especially caused by *Pseudomonas aeruginosa*): IV: 2 g q6–8hrs; maximum: 8 g/d
  - dosing adjustment in renal impairment
    - □ Clcr 30–50 ml/min: administer q12hrs
    - □ Clcr 10–30 ml/min: administer q24hrs
    - □ Clcr < 10 ml/min: administer q48hrs
  - hemodialysis: moderately dialyzable (20–50%); administer dose postdialysis or supplemental dose of 500 mg after dialysis
  - peritoneal dialysis: administer as for Clcr < 10 ml/min
  - continuous arteriovenous or venovenous hemofiltration (CAVH/CAVHD)
    - □ removes 50 mg of aztreonam per liter of filtrate per day
- ■ Pharmacokinetics
  - absorption: IM: well absorbed; IM and IV doses produce comparable serum concentration
  - distribution: relative diffusion of antimicrobial agents from blood into CSF
    - □ good only with inflammation (exceeds usual MICs)
    - □ ratio of CSF to blood level (%)
      - ▽ inflamed meninges: 8–40
      - ▽ normal meninges: ~1
  - volume of distribution
    - □ children: 0.2–0.29 L/kg
    - □ adults: 0.2 L/kg
  - protein binding: 56%
  - metabolism: partial
  - half-life
    - □ children 2 mos–12 yrs: 1.7 hrs
    - □ normal renal function: 1.7–2.9 hrs
    - □ end-stage renal disease: 6–8 hrs
  - time to peak: within 60 min (IM, IV push) and 90 min (IV infusion)
  - elimination: 60–70% excreted unchanged in urine and partially in feces
- ■ Adverse reactions
  - dermatologic: rash
  - gastrointestinal: diarrhea, nausea, vomiting, pseudomembranous colitis, abnormal taste, numb tongue
  - local: thrombophlebitis, pain at injection site
  - cardiovascular: hypotension
  - CNS: seizures, confusion, headache, vertigo, insomnia, dizziness, fever, diplopia, tinnitus
  - genitourinary: vaginitis
  - hepatic: hepatitis, jaundice, elevation of liver enzymes
  - hematologic: thrombocytopenia, eosinophilia, leukopenia, neutropenia
  - neuromuscular and skeletal: myalgia, weakness
  - miscellaneous: anaphylaxis
- ■ Pharmacy issues
  - administer by IVP over 3–5 min or by intermittent infusion over 20–60 min at a final concentration not to exceed 20 mg/ml
  - administer around the clock rather than 3 times/d to promote less variation in peak and trough serum levels
  - symptoms of overdose include seizures; if necessary, dialysis can reduce the drug concentration in the blood
  - monitor periodic liver function test
- ■ Nursing considerations
  - test interaction with urine glucose (Clinitest)
  - assess patient for allergies to penicillins or cephalosporins
  - anticipate dose reduction in patients with renal dysfunction
  - teach patient may experience alterations in taste during therapy; report if eating is impaired

DRUG: ACYCLOVIR

- ■ Other name: Zovirax
- ■ Uses
  - antiviral agent, used in treatment of initial and prophylaxis of recurrent mucosal and cutaneous herpes simplex (HSV-1 and HSV-2) infections
  - herpes simplex encephalitis
  - herpes zoster
    - □ acyclovir should be started within 72 hrs of the appearance of the rash to be effective
    - □ will not prevent postherpetic neuralgias
  - varicella-zoster infections in healthy, nonpregnant persons > 13 yrs of age, children > 12 mos of age who have a chronic skin or lung disorder or are receiving long-term aspirin therapy
  - immunocompromised patients
- ■ Mechanism of action
  - inhibits DNA synthesis and viral replication by competing with deoxyguanosine triphosphate for viral DNA polymerase and being incorporated into viral DNA
- ■ Dosing
  - dosing weight should be based on the smaller of lean body weight or total body weight
    - □ adult determination of lean body weight (LBW) in kg
      - ▽ LBW males: 50 kg + (2.3 kg × inches > 5 feet)
      - ▽ LBW females: 45 kg + (2.3kg × inches > 5 feet)
  - treatment of herpes simplex virus infections
    - □ children and adults: IV
      - ▽ mucocutaneous HSV infection: 750 $mg/m^2/d$ divided q8hrs or 5 mg/kg/dose q8hrs for 5–10 days
      - ▽ HSV encephalitis: 1,500 $mg/m^2/d$ divided q8hrs for 5–10 days
    - □ adults: oral
      - ▽ treatment of herpes simplex virus infections: 200 mg q4hrs while awake (5 times/d)
  - treatment of varicella-zoster virus (chicken pox) infections
    - □ oral
      - ▽ children: 10–20 mg/kg/dose (up to 800 mg) 4 times/d for 5 days; begin treatment within the first 24 hrs of rash onset
      - ▽ adults: 600–800 mg/dose q4hrs while awake (5 times/d) for 7–10 days or 1,000 mg q6hrs for 5 days
    - □ IV
      - ▽ children and adults: 1,500 $mg/m^2/d$ divided q8hrs or 10 mg/kg/dose q8hrs for 7 days
  - treatment of herpes zoster infections
    - □ oral
      - ▽ children (immunocompromised): 250–600 mg/m^2/dose 4–5 times/d for 7–10 days
      - ▽ adults (immunocompromised): 800 mg q4hrs (5 times/d) for 7–10 days
    - □ IV
      - ▽ children and adults (immunocompromised): 10–12 mg/kg/dose q8hrs
      - ▽ older adults (immunocompromised): 7.5 mg/kg/dose q8hrs; if nephrotoxicity occurs: 5 mg/kg/dose q8hrs
  - prophylaxis in immunocompromised patients
      - ▽ varicella zoster or herpes zoster in HIV-positive patients: adults: oral: 400 mg q4hrs (5 times/d) for 7–10 days
      - ▽ bone marrow transplant recipients: adults: 200 mg po tid or 2 mg/kg IV bid
      - ▽ autologous/allogeneic patients who are HSV seropositive: 150 mg/m^2/dose (5 mg/kg) q12hrs; with clinical symptoms of herpes simplex: 150 mg/m^2/dose q8hrs
      - ▽ autologous/allogeneic patients who are CMV seropositive: 500 mg/m^2/dose (10 mg/kg) q8hrs; for clinically symptomatic CMV infection, replace acyclovir with ganciclovir
  - prophylaxis of herpes simplex virus infections: adults: 200 mg 3–4 times/d or 400 mg twice daily
  - dosing adjustment in renal impairment
    - □ oral: HSV/varicella-zoster
      - ▽ Clcr 10–25 ml/min: administer dose q8hrs

- ▽ Clcr < 10 ml/min: administer dose q12hrs
- □ IV
  - ▽ Clcr 25–50 ml/min: 5–10 mg/kg/dose: administer q12hrs
  - ▽ Clcr 10–25 ml/min: 5–10 mg/kg/dose: administer q24hrs
  - ▽ Clcr < 10 ml/min: 2.5–5 mg/kg/dose: administer q24hrs
  - ▽ hemodialysis: dialyzable (50–100%): administer dose post-dialysis
  - ▽ peritoneal dialysis: dose as for Clcr < 10 ml/min
  - ▽ continuous arteriovenous or venovenous hemofiltration (CAVH/CAVHD) effects: dose as for Clcr < 10 ml/min

- ■ Pharmacokinetics
  - absorption: oral: 15–30%; food does not appear to affect absorption
  - distribution: widely distributed throughout the body including brain, kidney, lungs, liver, spleen, muscle, uterus, vagina, and CSF
  - protein binding: < 30%
  - metabolism: small amount of hepatic metabolism
  - half-life, terminal phase
    - □ neonates: 4 hrs
    - □ children 1–12 yrs: 2–3 hrs
    - □ adults: 3 hrs
  - time to peak serum concentration
    - □ oral: within 1.5–2 hrs
    - □ IV: within 1 hr
  - elimination: primary route is the kidney (30–90% of a dose excreted unchanged); hemodialysis removes ~60% of the dose while removal by peritoneal dialysis is to a much lesser extent (supplemental dose recommended)
- ■ Adverse reactions
  - CNS: headache, lethargy, dizziness, seizures, confusion, agitation, mental depression, insomnia, coma
  - local: inflammation at injection site
  - dermatologic: rash
  - gastrointestinal: nausea, vomiting
  - neuromuscular and skeletal: tremor
  - renal: impaired renal function, crystalluria
  - gastrointestinal: anorexia
  - hepatic: LFT elevation
- ■ Pharmacy issues
  - infuse over 1 hr; maintain adequate hydration of patient
  - use with caution in patients with preexisting renal disease or in those receiving other nephrotoxic drugs concurrently
  - maintain adequate urine output during the first 2 hrs after IV infusion
  - use with caution in patients with underlying neurologic abnormalities, serious hepatic or electrolyte abnormalities, or substantial hypoxia
  - drug interactions: increased CNS side effects with zidovudine and probenecid
- ■ Nursing considerations
  - patients should be encouraged to drink 2–3 L of fluids (especially during parenteral therapy), to prevent renal toxicity and crystalluria
  - teach patient to report burning, stinging, itching, and rash

DRUG: VALACYCLOVIR HYDROCHLORIDE

- ■ Other name: Valtrex
- ■ Uses
  - indicated for the treatment of herpes zoster (shingles) and genital herpes
- ■ Mechanism of action
  - valacyclovir hydrochloride is rapidly converted to acyclovir
  - acyclovir's highest antiviral activity in cell culture is against HSV-1, followed in decreasing order of potency against HSV-2 and VZV
  - inhibitory activity of acyclovir is highly selective due to its affinity for the enzyme thymidine kinase (TK) encoded by HSV, VZV, and EBV
  - the greater antiviral activity of acyclovir against HSV compared to VZV is due to its more efficient phosphorylation by the viral TK
  - acyclovir stops replication of herpes viral DNA in three ways
    - □ competitive inhibition of viral DNA polymerase
    - □ incorporation and termination of the growing viral DNA chain
    - □ inactivation of the viral DNA polymerase
- ■ Dosing
  - herpes zoster: 1 g po 3 times a day for 7 days
    - □ initiate at the earliest sign or symptom of herpes zoster
    - □ most effective when started within 48 hrs of the onset of rash
  - genital herpes: initial episode: 1 g po 2 times a day for 10 days
    - □ recurrent episode: 500 mg po 2 times a day for 5 days
  - suppressive therapy: 1 g once daily
  - dose adjustment necessary for renal impairment
- ■ Pharmacokinetics
  - absorption: valacyclovir hydrochloride is rapidly absorbed from the gastrointestinal tract
  - bioavailabilty: 45.4–63.6% of valacyclovir is converted to acyclovir and L-valine by first-pass intestinal and/or hepatic metabolism
  - distribution: 13.5–17.9% bound to plasma proteins
  - half-life: 2.5–3.3 hrs
  - elimination: in urine and feces as acyclovir and inactive metobolites
- ■ Adverse reaction
  - gastrointestinal: nausea, vomiting, abdominal pain, diarrhea
  - CNS: headache, dizziness, confusion, agitation, hallucinations (auditory and visual), aggressive behavior, mania
  - dermatologic: rash, urticaria, pruritus, dysnea, angioedema, anaphylaxis
  - hematologic: anemia, leukopenia, thrombocytopenia, aplastic anemia
  - renal: elevated creatinine, renal failure
  - hepatic: elevated AST (SGOT)
  - general: facial edema, hypertension, tachycardia
- ■ Pharmacy issues
  - availability: oral tablets: 500 mg and 1 g
  - avoid overdosage because precipitaton of acyclovir in renal tubules may occur when the solubility (2.5 mg/ml) is exceeded in the intratubular fluid
  - may be given without regard to meals
  - hemodialysis: administer dose after dialysis (about one-third of acyclovir in body removed by a 4 hr dialysis period)
- ■ Nursing considerations
  - dose is likely to be reduced if creatinine clearance < 50 ml/min
  - teach patient to take medication exactly as prescribed

DRUG: GANCICLOVIR (DHPG SODIUM, GCV SODIUM, NOREOXYGUANOSINE)

- ■ Other names: Cytovene, Vitrasert
- ■ Uses
  - IV: treatment of CMV retinitis in immunocompromised individuals
    - □ patients with acquired immunodeficiency syndrome
  - treatment of CMV pneumonia in marrow transplant recipients and AIDS patients
  - prophylaxis and treatment in organ transplant recipients with CMV
    - □ colitis
    - □ pneumonitis
    - □ multiorgan involvement
    - □ bone marrow transplant patients when given in combination with IVIG or CMV hyperimmune globulin
  - oral: alternative to the IV formulation for maintenance treatment of CMV retinitis in immunocompromised patients
    - □ including patients with AIDS, in whom retinitis is stable following appropriate induction therapy
    - □ patients for whom the risk of more rapid progression is balanced by the benefit associated with avoiding daily IV infusions
- ■ Mechanism of action
  - ganciclovir is phosphorylated to a substrate that competitively inhibits the binding of deoxyguanosine triphosphate to DNA polymerase resulting in inhibition of viral DNA synthesis
- ■ Dosing
  - slow IV infusion (dosing is based on total body weight): children > 3 mos and adults

  - induction therapy: 5 mg/kg/dose q12hrs for 14–21 days followed by maintenance therapy
  - maintenance therapy: 5 mg/kg/d as a single daily dose for 7 days/wk or 6 mg/kg/d for 5 days/wk
- oral: 1,000 mg 3 times/d with food or 500 mg 6 times/d with food
- dosing adjustment in renal impairment
  - IV
    - Clcr 50–79 ml/min: administer 2.5 mg/kg/dose q12hrs
    - Clcr 25–49 ml/min: administer 2.5 mg/kg/dose q24hrs
    - Clcr < 25 ml/min: administer 1.25 mg/kg/dose q24hrs
  - Oral
    - Clcr 50–69 ml/min: administer 1,500 mg/d or 500 mg 3 times/d
    - Clcr 25–49 ml/min: administer 1,000 mg/d or 500 mg 2 times/d
    - Clcr 10–24 ml/min: administer 500 mg/d
    - Clcr < 10 ml/min: administer 500 mg 3 times/wk following hemodialysis
    - hemodialysis: (50%) dialyzable administer dose postdialysis
    - peritoneal dialysis: dose as for Clcr < 10 ml/min
    - continuous arteriovenous or venovenous hemofiltration (CAVH/CAVHD): administer 2.5 mg/kg/dose q24hrs

- Pharmacokinetics
  - absorption: oral: absolute bioavailability under fasting conditions: 5%; following food: 6–9%; following fatty meal: 28–31%
  - protein binding: 1–2%
  - half-life: 1.7–5.8 hrs; increases with impaired renal function
    - end-stage renal disease: 3.6 hrs
  - elimination: majority (94–99%) excreted as unchanged drug in the urine
- Adverse reactions
  - CNS: headache, confusion, fever, ataxia, dizziness, nervousness, psychosis, malaise
  - hematologic: granulocytopenia, thrombocytopenia, anemia, eosinophilia, hemorrhage
  - dermatologic: rash, alopecia, pruritis, urticaria
  - hepatic: abnormal liver function values
  - cardiovascular: arrhythmia, hypertension, hypotension, edema
  - gastrointestinal: nausea, vomiting, diarrhea, abdominal pain
  - local: inflammation or pain at injection site
  - neuromuscular and skeletal: paresthesia, tremor
  - respiratory: dyspnea
- Pharmacy issues
  - the same precautions utilized with antineoplastic agents should be followed with ganciclovir administration
  - ganciclovir should be administered by slow IV infusion over at least 1 hr at a final concentration not to exceed 10 mg/ml
  - oral ganciclovir should be administered with food to inhance absorption
  - symptoms of overdose include neutropenia, vomiting, hypersalivation, bloody diarrhea, cytopenia, testicular atrophy
  - must be prepared in vertical flow hood
    - use chemotherapy precautions during administration
    - discard appropriately
- Nursing considerations
  - use cautiously in patients with renal dysfunction
  - do not administer IM or SubQ
  - granulocytopenia major toxicity; should not be administered if neutrophil count drops $< 500/mm^3$ or platelet count is $< 25{,}000$
  - hydrate patient adequately before and during infusion
  - teach patient to report dizziness, confusion, and seizures

DRUG: FAMCICLOVIR

- Other name: Famvir
- Uses
  - management of acute herpes zoster (shingles)
  - treatment of recurrent herpes simplex in immunocompetent patients
  - has not been studied in immunocompromised patients or patients with ophthalmic or disseminated zoster
- Mechanism of action
  - must undergo rapid biotransformation to the active compound penciclovir in vivo
  - famciclovir is phosphorylated by viral thymidine kinase in HSV-1, HSV-2, and VZV-infected cells to a monophosphate form
  - converted penciclovir triphosphate competes with deoxyguanosine triphosphate to inhibit HSV-2 polymerase (i.e., herpes viral DNA synthesis/replication is selectively inhibited)
- Dosing
  - adults: oral
    - acute herpes zoster: 500 mg q8hrs for 7 days
    - recurrent herpes simplex in immunocompetent patients: 125 mg twice daily for 5 days
    - dosing interval in renal impairment
      - Clcr > 60 ml/min: administer 500 mg q8hrs
      - Clcr 40–59 ml/min: administer 500 mg q12hrs
      - Clcr 20–39 ml/min: administer 500 mg q24hrs
      - Clcr < 20 ml/min: unknown
- Pharmacokinetics
  - absorption: food decreases the maximum peak concentration and delays the time to peak
    - AUC remains the same
  - distribution: Vdss: 0.98–1.08 L/kg
  - protein binding: 20%
  - metabolism: rapidly deacetylated and oxidized to penciclovir (not by cytochrome P-450)
  - bioavailability: 77%; Tmax: 0.9 hrs
  - half-life: penciclovir: 2–3 hrs (10, 20, and 7 hrs in HSV-1, HSV-2, and VZV-infected cells)
    - linearly decreased with reductions in renal failure
  - elimination: $> 90\%$ of penciclovir is eliminated unchanged in urine
    - Cmax and Tmax are decreased and prolonged, respectively, in patients with noncompensated hepatic impairment
- Adverse reactions
  - CNS: headache, fatigue, fever, dizziness, somnolence
  - gastrointestinal: nausea, diarrhea, vomiting, constipation, anorexia, abdominal pain
  - neuromuscular and skeletal: rigors, paresthesia
- Pharmacy issues
  - initiate therapy as soon as herpes zoster is diagnosed
    - most effective if initiated within 72 hrs of initial lesion
  - may take medication with food or on an empty stomach
  - dosage adjustment is required in patients
    - with renal insufficiency (CrCl < 60 ml/min)
    - in patients with noncompensated hepatic disease
  - safety and efficacy have not been established in children < 18 yrs of age
  - animal studies indicated increases in incidence of carcinomas, mutagenic changes, and decreases in fertility with extremely large doses
- Nursing considerations
  - teach infection control measures that will prevent infection transmission to family members
  - report early symptoms of herpes infection such as tingling, itching, or pain

DRUG: FOSCARNET SODIUM

- Other names: Foscavir, PFA, phosphonoformate, phosphonoformic acid
- Uses
  - antiviral agent (parenteral)
  - FDA approved in adult patients
    - herpes virus infections suspected to be caused by acyclovir (HSV, VZV) resistant strains
    - Ganciclovir (CMV) resistant strains: this occurs almost exclusively in

immunocompromised persons (e.g., advanced AIDS), who have received prolonged treatment for a herpes virus infection
  - □ CMV retinitis in persons with AIDS
  - □ other CMV infections in persons unable to tolerate ganciclovir
- ■ Mechanism of action
  - pyrophosphate analogue, which acts as a noncompetitive inhibitor of many viral RNA and DNA polymerases as well as HIV reverse transcriptase
  - inhibitory effects occur at concentrations that do not affect host cellular DNA polymerases
    - □ some human cell growth suppression has been observed with high in vitro concentrations
  - similar to ganciclovir, foscarnet is a virostatic agent
  - foscarnet does not require activation by thymidine kinase
- ■ Dosing
  - adolescents and adults: IV
    - □ CMV retinitis
      - ▽ induction treatment: 60 mg/kg/dose q8hrs for 14–21 days
      - ▽ maintenance therapy: 90–120 mg/kg/d as a single infusion
    - □ acyclovir-resistant HSV induction treatment: 40 mg/kg/dose q8–12hrs for 14–21 days
- ■ Pharmacokinetics
  - absorption: oral: poorly absorbed; IV therapy is needed for the treatment of viral infections in AIDS patients
  - distribution: up to 28% of cumulative IV dose may be deposited in bone
  - metabolism: biotransformation does not occur
  - half-life: ~3 hrs
  - elimination: up to 80–90% excreted unchanged in urine
- ■ Adverse reactions
  - CNS: fever, headache, seizures, fatigue, malaise, dizziness, hypoesthesia, depression, confusion, anxiety
  - gastrointestinal: nausea, diarrhea, vomiting, anorexia
  - hematologic: anemia, granulocytopenia, leukopenia
  - renal: abnormal renal function, decreased creatinine clearance
  - dermatologic: rash
  - endocrine and metabolic: electrolyte imbalance
  - local: injection site pain
  - neuromuscular and skeletal: paresthesia, involuntary muscle contractions, rigors, neuropathy (peripheral), weakness
  - ocular: vision abnormalities
  - respiratory: coughing, dyspnea
  - miscellaneous: sepsis, diaphoresis (increased)
  - cardiovascular: cardiac failure, bradycardia, arrhythmias, cerebral edema, leg edema, peripheral edema, syncope, substernal chest pain
- ■ Pharmacy issues
  - foscarnet should be diluted in D_5W or NS and transferred to PVC containers; stable for 24 hrs at room temperature or refrigeration
  - for peripheral line administration, foscarnet must be diluted to 12 mg/ml
  - for central line administration, foscarnet may be administered undiluted
  - incompatible with dextrose 30%, IV solutions containing calcium, magnesium, vancomycin, TPN
  - renal impairment occurs to some degree in the majority of patients treated with foscarnet
    - □ renal impairment may occur at any time and is usually reversible within 1 wk following dose adjustment or discontinuation of therapy
    - □ several patients have died with renal failure within 4 wks of stopping foscarnet
    - □ renal function should be closely monitored
  - foscarnet is deposited in teeth and bone of young growing animals
    - □ adversely affected tooth enamel development in rats
    - □ safety and effectiveness in children have not been studied
  - imbalance of serum electrolytes or minerals occurs in 6–18% of patients (hypocalcemia, low ionized calcium, hypo- or hyerphosphatemia, hypomagnesemia or hypokalemia)
  - seizures have been experienced by up to 10% of AIDS patients
    - □ risk factors for seizures include a low baseline ANC
    - □ impaired baseline renal function
    - □ low total serum calcium
- ■ Nursing considerations
  - some degree of nephrotoxicity occurs
    - □ use cautiously in patients with renal dysfunction; toxicity may be enhanced
  - dose must be individualized according to renal function
  - hydrate patient adequately before and during infusion
  - evaluate electrolyte values and creatinine clearance prior to initiation of therapy
    - □ obtain 2–3 times/wk during induction therapy and at least once q1–2wks during maintenance
  - assess patient for tetany and seizures associated with electrolyte imbalance
  - teach patient to report perioral tingling, numbness, and paresthesia

DRUG: TRIMETHOPRIM-SULFAMETHOXAZOLE, CO-TRIMOXAZOLE

- ■ Other names: Bactrim, Septra, Cotrim, Sulfatrim
- ■ Uses
  - oral
    - □ oral treatment of urinary tract infections due to *E. coli,* Klebsiella, and enterobacter sp, *M. morganii, P. mirabilis,* and *P. vulgaris*
    - □ prophylaxis of pneumocystis carinii pneumonia (PCP)
  - IV
    - □ treatment of severe or complicated infections when oral therapy is not feasible
    - □ documented PCP
    - □ empiric treatment of PCP in immunocompromised patients
    - □ treatment of documented or suspected shigellosis, Nocardia asteroides infection, or other infections caused by susceptible bacteria
- ■ Mechanism of action
  - sulfamethoxazole interferes with bacterial folic acid synthesis and growth via inhibition of dihydrofolic acid formation from para-aminobenzoic acid
  - trimethoprim inhibits dihydrofolic acid reduction to tetrahydrofolate resulting in sequential inhibition of enzymes of the folic acid pathway
  - co-trimoxazole is usually bactericidal
- ■ Dosing
  - dosage recommendations are based on the trimethoprim component
  - available in oral or parenteral form
  - UTI/chronic bronchitis (adults): oral 1 double-strength tablet q12hrs for 10–14 days
  - sepsis: IV 20 mg TMP/kg/d divided q6hrs
  - pneumocystis carinii: prophylaxis: oral, IV: 10 mg TMP/kg/d divided q12hrs for 3 days/wk
    - □ treatment: IV: 20 mg TMP/kg/d divided q6hrs
  - dosing interval/adjustment recommended in renal failure
- ■ Pharmacokinetics
  - absorption: oral 90–100%
  - distribution: crosses the placenta; distributes into breast milk
  - protein binding: SMX 68%, TMP 68%
  - metabolism: SMX is N-acetylated and glucuronidated, TMP is metabolized to oxide and hydroxylated to metabolites
  - half-life: SMX 9 hrs, TMP 6–17 hrs
  - time to peak concentrations: within 1–4 hrs
  - elimination: in urine as metabolites and unchanged drug
- ■ Adverse reactions
  - dermatologic: allergic skin reactions including rashes and urticaria, photosensitivity, Stevens-Johnson syndrome, toxic epidermal necrolysis, erythema multiforme
  - gastrointestinal: nausea, vomiting, anorexia, stomatitis, diarrhea, pseudomembranous colitis
  - hematologic: blood dyscrasias, thrombocytopenia, megaloblastic anemia, granu-

locytopenia, aplastic anemia, hemolysis (with G-6-PD deficiency)
- hepatic: hepatitis
- CNS: confusion, depression, hallucinations, seizures, fever, ataxia, kernicterus in neonates
- renal: interstitial nephritis
- miscellaneous: serum sickness

■ Pharmacy issues
- infuse over 60–90 min
- must be diluted prior to administration. May be given 5 ml/50 ml in D_5W or NS through central line
- maintain adequate fluid intake to prevent crystalluria
- co-trimoxazole causes
  - □ decreased effect: cyclosporines
  - □ increased effect: sulfonylureas and oral anticoagulants
  - □ increased toxicity: phenytoin, cyclosporines (nephrotoxicity), methotrexate (displaced from binding sites)

■ Nursing considerations
- do not refrigerate
- do not mix with other drugs
- drug should never be administered IM
- use cautiously in patients with impaired hepatic or renal function
- anticipate reduced dose with renal dysfunction
- assess
  - □ hypersensitivity reactions, rash, and fevers can occur; seen more frequently in AIDS patients
  - □ leukopenia and granulocytopenia
  - □ megaloblastic anemia due to folate deficiency is a contraindication because drug inhibits ability to produce folinic acid
- baseline lab data prior to administration
  - □ evaluate cultures
  - □ liver and renal function
- patient information
  - □ take oral medicine with 8 oz water on an empty stomach 1 hr before or 2 hrs after meals
  - □ report any skin rashes immediately
  - □ finish all medication
  - □ do not skip doses

DRUG: DAPSONE

■ Other name: Avlosulfon

■ Uses
- treatment of leprosy and dermatitis herpetiformis (infections caused by mycobacterium leprae)
- alternative agent for pneumocystis carinii pneumonia (PCP) prophylaxis (given alone)
- treatment for PCP (given with trimethoprim)

■ Mechanism of action
- dapsone is a sulfone antimicrobial
- usually bacteriostatic in action
- mechanism of action of the sulfones is similar to that of the sulfonamides
- sulfonamides are competitive antagonists of para-aminobenzoic acid (PABA) and prevent normal bacterial utilization of PABA for the synthesis of folic acid

■ Dosing
- available in 25 mg and 100 mg oral tablets
- prophylaxis of PCP: children > 1 mo: 1 mg/kg/d; maximum: 100 mg
- treatment of PCP: adults: 100 mg/d in combination with trimethoprim (20 mg/kg/d) for 21 days
- dosing adjustment in renal failure is recommended

■ Pharmacokinetics
- absorption: oral: well absorbed from the GI tract
  - □ trace amounts may be found in serum for 8–12 days after oral administration of a single 200 mg dose
- distribution: 1.5 L/kg; throughout total body water and present in all tissues, especially liver and kidney
- protein binding: 50–90% bound to plasma proteins
  - □ the major metabolite of dapsone, monoacetyldapsone, is almost completely bound to plasma proteins
- metabolism: dapsone is acetylated in the liver to monoacetyldapsone (MADDS)
  - □ also is hydroxylated in the liver to hydroxylamine dapsone (NOH-DDS)
  - □ NOH-DDS appears to be responsible for methemoglobinemia and hemolysis induced by the drug
- half-life: may range from 10–83 hrs and averages 20–30 hrs
- time to peak concentrations: within 2–8 hrs
- elimination: in urine as metabolites 70–85% and unchanged drug 20% and small amount in feces

■ Adverse reactions
- CNS: reactional states, insomnia, headache, blurred vision, tinnitus
- hematologic: dose-related hemolysis, methemoglobinemia with cyanosis, hemolytic anemia, methemoglobinemia, leukopenia, agranulocytosis
- dermatologic: exfoliative dermatitis
- gastrointestinal: nausea, vomiting
- hepatic: hepatitis, cholestatic jaundice
- neuromuscular and skeletal: peripheral neuropathy

■ Pharmacy issues
- monitor patient for signs of jaundice and hemolysis
- cytochrome P-450 3A enzyme substrate
- decreased effect/levels: para-aminobenzoic acid and rifampin
- increased toxicity: folic acid antagonists

■ Nursing considerations
- use cautiously in patients with chronic renal, hepatic, CV disease, and refractory types of anemia
- CBC should be monitored weekly for the first month and then monthly for 6 mos; semiannually thereafter
- anticipate reduced dose or temporary discontinuation if hemoglobin falls below 9, if WBC below 5,000, or RBC below 2.5 or remains low
- administer antihistamines as ordered to combat dapsone-induced allergic dermatitis
- assess baseline lab data prior to administration
- teach patient to take medication exactly as ordered
- report allergic dermatitis
  - □ usually appears before week 10 of therapy
  - □ possibility of developing into fatal exfoliative dermatitis
- patient information
  - □ frequent blood tests are required during early therapy
  - □ discontinue if rash develops
  - □ contact physician if persistent sore throat, fever, malaise, or fatigue occurs
  - □ may cause photosensitivity

DRUG: IMMUNE GLOBULIN (IVIG)

■ Other names: Gamimune N; Gammagard; Gammagard S/D; Gammar-P IV; Polygam; Polygam S/D; Sandoglobulin; Venoglobulin-I; Venoglobulin-S

■ Uses
- treatment of immunodeficiency sufficiency (hypogammaglobulinemia, agammaglobulinemia)
- IgG subclass deficiencies
  - □ severe combined immunodeficiency syndromes (SCIDS)
  - □ Wiskott-Aldrich syndrome
  - □ idiopathic thrombocytopenic purpura
- in conjunction with appropriate anti-infective therapy to prevent or modify acute bacterial or viral infections in patients with iatrogenically induced or disease-associated immunosuppression
  - □ chronic lymphocytic leukemia (CLL): chronic prophylaxis autoimmune neutropenia
  - □ bone marrow transplantation patients
  - □ autoimmune hemolytic anemia or neutropenia
  - □ refractory dermatomyositis/polymyositis
  - □ autoimmune diseases (myasthenia gravis, SLE, bullous pemphigoid, severe rheumatoid arthritis)
  - □ Kawasaki disease, Guillain-Barré syndrome
- therapy should be guided by clinical observation and serial determination of serum IgG levels

- Mechanism of action
  - replacement therapy for primary and secondary immunodeficiencies
  - interference with Fc receptors on the cells of the reticuloendothelial system for autoimmune cytopenias and ITP; possible role of contained antiviral-type antibodies
- Dosing
  - children and adults: IV
    - □ dosages should be based on ideal body weight and not actual body weight in morbidly obese patients
  - primary immunodeficiency disorders: 200–400 mg/kg q4wks or as per monitored serum IgG concentrations
  - chronic lymphocytic leukemia (CLL): 400 mg/kg/dose q3wks
  - idiopathic thrombocytopenic purpura (ITP)
    - □ maintenance dose
      - ▽ 400 mg/kg/d for 5 consecutive days
      - ▽ 800 mg/kg/d for 2 consecutive days
    - □ chronic ITP: 400–1,000 mg/kg/dose every 7 or 14 days
    - □ Kawasaki disease
      - ▽ 400 mg/kg/d for 4 days within 10 days of onset of fever
      - ▽ 800 mg/kg/d for 1–2 days within 10 days of onset of fever
      - ▽ 2 g/kg for one dose only
    - □ acquired immunodeficiency syndrome (patients must be symptomatic)
      - ▽ 200–250 mg/kg/dose q2wks
      - ▽ 400–500 mg/kg/dose every month or q4wks
    - □ autoimmune hemolytic anemia and neutropenia: 1,000 mg/kg/dose for 2–3 days
    - □ autoimmune diseases: 400 mg/kg/d for 4 days
    - □ postallogeneic bone marrow transplant: 500 mg/kg/wk for 4 mos post transplant
    - □ adjuvant to severe cytomegalovirus infections: 500 mg/kg/dose every other day for 7 doses
    - □ severe systemic viral and bacterial infections: children: 500–1,000 mg/kg/week
    - □ Guillain-Barré syndrome
      - ▽ 400 mg/kg/d for 4 days
      - ▽ 1,000 mg/kg/d for 2 days
      - ▽ 2,000 mg/kg/d for 1 day
    - □ dosing adjustment/comments in renal impairment: Clcr < 10 ml/min: avoid use
- Pharmacokinetics
  - IV provides immediate antibody level
  - half-life: 21–24 days
- Adverse reactions
  - cardiovascular: flushing of the face, tachycardia, hypotension, tightness in the chest
  - CNS: chills, dizziness, fever, headache
  - gastrointestinal: nausea
  - respiratory: dyspnea
  - miscellaneous: diaphoresis, hypersensitivity reactions
- Pharmacy issues
  - administration IV use only
    - □ initial treatment
      - ▽ lower concentration and/or a slower rate of infusion should be used
    - □ administer through separate lumen
      - ▽ should not be mixed with other drugs or blood products
  - stability and dilution dependent on the manufacturer and brand
  - increased toxicity with live virus, vaccines (measles, mumps, rubella)
    - □ do not administer within 3 mos after administration of these vaccines
  - anaphylactic hypersensitivity reactions can occur, especially in IgA-deficient patients
    - □ studies indicate that the currently available products have no discernible risk of transmitting HIV or hepatitis B
- Nursing considerations
  - possibility of anaphylaxis; epinephrine 1:1,000 should be available
  - monitor vital signs during infusion; hypotension will subside if rate of infusion is decreased or interrupted
  - assess
    - □ history of allergies and reaction to immunizations
    - □ past history of idiopathic thrombocytopenia purpura (ITP); these patients require close hematologic monitoring
    - □ inform patient to report side effects of nausea/vomiting, fevers, chills, flushing, lightheadedness, and tightness of chest; these may be related to the dosage or rate of infusion

DRUG: FILGRASTIM, G-CSF; GRANULOCYTE COLONY STIMULATING FACTOR

- Other name: Neupogen
- Uses
  - indicated to decrease the incidence of infection, as manifested by febrile neutropenia
  - FDA approved
    - □ patients with nonmyeloid malignancies receiving myelosuppressive anticancer drugs associated with a significant incidence of neutropenia
    - □ cancer patients receiving bone marrow transplant (BMT)
    - □ patients with severe chronic neutropenia (SCN)
    - □ patients undergoing peripheral blood progenitor cell (PBPC) collection
- Mechanism of action
  - stimulates the production, maturation, and activation of neutrophils
  - G-CSF activates neutrophils to increase both their migration and cytotoxicity
- Dosing
  - dosage should be based on actual body weight (even in morbidly obese patients)
  - existing clinical data suggest that starting G-CSF between 24 and 72 hrs subsequent to chemotherapy may provide optimal neutrophil recovery
  - continue therapy until the occurrence of an absolute neutrophil count of 1,500 to 10,000/mm^3 after the neutrophil nadir
  - myelosuppressive chemotherapy SubQ injection 5 mcg/kg/d
  - doses may be increased in increments of 5 mcg/kg for each chemotherapy cycle, according to the duration and severity of the absolute neutrophil count (ANC) nadir
- Pharmacokinetics
  - onset of action: rapid elevation in neutrophil counts within the first 24 hrs, reaching a plateau in 3–5 days
  - duration: ANC decreases by 50% within 2 days after discontinuing G-CSF
    - □ white count returns to normal range in 4–7 days
  - absorption: SubQ 100% absorbed
    - □ peak plasma levels can be maintained for up to 12 hrs
  - distribution: Vd: 150 ml/kg
    - □ no evidence of drug accumulation over an 11–20 day period
  - metabolism: systemically metabolized
  - bioavailability: oral: not bioavailable
  - half-life: 1.8–3.5 hrs
  - time to peak serum concentration: SubQ: 2–6 hrs
- Adverse reactions
  - effects are generally mild and dose related
    - □ CNS: neutropenic fever, headache, fever
    - □ dermatologic: alopecia, skin rash
    - □ gastrointestinal: nausea, vomiting, diarrhea, mucositis, anorexia, constipation
    - □ splenomegaly more common in patients with cyclic neutropenia/congenital agranulocytosis who received SubQ injections for a prolonged (> 14 days) period of time
      - ▽ ~33% of these patients experience subclinical splenomegaly (detected by MRI or CT scan)
      - ▽ ~3% of these patients experience clinical splenomegaly
    - □ neuromuscular and skeletal: medullary bone pain (24% incidence)
      - ▽ most commonly occurs in lower back, posterior iliac crest, and sternum
      - ▽ controlled with non-narcotic analgesic
    - □ cardiovascular: chest pain, fluid retention, transient supraventricular arrhythmia, pericarditis
    - □ hematologic: leukocytosis
    - □ local: pain at injection site
    - □ neuromuscular and skeletal: weakness
    - □ respiratory: dyspnea, cough, sore throat

- □ miscellaneous: anaphylactic reaction

- ■ Pharmacy issues
  - do not give to patients with known hypersensitivy to *E. coli*–derived proteins or G-CSF
  - filgrastim is a clear, colorless solution
    - □ stored under refrigeration at 2–8° C (36–46° F)
    - □ protect from direct sunlight
    - □ protect from freezing and temperatures > 30° C to avoid aggregation
  - the solution should not be shaken, since bubbles and/or foam may form
    - □ if foaming occurs, the solution should be left undisturbed for a few min until bubbles dissipate
  - filgrastim is stable for 24 hrs at 9–30° C
  - the product is packaged as single-use vial without a preservative
  - undiluted filgrastim is stable for 24 hrs at 15–30° C and 7 days at 2–8° C in tuberculin syringes
    - □ however, refrigeration and use within 24 hrs are recommended because of concern for bacterial contamination
- ■ Nursing considerations
  - vials are for single dose use and contain no preservatives
  - do not give drug within 24 hrs of cytotoxic chemotherapy
  - counts should be performed twice weekly; transiently increased neutrophil count is common 1–2 days after initiation of therapy
  - give daily for up to 2 wks or until ANC has returned to 1,500–10,000/mm^3 after expected chemotherapy-induced neutrophil nadir

DRUG: SARGRAMOSTIM, GM-CSF; GRANULOCYTE-MACROPHAGE COLONY STIMULATING FACTOR; RGM-CSF

- ■ Other names: Prokine, Leukine
- ■ Uses
  - sargramostim is a recombinant granulocyte-macrophage colony stimulating factor (rhu GM-CSF)
  - produced by recombinant DNA technology in a yeast *(S. cerevisiae)* expression system
  - indicated for acceleration of myeloid recovery in patients with
    - □ non-Hodgkin's lymphoma (NHL)
    - □ acute lymphoblastic leukemia (ALL)
    - □ Hodgkin's lymphoma
    - □ autologous bone marrow transplantation (BMT)
    - □ allogeneic bone marrow transplantation
    - □ peripheral stem cell transplantation
    - □ acute myelogenous leukemia (AML)
    - □ metastatic breast cancer
    - □ multiple myeloma
- ■ Mechanism of action
  - sargramostim is a hematopoietic growth factor
  - stimulates proliferation, development, and functional activation of all granulocytes
    - □ neutrophils
    - □ monocytes
    - □ eosinophils
    - □ macrophages
    - □ megakaryocytes
    - □ erythroid cells
  - activates monocyte-macrophages to produce cytokines
    - □ tumor necrosis factor
    - □ interleukin
- ■ Dosing
  - children and adults: SubQ or IV infusion over > 2 hrs
  - initiation of GM-CSF between 24 and 72 hrs subsequent to chemotherapy may provide optimal neutrophil recovery based on existing clinical data
  - continue therapy until the occurrence of an absolute neutrophil count of 10,000/mm^3 after the neutrophil nadir
  - myeloid reconstitution after peripheral stem cell, allogeneic or autologous bone marrow transplant
  - SubQ or IV
    - □ 250 mcg/m^2/d to begin 2–4 hrs after the marrow infusion on day 0 of autologous bone marrow transplant or > 24 hrs after chemotherapy or 12 hrs after last dose of radiotherapy
    - □ if significant adverse effects or "first dose" reaction is seen at this dose, discontinue the drug until toxicity resolves
      - ▽ restart at a reduced dose of 125 mcg/m^2/d
  - length of therapy: bone marrow transplant patients
    - ▽ GM-CSF should be administered daily for up to 30 days or until the ANC has reached 1,500 mm^3 for 3 consecutive days following the expected chemotherapy-induced neutrophil nadir
  - cancer chemotherapy recovery: SubQ or IV: 3–15 mcg/kg/d for 14–21 days
    - □ maximum daily dose is 15 mcg/kg/d due to dose-related adverse effects
    - □ discontinue therapy if the ANC count is > 20,000/mm^3
- ■ Pharmacokinetics
  - onset of action: increase in WBC in 7–14 days
  - duration: WBC will return to baseline within 1 wk after discontinuing drug
  - half-life: 2 hrs
  - time to peak serum concentration: SubQ: within 1–2 hrs
  - metabolism: undetermined
  - excretion: unknown
- ■ Adverse reactions
  - "first-dose" effects: fever, hypotension, tachycardia, rigors, flushing, nausea, vomiting, dyspnea
  - CNS: neutropenic fever, headache, malaise, fever
  - dermatologic: alopecia, rash
  - endocrine and metabolic: polydipsia, fluid retention
  - gastrointestinal: nausea, vomiting, diarrhea, stomatitis, GI hemorrhage, mucositis, anorexia, sore throat
  - neuromuscular and skeletal: bone pain, myalgia, weakness, rigors
  - cardiovascular: chest pain, peripheral edema, capillary leak syndrome, hypotension, flushing, pericardial effusion, transient supraventricular arrhythmias, pericarditis
  - hematologic: leukocytosis
  - local: pain at injection site
  - respiratory: dyspnea, cough
  - miscellaneous: anaphylactic reaction
- ■ Pharmacy issues
  - increased toxicity: lithium, corticosteroids may potentiate myeloproliferative effects
  - administer by SubQ (undiluted)
  - can premedicate with analgesics and antipyretics
  - control bone pain with non-narcotic analgesics
  - do not shake solution
  - rotate injection sites when administering GM-CSF SubQ
- ■ Nursing considerations
  - monitor neutrophil count and platelets closely
  - obtain baseline CBC, liver and renal functions
  - use cautiously in patients with preexisting cardiac disease or fluid retention, hypoxia, pulmonary infiltrates, CHF, or impaired renal or hepatic functions; these conditions could be exacerbated
  - document all therapy (drugs or radiation) the patient is receiving
    - □ drug should not be administered 24 hrs preceding or following chemotherapy
    - □ drug should not be administered within 12 hrs preceding or following radiation therapy
  - vials are for single dose use and contain no preservatives
  - assess for rash and local reactions at injection site

Hypercalcemia of Malignancy

S. G. E. Mezitis, M. L. Adler, L. Haser, and R. J. Robbins

OVERVIEW

■ Hypercalcemia is the most common life-threatening metabolic complication in cancer patients, affecting 10–20% of all cancer patients during the course of the disease
- hypercalcemia of malignancy is usually an indication of advanced disease (mean life span is < 1 yr)

■ Hypercalcemia most commonly occurs in epidermoid neoplasms of the oropharynx, lung, and genitourinary tract

■ It can occur in any cancer but is more common in breast cancer, multiple myeloma, lymphomas, and some leukemias

PATHOPHYSIOLOGY

■ Calcium balance is maintained by dietary intake, intestinal absorption, bone resorption and formation, as well as renal excretion and reabsorption

■ Serum calcium is tightly regulated by an interacting network of hormones that includes parathyroid hormone (PTH), 1,25 $(OH)_2$ vitamin D3 (D3), calcitonin, and cortisol

■ Overproduction of PTH, D3, or the tumor-derived PTH-related peptide (PTHRP) can cause hypercalcemia

■ Local osteolytic hypercalcemia (LOH) results from activation of osteoclasts by local cytokines that may be released by tumor cells or normal marrow elements

DIAGNOSIS AND PREVENTION

■ Differential diagnosis
- primary hyperparathyroidism (usually due to an adenoma)
- excess D3 production by tumoral 1α hydroxylase (e.g., lymphoma)
- humoral hypercalcemia of malignancy (HHM) due to PTHRP
- immobilization (especially teenagers and Paget's disease)
- endocrine disorders (hyperthyroidism or adrenal insufficiency)
- familial hypocalciuric hypercalcemia
- drug induced (e.g., lithium, thiazides, excess vitamin D)

■ Diagnostic evaluation
- total calcium and albumin (ionized calcium if necessary)
- electrolytes, renal function, phosphorus, alkaline phosphatase, and urinary calcium and creatinine
- ECG to measure QTc interval
- PTH, PTHRP, and D3 levels if indicated

THERAPY

■ Generally, therapy includes treatment of the underlying malignancy, surgery for parathyroid adenoma, or discontinuation of offending medication
- IV hydration with 200–300 ml/hr of isotonic saline
  - □ after adequate rehydration, the loop diuretic furosemide 40 mg IV q2–6hrs may be used to promote urinary excretion of calcium and to prevent volume overload
- bisphosphonates
  - □ treatment with bisphosphonates is effective within a few days
- calcitonin (usually reserved for very severe hypercalcemia, i.e., ≥18 mg%)
- plicamycin (mithramycin)
- glucocorticoids
- gallium nitrate

■ Specific drugs
- pamidronate (Aredia)
  - □ in breast cancer and multiple myeloma, pamidronate reduces bone pain, fractures, and may slow progression of disease
- calcitonin
- plicamycin (mithramycin)
- glucocorticoids
- gallium nitrate

KEY REFERENCES

Bilezikian JP: Management of acute hypercalcemia. N Engl J Med 1992; 326(18): 1196–1203

Chrisholm MA, Mulloy AL, Taylor AT: Acute management of cancer-related hypercalcemia. Ann Pharmacother 1996; 30:507–13

DRUG: PAMIDRONATE DISODIUM

■ Other name: Aredia

■ Uses
- approved by the FDA for treatment of hypercalcemia of malignancy, Paget's disease, osteolytic bone metastases of breast cancer, and osteolytic lesions of multiple myeloma

■ Mechanism of action
- a bisphosphonate that inhibits bone resorption. Effect is a result of inhibition of osteoclast hyperactivity. It may directly block dissolution of calcium phosphate (hydroxyapatite) crystals by absorbing to this mineral component of bone

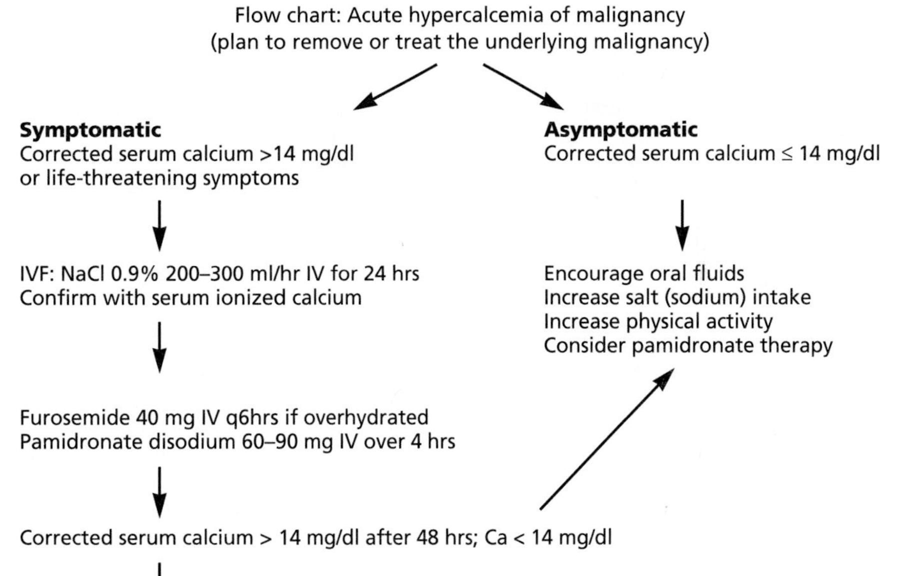

Second-line agents:
Calcitonin (salmon) 100 IU SubQ q6hrs for 8 doses
Hydrocortisone 200–300 mg IV daily for 3–5 days in lymphomatous disease and breast cancer
Gallium nitrate 200 mg/m²/d over 24 hrs for 5 days

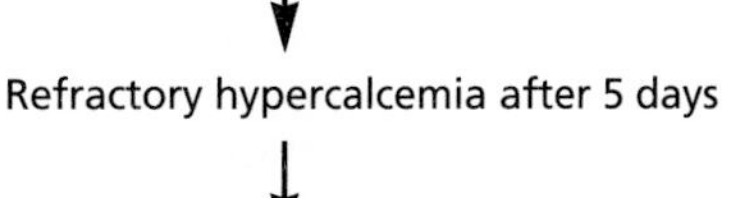

Refractory hypercalcemia after 5 days

Third-line agent:
Plicamycin 30 mcg/kg/d over 4–6 hrs for 4 days

Note: Pamidronate monotherapy can be considered for treatment of more mild hypercalcemia of malignancy.

- Dosing
  - available only in parenteral form in 30 mg, 60 mg, and 90 mg vials
  - the lyophilized pamidronate disodium is diluted before use in sterile 0.45% or 0.9% sodium chloride or 5% dextrose injection that is stable for IV use for up to 24 hrs at room temperature
  - the recommended dose of pamidronate disodium in moderate hypercalcemia (corrected seum calcium 12–13.5 mg/dl) is an initial single dose of 60 mg diluted in 1,000 ml administered as IV infusion over at least 4 hrs. For severe hypercalcemia (corrected serum calcium > 13.5 mg/dl), the 90 mg dose must be given by an initial single dose of 1,000 ml IV infusion over 4–6 hrs
  - retreatment identical to initial therapy must be after at least 7 days to allow for full response to the initial dose and can be repeated as needed
  - the recommended dose of pamidronate disodium in patients with osteolytic bone lesions of multiple myeloma or breast cancer is 90 mg diluted in 500 ml and administered as a 3–4 hr infusion given q3–4wks
- Pharmacokinetics
  - pamidronate is not metabolized and is exclusively eliminated by renal excretion.The elimination half-life is 28 ± 7 hrs
  - following parenteral administration of 90 mg over 24 hrs, Cmax is 1.38 mcg/ml and percentage of drug excreted unchanged in urine within 120 hrs is 47.5%
  - in patients with serum creatinine > 2.5 mg/dl given the maximum 90 mg over 4 hrs on a monthly basis, excessive accumulation of pamidronate was not observed
  - phosphate levels decrease after administration of pamidronate because of decreased release from bone and increased renal excretion as suppressed parathyroid levels return to normal. Thirty percent of patients treated with pamidronate need phosphate replacement for 7–10 days
  - no human pharmacokinetic data available with pamidronate and drug interactions or in patients with hepatic insufficiency
  - pamidronate normalizes serum calcium concentration in 60–100% of hypercalcemic patients
- Side effects
  - fever after initial dose (34%)
  - catheter site soft tissue symptoms: redness, swelling or induration, pain on palpation (18%)
  - fluid overload, hypertension, abdominal pain, anorexia, nausea, bone pain (15%)
  - urinary tract infection (15%)
  - anemia, hypocalcemia, hypomagnesemia, hypophosphatemia (15%)
- Nursing considerations
  - monitor IV site carefully during administration for infusion site reaction (redness, pain, swelling)
  - monitor electrolytes regularly. Patient may require phosphate replacement
  - assess
    - □ for increasing weakness and fatigue; this could either be drug and/or disease related
    - □ for generalized bone pain. Patient may experience a decrease in analgesia requirements after first or second dose
    - □ nutritional status for alterations related to nausea, vomiting, lack of appetite
  - teach patient
    - □ instruct patient of possible occurrence of joint/muscle pain for up to 1–3 days following the first or second treatment
    - □ report fever

DRUG: ETIDRONATE DISODIUM

- Other name: Didronel
- Uses
  - approved by the FDA for hypercalcemia, Paget's disease, and bone pain
- Mechanism of action
  - a bisphosphonate that inhibits osteoclastic hyperactivity in bone disease
- Dosing
  - available in oral and parenteral form
  - the recommended dose for acute hypercalcemia is 7.5 mg/kg IV infused over 2–4 hrs daily for 3–7 days
- Pharmacokinetics
  - etidronate is not metabolized
  - the plasma half-life is 6 ± 0.7 hrs. The half-life in bone is in excess of 90 days
  - a large fraction of the infused dose is excreted rapidly and unchanged in the urine
  - do not use in patients with serum creatinine > 2.5 mg/dl
  - clinical trials indicate that etidronate normalized serum calcium concentrations in 40–92% of patients
  - risk of osteomalacia with repeated dosing due to inhibition of bone formation
- Side effects
  - renal insufficiency (10%)
  - change in taste (5%)
  - transient fever, rash, nausea (< 1%)
  - hypocalcemia (18%)
  - hyperphosphatemia is possible due to increased renal tubular reabsorption
- Other considerations
  - advantages of pamidronate over etidronate include its use as a single-dose agent and its greater effectiveness demonstrated by percentage of patients achieving normocalcemia by day 7 after initiation of treatment (70% vs. 41%)
  - other bisphosphonates that may soon become available for treatment of hypercalcemia include clodronate, zolendronate, and alendronate that may have greater ease of administration, greater effectiveness, fewer adverse effects, and lower cost
- Nursing considerations
  - administer drug with vigorous hydration and over multiple days for maximum effect
  - provide safe environment for patient, since the calcium level is decreased gradually over multiple days
  - do not use in combination with NSAIDs or diuretics. This may contribute to renal failure
  - assess
    - □ monitor renal function; monitor electrolytes
    - □ assess for fluid overload; monitor I/O and daily weights
  - teach patient
    - □ to drink 2–3 L of fluids per day unless contraindicated
    - □ to report any decrease or absence of appetite, nausea, vomiting, constipation, fatigue, weakness, or thirst
    - □ etidronate prevents bone mineralization; instruct patient/caregiver not to overstress bones and to be gentle when assisting patient; they should not pull on arms, legs, or squeeze ribs
    - □ encourage mobilization or isometric exercises to tolerance

DRUG: CALCITONIN (SALMON)

- Other names: Calcimar, Miacalcin, Osteocalcin
- Uses
  - approved by the FDA for the treatment of hypercalcemia, symptomatic Paget's disease of bone, and postmenopausal osteoporosis
- Mechanism of action
  - calcitonin (salmon) is a synthetic polypeptide of 32 amino acids
  - acts primarily on bone and causes a marked transient inhibition of bone resorption by decreasing the number of osteoclasts and their resorptive activity. Bone formation may be augmented through increased osteoblastic activity
  - calcitonin also increases the renal excretion of filtered calcium, phosphate, and sodium by decreasing their tubular reabsorption
- Dosing
  - available in SubQ, IM injection (200 units/ml) and nasal spray forms
  - injection is the recommended route of administration in hypercalcemia
  - possible anaphylaxis requires initial test dosing, especially in those patients with prior exposure
  - the starting dose is 4 IU/kg body weight q12hrs
  - if the response is unsatisfactory, the dose may be increased to 8 IU/kg q12hrs to a

maximum of 8 IU/kg q6hrs and given for a maximum of 8 consecutive doses
- it may be added to existing therapeutic regimens for hypercalcemia

- Pharmacokinetics
  - calcitonin (salmon) has a greater potency per mg and a longer duration of action than mammalian calcitonin
  - the decrease of calcium occurs about 2 hrs after the first injection and lasts for ~6–8 hrs
  - after 5–8 days of calcitonin-salmon injection q12hrs, the calcium lowering effect is ~9%
  - animal studies suggest that calcitonin is rapidly metabolized to inactive fragments primarily in the kidneys
  - normocalcemia is achieved in 31% of patients and its mean duration is 1 day
  - serum calcium concentrations may decline by 2–3 mg/dl within a few hrs and the nadir can be reached within 24 hrs
- Side effects
  - nausea, vomiting, inflammatory reaction at injection site (10%)
  - flushing of face or hands (2–5%)
  - isolated cases of skin rash, nocturia, fever, eye pain, salty taste, poor appetite, abdominal pain, and foot edema
  - rare cases of anaphylactic reactions
- Other considerations
  - long-term efficacy is limited by antibody production when calcitonin is given parenterally after weeks to months of treatment
- Nursing considerations
  - test dose of one unit SubQ is recommended; potential for anaphylaxis; risk is greater in patients previously exposed to drug
  - long-term efficacy of drug is limited with prolonged parenteral administration
  - best responses are seen with patients with multiple myeloma and other hematologic malignancies
  - treatment is more effective when combined with glucocorticoids
  - treatment is very expensive and is of short duration
  - assess
    - □ although rare; assess for abdominal pain, poor appetite, pedal edema, fever, and eye pain
    - □ for localized skin reaction at the site of injection
  - teach patient
    - □ instruct patient for potential of nausea, vomiting, and facial flushing

Osteoporosis/Osteopenia

R. L. Theriault, S. Noble Kempin, and G. N. Hortobagyi

OVERVIEW

- Osteoporosis is the most common metabolic bone disease
- Characteristics of osteoporosis and osteopenia
  - low bone mass
  - microarchitectural destruction of bone tissue, leading to fragility
  - altered tensile strength and clinical susceptibility to fracture
- Populations at risk
  - menopausal women
  - Caucasian or Asian race
  - a sedentary lifestyle
  - family history of osteoporosis
  - prolonged calcium-deficient diet
  - excessive alcohol intake
  - long-term use of medication, such as glucocorticoids and thyroid hormone preparations
- Bone fracture is the most important clinical complication of osteoporosis and osteopenia
  - fractures occur at sites of low bone mass, most commonly of the wrist, vertebrae, and hip
  - ~1.5 million fractures occur each year in the United States
  - hip fractures have a 12–25% mortality rate per year
  - vertebral fractures may result in spinal deformity, nerve-root entrapment, and chronic pain

PATHOPHYSIOLOGY

- Bone integrity is maintained by the coupling function of the osteoblast and osteoclast, which constantly remodel bone
  - reduction of osteoblast function or excessive osteoclast activity results in destruction of bone
  - estrogen inhibits osteoclast function and maintains osteoblast integrity; estrogen deficiency leads to excessive osteoclast activity
- Deficiencies in appropriate nutrients, such as calcium, also may result in defective bone remodeling
  - medications that increase osteoclast activity, such as glucocorticoids and thyroid hormone, will result in bone loss

DIAGNOSIS AND PREVENTION

- Prevention
  - identify those at risk
    - □ counsel those people about lifestyle changes, such as cessation of smoking, limiting alcohol intake, and a regular exercise program
  - suggest diet with appropriate amounts of calcium and vitamin D
- Diagnostic measures
  - dual-energy x-ray absorptiometry (DEXA)
    - □ preferred method, since it can measure spine, proximal femurs, or whole body bone mineral density
    - □ it has a scan time of < 5 min
    - □ it is highly precise and accurate, with high resolution and low radiation
  - single-energy x-ray absorptiometry
  - quantitative-computed tomography
  - ultrasound
- Diagnostic criteria
  - osteopenia: bone mineral density value of > 1 standard deviation but < 2.5 below young adult mean value
  - osteoporosis: bone mineral density value of ≥2.5 standard deviation below the young adult mean value
  - for DEXA, normal adult mean value is reported as T score; age and sex match control subjects are reported as Z scores. For each 10% decrease in bone mineral density, the risk of fracture is approximately doubled

THERAPY

- Estrogen replacement therapy (ERT)
  - oral conjugated estrogens, such as Premarin tablets
  - estrogen/progestin combinations, such as Prempro and Premphase
  - estrogen administration is absolutely contraindicated during pregnancy
- Dietary or supplemental calcium
  - without ERT, 1,500 mg per day
  - with ERT, 1,000 mg per day
- Bisphosphonates
  - alendronate sodium: 5 and 10 mg tablets
  - clodronate (currently unavailable in United States)
- Calcitonin: available as a parenteral preparation or as nasal spray
- Raloxifene: available as a 60 mg tablet

KEY REFERENCES

Baran DT, Faulkner KG, Genant HK, Miller PD, Pacifici R: Diagnosis and management of osteoporosis: guidelines for the utilization of bone densitometry. [review] Calcified Tissue International 1997; 61(6):433–40

Miller PD: Management of osteoporosis. [review] Adv Int Med 1999; 44:175–207

Prestwood KM, Kenny AM: Osteoporosis: pathogenesis, diagnosis, and treatment in older adults. [review] Clin in Geriatric Med 1998; 14(3):577–99

Rosen CJ, Kessenich CR: Comparative clinical pharmacology and therapeutic use of bisphosphonates in metabolic bone diseases. [review] Drugs 1996; 51(4):537–51

DRUG: CALCITONIN SALMON NASAL SPRAY

- Other name: Miacalcin
- Uses
  - miacalcin is indicated for treatment of postmenopausal osteoporosis for women who are unable or unwilling to take hormone replacement therapy
  - calcitonin appears to exert an antiosteoclast effect through a direct receptor mechanism
  - inhibition of osteoclast results in decreased bone resorption
- Dosing
  - calcitonin salmon nasal spray is administered 200 units per day; 1 intranasal administration daily, alternating nostrils
- Pharmacokinetics
  - calcitonin salmon is absorbed rapidly through the nasal mucosa
  - peak plasma concentration 30–40 min after nasal administration
  - ~3% of nasally administered drug is bioavailable
  - half-life of elimination is estimated to be 43 min
  - no drug accumulation upon repeated nasal administration
- Toxicity
  - nasal adverse reactions including rhinitis, nasal crusts, dryness, redness, or erythema are most frequent occurring in ~22%
  - only 5% of these reactions were considered severe
  - other adverse events reported include back pain, arthralgia, epistaxis, and cephalgia
- Pharmacy issues
  - metered dose 2 ml fill glass bottles, 200 IU per activation
- Nursing considerations
  - do not freeze; store under refrigeration until open, then store in upright position at room temperature; drug is stable at room temperature for 30 days
  - contraindicated in persons with fish hypersensitivity
  - systemic reactions may occur; skin testing should be considered prior to initiation of therapy; epinephrine should be available; do not administer if erythema or wheal appears within 15 min; notify physician
  - calcium and vitamin D supplements should be given to patients
- Assess
  - □ for symptoms of hypo or hypercalcemia; monitor serum calcium levels at regular intervals
  - □ for signs of nasal irritation; assess nasal mucosa regularly
  - teach patient
    - □ instruct on proper activation of spray pump and administration of nasal spray in alternating nostrils daily
    - □ provide recommendations for symptomatic treatment of nasal irritation
    - □ self-administration of calcium and vitamin D supplements
    - □ expected side effects and the need to report symptoms of hypo or hypercalcemia

DRUG: ALENDRONATE SODIUM TABLETS

- Other name: Fosamax
- Mechanism of action

  - alendronate preferentially localizes in sites of bone resorption and specifically interferes with osteoclast function
  - alendronate interferes with osteoclast lysosomal activity at bone surface
  - it is reported to inhibit osteoclast recruitment from monocyte/macrophage cell line
- Dosing
  - alendronate is available in 5 and 10 mg tablets
  - it must be taken 1 hr before first food, beverage, or medication of the day with water only
  - patients taking alendronate should not lie down for at least 30 min and only after their first food of the day
  - alendronate should not be taken at bedtime or before arising for day
- Pharmacokinetics
  - oral bioavailability of alendronate is 0.7% for doses of 5–40 mg
  - bioavailability is substantially decreased when administered with other medications or meals
  - bioavailability was near 0 with alendronate administered with or up to 2 hrs after a standardized meal
  - both coffee and orange juice reduce bioavailability by 60%
- Metabolism
  - no evidence of metabolism of alendronate has been documented in animals or humans
  - the terminal half-life in humans is estimated to exceed 10 yrs
- Toxicity
  - adverse experiences include gastrointestinal, musculoskeletal, nervous system, and special sense toxicity
  - gastrointestinal toxicity is most common and includes abdominal pain, nausea, dyspepsia, diarrhea, flatulence, esophageal ulceration, acid reflux
  - musculoskeletal adverse events include muscle or joint or bone pain
  - nervous system includes headache and occasional dizziness. Taste perversion has been reported
- Nursing considerations
  - treat overdoses with milk or antacids
  - drug interactions include aluminum hydroxide, antacids, ranitidine, anti-inflammatory drugs, calcium, iron and magnesium salts
  - calcium and vitamin D supplements should be given to patients
  - assess
    - □ monitor serum calcium and phosphorus values during therapy
    - □ baseline medical history to identify patients for presence of gastroesophageal disturbances, reflux or hiatal hernia; monitor these patients closely
  - teach patient
    - □ importance of proper administration of medication to improve absorption and efficacy; to swallow tablets with a full glass of plain water only *(not mineral water)* prior to first food, beverage, or other medication without lying down for 30 min or consuming food, beverage, or medication within 1 hr
    - □ report chest pain or burning, difficulty swallowing, or tarry stools
    - □ self-administration of calcium and vitamin D supplements
    - □ avoidance of the above drugs that have a potential for drug interaction

DRUG: RALOXIFENE

- Other name: Evista
- Indications
  - approved by the FDA for the prevention of osteoporosis in postmenopausal women
- Mechanism of action
  - raloxifene is a selective estrogen receptor modulator belonging to the benzothiophene class of compounds
  - raloxifene reduces resorption of bone and decreases overall bone turnover
  - raloxifene biologic actions are mediated by binding to estrogen receptors. Clinical data indicate that this binding results in estrogenlike effects on bone resulting in increased bone mineral density
- Dosing
  - raloxifene is available in 60 mg tablets. Recommended dose is one 60 mg tablet daily administered without regard to meals
- Pharmacokinetics
  - 60% of an oral dose is absorbed; however, absolute bioavailability is only 2%
- Metabolism
  - raloxifene is biotransformed with extensive first-pass metabolism to glucuronide conjugates
- Excretion
  - raloxifene is primarily excreted in feces with < 6% administered dose eliminated in urine as glucuronide conjugates. Volume of distribution is large; ~2,348 L/kg, not dose dependent
- Side effects
  - common adverse events include hot flashes and leg cramps
- Nursing considerations
  - concomitant use with systemic hormone replacement therapy is not recommended
  - risk of thromboembolic disease is similar to that associated with hormone replacement
  - calcium and vitamin D supplements should be given to patients
  - associated risk of endometrial or breast tumors
  - assess
    - □ for unusual uterine bleeding
    - □ history of and risk factors for development of venous thromboembolic disease; encourage smoking cessation
  - teach patient
    - □ to report symptoms of headaches, blurred vision, numbness, weakness of extremities, shortness of breath, or calf pain
    - □ may experience hot flashes; recommend dietary modifications or other measures for symptomatic relief
    - □ self breast examinations
    - □ self-administration of calcium and vitamin D supplements
    - □ drug may be taken with or without food

DRUG: CALCITONIN INJECTION

- Other names: Miacalcin Synthetic, Calcimar
- Uses
  - salmon calcitonin injection is indicated for the treatment of Paget's disease of bone, hypercalcemia, and treatment of postmenopausal osteoporosis
- Mechanism of action
  - a single injection decreases ongoing bone resorption. Repeated administration results in prolonged inhibition of bone resorption with decreased osteolytic activity
- Dosing
  - the minimum effective dose of salmon calcitonin for prevention of vertebral bone loss has not been established. Recommended dose is 100 IU SubQ or IM every other day
- Pharmacokinetics
  - metabolism of parenteral salmon calcitonin has not been studied. Animal data suggest that parenteral administration results in rapid bone metabolism with a small amount of unchanged hormone and metabolites excreted in the urine
- Adverse reactions
  - systemic allergic reactions are possible including bronchospasm, anaphylactic shock, and swelling of tongue or throat. It is possible that administration may lead to hypocalcemia and/or tetany
  - gastrointestinal adverse reactions include nausea, with or without vomiting
  - skin reactions include local inflammation at the site of administration, as well as skin rash including flushing of face and hands
- Availability
  - 2 ml vial, 200 IU/ml
- Nursing considerations
  - store under refrigeration; do not freeze
  - contraindicated in patients with fish hypersensitivity
  - systemic reactions may occur; skin testing should be considered prior to initiation of therapy; do not administer if patient develops a systemic reaction, if erythema or wheal appears within 15

min; notify physician; epinephrine should be available
- calcium and vitamin D supplements must be given to patients
- assess
  - □ for symptoms of hypo or hypercalcemia; monitor serum calcium levels at regular intervals
- teach patient
  - □ that taking drug at bedtime may alleviate nausea and vomiting
  - □ facial flushing may occur and last up to 1 hr after administration
  - □ self-administration of calcium and vitamin D supplements
  - □ expected side effects and the need to report symptoms of hypo or hypercalcemia

DRUG: ESTROGEN

- Other names: Premarin, Premphase, Prempro
- Indications
  - estrogen is indicated for the treatment and prevention of postmenopausal osteoporosis
- Dosage and administration
  - Premarin is available in tablets 0.3 mg, 0.625 mg, 0.9 mg, 1.25 mg, and 2.5 mg
  - Premphase: conjugated estrogens plus medroxyprogesterone acetate consist of Premarin 0.625 mg tablets taken days 1–14, followed by 0.625 mg conjugated estrogens with 5 mg of medroxyprogesterone acetate taken on days 15–28
  - Prempro: 0.625 mg conjugated estrogen and 2.5 mg medroxyprogesterone acetate: 1 tablet daily
- Pharmacokinetics
  - the effects of conjugated estrogens are similar to endogenous estrogens and they have broad physiologic effects
  - these include maintenance of the integrity of the genitourinary epithelium, stimulation of the endometrial lining of uterus, and the maintenance of bone integrity
  - they are metabolized and inactivated in the liver after gastrointestinal absorption
  - maximum plasma levels are obtained ~4–10 hrs after oral administration. Conjugated estrogens are primarily bound to albumin, unconjugated estrogens are bound to albumin and sex hormone globulin
- Adverse reactions
  - genitourinary symptoms including vaginal bleeding, increased frequency of candidiasis, an alteration in vaginal secretions, breast tenderness and enlargement, nausea, vomiting, abdominal cramping, and increased incidence of cholelithiasis, potential for headache, dizziness, and mental depression
- Contraindications
  - known or suspected primary breast cancer or other estrogen-dependent neoplasm, undiagnosed abnormal genital bleeding, thromboembolic disorders
  - estrogen administration is absolutely contraindicated during pregnancy
- Nursing considerations
  - should not be administered concomitantly with tamoxifen
  - contraindicated in patients with estrogen-dependent tumors and in patients with a history of thrombophlebitis and thromboembolic disorders
  - associated risk of endometrial or breast tumors
  - use cautiously in patients with a history of migraine headaches
  - pathology specimens should indicate that patient is receiving estrogen replacement
  - assess
    - □ for unusual uterine bleeding
    - □ history of and risk factors for development of venous thromboembolic disease; encourage smoking cessation
  - teach patient
    - □ to report symptoms of headaches, blurred vision, numbness, weakness of extremities, shortness of breath, or calf pain
    - □ self breast examinations
    - □ potential for photosensitivity; use caution with sun exposure until tolerance is established

Cachexia and Anorexia

E. L. Paxton, J. Geick Miller, and J. M. Mirtallo

OVERVIEW

- Wasting disorders, such as anorexia and cachexia, involve involuntary weight loss of lean muscle during chronic illness. Several studies have demonstrated a direct relationship between mortality and loss of lean muscle mass
- Cachexia is seen in 15% of all oncology patients and usually associated with a decrease in the quality of life, as well as increase in morbidity
- Weight loss is dependent on the type of cancer, extent of disease, and response to therapy
- Nutrition support in oncology patients with anorexia or cachexia remains a challenge for clinicians
- Cachexia is different from starvation in that there is equal loss of muscle and fat, which is usually characterized by increased catabolism and decreased protein synthesis

PATHOPHYSIOLOGY

- Malabsorption of nutrients due to gastrointestinal obstruction, increased catabolism, and abnormal macronutrient metabolism can contribute to cachexia and anorexia in cancer patients
  - bowel stasis or obstruction
  - postoperative ileus
  - chemotherapy-induced nausea, vomiting, mucosis
  - radiation-attributed changes, such as enteritis
  - delayed reactions: persistent mucosal inflammation and intestinal fibrosis and strictures
- Macronutrient metabolism abnormalities are caused by alterations in regulatory hormones and cytokines
  - neutralization of cytokines with antibodies in animal models of wasting has suggested the validity of an anticytokine therapy to combat cachexia
  - animal studies also have shown that no single cytokine is responsible for all abnormalities contributing to cachexia
- Cytokines contribute to cancer cachexia and a hypermetabolic state
  - tumor necrosis factor-alfa (TNF-α) increases body temperature, oxygen consumption, and protein turnover; TNT-α also increases glucose uptake and peripheral insulin resistance
  - interleukin-1 (IL-1) causes fever, anorexia, and decreased food intake; interleukin-6 (IL-α) mediates cachexia and regulates the hepatic acute phase response in cancer patients
  - interferon-gamma (INF-γ) inhibits lipoprotein lipase and acts in conjunction with TNF-α to cause cachexia

DIAGNOSIS AND PREVENTION

- The normal, adaptive response to starvation is to rely on body energy reserves and deplete energy-dense lipid stores while sparing protein, which results in the loss of fat and relative preservation of lean tissue
- Cachexia patients experience severe and incapacitating muscle wasting with a relative sparing of adipose tissue
- Signs and symptoms of cachexia
  - anorexia, decreased intake, or early satiety
  - significant body composition changes with associated weight loss
  - depletion of adipose tissue and muscle
  - generalized weakness and declining attention span and cognitive abilities

THERAPY

- The goal of nutrition support in cancer patients is to reverse cachexia, improve or maintain protein stores (lean body mass), and/or increase weight with minimal side effects
  - nutritional supplementation that increases oral intake with food, enteral, or parenteral nutrition alone will not correct the underlying metabolic problems associated with cachexia or anorexia
  - weight gain with supplementation or pharmacologic agents is often due to an increase in body fat deposition and increased body water, not an increase in lean body mass
- The pharmacologic management of cachexia is directed toward appetite stimulation or suppressing the effects of cytokines
  - long-term administration of anticytokines is unlikely to be a practical option
  - the ideal pharmacologic agent would be orally administered and well tolerated
  - the agents studied for AIDS or cancer-related cachexia were not developed to treat anorexia or cachexia—nor FDA approved for such—but rather, the extension of these agents resulted in weight gain as an unintended characteristic or response; these agents are being studied for off-label use in clinical trial. Such agents include thalidomide, melatonin, anabolic steroids, and human growth factor
  - the efficacy reported in several of these agents has not been remarkable; however, they are demonstrating promise in advances toward better treatment options for patients

KEY REFERENCES

Goldberg RM, Loprinzi CL, Mailliard JA, O'Fallon JR, Krook JE, Ghosh C, Hestorff RD, Chong SF, Reuter NF, Shanahan TG: Pentoxifylline for treatment of cancer anorexia and cachexia? A randomized double-blind, placebo-controlled trial. J Clin Oncol 1995; 13: 2856–9

Herrington AM, Herrington JD, Church CA: Pharmacologic options for the treatment of cachexia. Nutr Clin Pract 1997; 12:101–13

Herrman VM, Fuhrman P, Borum PR: Wasting diseases. *The ASPEN Nutrition Support Practice Manual.* Silver Spring, MD: ASPEN Publications, 1998

Kardinal CG, Loprinzi CL, Schaid DJ, et al.: A controlled trial of cyproheptadine in cancer patients with anorexia and/or cachexia. Cancer 1990; 65:2657–62

Klein S, Kinney J, Jeejeebhoy K, Aplers D, et al.: Nutrition support in clinical practice: review of published data and recommendations for future directions. JPEN 1997; 21:133–55

Ottery FD, Walsh D, Strawford A: Pharmacologic management of anorexia/cachexia. Semin Oncol 1998; 25:35–44

DRUG: MEGESTROL ACETATE

- Other name: Megace
- Uses
  - palliative treatment of breast and endometrial carcinomas
  - appetite stimulation and promotion of weight gain in cachexia
  - FDA has approved its use to treat cachexia in head and neck cancer, non–small cell lung cancer patients, or patients with gastrointestinal cancer
- Mechanism of action
  - unknown, but causes both appetite stimulation and anabolic effects
- Dosing
  - available in suspension 40 mg/ml and tablets 20 mg and 40 mg
  - recommended dosage range is 400–800 mg/d
    - at least 2 mos of continuous therapy is necessary
- Pharmacokinetics
  - absorption: well absorbed orally
  - metabolism: completely metabolized in the liver to free steroids and glucuronide conjugates
    - time to peak concentration 1–3 hrs after ingestion
    - half-life, elimination: in urine as steroid metabolites and inactive compound, some in feces and bile
- Side effects
  - edema and weakness > 10%
  - insomnia, depression, fever, headache, allergic rash, melasma or chloasma, fluid retention, hyperglycemia, weight gain, nausea, vomiting, stomach cramps, cholestatic jaundice, hepatotoxicity and thrombophlebitis, and hyperpnea 1–10%
  - women: breakthrough bleeding and spotting, changes in menstrual flow > 10%
  - breast tenderness, changes in cervical erosion and secretions, and increased breast tenderness 1–10%

- Other considerations
  - use with caution in patients with a history of thrombophlebitis. Elderly women may have vaginal bleeding or discharge and need to be forewarned of this side effect and inconvenience
- Nursing considerations
  - FDA currently recommends that procedures for proper handling and disposal of antineoplastic agents be considered
  - assess baseline peripheral vascular status and monitor during therapy
  - expected side effects and self-care measures

DRUG: MEDROXYPROGESTERONE ACETATE

- Other names: Amen, Curretab, Cycrin, Depo-Provera, Provera
- Mechanism of action
  - unclear: appetite stimulation and anabolic effects when given in high doses
  - weight gain and appetite stimulation maintained at 6–12 wks when compared to placebo
- Dosing
  - available in injection, suspension: 100 mg/ml, 150 mg/ml, 400 mg/ml
  - oral tablets: 2.5 mg, 5 mg, and 10 mg
  - 100 mg 3 times daily
  - 500 mg twice daily
- Pharmacokinetics
  - absorption: IM: slow
  - metabolism: oral: hepatic
  - elimination: oral: urine and feces
- Side effects
  - edema and weakness > 10%
  - embolism, central thrombosis, mental depression, fever, insomnia, melasma or chloasma, allergic rash, weight gain or loss, cholestatic jaundice 1–10%
  - women: breakthrough bleeding, spotting, changes in menstrual flow, and amenorrhea > 1%
  - changes in cervical erosion and secretions, increased breast tenderness 1–10%
- Other considerations
  - dosage reduction recommended in hepatic insufficiency
  - due to safety of injection form, oral administration only is recommended
- Nursing considerations
  - monitor for loss of vision, sudden-onset proptosis, diplopia, migraine, and signs and symptoms of thromboembolic disorders

DRUG: CORTICOSTEROIDS: DEXAMETHASONE, METHYLPREDNISOLONE, AND PREDNISOLONE

- Mechanism of action
  - temporary increase in appetite stimulation attributed to the euphoric and anti-inflammatory side effects of the drug
- Dosing
  - available in oral (tablet and elixir) and parenteral formulations
  - dexamethasone: oral: elixir, and concentrated solution: 0.5 mg/ml (30% alcohol); regular solution: 0.5 mg/5 ml; tablets: 0.25 mg, 0.5 mg, 0.75 mg, 1 mg, 1.5 mg, 2 mg, 4 mg, and 6 mg
  - dexamethasone: injection: as acetate suspension: 8 mg/ml and 16 mg/ml; as sodium phosphate: 4 mg/ml, 10 mg/ml, 20 mg/ml, and 24 mg/ml; 0.75 mg–1.5 mg 4 times daily
  - methylprednisolone: oral tablets: 2 mg, 4 mg, 8 mg, 16 mg, 24 mg, and 32 mg injection: as acetate: 20 mg/ml, 40 mg/ml, and 80 mg/ml; as sodium succinate: 40 mg, 125 mg, 500 mg, and 1,000 mg, 16 mg twice daily
  - prednisolone: oral liquid: as sodium phosphate: 5 mg/ml; syrup: 15 mg/ml, tablets: 5 mg
  - prednisolone: injection: as acetate: 25 mg/ml and 50 mg/ml; as sodium phosphate: 20 mg/ml; as tebutate: 20 mg/ml; 5 mg 3 times daily
- Pharmacokinetics
  - absorption: readily absorbed when administered as free alcohols, ketones, or acetates; rapid when given IM as sodium succinate and phosphate
  - metabolism is mostly by the liver via cytochrome P-450 3A substrate to inactive metabolites, small amounts excreted in the urine and by hepatic; elimination: urine and bile
- Side effects
  - adrenal insufficiency when given for prolonged periods
  - muscle wasting
  - osteoporosis
  - increased susceptibility to infection
  - fluid and electrolyte disturbance: edema, hypertension, sodium retention, hypokalemia
  - cataracts and glaucoma
  - endocrine abnormalities: Cushing's syndrome, hyperglycemia, amenorrhea, diabetes mellitus
  - GI effects: nausea, vomiting, anorexia, increased appetite, pancreatitis, gastric ulcers, and ulcerative esophagitis
  - CNS: headache, insomnia, vertigo, seizures, euphoria, mood swings, depression, anxiety, and frank psychoses
  - dermatologic: acne, skin atrophy, skin thinning, delayed wound healing, striae, hirsutism, easy bruising
- Other considerations
  - use with caution in patients with peptic ulcer disease, hypertension, osteoporosis, diabetes, hyperthyroidism, thrombophlebitis, cirrhosis, myasthenia gravis, CHF, and acute adrenal insufficiency
  - recommend use of immediate-release formulations only
- Nursing considerations
  - monitor blood pressure, electrolytes, blood glucose, signs and symptoms of steroid withdrawal syndrome: anorexia, nausea, vomiting, lethargy, headache, fever, joint pain, myalgias, weight loss, and hypertension
  - instruct patient to take oral pills with food or milk

DRUG: CYPROHEPTADINE

- Other name: Periactin
- Mechanism of action
  - serotonin antagonism
- Dosing
  - syrup: 2 mg/5 ml
  - tablet: 4 mg
  - 8 mg 3 times daily
- Pharmacokinetics
  - well absorbed orally
  - almost completely metabolized in the liver
  - metabolites excreted in the urine and feces
- Side effects
  - drowsiness and thickening of bronchial secretion > 10%
  - headache, fatigue, nervousness, dizziness, appetite stimulation, nausea, diarrhea, abdominal pain, xerostomia, arthralgia, and pharyngitis 1–10%
  - tachycardia, seizures, hemolytic anemia, leukopenia, thrombocytopenia, hepatitis, and epistaxis < 1%
- Other considerations
  - dosing should be adjusted in hepatic insufficiency
  - syrup contains 5% alcohol
- Nursing considerations
  - monitor mental status changes, weight
  - use syrup with caution in patients with mucositis
  - instruct patients to take pill with food to decrease incidence of upset stomach
  - instruct patients to avoid other medications that may make them drowsy

Tumor Lysis Syndrome

P. J. Bierman and D. Berg

OVERVIEW

- Tumor lysis syndrome (TLS) is a potentially life-threatening complication of cancer treatment. Prevention and aggressive treatment make serious complications unusual. Complications are usually reversible if they do occur
- TLS is a constellation of metabolic abnormalities related to rapid release of intracellular products when tumors undergo death or necrosis
- TLS usually occurs after chemotherapy, but can occur after steroids, radiation, hormonal therapy, biologic response modifiers, or spontaneously
  - TLS is most commonly associated with rapidly growing hematologic malignancies, such as Burkitt's lymphoma, other high-grade lymphomas, and acute lymphoblastic leukemia
  - it can also occur with low-grade lymphomas and chronic leukemia, and has been described after treatment of solid tumors, such as small cell lung carcinoma, breast carcinoma, and neuroblastoma
- Laboratory findings consistent with TLS may be seen in 50% of patients undergoing therapy for hematologic neoplasms, although clinical findings are much less frequent
  - laboratory findings include hyperuricemia, hyperkalemia, hyperphosphatemia, hypocalcemia, azotemia, and acidosis. Arrhythmias and renal failure may occur

PATHOPHYSIOLOGY

- Sudden tumor cell death leads to release of intracellular potassium, phosphate, and nucleic acids, which overload buffering systems and renal excretion mechanisms
- Hyperkalemia may result in acidosis, renal insufficiency, and arrhythmias
- Hyperphosphatemia may lead to calcium salt deposition and hypocalcemia
- Renal failure is due to dehydration, uric acid precipitation, and calcium phosphate precipitation

DIAGNOSIS AND PREVENTION

- Risk factors for the development of TLS include preexisting renal insufficiency, high tumor bulk, and elevated lactate dehydrogenase levels
- Abnormalities usually occur within 24–48 hrs of starting therapy, but may be seen after several days
- Signs and symptoms include nausea and vomiting, lethargy, urine cloudiness, and renal colic
- Maintain a high index of suspicion
  - avoid IV contrast or other nephrotoxic agents, especially if patient is volume depleted
  - consider delaying the start of therapy until volume depletion, mild renal insufficiency, hyperuricemia, and electrolyte abnormalities are corrected
  - administer allopurinol at 300–600 mg/d for 1–2 days in adults, followed by 300 mg/d for several more days
  - maintain hydration to keep urine output at 3–4 L/d
    - □ uric acid excretion can be increased by alkalinization of the urine to a pH of 7–7.5
    - □ 50–100 meq $NaHCO_3$ can be added to a liter of D_5W or D_5W + 0.25% NS
    - □ urinary alkalinization in the setting of hyperphosphatemia may increase the likelihood of calcium phosphate precipitation and hypocalcemia

THERAPY

- Monitor electrolytes and chemistry values frequently. Consider the possibility that dialysis may be necessary
- Monitor volume status, renal function, and cardiac rhythm
- Hyperkalemia can be treated with sodium polystyrene sulfonate, furosemide, $NaHCO_3$, and dextrose and insulin. Dialysis may be required
- Hyperphosphatemia can be treated with aluminum hydroxide
- Calcium gluconate can be used for significant hypocalcemia and arrhythmias
- Indications for dialysis include severe or unresponsive hyperkalemia, volume overload, hyperphosphatemia, hyperuricemia, hypocalcemia, and uremia

SPECIAL NURSING CONSIDERATIONS

- Recognize patients at risk and institute preventive measures early
- Assess
  - physical signs of potential syndrome: weakness, muscle twitching, paresthesia, nausea and vomiting, decreased urinary output; EKG changes
  - monitor fluid balance; measure I/O and weight
  - pulmonary status baseline and during therapy; evaluate breath sounds, shortness of breath, and edema
  - for allopurinol-induced side effects

KEY REFERENCES

Arrambide K, Toto R: Tumor lysis syndrome. Semin Nephrol 1993; 13:273–80

Hande K, Garrow G: Acute tumor lysis syndrome in patients with high-grade non-Hodgkin's lymphoma. Am J Med 1993; 94:133–9

Kalemkerian G, Darwish B, Varterasian M: Tumor lysis syndrome in small cell carcinoma and other solid tumors. Am J Med 1997; 103:363–7

DRUG: ALLOPURINOL

- Other name: Zyloprim
- Uses
  - approved by the FDA for management of patients with signs and symptoms of primary or secondary gout, the management of patients with leukemia, lymphoma, and malignancies who are receiving cancer therapy which causes elevations of serum and urinary uric acid levels, and the management of patients with recurrent calcium oxalate calculi
  - useful in combination with other agents for treatment of leishmaniasis and may be useful when added to quinine for treatment of malaria
  - useful as adjunctive therapy in patients with refractory epilepsy
  - may be useful in prevention of ischemic tissue damage
  - may possibly be effective in the treatment of carbon monoxide poisoning, chronic Chagas's disease, 5-fluorouracil-induced stomatitis, and prostatitis
- Mechanism of action
  - xanthine oxidase inhibitor
- Dosing
  - available in 100 mg or 300 mg tablets
  - an injectable dosage form is available from the manufacturer (Glaxo Wellcome) on a compassionate use basis
  - an oral suspension may be prepared using crushed tablets in cherry syrup
  - doses of 100–800 mg/d have been recommended in various situations
- Pharmacokinetics
  - ~80–90% absorbed after oral administration, with peak plasma concentration in 30–60 min
  - plasma half-life of 2–3 hrs resulting from conversion to alloxanthine (oxipurinol)
  - ~20% is excreted in the feces in 48–72 hrs, and ~30% is excreted unchanged in the urine during chronic administration
  - ~45–65% of a dose is excreted in the urine as alloxanthine, with a plasma half-time of 18–30 hrs
  - allopurinol and alloxanthine are distributed in total tissue water and are not protein-bound
- Side effects
  - attacks of acute gouty arthritis can be precipitated upon initiation of therapy
  - the most frequent adverse reaction is skin rash. Hypersensitivity reactions may occur after prolonged periods of administration. The incidence of skin reactions is <5%; however severe and fatal Stevens-Johnson syndrome and exfoliative reactions have been described
  - gastrointestinal side effects such as nausea, diarrhea, and abnormal liver function tests may be seen

Tumor Lysis Syndrome *(Continued)*

- Precautions
  - dose adjustments are required for patients with impaired renal function
  - caution is required when administering allopurinol with 6-mercaptopurine and azathioprine, and dose adjustments are required
- Nursing considerations
  - in patients with history of gout, acute exacerbations may be precipitated on initiation of allopurinol therapy
  - dose should be reduced in patients with moderate to severe renal impairment to prevent significant drug accumulation
  - can be hepatotoxic in patients receiving diuretics or in those with compromised renal failure
  - ocular lesions, alopecia, slight bone marrow suppression, drowsiness, peripheral neuropathy, and GI upsets have been reported

Chapter 13

DRUG–DISEASE INTERACTIONS

Diabetes Mellitus

J. H. Ward

OVERVIEW OF UNDERLYING DISEASE

■ Diabetes mellitus is a common disorder and a frequent comorbid condition in patients with cancer
- diabetes can affect the host response to surgery and radiation, and antineoplastic agents can lead to difficulty in controlling diabetes
- depending on the patient's life expectancy and quality of life, an early decision should be made about how tightly blood glucose should be monitored
- the problems of hypoglycemia in tightly regulated patients who are unable to eat may be more severe than those of hyperglycemia

■ Cancer in patients with diabetes may be associated with a higher mortality

GENERAL PRINCIPLES

■ Anorexia, mucositis, nausea, vomiting, and diarrhea may all cause inconsistent caloric intake and complicate management of blood glucose

■ The renal function of the diabetic patient always should be evaluated before dosing with drugs with prominent renal excretion

■ Ectopic ACTH syndrome is associated with new or worsened diabetes two-thirds of the time

RECOMMENDATIONS AND PRECAUTIONS FOR TREATMENT

■ Glucocorticoids are ubiquitous in the management of cancer patients
- they promote glucose intolerance; thus it is imperative to monitor blood glucose in diabetics receiving steroids
  - □ since these can be used episodically or in pulses, this can be a serious challenge
- steroids are commonly used as components of regimens to treat myeloma, lymphoma, acute lymphoblastic leukemia
  - □ steroids are used in the treatment of radiation pneumonitis, spinal cord compression, brain metastases, and associated immune-mediated hemolytic anemia or thrombocytopenia
- steroids and serotonin receptor antagonists are regularly used as pretreatment antiemetic regimens
  - □ they are used as premedication for the taxanes: paclitaxel and docetaxel
- steroids are part of most regimens to control delayed nausea and vomiting

■ Other hormonal agents
- ketoconazole can improve the hyperglycemia of ectopic ACTH syndrome
- tamoxifen has been associated with vulva-vaginal candidiasis, which in turn is more common in diabetics
- octreotide may be associated with hyper- or hypoglycemia, requiring adjustment of insulin dose
- aminoglutethimide can cause hypoglycemia in high doses or in overdose

■ Chemotherapeutic agents associated with blood glucose aberrations
- L-asparaginase, pegaspargase may cause hyperglycemia
- procarbazine may enhance hypoglycemic effects of oral hypoglycemics or insulin
- streptozocin may cause hypoglycemia due to sudden release of insulin
- PALA (N-phosphonacetyl-L-aspartic acid), an experimental modulator of 5-fluorouracil, may cause severe hyperglycemia
- cisplatin must be used with care in patients with diabetes who have concurrent renal insufficiency
- vinca alkaloids may exacerbate diabetic neuropathy

■ Indirect effects of chemotherapy-related side effects on diabetes mellitus
- nausea and vomiting
  - □ poor oral intake leads to the risk of hypoglycemia
- infection, particularly in the presence of neutropenia, may lead to loss of diabetic control, and increase the risk of diabetic ketoacidosis
- diabetes may predispose cancer patients to oral candidiasis, particularly when receiving concurrent glucocorticoids

■ Effects of diabetes on other aspects of cancer care
- total parenteral nutrition, if required for management of such cancer complications as severe mucositis or bowel obstruction, will exacerbate hyperglycemia
- patients with diabetes are more likely to have postoperative complications following lung cancer or colorectal cancer surgery, and those recovering from surgery in the face of diabetes mellitus may have poor wound healing
- radiation-induced GI toxicity is worse in patients with diabetes mellitus
- radiation skin sensitivity may be worse in individuals with diabetes mellitus
- IV contrast for radiologic procedures must be given with caution in patients with renal insufficiency, a common complication of diabetes
- in confused cancer patients with diabetes, hypoglycemia must always be considered in the differential diagnosis

KEY REFERENCES

Levine W, Dyer AR, Shekelle RB, Schoenberger JA, Stamler J: Post-load plasma glucose and cancer mortality in middle-aged men and women. 12 year follow-up findings of the Chicago Heart Association Detection Project in industry. Am J Epidemiol 1990; 131:254–62

Poulson J: The management of diabetes in patients with advanced cancer. J Pain Symptom Manage 1997; 13:339–46

Winquist EW, Laskey J, Crump M, Khamsi F, Shepherd FA: Ketoconazole in the management of paraneoplastic Cushing's syndrome secondary to ectopic adrenocorticotropin production. J Clin Oncol 1995; 13:157–64

Chronic Renal Insufficiency

C. F. Stewart

OVERVIEW OF UNDERLYING DISEASE

- Clinical course of progressive renal disease is divided into four stages
  - *loss of renal reserve:* typically without symptoms, glomerular filtration rate may decrease 50% before plasma creatinine or BUN increase
  - *renal insufficiency:* corresponds to creatinine clearance of 30–50 ml/min
  - *chronic renal failure:* creatinine clearance below 30 ml/min, symptomatic and laboratory abnormalities (phosphorous, calcium, potassium, anemia, metabolic acidosis)
  - *end-stage renal disease:* patient requires chronic dialysis or transplantation
- Increased frequency of chronic renal failure is seen for the following reasons
  - an increased incidence of cancer in older patients in whom decreased renal function is directly related to the aging process
  - certain types of malignancies or pathophysiologic processes related to malignancies can cause impaired renal function
  - decreased renal function can result from many of the anticancer drugs used
- Indices of renal function
  - serum creatinine is not always a good measure of renal function
  - insulin clearance measures glomerular filtration rate (GFR) but is tedious and difficult for routine use
  - creatinine clearance (CrCl) approximates GFR and is calculated from urine collection and serum creatinine
  - creatinine clearance can be estimated by equations that incorporate patient-specific variables (i.e., Cockroft and Gault)
    - □ men: CrCl = (weight × (140 – age)/ Serum creatinine × 72)
    - □ women: CrCl = (CrCl male × 0.85)
  - serum clearance of radioactive tracers (e.g., ^{99m}Tc DTPA) are a reliable, clinically feasible measure of GFR

GENERAL PRINCIPLES

- Possible effects of chronic renal disease on drug disposition
  - absorption
    - □ oral absorption of drugs may be decreased, but very few studies exist that document this for anticancer drugs
    - □ changes in other pharmacokinetic parameters could mask the impact of renal disease on oral absorption
  - distribution and protein binding
    - □ plasma protein binding of acidic drugs reduced in patients with severe renal failure; however, effect of mild or moderate renal failure is unknown
    - □ reduced protein binding will result in an increase in the apparent distribution volume
    - □ less is known about the effect of renal disease on the binding of basic drugs
    - □ apparent volume of distribution at steady state may be affected by changes in plasma protein binding, as well as alterations in tissue binding
  - metabolism
    - □ chronic renal failure may have an effect on nonrenal clearance mechanisms
    - □ this may have an effect on many nonrenal pathways, including deacetylation, hydroxylation, O-demethylation, N-demethylation, sulfoxidation, and glucuronidation
    - □ although a decrease in nonrenal pathway may be seen, it usually is not to the same extent as the reduction in renal clearance
  - drug excretion
    - □ principal excretory mechanisms of the kidneys include glomerular filtration, tubular secretion (active and passive), and reabsorption
    - □ active tubular secretion of a drug consists of anionic and cationic substrate-specific pathways
    - □ activity depends on affinity of drug molecule for tubular transport site, the capacity of the site, and renal blood flow
    - □ secretion can be so extensive that virtually all drug is removed from the blood (i.e., tubular secretion is greater than glomerular filtration)
    - □ passive tubular reabsorption of a drug is determined by its degree of lipophilicity, degree of ionization, and urine flow rate
    - □ it is difficult to determine the type and extent of renal tissue damage caused by nephrotoxins and kidney diseases, and how that damage will alter drug excretion

RECOMMENDATIONS AND PRECAUTIONS FOR TREATMENT

- Precautions
  - few published studies are available describing the effect of altered renal function on anticancer drug therapy, thus dosing guidelines for many drugs are not available
    - □ this is especially a problem for anticancer drugs, which have a narrow therapeutic index
  - arbitrary dosage reductions based solely on renal function, without regard to pharmacologic effect, can lead to overdosing and toxicity, or to underdosing and inadequate tumor kill
  - for many drugs, nomograms and equations have been developed to adjust drug dosage in the presence of renal insufficiency, but these approaches have not been validated for most anticancer drugs
  - anticancer drugs can be used for curative (i.e., aggressive) as well as palliative intent, and in this case the extent of dosage adjustment for renal insufficiency requires the oncologist's clinical judgment, based on guidelines suggested in the next section
- Specific drug dosage recommendations for patients with renal insufficiency
  - alkylating agents
    - □ cyclophosphamide: no dosage adjustment is necessary for patients with CrCl > 10 ml/min
    - □ ifosfamide: CrCl < 30 ml/min = 70% of dose can be administered; 31–45 ml/min = 75% of dose; 46–60 ml/min = 80% of dose
    - □ melphalan: CrCl < 30 ml/min = 70% of dose can be administered; 31–45 ml/min = 75% of dose; 46–60 ml/min = 85% of dose
  - antimetabolites
    - □ cytarabine (1–3 g/m^2): CrCl < 30 ml/min = use not recommended; 31–45 ml/min = 50% of dose; 46–60 ml/min = 60% of dose
    - □ fludarabine: CrCl < 30 ml/min = 65% of dose can be administered; 31–45 ml/min = 75% of dose; 46–60 ml/min = 80% of dose
    - □ 5-fluorouracil: no dosage adjustment is necessary for patients with CrCl > 10 ml/min
    - □ methotrexate: CrCl < 30 ml/min = use not recommended; 31–45 ml/min = 50% of dose; 46–60 ml/min = 65% of dose
    - □ pentostatin: CrCl < 30 ml/min = use not recommended; 31–45 ml/min = 60% of dose; 46–60 ml/min = 70% of dose
  - antitumor antibiotics
    - □ daunorubicin and doxorubicin: no dosage adjustment recommended for patients with renal insufficiency
    - □ mithramycin: CrCl < 30 ml/min = 50–75% of the dose can be administered; 31–60 ml/min = 75% of dose
    - □ mitomycin: CrCl < 30 ml/min = 50–75% of the dose can be administered; 31–60 ml/min = 75% of dose
  - nitrosoureas
    - □ carmustine: CrCl < 30 ml/min = use not recommended; 31–45 ml/min = 75% of dose; 46–60 ml/min = 80% of dose
    - □ lomustine: CrCl < 30 ml/min = use not recommended; 31–45 ml/min = 70% of dose; 46–60 ml/min = 75% of dose

- semustine: CrCl < 30 ml/min = use not recommended; 31–30 ml/min = 70% of dose
- streptozotocin: CrCl < 30 ml/min = 50 to 75% of the dose can be administered; 31–60 ml/min = 75% of dose

– topoisomerase interactive agents
  - etoposide: CrCl < 30 ml/min = 75% of the dose can be administered; 31–45 ml/min = 80% of dose; 46–60 ml/min = 85% of dose
  - topotecan: CrCl < 30 ml/min = 70% of the dose can be administered; 31–45 ml/min = 75% of dose; 46–60 ml/min = 80% of dose

- Miscellaneous agents
  - bleomycin: CrCl < 30 ml/min = use not recommended; 31–45 ml/min = 60% of dose; 46–60 ml/min = 70% of dose
  - dacarbazine: CrCl < 30 ml/min = 70% of the dose can be administered; 31–45 ml/min = 75% of dose; 46–60 ml/min = 80% of dose
  - hydroxyurea: CrCl < 30 ml/min = 75% of the dose can be administered; 31–45 ml/min = 80% of dose; 46–60 ml/min = 85% of dose
  - vinca alkaloids (vincristine and vinblastine): no dosage adjustment is necessary for patients with CrCl > 10 ml/min
- Platinum-containing agents
  - carboplatin: CrCl < 15 ml/min = no data; 16–40 ml/min = 200 mg/m^2; 41–59 ml/min = 250 mg/m^2 (alternatively, the dose [mg] = desired area under the plasma concentration time curve [AUC] in mg/ml/min multiplied by GFR [or CrCl] + 25)
  - cisplatin: CrCl < 30 ml/min = use not recommended; 31–45 ml/min = 50% of dose can be administered; 46–60 ml/min = 75% of dose

KEY REFERENCES

Kintzel PE, Dorr RT: Anticancer drug renal toxicity and elimination: dosing guidelines for altered renal function. Cancer Treatment Rev 1995; 21:33–64

Patterson WP, Reams GP: Renal toxicities of chemotherapy. Semin Oncol 1992; 19: 521–8

Powis G: Effect of human renal and hepatic disease on the pharmacokinetics of anticancer drugs. Cancer Treatment Rev 1982; 9:85–124

Stewart CF, Fleming RA, Madden T: Chemotherapy drugs. In: RW Schrier and JG

Liver Dysfunction

A. P. Venook

OVERVIEW OF UNDERLYING DISEASE

- The liver plays a critical role in the handling of most pharmaceuticals, from the activation of pro-drugs to the metabolism and clearance of active agents
- Little data exist that guide dosing decision making for chemotherapy, reflecting several complicating clinical issues
  - absence of reliable measures of degrees of hepatic dysfunction
  - heterogeneous causes of hepatic dysfunction in cancer patients
  - secondary manifestations of liver disease that may alter the pharmacodynamics of patient–drug interactions
  - standard use of combination chemotherapy confuses the applicability of data on single-agent pharmacokinetics
- Dosing decisions must be made on a case-by-case basis, with careful, balanced attention paid to organ function and therapeutic goals
  - the tendency to reduce chemotherapeutic dosage in patients with liver disease will sometimes be incorrect, although, in general, it would be a reasonable practice

GENERAL PRINCIPLES

- The diagnostic tools most often used—transaminase, alkaline phosphatase and bilirubin levels, prothrombin time, albumin—are neither specific for liver function nor absolutely predictive of drug handling
- The rate of hepatic blood flow is a critical determinant of the rate and amount of drugs processed by the liver, making it difficult to predict drug handling in cancer patients
  - patients with viral hepatitis may have increased hepatic blood flow; patients with alcoholic hepatitis may have diminished blood flow
  - patients with hepatocellular carcinoma may have altered blood flow due to their underlying liver disease, as well as changes in flow, secondary to portal vein occlusion or mass effect
- Functional hepatocyte mass is a determinant of hepatic extraction of a drug
  - generally, patients with liver disease have reduced hepatocyte mass, although quantification is unreliable
- Secondary manifestations of liver disease and cirrhosis can affect the therapeutic index of chemotherapeutics
  - anasarca may alter gastrointestinal absorption of oral agents while concomitant decreases in kidney blood flow may change the contribution that renal clearance makes to drug handling
  - hepatitis B viral disease may alter bone marrow function and accentuate the effects of chemotherapeutic agents, independent of drug handling
  - although difficult to evaluate, altered plasma proteins—diminished production, for example—may alter systemic clearance of a drug because of the differential amounts of unbound, as compared to bound, drug
- Patients with hepatic tumor involvement or transaminitis without gross anatomic changes associated with cirrhosis may have alterations in hepatic blood flow, functional hepatocyte mass, and/or plasma protein binding
  - these effects on drug handling may be unpredictable
  - these patients may also have mild variance in glucuronidation with no substantial change in liver function

RECOMMENDATIONS AND PRECAUTIONS FOR TREATMENT

- Some recommendations are based on observational data, others on the absence of observational data, and a few on prospective studies carried out to address the specific issues
- Specific recommendations for dosing of chemotherapeutics in the presence of liver dysfunction can be made for only a few agents
  - 5-fluorouracil
    - □ generally, despite animal model data, most clinicians would not adjust dosing of this drug in the presence of abnormal liver function tests or cirrhosis
  - cyclophosphamide
    - □ impaired liver function significantly affects the pharmacokinetics of this drug, which is metabolized to its active form by the cytochrome P-450 oxidase system
    - □ while parent compound clearance may be diminished in such patients, so too might the conversion of the pro-drug to the active aldophosphamide
    - □ for these reasons, the reflexive dose reduction applied to patients with liver dysfunction may be incorrect
  - vincristine
    - □ vinca alkaloids are metabolized by the liver and excreted in the bile
    - □ the area under the curve is increased in patients with elevations of alkaline phosphatase, and this alteration in clearance increases the incidence of neurotoxicity
    - □ generally, dosing of vinca alkaloids should be reduced in patients with evidence of decreased hepatic clearance, although precise parameters have not been defined
  - doxorubicin
    - □ this drug and its active metabolite, doxorubicinol, are eliminated mainly by the biliary route
    - □ numerous studies have documented increased toxicity of these agents in patients with evidence of liver disease, and specific dose-reduction parameters are available
    - □ at least some conflicting data, however, suggests that dose reductions may inhibit antitumor efficacy
  - paclitaxel
    - □ prospective studies have indicated that hepatic metabolism is critical for the clearance of the taxanes and the dosing of this drug in patients with varying degrees of hepatic dysfunction
    - □ treatment and dosing cohorts were based on transaminase or bilirubin abnormalities
    - □ while increased myelosuppression and other toxicities were seen in patients with hepatic dysfunction, the confounding of results could be caused by prior treatment, tumor type, or other factors
    - □ pharmacokinetic sampling identified diminished drug clearance as a possible mechanism for increased toxicity in patients treated with a 3 hr infusion

KEY REFERENCES

Benjamin RS, Wiernik PH, Bachur NR: Adriamycin chemotherapy—efficacy, safety, and pharmacologic basis of an intermittent single high-dosage schedule. Cancer 1974; 33:19–27

Johnson PJ, Alexopoulos A, Johnson RD, Williams R: Significance of serum bilirubin level in response of hepatocellular carcinoma to doxorubicin. J Hepatol 1986; 3:149–53

Koren G, Beatty K, Seta A, Einarson TR, Lishner M: The effects of impaired liver function on the elimination of antineoplastic agents. Ann Pharmacother 1992; 26:363–71

Morgan DJ, McLean AJ: Clinical pharmacokinetic and pharmacodynamic considerations in patients with liver disease. Clin Pharmacokinet 1995; 29:370–91

Van den Berg HW, Desai ZR, Wilson R, Kennedy G, Bridges JM, Shanks RG: The pharmacokinetics of vincristine in man: reduced drug clearance associated with raised serum alkaline phosphatase and dose-limiting elimination. Cancer Chemother Pharmacol 1982; 8:215–9

Venook AP, Egorin MJ, Rosner GL, Brown TD, Jahan TM, Batist G, Hohl R, Budman D, Ratain MJ, Kearns CM, Schilsky RL: Phase I and pharmacokinetic trial of paclitaxel in patients with hepatic dysfunction: Cancer and Leukemia Group B 9264. J Clin Oncol 1998; 16:1811–9

Congestive Heart Failure

S. Chittoor and S. Swain

OVERVIEW OF UNDERLYING DISEASE

- Congestive heart failure is a general condition in which the heart is unable to pump enough blood to meet the needs of the body's other organs
  - common causes include coronary artery disease, cardiomyopathy, and congenital heart disease
- Cardiotoxicity related to chemotherapy can manifest as rhythm disturbances, decreased myocardial contractility, or coronary vasospasm
- ~10% of patients with cancer have metastatic involvement of the cardiac structures
  - this complication might be predictable and reversible and can exacerbate underlying cardiovascular disease

GENERAL PRINCIPLES

- A complete pretreatment history and physical evaluation is vital before administering cancer drugs
  - symptoms of chest pain, dyspnea, palpitations
  - cardiac auscultation, evaluation for orthostasis, bruits, and manifestations of cardiovascular disease in target organs, i.e., eyes, brain, lungs, and abdomen
  - a standard EKG and a two-dimensional echocardiogram or a MUGA scan

RECOMMENDATIONS AND PRECAUTIONS FOR TREATMENT

- Anthracycline antitumor antibiotic: doxorubicin
  - conclusive data are not available on preexisting heart disease as a cofactor for increased risk of doxorubicin-induced cardiac toxicity
    - □ preliminary data suggest that cardiac toxicity may occur at doses lower than the recommended cumulative limit
    - □ risk of cardiotoxicity is reduced by low-dose weekly administration of doxorubicin or prolonged 48–96 hr continuous IV infusion
  - doxorubicin treatment is contraindicated in patients who have received previous treatment with complete, cumulative doses of doxorubicin, daunorubicin, or other anthracyclines and anthracenes
  - acute toxicity occurs during or within hours of administration, manifesting as dysrhythmias or as non-specific EKG changes
  - chronic toxicity occurs weeks or months after administration and is related to the cumulative dose
  - risk factors include children and elderly (age > 70 yrs), prior mediastinal irradiation, and conditions associated with increased left ventricular wall tension
  - dexrazoxane is effective when given to patients who have already received 300 mg/m^2 of doxorubicin in patients with breast cancer
  - deteriorating cardiac function in adults may be avoided by stopping doxorubicin when there is a 10% decline in the LVEF to below the lower limit of normal, an absolute LVEF of 45%, or a 20% decline in the LVEF at any level. However, MUGA scans and echo scans are not always sensitive to predict congestive heart failure
  - endomyocardial biopsy grade of > 1.5 predicts congestive heart failure
    - □ consider endomyocardial biopsy in patients who do not have clinical symptoms and have received 400–500 mg/m^2 of anthracycline
  - crossing from one anthracycline agent to another does not offer cardioprotection
  - probability of clinical congestive cardiac failure with mitoxantrone is 2.6% in patients who received up to 140 mg/m^2
  - management of cardiac complications from doxorubicin
    - □ treatment of anthracycline- or anthracendione-associated cardiomyopathy is similar to that of cardiomyopathies caused by other etiologies
    - □ discontinue agent
    - □ restrict fluids and activity
    - □ use diuretics and morphine sulfate as needed
    - □ oxygen prn
    - □ use agents that reduce afterload, such as captopril or enalapril
    - □ digoxin
    - □ anticoagulation or antiplatelet therapy
    - □ admit to intensive care unit if vasopressors are indicated
- Antitumor antibiotics: mitomycin-C
  - may enhance the cardiotoxicity of anthracyclines
  - cardiac evaluation and prospective cardiac function monitoring if patients received prior anthracycline therapy
- Antimetabolites: 5-fluorouracil (5-FU)
  - coronary vasospasm can occur immediately, or up to 18 hrs after 5-FU administration
  - 5-FU can cause decompensation in patients with congestive heart failure
  - long-acting nitrates or calcium channel blockers may prevent angina
- Alkylating agents: cyclophosphamide
  - cardiotoxicity is seen after high doses (120–270 mg/kg) and is not related to cumulative dose
    - □ onset is acute and death occurs within 15 days, although milder presentations may be reversible
  - prior mediastinal irradiation and anthracycline administration may be risk factors
- Taxanes
  - docetaxel
    - □ use diuretics at the first sign of peripheral edema
    - □ fluid retention, despite premedication with dexamethasone, may precipitate heart failure in patients with history of cardiovascular disease
  - paclitaxel
    - □ in patients with congestive heart failure, bradycardia could lead to cardiac decompensation
    - □ asymptomatic EKG changes unrelated to prior anthracycline therapy occur in ~20% of all patients
    - □ continuous cardiac monitoring for patients with serious conduction abnormalities
    - □ when doxorubicin is followed immediately by 3 hrs of paclitaxel, cardiotoxicity is increased due to decreased clearance of doxorubicin by 30%
    - □ delay the administration of paclitaxel for up to 24 hrs following doxorubicin, or limit the total cumulative doxorubicin dose to avoid cardiotoxicity
- Biological response modifiers
  - interferons (IFN) should be used with caution in patients with heart failure
  - IFN in a dose-dependent manner can cause tachypnea, tachycardia, nonspecific EKG changes, and rare myocardial infarction
  - interleukin-2 causes capillary leak syndrome when given in doses over 100,000 U/kg, resulting in hypotension and occasional supraventricular tachyarrhythmia
    - □ when complications arise, admit to ICU
    - □ high Fowler position
    - □ oxygen prn
    - □ restrict fluids and diet
    - □ use diuretics and morphine sulfate, as needed
    - □ ensure accurate fluid intake and output
    - □ use ventilatory support if necessary
- Other considerations
  - cisplatin may be associated with dysrhythmias caused or exacerbated by electrolyte abnormalities from hydration and diuresis
  - transretinoic acid may cause pericardial effusions and myocardial dysfunction, which is reversible with dexamethasone
  - trastuzumab administration can result in the development of ventricular dysfunction
    - □ the incidence and severity is particularly high when administered in combination with cyclophosphamide and anthracyclines
    - □ frequent cardiac monitoring is recommended

KEY REFERENCES

Alexander J, Dainiak N, Berger HJ, Goldman L, Johnstone D, Reduto L, Duffy T, Schwartz P, Gottschalk A, Zaret BL: Serial assessment of doxorubicin cardiotoxicity with quantitative radionuclide angiocardiography. N Engl J Med 1979; 300:278–83

Allen A: The cardiotoxicity of chemotherapeutic drugs. Semin Oncol 1992; 19:529–42

Gianni L, Vigano L, Locatelli A, Locatelli A, Capri G, Giani A, Tarenzi E, Bonadonna G: Human pharmacokinetic characterization and in vitro study of the interaction between doxorubicin and paclitaxel in patients with breast cancer. J Clin Oncol 1997; 15: 1906–15

Legha SS, Benjamin RS, Mackay B, Ewer M, Wallace S, Valdivieso M, Rasmussen SL, Blumenschein GR, Freireich EJ: Reduction of doxorubicin cardiotoxicity by prolonged continuous intravenous infusion. Ann Intern Med 1982; 96:133–9

Lee R, Lotze M, Skibber J, Tucker E, Bonow RO, Ognibene FP, Carrasquillo JA, Shelhamer JH, Parrillo JE, Rosenberg SA: Cardiorespiratory effects of immunotherapy with interleukin-2. J Clin Oncol 1989; 7:7–20

Porembka DT, Lowder JN, Orlowski JP, Bastulli J, Lockrem J: Etiology and management of doxorubicin cardiotoxicity. Crit Care Med 1989; 17:569

Swain SM, Whaley FS, Gerber MC, Ewer MS, Bianchine JR, Gams RA: Delayed administration of dexrazoxane provides cardioprotection for patients with advanced breast cancer treated with doxorubicin containing therapy. J Clin Oncol 1997; 15:1333–40

Management of AIDS-Associated Malignancies

J. A. Sparano and G. Kalkut

KAPOSI'S SARCOMA

- Prevalence
  - risk elevated ~40,000-fold compared with the general population
  - occurs in 20–30% of HIV-infected individuals
- Clinical presentation
  - involves skin, mucous membranes, viscera, and lymph nodes
  - skin involvement almost always present
    - painless, nonpruritic macules or nodules
    - may be violaceous, red, or brown, and may be difficult to appreciate in dark-skinned individuals
    - a few to hundreds of lesions may occur
    - skin lesions may coalesce to form plaques
    - may be associated with significant edema
  - mucosal involvement common
    - oral cavity (hard and soft palate, gingiva)
    - conjunctiva
    - gastrointestinal tract is usually asymptomatic
  - pulmonary involvement requires therapy
    - may be rapidly fatal and usually requires prompt therapy
    - chest radiography: may be difficult to distinguish from pulmonary infection on chest x-ray or computerized tomography
    - combination of gallium scan (positive in infection) and thallium scan (positive in KS) may be useful
    - bronchoscopy usually reveals characteristic blue-violet submucosal lesions; transbronchial biopsy is usually not necessary
- Diagnosis and pathogenesis
  - skin lesions may be confused with bacillary angiomatosis
  - biopsy of skin or other sites is recommended to confirm the diagnosis
  - biopsy shows proliferation of spindle cells and infiltration by red cells and mononuclear cells
  - cell of origin is likely a mesenchymal progenitor of lymphatic or endothelial cell origin
  - human herpes virus-8 infection is postulated to be causative
- Treatment and prognosis
  - disease may regress with reduction in HIV burden after antiretroviral therapy
  - a staging system has been proposed that has prognostic value. Poor prognostic features include
    - low CD4 count (< 200/mcl)
    - advanced tumor
      - edema or ulceration
      - GI, visceral, or extensive mucosal involvement
    - systemic illness
      - history of opportunistic infection or thrush
      - B symptoms
      - other HIV-associated illnesses
      - poor performance status (KPS < 70%)
    - indications for systemic therapy
      - pulmonary involvement
      - palliation of advanced, symptomatic disease
      - cosmetic considerations
    - systemic therapy options
      - cytotoxic agents: liposomal anthracyclines, paclitaxel
      - alpha-interferon plus antiretroviral therapy
      - anti-angiogenic agents (e.g., thalidomide)

DHHS Guidelines: Indications for initiating antiretroviral therapy (January 28, 2000)

Clinical Category	CD4+ T-cell Count and HIV RNA	Recommendation
Symptomatic (AIDS, thrush, unexplained fever)	Any value	Treat
Asymptomatic	CD4+ T cells < 500/mm^3 *or* HIV RNA > 10,000 (bDNA)* *or* > 20,000 (RT-PCR)*	Treatment should be offered
Asymptomatic	CD4+ T cells > 500/mm^3 *and* HIV RNA < 10,000 (bDNA) or < 20,000 (RT-PCR)*	Many experts would delay therapy and observe; however, some experts would treat

* bDNA and RT-PCR are different commercially available methods of HIV quantitation.

DHHS Guidelines for antiretroviral therapy (January 28, 2000)

Column A	Column B
Strongly Recommended	
Efavirenz	Stavudine + lamivudine
Indinavir	Stavudine + didanosine
Nelfinavir	Zidovudine + lamivudine
Ritonavir + Saquinavir [SGC or HGC]	Zidovudine + didanosine
Recommended as an Alternative	
Abacavir	Didanosine + lamivudine
Amprenavir	Zidovudine + zalcitabine
Delavirdine	
Nelfinavir + Saquinavir-SGC	
Nevirapine	
Ritonavir	
Saquinavir	

Drugs listed alphabetically, not in order of priority.

Non-nucleoside reverse transcriptase inhibitors (Column A)

Drug	Adult dose and preparation	Toxicity
Nevirapine [Viramune]	200 mg qd × 14 days, then 200 mg bid if no rash Tablets (200 mg) Oral suspension (50 mg/5 ml)	Skin rash (8%) may progress to severe or life-threatening conditions (discontinue if severe rash or rash with constitutional symptoms); LFT abnormalities
Delavirdine [Rescriptor]	400 mg tid (4–100 mg tablets in 3 oz of water to produce a slurry) Tablets (100 mg) Separate dosing with ddI or antacids by at least 1 hr	Skin rash, headaches
Efavirenz [Sustiva]	600 mg qhs Capsules (50, 100, 200 mg)	Rash, central nervous system symptoms, increased transaminase levels, false positive cannabinoid test

Protease inhibitors (Column A)

Drug*	Adult dose and preparation	Toxicity*
Nelfinavir [Viracept]	750 mg tid or 1,250 mg bid Take with food (meal or light snack) Tablets (250 mg); powder (50 mg/g)	Diarrhea, hyperglycemia
Indinavir [Crixivan]	800 mg q8h Take 1 hr before or 2 hrs after meals; may take with skim milk or low-fat meal; separate dosing with ddI by 1 hr Capsules (200, 333, 400 mg)	Nephrolithiasis, asymptomatic hyperbilirubinemia, rash, dry skin, pharyngitis, taste perversion, abdominal pain, nausea, vomiting, headache
Amprenavir [Agenerase]	1,200 mg bid Tablets (50, 150 mg) Oral solution (15 mg/ml) (tablets and solution not interchangeable on a mg per mg basis) Can be taken with or without food, but high-fat meal should be avoided	Nausea, diarrhea, rash, headache, paresthesias, increased liver function tests
Ritonavir [Norvir]	600 mg q12h (or bid with Invirase) Take after meals; taste of the oral solution may be improved by mixing with chocolate milk, Ensure, or Advera within 1 hr of dosing Capsules (100 mg) should be refrigerated Solution (600 mg/7.5 cc) should *not* be refrigerated	Nausea, vomiting, anorexia, diarrhea, abdominal pain, taste perversion, circumoral and peripheral paresthesias, asymptomatic increase in SGOT/SGPT
Saquinavir [Invirase] [Fortovase]	Hard gelatin capsules (200 mg): Invirase 400 mg bid with ritonavir (otherwise not recommended) Take within 2 hrs of a meal Soft gelatin capsule (200 mg): Fortovase 1,200 mg tid Take with large meal	Diarrhea, abdominal discomfort, nausea, headache, elevated aminotransferase levels, hyperglycemia

*All protease inhibitors may cause hypertriglyceridemia and a lipodystrophy syndrome.

Nucleoside reverse transcriptase inhibitors (Column B)

Drug	Adult dose and preparation	Toxicity
Zidovudine (AZT) [Retrovir]	200 mg tid or 300 mg bid Capsules (100 mg), tablets (300 mg) Syrup (50 mg/5 ml; 240 ml bottle)	Anemia, granulocytopenia, headache, malaise, anorexia, nausea, vomiting, myopathy, hepatic steatosis/failure, lactic acidosis
Lamivudine (3TC) [Epivir]	150 mg bid Tablets (150 mg) Oral solution (10 mg/ml) Combivir: 1 tablet contains 300 mg zidovudine + 150 mg lamivudine	Neuropathy, pancreatitis, hepatic steatosis/failure, lactic acidosis
Didanosine (ddI) [Videx]	Doses for tablets/powder: ≥60 kg: 400 mg qd or 200 mg bid <60 kg: 250 mg qd or 125 mg bid Take 30 min before or 1 hr after meals Tablets (25, 50, 100, 150, 200 mg) Powder (100, 167, 250 mg per packet) Pediatric powder (2 g bottle; 4 g bottle)	Neuropathy, pancreatitis, diarrhea, hyperuricemia, hepatic steatosis/failure, lactic acidosis, retinal depigmentation
Stavudine (d4T) [Zerit]	≥60 kg: 40 mg bid <60 kg: 30 mg bid (If neuropathy, reduce dose 50%) Capsules (15, 20, 30, 40 mg) Oral solution (1 mg/ml)	Neuropathy, increased SGOT/SGPT, pancreatitis, hepatic steatosis/failure, lactic acidosis
Abacavir [Ziagen]	300 mg bid Tablets (300 mg) Oral solution (20 mg/ml; 240 ml bottle)	Hypersensitivity reactions, nausea, vomiting, headache, fever, anorexia. Should not be restarted after a reaction—symptoms will recur within hours and may be fatal
Zalcitabine (ddC) [Hivid]	0.75 mg tid Tablets (0.375, 0.75 mg)	Neuropathy, pancreatitis, oral/esophageal ulcers, hepatic steatosis/failure

USPHS/IDSA infection prophylaxis guidelines: strongly recommended as standard of care

Infection	Indication	Preferred Agent
Pneumocystis carinii	CD4 < 200/μL *or* oropharyngeal candidiasis	TMP-SMZ 1 DS tablet qd or 1 SS tablet qd
Toxoplasma gondii	CD4 < 100/μL; IgG seropositive	TMP-SMZ 1 DS qd
MAI Complex	CD4 < 50/μL	Azithromycin 1,200 mg once weekly *or* Clarithromycin 500 mg bid
Mycobacterium tuberculosis	TST reaction ≥ 5 mm *or* Prior + TST without therapy *or* Contact with a TB	**INH-sensitive** Isoniazid 300 mg qd + pyridoxine 50 mg qd × 9 mos **INH-resistant** Rifampin 600 mg qd + Pyrazinamide 20 mg/kg qd × 2 mos **Multidrug-resistant** Consult local public health official

1999 USPHS/ISDA Guidelines

Abbreviations: TMP-SMZ: trimethoprim/sulfamethoxazole; TST: tuberculin skin test.

Potential drug interactions and overlapping toxicity: antiretroviral and cytotoxic agents

Metabolic or toxic effect of antiretroviral drug	Antiretroviral drug	Potential interaction or additive toxicity with cytotoxic therapy
Inhibits cytochrome P-450 Most potent inhibition Less potent inhibition	 Ritonavir Indinavir, Nelfinavir, saquinavir, and delavirdine	Expect *increased* serum concentration of drugs that are metabolized by cytochrome P-450 such as: Alkylators (cyclophosphamide) Anthracyclines (doxorubicin, daunorubicin) Epipodphyllotoxins (etoposide) Taxanes (paclitaxel, docetaxel) Vinca alkaloids (vincristine, vinblastine)
Induces cytochrome P-450	Nevirapine	Expect *decreased* serum concentration of drugs that are metabolized by cytochrome P-450
Myelosuppression	Zidovudine	Potential for additive myelosuppression with regimens associated with moderately severe or severe myelosuppression
Peripheral neuropathy	Didanosine, stavudine, zalcitabine	Potential for additive neurotoxicity with vinca alkaloids and taxanes
Mucositis	Zalcitabine	Potential for additive mucosal toxicity
Gastrointestinal toxicity	Didanosine, ritonavir, indinavir, saquinavir	Potential for poor antiretroviral compliance with cytotoxic agents that are emetogenic

Supportive care for the patient with AIDS and cancer

	Drug(s)
1. Primary Infection Prophylaxis	
Pneumocystis carinii pneumonia and Toxoplasma gondii	TMP-SMZ 1 DS qd
Oral and/or esophageal candidiasis	Fluconazole 100 mg qd (if myelosuppressive therapy)
2. Secondary Infection Prophylaxis	
Herpes simplex infections	Acyclovir 400 mg bid or 200 mg tid
Cytomegalovirus infection	Gancyclovir 1 g tid
Mycobacterium-avium complex	Clarithromycin 500 mg bid *plus* one or more of the following: ciprofloxacin 500–750 mg bid, ethambutol 15 mg/kg qd, clofazimine 100 mg qd, rifabutin 300 mg qd
Toxoplasma gondii	Sulfadiazine 1–1.5 g q6hrs *plus* pyrimethamine 25–75 mg qd *plus* leucovorin 10–25 mg qd
Cryptococcus neoformans, Coccidiodes immites	Fluconazole 200 mg qd
Histoplasma capsulatum	Itraconazole 200 mg bid
Salmonella species	Ciprofloxacin 500 mg bid
3. Hematopoietic Growth Factors	
For selected patients in whom the risk of febrile neutropenia ≥40%	G-CSF 5 mcg/kg or GM-CSF 250 mcg/m² SubQ daily beginning after completion of chemotherapy and continue until neutrophil recovery
4. Antiretroviral Therapy	As per standard recommendations

Management of AIDS-Associated Malignancies *(Continued)*

SYSTEMIC NON-HODGKIN'S LYMPHOMA

- Prevalence (of systemic and CNS lymphoma)
  - risk elevated about 200-fold compared with the general population
  - occurs in 5–6% of HIV-infected individuals
- Clinical presentation
  - extranodal involvement occurs in > 80%, including the gastrointestinal tract, bone marrow, liver, lungs, meninges, skin, oral cavity, rectum, body cavity, and unusual sites
  - histology most commonly diffuse large cell, immunoblastic, or small noncleaved cell
- Treatment and prognosis
  - stage IE disease: CHOP for 3 cycles plus local irradiation
  - stage II–IV disease: CHOP or other standard combinations for intermediate–high grade lymphoma
    - □ some experts recommend a 25–50% reduction in chemotherapy doses, whereas others recommend full-dose therapy with hematopoietic growth factor support
    - □ some evidence suggests that infusional cyclophosphamide, doxorubicin, and etoposide (96 hr infusion) is more effective, although randomized studies demonstrating this are lacking
  - CNS prophylaxis
    - □ indicated because of the high rate of meningeal relapse (4 injections of intrathecal cytarabine or methotrexate commonly used)
    - □ some experts recommend prophylaxis for all patients, whereas others recommend prophylaxis only if there is small, noncleaved cell lymphoma, bone marrow involvement, or other high-risk sites (e.g., sinus involvement)
  - low CD4 lymphocyte count (< 100/mcl) the most significant adverse prognostic factor

PRIMARY CENTRAL NERVOUS SYSTEM LYMPHOMA

- Clinical presentation
  - seizures, altered mental status, focal neurologic findings, or subtle neurologic symptoms
  - CD4 count usually < 50/mcl
  - CT scan of the brain with contrast usually reveals
    - □ solitary (50%) or multiple (50%) lesions
    - □ lesions usually isodense or hyperdense
    - □ lesions usually relatively large (2–4 cm) with edema
    - □ located in the cerebral hemispheres, cerebellum, or periventricular regions (basal ganglia, thalamus, corpus collosum, or brain stem)
    - □ lesions enhance after contrast injection about 90% of the time, with ring enhancement in 50%
    - □ radiographically indistinguishable from CNS toxoplasmosis and other infections
    - □ ~ 10% of patients may have a normal CT scan
  - histology most commonly diffuse large cell, immunoblastic, or small noncleaved cell
- Diagnosis
  - definitive
    - □ brain biopsy confirming lymphoma usually performed to confirm the diagnosis after failure to improve clinically or radiographically after a 1–3 wk course of antitoxoplasmosis therapy
    - □ CSF cytology revealing malignant cells occurs in ~ 20%
  - highly likely
    - □ positive CSF analysis for Epstein-Barr virus DNA by PCR: 80% sensitive and 95% specific for CNS lymphoma
    - □ positive Thallium-201 SPECT scan: 90% sensitive and 90% specific for CNS lymphoma in some studies
    - □ combination of positive CSF EBV DNA and/or Thallium-201 SPECT has a very high sensitivity, specificity, and predictive value
- Treatment and prognosis
  - whole brain irradiation may palliate symptoms and result in occasional (~ 15%) survivors beyond 1 yr
  - prolonged survival associated with good performance status and absence of prior opportunistic infections
  - systemic chemotherapy not of proven value
  - anecdotal reports of spontaneous remission associated with highly active antiretroviral therapy

KEY REFERENCES

AIDS-Associated Malignancies

Antinori A, DeRossi G, Ammassari A, Cingolani A, Murri R, DiGiuda D, DeLuca A, Pierconti F, Tartaglione T, Scerrati M, Larocca LM, Ortona L: Value of combined approach with thallium-201 single-photon emission computed tomography and Epstein-Barr virus DNA polymerase chain reaction in CSF for the diagnosis of AIDS-related primary CNS lymphoma. J Clin Oncol 1999; 17:554–60

Fine HA, Mayer RJ: Primary central nervous system lymphoma. Ann Intern Med 1993; 119:1093–1104

Kaplan, LD, Kahn, JO, Crowe, S, Northfelt D, Neville P, Grossberg H, Abrams DI, Tracey J, Mills J, Volberding P: Clinical and virologic effects of recombinant human granulocyte-macrophage colony-stimulating factor in patients receiving chemotherapy for human immunodeficiency virus–related non-Hodgkin's lymphoma: results of a randomized trial. J Clin Oncol 1990; 9:929–40

Levine AM: AIDS-related malignancies: the emerging epidemic. J Natl Cancer Inst 1993; 85:1382–97

Sparano JA, Hu X, Wiernik PH, Sarta C, Schwartz EL, Soeiro R, Henry DH, Mason B, Ratech H, Dutcher JP: A pilot trial of infusional cyclophosphamide, doxorubicin, and etoposide plus didanosine and granulocyte colony stimulating factor in patients with HIV-associated non-Hodgkin's lymphoma. J Clin Oncol 1996; 14:3026–35

Von Roenn JH: Kaposi's sarcoma: evaluation and treatment. In *American Society of Clinical Oncology Educational Book,* M Perry (ed) (pp. 76–86). Philadelphia: WB Saunders Company, 1998

Antiretroviral Therapy and Supportive Care

HIV/AIDS Treatment Information Service
Phone: 800-448-0440
Fax: 301-519-6616
http://www.hivatis.org

Chapter 14

ACCESS DEVICES AND PUMPS: OPTIONS IN ADMINISTRATION

Introduction

Consuelo Skosey

■ In recent years there has been remarkable growth in the development and introduction of vascular access devices (VADs) that are employed for drug delivery. First introduced in the 1970s, these short-term and long-term devices are used in adults and children and more than 500,000 are placed yearly (Fulton, 1997). Countless devices such as nontunneled catheters, tunneled catheters, implantable ports, and pumps are currently on the market

■ The availability of so many devices has led to some confusion about which may be the best to use (Winston et al., 1995). VADs are used for treatment delivery, pain control, parenteral nutrition, blood component therapy, and blood withdrawal. They enable physicians to deliver high concentrations of drug directly to the site of disease as in the case of some hepatic tumors and have influenced the treatment approach to intra-abdominal tumors like ovarian cancer. VADs afford advantages to nurses by providing a safe reliable method for delivering long-term, continuous, and/or frequent infusions to patients in the hospital, ambulatory/office facility, and/or home care setting

■ Cancer therapy has been transformed by the many different devices available because they allow flexibility in choosing a device that meets individual patient needs, thereby enhancing the patient's quality of life. As their use increases, new approaches in catheter care and maintenance, insertion techniques, and in the management of complications continue to evolve

NURSING CONSIDERATIONS

- ■ Complications
  - occlusions
    - □ Gabriel et al. (1997)
      - ▽ associated persistent withdrawal occlusion with VADs more common with devices left in place for > 7 days
      - ▽ addresses potential causes and describes how fibrin sheath formation, the most common cause, can be remedied
    - □ Eastbridge and Lefor (1995)
      - ▽ found the incidence of thrombotic complications in patients with triple-lumen catheters compared to those with double lumens as well as a significantly ($p < .05$) decreased mean time until catheter failure (40 vs. 146 days)
      - ▽ observed a significant increase in the rate of thrombosis in patients with a catheter tip above T3 level
      - ▽ authors recommend use of fluoroscopy at time of placement to assure adequate catheter length and tip position and the use of triple catheters only when necessary for concurrent drug administration
  - infections
    - □ Darouiche and Raad (1997) found two approaches that can be used nonexclusively for successful prevention of these infections
      - ▽ the first approach includes measures such as placement and maintenance of vascular catheters by a skilled infusion therapy team
      - ▽ the second approach uses antimicrobial agents and involves the application of topical disinfectants such as chlorhexidine, use of silver-impregnated SubQ cuffs (for short-term central venous catheters), flushing catheters with a combination of antimicrobial and antithrombotic agents, and coating of catheters impregnated with either minocycline and rifampin or chlorhexidine and silver sulfadiazine
    - □ Darouiche et al. (1999)
      - ▽ conducted a comparison study with two antimicrobial-impregnated central venous catheters in 12 university-affiliated hospitals
      - ▽ authors conclude that the use of central venous catheters impregnated with minocycline and rifampin is associated with a lower rate of infection than the use of catheters impregnated with chlorhexidine and silver sulfadiazine
    - □ Rumsey and Richardson (1995); Gabriel (1997)
      - ▽ examined etiology, assessment, diagnosis, and management of infections and occlusions; investigators determined that although several strategies have been attempted to prevent and treat infections and occlusions, one specific method has yet to be determined and thus there exist controversies in the best way to manage these complications
    - □ researchers continue to investigate issues related to these areas; however, the rates of infection and occlusion remain essentially unchanged (Herbst, 1993)
  - less frequent complications
    - □ catheter becoming pinched
    - □ malposition or migration of the catheter
    - □ cardiac perforation
    - □ extravasation of the infusion
    - □ breakage of some portion of the catheter, or a defective device
  - care
    - □ aseptic technique, proper access, and appropriate heparinization provide safe yet rapid vascular access with minimal patient discomfort or risk of complication (Johnson, 1994)
    - □ nurses are key in decreasing complications with these devices and in providing optimal safe care; there are many debatable practice issues regarding the management and care of these devices (Ryder, 1993)
    - □ familiarity with institutional policies and procedures is necessary (i.e., catheter flushing, use of anticoagulant and thrombolytic therapy), conscientious adherence to established protocols for VAD care is mandatory (Rumsey and Richardson, 1995; Gabriel, 1997)
    - □ continual assessment of the device is important in identifying catheter prob-

lems promptly, followed by implementation of early and appropriate intervention(s) (Almadrones et al., 1995; Ingle, 1995)
- selection
  - □ be cognizant of the patient's infusion requirements that include frequency of venous access, type of treatment, duration of therapy, mode of administration, drug stability, venous integrity, cost, patient support system, and patient preference
  - □ nurses must be knowledgeable of the anatomic position of the catheter and the vessels involved, as well as the advantages and disadvantages of each VAD (Hadaway, 1995), to ensure appropriate selection that meets the needs of the patient
  - □ the Intravenous Nurses Society (INS) asserts that registered IV nurses, as the definitive end users of VADs, are the most qualified for their selection (INS, 1997)

COMPETENCY

■ Proficiency must be continuously assessed; device maintenance and care can be similar with regard to dressing changes and need for aseptic technique but can be very dissimilar in their flushing techniques, catheter clamping and capping, administration of solutions, and in their repair

■ Adherence to specific guidelines that apply to each device will improve their integrity; nurses should be aware of those guidelines

■ Institutions should assess competency annually and as procedural changes are implemented (Moore et al., 1996)

■ It is essential for nurses to remain current by reading journal articles, attending conferences, and seeking out education and training opportunities

■ The liability of nurses has increased, and awareness of statutes that govern nursing practice is essential (Ryder, 1993); nurses should be aware of their legal responsibilities with regard to their competency, assessment, and education of the patient/family, all aspects of chemotherapy administration (e.g., routes, prevention and detection of extravasation, etc.), chemotherapy delivery systems, and competent documentation

■ Accurate and timely documentation is important; devices must be consistently monitored and findings and interventions accurately documented

■ As health care delivery continues to move from the hospital to outpatient facility and home, nurses will find themselves assuming more responsibilities outside the protection previously provided by the hospital; some authorities feel it is important for nurses to carry individual professional liability insurance

SAFETY

■ Utilizing VADs for cytotoxic drug administration carries the potential hazard of drug exposure to health care professionals

■ All personnel preparing antineoplastic agents must receive specific training on safety measures that will protect them in preparation, administration, and disposal

■ Guidelines to prevent cytotoxic exposure have been established by the Occupational Safety and Health Administration (OSHA), Oncology Nursing Society (ONS), and the American Society of Hospital Pharmacists

■ The section of "Safety Precautions During Chemotherapy Administration" from the ONS "Cancer Chemotherapy Guidelines Recommendations for Practice" is listed in Appendix A, "Considerations for Health Professionals"

PATIENT TEACHING

■ Dougherty determined that routine maintenance of a device is a shared responsibility between the nurse and the patient (Dougherty, 1998)

■ Gorski and Grothman (1996) examined issues related to an effective home infusion therapy program for cancer patients
- they conclude that a competent and experienced nurse is key to a successful home infusion program and can increase benefits and decrease serious complications

■ Age, physical and emotional status, willingness/readiness to learn, cost, educational level, and availability of support system will affect patient teaching (McDermott, 1995)

■ Teaching must be clear, individualized, and reinforced. A return demonstration of the teaching should be ascertained

■ Written literature and instructions should be provided

■ The need to have a family member or significant other present when educating is very important. Documentation of teaching and dates of reinforcement should be recorded

■ Patients and their families are at risk for drug exposure; procedures to prevent spills and undue exposure should be taught as well as corrective actions for potential complications and emergency procedures

■ A copy of "Spill Kit Procedure for Home Use" from "Home Chemotherapy Safety Procedures," C. Blecke, 1989, Oncology Nursing Forum, 16, p. 721, can be found in the back section of this book. Where applicable, nurses will find these procedures valuable to review with patients

CONCLUSION

■ Emerging technology continues to influence care issues surrounding VADs; therefore it is essential to be conscious of new advancements and progress with these devices. Continuous assessment of new information is integral for nurses to remain current and competent. As a result of the many practice care issues regarding these devices, nurses have an opportunity to develop research studies that can address these important questions. Continuing research efforts are needed to capture specific design features of the various devices that qualify performance, examine differences within patient subgroups, and address underrepresented patients and settings (Fulton, 1997)

■ This chapter is not intended to provide the reader with all of the available products or to be specific in their maintenance and care. The manufacturers of these devices are continually developing new VADs and making improvements with currently available ones. We have tried to include those devices that are most often used and likely to be seen in your practice. To avoid repetition, we have in some cases combined similar-type devices whose care and management are somewhat comparable. As institutions differ in their policies and procedures we have devised general guidelines, instructions, and considerations with regard to VADs. Adherence to established protocols for these devices is necessary. We do not constitute an endorsement of any product

KEY REFERENCES

Almadrones L, Campana P, Dantis EC: Arterial, peritoneal, and intraventricular access devices. Semin Oncol Nurs 1995; 11(3): 194–202

Darouiche RO, Raad II: Prevention of catheter-related infections: the skin. Nutrition 1997; 13(4 Suppl):26S–29S

Darouiche RO, Raad II, Heard SO, et al.: A comparison of two antimicrobial-impregnated central venous catheters. Catheter Study Group. N Engl J Med 1999; 340(1):1–8

Dougherty L: Maintaining vascular access devices: the nurse's role. Support Care Cancer 1998; 6(1):23–30

Eastbridge BJ, Lefor AT: Complications of indwelling venous access devices in cancer patients. J Clin Oncol 1995; 13(1):233–8

Fulton JS: Long term vascular access devices. Annu Rev Nurs Res 1997; 15:237–62

Gabriel J: Fibrin sheaths in vascular access devices. Nurs Times 1997; 93(10):56–7

Gorski LA, Grothman L: Home infusion therapy. Semin Oncol Nurs 1996; 12(3):193–201

Hadaway LC: Comparison of vascular access devices. Semin Oncol Nurs 1995; 11(3): 154–66

Herbst SF: Accumulation of blood products and drug precipitates in VADs: a setup for trouble. Journal of Vascular Access Networks 1993; 3(3):9–13

Ingle RJ: Rare complications of vascular access devices. Semin Oncol Nurs 1995; 11(3):184–93

The Intravenous Nurses Society (INS): The registered nurse's role in vascular access devices selection. J Intraven Nurs 1997; 20(2):71–2

Introduction *(Continued)*

Johnson JC: Complications of vascular access devices. Emerg Med Clin North Am 1994; 12(3):691–705
McDermott MK: Patient education and compliance issues associated with access devices. Semin Oncol Nurs 1995; 3(3):9–13
Moore C, Strong D, Childress J, et al.: Ambulatory infusional cancer chemotherapy: nursing role in patient management. The Cancer Center of Boston. J Infus Chemother 1996; 6(4):164–70
Rumsey KA, Richardson DK: Management of infection and occlusion associated with vascular access. Semin Oncol Nurs 1995; 11(3):174–83
Ryder MA: Peripherally inserted central venous catheters. Nurs Clin North Am 1993; 28(4):937–71
Winslow MN, Trammell L, Camp-Sorrell D: Selection of vascular access devices and nursing care. Semin Oncol Nurs 1995; 11(3):167–73

Device: Butterfly, Angiocatheter, Midline

Catherine Kefer

PERIPHERAL ACCESS DEVICES

■ These intravenous (IV) devices are the most commonly used to deliver chemotherapy. They allow for easy absorption of the drug, thus providing predictable blood levels

- *butterfly catheters* have needles made of rigid aluminum or stainless steel without a sheath attached to a plastic portion shaped like a butterfly or wings. A piece of flexible 3–12 inch tubing extends from the wings. They are also made with a vacutainer connector at the end for blood drawing. They come in gauges from 17–25 with a needle length that can vary from ½–1¼ inches. They are not recommended for the administration of viscous solutions or blood products
- *Angiocatheters* are also called over-the-needle catheters. They consist of an aluminum or stainless steel needle inside of a plastic catheter or sheath. A variety of them are available. The catheter length is available between ¾–2 inches in length with a needle gauge of 14–25. The needle is removed after insertion, and the flexible plastic sheath remains in place. Insertion can be more painful than with a butterfly, and a larger vein is required. These catheters can be left in place for 3–5 days depending on institutional policy and manufacturer guidelines
- *midline catheters* are similar to over-the-needle angiocatheters. They consist of a flexible catheter placed over or within a needle. Once inserted, the needle is either removed and the catheter is threaded into the vein, or with some models, the needle is a breakaway needle that is removed after insertion and the flexible catheter is threaded further along the vein. The midline catheter sheath length varies from 8–22 inches. A portion of the catheter remains outside the vein and is used to anchor the catheter to the skin. These catheters can be utilized for long-term therapy up to 6 wks and require use of large basilic or cephalic veins for placement

■ Four methods of IV administration

- IV push: administering the drug directly into the IV cannula
- IV piggyback: the drug is piggybacked into a main line
- IV sidearm technique: delivery through a main line directly into the cannula. This is the technique of choice when administering vesicants
- infusion: this method of administration delivers chemotherapy through a main line as an infusion over several minutes (bolus), several hours (intermittent), or 24 hrs a day (continuous) for ≥1 day

■ Indications for use: delivery of systemic short-term therapy

■ Advantages: provides quick, simple access to vascular system; may be used in all patient care settings; insertion costs are minimal when compared to other venous access procedures; available in single- or double-lumen design; consistent absorption; low risk for infection due to the short duration of use

RISKS/DISADVANTAGES

■ Short life span; discomfort with insertions; difficult to maintain in elderly patients; peripheral vessels can become irritated from the infusion of many products; this method is less desirable for giving vesicants; may require frequent site changes, thereby exhausting peripheral veins; potential for phlebitis

SURGICAL CONSIDERATIONS

MOHAMED YASSINE

■ Preoperation

- assess the patient and prepare for the procedure
- provide the patient with information regarding the procedure, maintenance care, and expected outcome
- involve the patient in the decision making. This facilitates the learning process and adaptation to the device after insertion
- careful vein selection is essential for patient comfort, ease of drug delivery, and prevention of extravasation
- always use veins that are smooth and pliable, not inflamed, sclerosed, phlebitic, or bruised. Avoid areas with decreased circulation or impaired lymphatic drainage, as well as veins in the legs and feet
- the size and anatomic location of the appropriate vein is dependent on the chemotherapy agent, fluids, and blood products to be administered and the length of the infusion
- discuss different insertion site options with the patient so convenience and quality of life is minimally affected

■ Postoperation

- confirm placement by flushing with 5 ml normal saline. Observe swelling and pain at the insertion site or along the vein
- stabilize the line with a dressing to help prevent trauma, drainage, and infection
- use at least 20 ml of saline to flush after every use; this will help prevent drug precipitation, which is due to sudden pH changes
- avoid applying pressure when flushing to minimize catheter and vein damage

CLINICAL ASSESSMENT/ INTERVENTIONS/IMPLICATIONS

■ Patient assessment: includes examination of the catheter and insertion site

- monitor temperature
- inspect for erythema, swelling, and drainage at insertion site
- check for blood return before, during, and after administration of drugs
- assess for pain or tenderness at insertion site; assess for pain along the vein with drug delivery
- flush catheter to assess flow, swelling, resistance
- assess patient for side effects related to the drug administered

■ Maintenance requires aseptic technique. Cleanse the skin beginning at the insertion site, and move outward in a circular motion using betadine or alcohol. Tape all junctures and tubing to avoid local trauma and dislodgement. A heplock flush and cap is required if left in place for a few days

■ Flushing: these catheters require flushing before and after each medication with normal saline to prevent drug mixture precipitation and vein damage. Angiocatheters require a heplock flush daily or with each use if they are left in place for 3–5 days. Refer to institutional policies

- flush catheter before and after each medication with normal saline
- flush with 2–3 cc of heparin solution (10–1,000 units/ml) once or twice a day
- flush with 10–20 ml of normal saline followed by the heparin flush when blood is drawn from the catheter

■ Catheter care/dressing requirements

- requires aseptic technique: transparent or gauze dressing should be changed q3days and whenever they become wet, soiled, or loose
- butterfly catheters require no dressing changes because they are removed after each use

■ Management of complications

- occlusion: the inability to withdraw or infuse solutions; commonly caused by a blood clot or dislodgement from the vein. To prevent/minimize this
  - □ use larger veins if possible
  - □ rotate sites to avoid trauma to veins
  - □ infuse solutions/agents slowly
  - □ avoid excessive manipulation of catheter
  - □ flush with sterile saline after blood products
  - □ flush catheter after each agent is administered
  - □ inspect solutions to be administered for visible precipitants
  - □ limit ROM in the extremity during administration
- infection
  - □ infection can occur locally at the insertion site. Signs and symptoms include skin warm to the touch, erythematous, with or without visual exudate
  - □ the patient may experience discomfort

    - □ management includes obtaining a culture of the site and administration of antibiotics
  - other complications include
    - □ a kinked line, malposition due to manipulation, a catheter that is severed, punctured, split, or separated
    - □ infiltration/extravasation can occur when the catheter becomes dislodged from the vein or the vein is perforated
    - □ *do not use device if function is questionable*
  - home infusions (if catheter heplocked)
    - □ use aseptic technique
    - □ clean insertion site using skin-cleansing agents; begin at the insertion site and cleanse outward in a circular motion
    - □ flush daily and between drugs
    - □ inspect home environment for sources of infection
- ■ Special considerations
  - inspect all fluids being administered for visible precipitants to avoid complications
- ■ Document procedure, findings, and interventions

ISSUES FOR PATIENT AND FAMILY TEACHING

- ■ Name of the device: butterfly, angiocatheter, or midline catheter
- ■ Frequency and procedure for dressings, flushing, and clamping
- ■ Provide verbal and written review of care with patient and family
- ■ Instruct patient to report fever, tenderness, irritation, drainage at catheter site, and difficulty in flushing
- ■ Provide telephone numbers of physician and nurse
- ■ Showering and bathing is not permitted
- ■ Routine assessment of compliance with recommendations for care

KEY REFERENCES

Access Device Guidelines: Recommendations for Nursing Practice and Education, D Camp-Sorrell (ed). Pittsburgh: Oncology Nursing Society, n.d.

Adverse reactions associated with midline catheters—United States, 1992–1995. From the Centers for Disease Control and Prevention. JAMA 1996; 749–50

Alexander HR: Vascular access and specialized techniques of drug delivery. In *Cancer: Principles and Practice of Oncology* (5th ed., pp. 725–34), V DeVita Jr, S Hellman, SA Rosenberg (eds). Philadelphia: Lippincott-Raven, 1997

Berg D: Drug delivery system. In *Cancer Chemotherapy: A Nursing Process Approach* (2nd ed., pp. 561–95), M Burke, G Wilkes, K Ingwersen (eds). London: Jones and Bartlett, 1996

Goetz AM, Miller J, Wagener MM, et al.: Complication related to intravenous midline catheter usage. A 2-year study. J Intraven Nurs 1998; 21(2):76–80

Martin V: Delivery of cancer chemotherapy. In *Cancer Nursing A Comprehensive Textbook* (2nd ed., pp. 395–433), R McCorkle, M Grant, M Frank-Stromborg (eds). Philadelphia: WB Saunders, 1996

Reyman P: Chemotherapy: principles and practice. In *Cancer Nursing Principles and Practice* (3rd ed., pp. 293–330), S Groenwald, M Frogge, M Goodman, et al. (eds). London: Jones and Bartlett, 1993

Silverstein B, Witkin KM, Frankos VH, et al.: *Assessing the role of the biomaterial Aquavene in patient reaction to Landmark midline catheters.* Regul Toxicol Pharmacol 1997; 25(1):60–7

Device: Quinton, Subclavian, Pheresis

Catherine Kefer

MULTIPLE MANUFACTURERS

TYPE: NONTUNNELED CATHETERS

■ Description: these catheters are made of polyurethane and are typically rigid. They are inserted using local anesthesia. The right internal jugular vein and the left subclavian vein are the preferred sites of insertion. The tip is threaded into the superior vena cava just outside the atrium. They are available in single, double, or triple lumens

■ Indications for use: the catheters have a large-bore lumen and can be used for large-volume exchanges like dialysis and pheresis

■ Advantages: nontunneled catheters are less costly than surgically implanted devices. Delays while waiting for surgical placement can be avoided. The devices can be inserted at the bedside or with same day surgery. They are effective for short-duration therapies and can be removed at the bedside

RISKS/DISADVANTAGES

■ Maintenance costs are higher because the catheter needs to be changed q7d. Infection rate may be higher and lines can dislodge if located in areas where securing the line is awkward. Requires frequent maintenance, and care and supplies are costly

SURGICAL CONSIDERATIONS

Mohamed Yassine

- Preoperation
  - provide patient and relatives with information on the procedure, maintenance care, and expected outcome
  - involve patient in decision making. This facilitates the learning process and adaptation to the device after surgery
  - consider placing a rolled towel beneath the neck and shoulders
  - position patient in 15 Trendelenburg position to distend the selected vein
- Postoperation
  - obtain chest x-ray for verification of placement in the superior vena cava and detection of pneumothorax
  - apply a sterile pressure dressing immediately after insertion
  - stabilize the line with a dressing to help prevent trauma, drainage, and infection
  - if the catheter is inserted medial to the midclavicular line, observe for intermittent positional occlusion "pinch-off syndrome," which occurs when the catheter becomes occluded between the clavicle and the first rib
  - if "pinch-off syndrome" is suspected, have patient roll shoulder or raise arm on the ipsilateral side. This will open the angle of the costoclavicular space (this is the hallmark of the syndrome)
  - observe for tip migration, especially in patients with excessive coughing, sneezing, and vomiting

CLINICAL ASSESSMENT/ INTERVENTIONS/IMPLICATIONS

- Patient assessment: includes examination of the catheter and insertion site
  - monitor temperature
  - inspect for erythema, swelling, and drainage at insertion site
  - examine lumens, connections, and clamps for visible leaks, cracks, or defects in the line
  - assess for pain or tenderness at insertion site, and pain along the vein when patient is breathing or coughing
  - flush lumens to assess flow and/or resistance
  - assess patient for side effects related to the drug(s) administered
- Maintenance: Flushing
  - daily and after each use with normal saline
  - if catheter is not being used, flush q72hrs with heplock 1.5 ml (5,000 units/ml = 7,500 units). Refer to institutional policies and procedures
  - flush with 10 ml of sterile saline before and after IV infusions to minimize catheter and vein damage; do not apply a great deal of pressure when flushing
  - avoid blood draws if possible; the large diameter of the catheter increases risk of infection. If the catheter must be used, flush with 10 ml of sterile saline
  - never directly clamp catheter, but if necessary use protective cover over catheter to avoid damage to the catheter
- Catheter care/dressing requirements
  - change cap weekly. May require more frequent changes depending on the number of punctures the cap has sustained
  - transparent tegaderm q3d to weekly; gauze dressings should be changed every other day or with catheter care

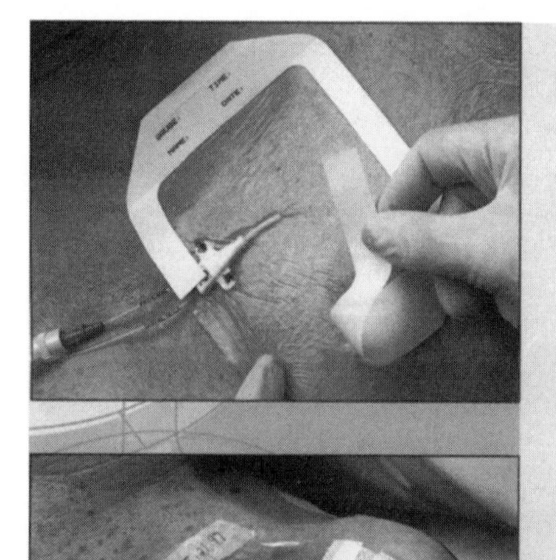

IV Applications

- use for effective, timesaving IV care
- provides a barrier from liquids and bacteria
- breathable—lets oxygen in and moisture vapor out, allowing skin to function normally
- clinically proven in numerous controlled studies
- helps to stabilize and properly secure the catheters
- allows the site to be monitored for early signs of complications
- can be worn much longer than gauze and tape
- special notched design with sterile tape strips for bulky catheters and jugular sites

Courtesy of 3M Health Care, St. Paul, Minnesota.

- observe insertion site for signs of infection or drainage; if present, obtain a culture of the site
- loop catheter securely with tape
- if crusting is present, cleanse with hydrogen peroxide using a cotton tip apparatus
- using sterile technique, cleanse the exit site and surrounding tissue with providine-iodine swab sticks. Using a spiral motion, begin at the exit site and work outward in a circular motion

■ Management of complications
- intraluminal occlusion: can create a sluggish flow or blood return or the inability to withdraw or infuse fluid. Commonly caused by a blood clot within the catheter or incompatible drugs or lipids. To prevent/minimize this
  - □ maintain positive pressure with the catheter when flushing
  - □ flush with at least 10–20 ml of sterile saline before and after infusions, blood products, and with 10 ml of saline between each drug
  - □ avoid excessive manipulation of external catheter
  - □ to declot catheter: take a 3 cc syringe and draw 5,000 units of streptokinase and instill into catheter. Clamp for 30 min. Attempt to aspirate. If unsuccessful, repeat procedure. If successful, flush with saline and use appropriately
- extraluminal occlusion: sluggish or partial occlusions could be due to a fibrin formation or thrombosis. With a partial occlusion the patient has no pain. Change the patient's position, raise the arms, and have the patient deep-breathe and/or cough. If flushing is easy but backflow is sluggish, flush with a thrombolytic agent of choice
- thrombosis
  - □ signs and symptoms related to impaired blood flow can include burning in neck, chest, shoulder; edema of neck, face, or arm; prominent superficial veins; numbness or tingling of extremity; tachycardia or shortness of breath; skin color or temperature change
  - □ treatment and management depend on the type and extent of the thrombus. Therapy with anticoagulants or thrombolytic agents should be used. Prophylactic administration of low-dose warfarin
  - □ adherence to recommended flushing protocols will decrease catheter-related thrombosis
- infection
  - □ infection can occur locally at the insertion site, in the catheter tunnel, and systemically. Signs and symptoms include warm skin, erythema, and possible exudate. The patient may have discomfort and a fever
  - □ management: obtain a culture of the site and lumens and blood cultures if a systemic infection is suspected. Administer antibiotics; increase frequency of dressing changes using meticulous site care. If infection does not resolve, consider replacement of catheter
  - □ remember: neutropenic patients typically will not have drainage from insertion site if infection is due to a decreased white count
- other complications
  - □ a kinked line, compression by tumor, compression between rib and clavicle, malposition due to manipulation, a catheter that is severed, punctured, split, or separated
  - □ use of the line with these complications can cause extravasation into the chest wall or thorax, which can result in severe deformity, loss of function, or death
  - □ *do not use device if function is questionable*

■ Home infusions
- use aseptic technique
- clean insertion site
- inspect home environment for potential sources of infection

■ Special considerations
- inspection of all fluids administered for visible signs of precipitants can prevent complications

■ Document procedure, findings, and interventions

ISSUES FOR PATIENT AND FAMILY TEACHING

■ Name of device: central venous catheter

■ Frequency and procedure for dressings, cap changes, flushing, and clamping

■ Instruct patient to report fever, tenderness, irritation, and drainage at catheter site; difficulty in flushing (should not force flush); pain in neck or chest; swelling of neck, face, or arm; numbness and tingling

■ Provide telephone numbers of physician and nurse

■ Provide verbal and written review of care with patient and family

■ Showering and bathing is not permitted

■ Routine assessment of compliance with recommendations for care

KEY REFERENCES

Access Device Guidelines: Recommendations for Nursing Practice and Education, D Camp-Sorrell (ed). Pittsburgh: Oncology Nursing Society, n.d.

Alexander HR: Vascular access and specialized techniques of drug delivery. In *Cancer: Principles and Practice of Oncology* (5th ed., pp. 725–34), V DeVita Jr, S Hellman, SA Rosenberg (eds). Philadelphia: Lippincott-Raven, 1997

Andris DA, Krzywda EA: Catheter pinch-off syndrome: recognition and management. Department of Surgery, Medical College of Wisconsin; J Intraven Nurs 1997; 20(5):233–7

Berg D: Drug delivery system. In *Cancer Chemotherapy: A Nursing Process Approach* (2nd ed., pp. 561–95), M Burke, G Wilkes, K Ingwersen (eds). London: Jones and Bartlett, 1996

Martin V: Delivery of cancer chemotherapy. In *Cancer Nursing: A Comprehensive Textbook* (2nd ed., pp. 395–433), R McCorkle, M Grant, M Frank-Stromborg, et al. (eds). Philadelphia: WB Saunders, 1996

Reyman P: Chemotherapy: principles and practice. In *Cancer Nursing Principles and Practice* (3rd ed., pp. 293–330), S Groenwald, M Frogge, M Goodman, et al. (eds). London: Jones and Bartlett, 1993

Device: Hickman and Broviac Catheters

Catherine Kefer and Patricia Sorokin

MULTIPLE MANUFACTURERS: BARD ACCESS SYSTEMS, COOK INC., HDC CORPORATION

TYPE: TUNNELED CATHETER

- Description: a silicone-tunneled central venous catheter (TCVC) with a large-bore lumen that is inserted in the cephalic, internal, or jugular vein with tip resting in the right atrium. The catheter has a Dacron cuff, providing safe, reliable, long-term access. Available in single, double, and triple lumens. The cuff (2 inches from the exit site) becomes enmeshed with scar tissue that secures the catheter in place, reducing the risk of organisms ascending the catheter
- Indications for use: long-term access device (months to years). This catheter is suitable for most hematology/oncology patients requiring continuous or intermittent chemotherapy, antibiotics, total parenteral nutrition (TPN), and blood products. Newer models have a special port that allows pheresis
- Advantages: the catheter has a low incidence of infection. It is larger and therefore more versatile. It is more flexible, less irritating, and allows easy administration of vesicants and irritants, decreasing the risk of extravasation. Fewer problems with flow rate

RISKS/DISADVANTAGES

- The catheter is costly because it requires surgical placement and removal. High maintenance requiring the use of syringes, heparin/saline, and dressing materials

SURGICAL CONSIDERATIONS

Mohamed Yassine

- Preoperation
  - provide patient and relatives with information on the procedure, maintenance care, and expected outcome
  - involve the patient in the decision making. This facilitates the learning process and adaptation to the device after surgery
  - discuss different insertion site options, if possible, so convenience and quality of life is minimally affected
- Postoperation
  - obtain chest x-ray study to confirm placement
  - observe for bleeding or drainage at the operation site
  - a suture is usually placed at the exit site to retain the catheter in place and is removed when granulation has occurred around the cuff
  - observe patient for signs of chest pain or shortness of breath for several hours after insertion
  - comply with sterile technique until the formation of granulation tissue around the cuff
  - observe for signs of infection
  - once granulation has occurred, site care involves bathing and securing the catheter with tape to prevent displacement

CLINICAL ASSESSMENT/ INTERVENTIONS/IMPLICATIONS

- Patient assessment: includes examination of the catheter and insertion site
  - monitor temperature
  - inspect for erythema, swelling, and drainage at insertion site
  - examine lumens, connections, and clamps for visible leaks, cracks, or defects in the line
  - assess for pain or tenderness at insertion site, and pain along the track when patient is breathing or coughing
  - flush lumens to assess flow and/or resistance
  - assess patient for side effects related to the drug(s) administered
- Maintenance: Flushing
  - catheter should be flushed when not in use and after each use
  - if drawing blood or giving medication through any of the lumens it will be necessary to flush with 3 ml of normal saline followed with a flush using a heparinized solution
  - each lumen must be flushed at least every day with 3 ml of heparin 100 units/ml
  - if clamping the lumen use protective covering to avoid damaging catheter
- Catheter care/dressing requirements
  - dressing changes require sterile technique in the hospital, clean technique for the home. Dressings should be changed whenever they become wet, soiled, or loose
  - observe insertion site for signs of infection and drainage. If present, obtain a culture of the site
  - dressings should be changed daily for first 10 days postinsertion or until exit site is well healed
  - frequency of dressing changes depends on material of choice and institutional policy
    - □ E-med strip: twice a week
    - □ transparent: 72 hrs or weekly
    - □ gauze coverlet: q24hrs
  - loop catheter securely with tape to avoid dislodgement
  - change caps weekly
  - if crusting is present cleanse with hydrogen peroxide using a cotton tip apparatus
  - cleanse exit site and surrounding tissue with providine-iodine swab sticks. Using a spiral motion, begin at the exit site and work outward in a circular motion
- Management of complications
  - intraluminal occlusion: can create a sluggish flow or sluggish blood return or the inability to withdraw or infuse solutions; commonly caused by a blood clot within the catheter or incompatible drugs or lipids. To prevent/minimize this
    - □ maintain positive pressure with the catheter when flushing
    - □ flush with at least 20 ml of sterile saline before and after blood products, infusions, and with 10 ml of saline between each drug
    - □ avoid excessive manipulation of external catheter
    - □ flush q8–12hrs when giving TPN and/or lipids
    - □ inspect TPN and IV fluids for visible precipitants
    - □ to declot catheter: take a 3 cc syringe and draw 5,000 units of streptokinase and instill into catheter. Clamp for 30 min. Attempt to aspirate. If unsuccessful repeat procedure. If successful, flush with saline and use appropriately
  - extraluminal occlusion: sluggish or partial occlusions could be due to a fibrin formation or thrombosis. With a partial occlusion the patient has no pain. Because catheter position can affect the flow, change the patient's position, raise the arms, and have patient deep-breathe and/or cough. If flushing is easy but backflow is sluggish, flush with thrombolytic agent of choice
  - thrombosis
    - □ signs and symptoms related to impaired blood flow can include edema of neck, face, shoulder, or arm due to impaired blood flow; prominent superficial veins; neck pain; tingling of neck, shoulder, or arm; skin color or temperature changes
    - □ a radiographic study can define the extent of the thrombosis
    - □ management depends on type and extent of the thrombus. Therapy with anticoagulants or thrombolytic agents are used (all lumens must be treated). Prophylactic administration of low-dose warfarin
    - □ adherence to recommended flushing protocols will decrease risk of catheter-related thrombosis
  - infection
    - □ infection can occur locally at the insertion site, in the catheter tunnel, and systemically. Signs and symptoms include warm skin, erythema, and possible exudate. The patient may have discomfort and a fever
    - □ management: obtain a culture of the site and lumens and blood cultures if a systemic infection is suspected. Administer antibiotics. Increase frequency of dressing changes using

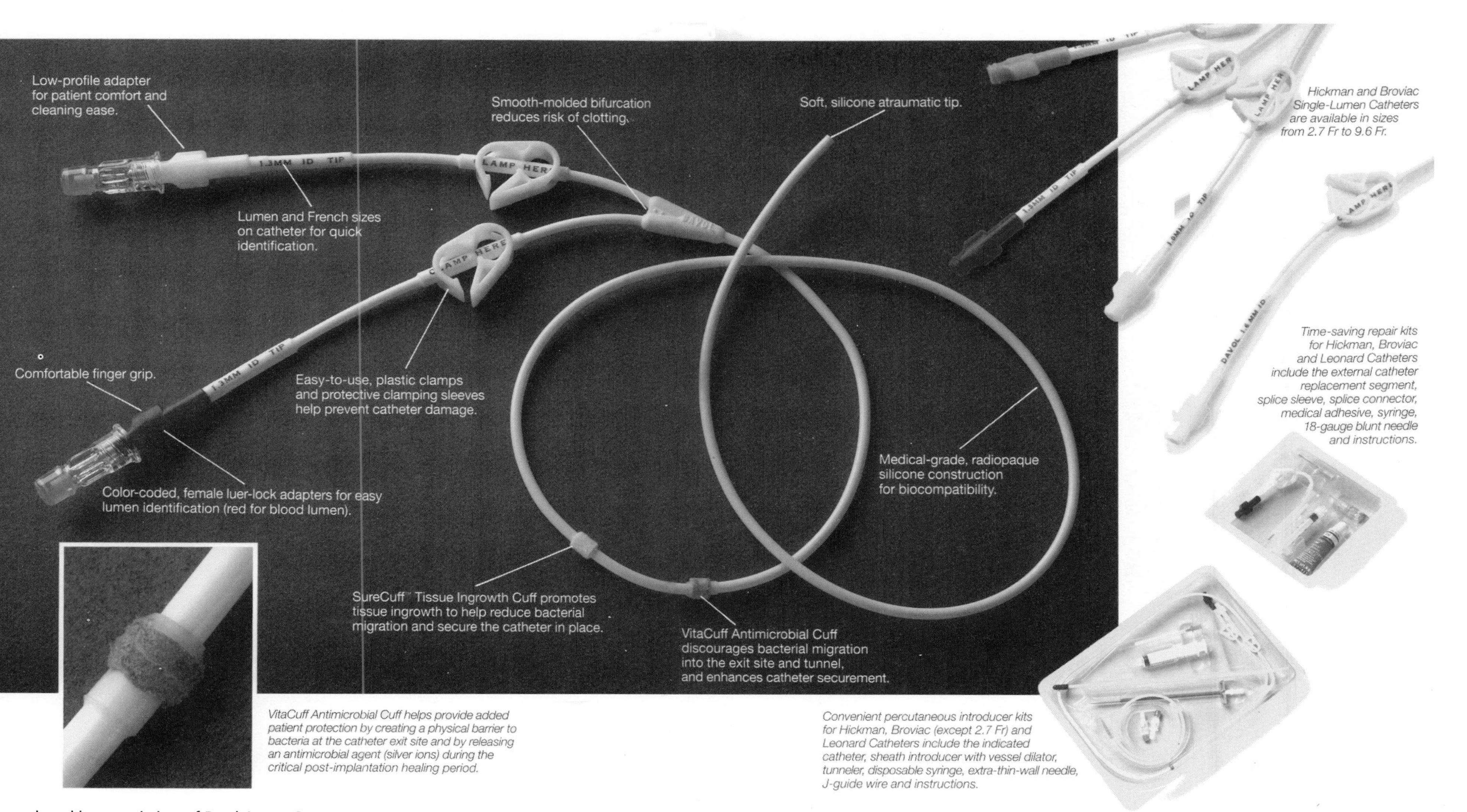

Reproduced by permission of Bard Access Systems.

meticulous site care. If infection does not resolve, consider replacement of catheter
  - □ remember: neutropenic patients typically will not have drainage from insertion site if infection is due to decreased white count
  - □ adherence to aseptic technique during maintenance will decrease the risk of infection
- – other complications may include:
  - □ a kinked line, compression by tumor, compression between rib and clavicle, malposition due to manipulation, a catheter becomes severed, punctured, split, or separated
  - □ use of the line with these complications can cause extravasation into the chest wall or thorax resulting in severe deformity, loss of function, or death
  - □ placement can be confirmed with an x-ray
  - □ *do not use device if function is questionable*

- Home infusions
  - – use aseptic/clean technique during care
  - – clean insertion site
  - – flush daily and between drugs
  - – ensure availability of needed supplies
  - – inspect home environment for potential sources of infection
- Special considerations
  - – inspection of all fluids administered for visible signs of precipitates can prevent complications
- Document procedure, findings, and interventions

ISSUES FOR PATIENT AND FAMILY TEACHING

- Name of device: Hickman
- Frequency and procedure for dressings, cap changes, flushing, and clamping
- Instruct patient to report fever, tenderness, irritation, and drainage at catheter site and difficulty in flushing, (should not force flush); pain in neck, chest, swelling of neck, face, or arm, and any numbness and tingling
- Provide telephone numbers of physician and nurse
- Provide verbal and written review of care with patient and family
- Showering and bathing is permitted with precautions
- Routine assessment of compliance with recommendations for care

KEY REFERENCES

Access Device Guidelines: Recommendations for Nursing Practice and Education, D Camp-Sorrell (ed). Pittsburgh: Oncology Nursing Society, n.d.

Alexander HR: Vascular access and specialized technique of drug delivery. In *Cancer: Principles and Practice of Oncology* (5th ed., pp. 725–34), V DeVita Jr, S Hellman, SA Rosenberg (eds). Philadelphia: Lippincott-Raven, 1997

Berg D: Drug delivery system. In *Cancer Chemotherapy: A Nursing Process Approach* (2nd ed., pp. 561–95), M Burke, G Wilkes, K Ingwersen (eds). London: Jones and Bartlett, 1996

Martin V: Delivery of cancer chemotherapy. In *Cancer Nursing: A Comprehensive Textbook* (2nd ed., pp. 395–433), R McCorkle, M Grant, M Frank-Stromborg, et al. (eds). Philadelphia: WB Saunders, 1996

Reyman P: Chemotherapy: practice and principles. In *Cancer Nursing Principles and Practice* (3rd ed., pp. 293–330), S Groenwald, M Frogge, M Goodman, et al. (eds). London: Jones and Bartlett, 1993

Device: Groshong Catheter

Catherine Kefer

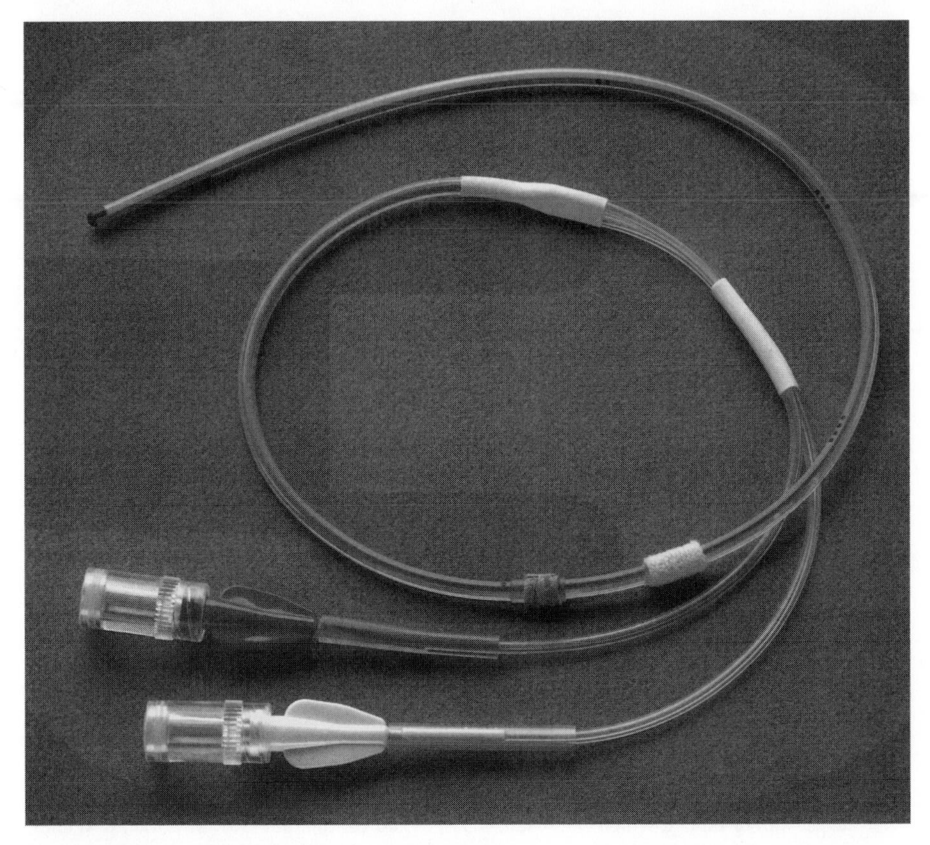

Reproduced by permission of Bard Access Systems.

MANUFACTURERS: BARD ACCESS SYSTEMS, COOK INC., HDC CORPORATION

TYPE: TUNNELED

■ Description: the catheter is made of silicone rubber and surgically placed using local or general anesthesia. Common insertion site is into the superior vena cava, with both an entry and exit site. This tunneled catheter has a Dacron cuff that anchors it SubQ and provides a barrier to infection. The Groshong has a slit valve at the distal end and is available in single and double lumens. The valve prevents backflow of blood into the catheter to prevent clotting

■ Indications for use: for patients requiring long-term treatment, including blood products and blood draws, chemotherapy, antibiotics, and parenteral nutrition

■ Advantages: the three-way valve within the lumen eliminates the need for daily heparin flushes, minimizes blood backflow problems, and reduces the risk of air embolism. The catheter may be removed when therapy is complete

RISKS/DISADVANTAGES

■ Dressings are required. Costly as they require surgical placement. Higher risk of infection, occlusion, breakage, or leakage. Can be difficult to aspirate blood or infuse fluids

SURGICAL CONSIDERATIONS

Mohamed Yassine

■ Preoperation
- provide patient and relatives with information on the procedure, maintenance care, and expected outcome
- involve the patient in the decision making. This facilitates the learning process and adaptation to the device after surgery
- discuss different insertion site options so convenience and quality of life is minimally affected

■ Postoperation
- a chest x-ray study should be performed to confirm placement
- observe for bleeding or drainage at the operation site
- a suture is usually placed at the exit site to retain the catheter in place and removed when granulation has occurred around the cuff
- observe patient for signs of chest pain or shortness of breath for few hours postinsertion
- comply with sterile technique until the formation of granulation tissue around the cuff
- observe for signs of infection
- once granulation has occurred, site care involves bathing and securing the catheter with tape to prevent displacement

CLINICAL ASSESSMENT/ INTERVENTIONS/IMPLICATIONS

■ Patient assessment: includes examination of the catheter and insertion site
- monitor temperature
- inspect for erythema, swelling, and drainage at insertion site
- examine lumens, connections, and clamps for visible leaks, cracks, or defects in the line
- assess for pain or tenderness at insertion site and pain along the track when patient is breathing or coughing
- flush lumens to assess flow and/or resistance
- assess patient for side effects related to the drug(s) administered

■ Maintenance: Flushing
- if the catheter is not being used, flush vigorously with 5–10 ml of normal saline weekly. (A study by Mayo et al. concluded that Groshong catheters flushed with heparinized saline decrease the likelihood of intraluminal clot formation and catheter malformation)
- after blood draws flush with 10–20 ml of normal saline
- Groshong catheters do not require clamping if the valve is functioning properly. If clamping is required, use a protective cover over the catheter to avoid damage to the catheter

■ Catheter care/dressing requirements
- change cap weekly according to use (e.g., number of punctures and blood in the cap)
- occlusive dressing is placed on the entry and exit sites after the catheter is inserted and left in place for 48 hrs (may need to reinforce if there is bleeding)
- use aseptic technique when changing dressings. Change gauze dressings every other day or transparent dressings q72hrs or weekly. Cleanse exit site and then apply a transparent dressing over a dry sterile dressing. Once healing has occurred apply only a plastic strip over the exit site
- observe insertion site for signs of infection or drainage. If present, obtain a culture of the site
- loop catheter securely with tape
- if crusting is present, cleanse with hydrogen peroxide using a cotton tip apparatus
- cleanse exit site and surrounding tissue with providine-iodine swab sticks. Using a spiral motion, begin at the exit site and work outward in a circular motion

- Management of complications
  - intraluminal occlusion: can create a sluggish flow or blood return or the inability to withdraw or infuse solutions. Commonly caused by a blood clot within the catheter or incompatible drugs or lipids. To prevent/minimize this
    - □ maintain positive pressure with the catheter when flushing
    - □ flush with at least 20 ml of sterile saline before and after blood products, infusions, and with 10 ml of saline between each drug
    - □ flush q8–12hrs when giving TPN or lipids
    - □ avoid excessive manipulation of external catheter
    - □ inspect TPN and IV fluids for visible precipitants
    - □ to declot catheter: take a 10 ml syringe and draw 5,000 units/ml of streptokinase and instill into catheter. Clamp for 30 min. Attempt to aspirate. If unsuccessful, repeat procedure. If successful, flush with saline and use appropriately
  - extraluminal occlusion: sluggish or partial occlusions could be due to a fibrin formation or thrombosis. With a partial occlusion the patient has no pain. Change the patient's position, raise the arms, and have patient deep-breathe and/or cough. If flushing is easy but backflow is sluggish, flush with a thrombolytic agent of choice
  - Thrombosis
    - □ signs and symptoms related to impaired blood flow include edema of neck, face, shoulder, or arm due to impaired blood flow; prominent superficial veins; neck pain; tingling of neck, shoulder, or arm; skin color or temperature changes
    - □ management depends on type and extent of thrombus. Therapy with anticoagulants or thrombolytic agents are used (all lumens must be treated). Prophylactic administration of low-dose warfarin
    - □ adherence to recommended flushing protocols will decrease risk of catheter-related thrombosis
  - infection
    - □ infection can occur locally at the insertion site, in the catheter tunnel, and systemically. Signs and symptoms include warm skin, erythema, and possible exudate. The patient may have discomfort and a fever
    - □ management: obtain a culture of the site and lumens, and blood cultures if a systemic infection is suspected. Administer antibiotics and increase frequency of dressing changes using meticulous site care. If infection does not resolve, consider replacement of catheter
    - □ remember: neutropenic patients typically will not have drainage from insertion site if infection is due to decreased white count
  - other complications
    - □ a kinked line, compression by tumor, compression between rib and clavicle, malposition due to manipulation, a catheter that is severed, punctured, split, or separated
    - □ use of the line with these complications can cause extravasation into the chest wall or thorax, which can result in severe deformity, loss of function, or death
    - □ *do not use device if function is questionable*
- Home infusions
  - use aseptic technique
  - clean insertion site
  - inspect home environment for potential sources of infection
- Document procedure, findings, and interventions

ISSUES FOR PATIENT AND FAMILY TEACHING

- Name of device: Groshong
- Frequency and procedure for dressings, cap changes, and flushing
- Instruct patient to report fever, tenderness, irritation, and drainage at catheter site, and difficulty in flushing (should not force flush); report pain in neck, chest, swelling of neck, face, or arm and any numbness or tingling
- If catheter is accidentally pulled out, instruct patient to cover with gauze and call physician
- Provide telephone numbers of physician and nurse
- Provide verbal and written review of care with patient and family
- Showering and bathing is permitted with precautions
- Routine assessment of compliance with recommendations for care

KEY REFERENCES

Access Device Guidelines: Recommendations for Nursing Practice and Education, D Camp-Sorrell (ed). Pittsburgh: Oncology Nursing Society, n.d.

Alexander HR: Vascular access and specialized technique of drug delivery. In *Cancer: Principles and Practice of Oncology* (5th ed., pp. 725–34), V DeVita Jr, S Hellman, SA Rosenberg (eds). Philadelphia: Lippincott-Raven, 1997

Berg D: Drug delivery system. In *Cancer Chemotherapy: A Nursing Process Approach* (2nd ed., pp. 561–95), M Burke, G Wilkes, K Ingwersen (eds). London: Jones and Bartlett, 1996

Martin V: Delivery of cancer chemotherapy. In *Cancer Nursing: A Comprehensive Textbook* (2nd ed., pp. 395–433), R McCorkle, M Grant, M Frank-Stromborg, et al. (eds). Philadelphia: WB Saunders, 1996

Mayo DJ, Horne MK III, Summers BL, et al.: The effects of heparin flush on patency of the Groshong catheter: a pilot study. Oncol Nurs Forum 1996; 23(9):1401–5

Reyman P: Chemotherapy: practice and principles. In *Cancer Nursing Principles and Practice* (3rd ed., pp. 293–330), S Groenwald, M Frogge, M Goodman, et al. (eds). London: Jones and Bartlett, 1993

Device: Peripherally Inserted Central Catheter: PICC

Patricia A. Sorokin

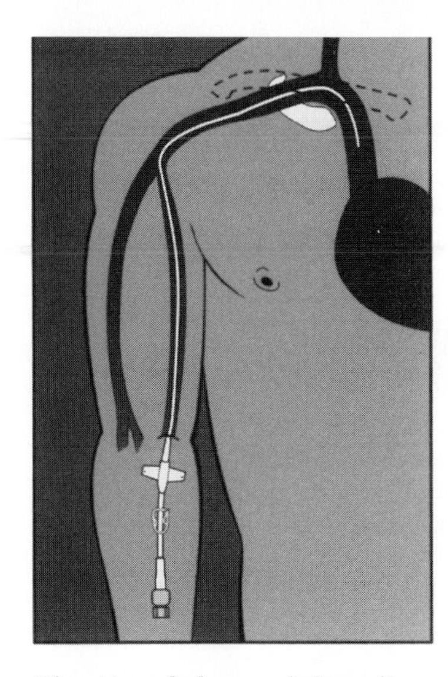

The tip of the peripherally inserted central catheter (PICC) resides in a central vein.

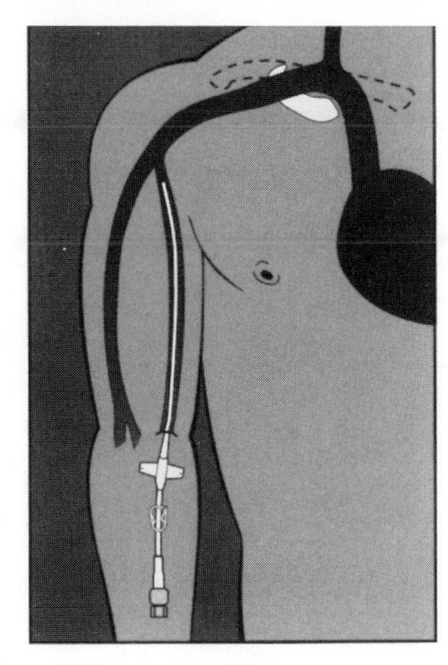

The tip of the Midline catheter is positioned in a peripheral vein.

Reproduced courtesy of SIMS Deltec, Inc., St. Paul, Minnesota

MULTIPLE MANUFACTURERS: BARD ACCESS SYSTEMS, COOK INC., HDC CORPORATION, SIMS DELTEC, INC.

TYPE: MAY BE A SINGLE OR DOUBLE LUMEN: MAY BE GROSHONG TIP

■ Description: these small gauge thin-walled catheters, made of silicone, polyurethane, or elastomeric, are inserted at the antecubital fossa into the basilic or cephalic vein. The catheter gauge ranges from 16–24 and can be a single or double lumen. The catheter is threaded through the vein and exits in the SVC

■ Indications for use: for patients who are to receive 6 mos of therapy or less. Can be used to infuse vesicant/nonvesicant chemotherapy, IV fluid, antibiotics, transfusion of blood products (through a large-bore lumen), and blood draws

■ Advantages: inexpensive placement. Excellent choice for patients who require therapy for >5 days in the hospital or in the home care setting. Ease with placement; does not require surgery. They may be placed by certified nurses at the bedside or under fluoroscopy by an interventional radiologist. Can be easily removed. Lower complication rate than with other types of access devices

RISKS/DISADVANTAGES

■ Supplies can be expensive. Phlebitis can occur as a result of the insertion. Arm movement may be limited due to placement in the antecubital fossa. May be unreliable for blood drawing. May be difficult to place and/or thread the catheter if peripheral access is poor

SURGICAL CONSIDERATIONS

Mohamed Yassine

- Preoperation
  - provide patient and relatives with information on the procedure, maintenance care, and expected outcome
  - involve the patient in the decision making. This facilitates the learning process and adaptation to the device after surgery
  - avoid the use of powdered gloves when preparing for the insertion of PICC. This minimizes the possibility of phlebitis
- Postoperation
  - obtain chest x-ray for verification of tip placement in the superior vena cava
  - apply a sterile pressure dressing immediately after insertion for the first 24 hrs, especially if the patient is thrombocytopenic
  - avoid use of the arm (with the catheter) for measuring blood pressure
  - stabilize the line with a dressing to help prevent trauma, drainage, and infection
  - use at least 20 ml of saline to flush after every use; this will help prevent drug precipitation, which is due to sudden pH changes
  - do not apply a great deal of pressure when flushing; this minimizes damage to catheter and vein
  - observe for tip migration, especially in patients with excessive coughing, sneezing, and vomiting

CLINICAL ASSESSMENT/ INTERVENTIONS/IMPLICATIONS

■ Patient assessment: includes examination of the catheter and insertion site
  - at baseline, determine the catheter length by measuring from the point of venipuncture over the course of the selected venous pathway across shoulder to the right side of the sternal notch and down to the third intercostal space
  - a chest x-ray should be obtained immediately after placement and prior to use if placed in the SVC
  - examination of the insertion site to assess for swelling, redness, discharge, pain/tenderness
  - assess for blood return and flow or resistance when flushing
  - examine lumens, connection, clamps, and catheter for visible leaks, cracks, defects in the line
  - measure upper arm circumference at baseline and weekly to assess for signs of swelling
  - assess patient for side effects related to the drug(s) administered
- Maintenance: Flushing
  - the Groshong PICC should only be flushed with 5–10 cc of normal saline or 10–20 cc after withdrawal/infusion
  - other catheter types should be flushed after each use (blood draw, medication, fluid administration) with 10–20 cc normal saline followed by 3 cc of 100 units/ml of heparin. Lumens not in use should be flushed with 3 cc of 100 units/ml of heparin once a day per institutional policy
- Catheter Care/dressing requirements
  - frequency of dressing change depends on material of choice and institutional policy
  - initial dressing change should be within 24 hrs of placement because of the likelihood for bloody drainage due to catheter insertion
  - when cleansing skin (alcohol, iodophors, chlorhexidene) begin at the insertion site and cleanse in an outward circular motion, using care not to return to a clean area with the same sponge or swab
  - frequency of dressing change depends on material of choice
    - □ E-med strip: twice a week
    - □ transparent: 72 hrs or weekly depending on institutional policy
    - □ gauze coverlet: q24hrs
  - if ointment is applied to insertion site, the dressing must be changed q48–72hrs
  - tape catheter securely

- change cap if any of the following occur: cap is removed, cap has not been changed in 7 days, or blood cannot be completely flushed from the cap

■ Management of complications
- migration/malposition: can occur and indicates that the catheter tip is no longer positioned in the lower one-third of the SVC. This can be due to a change in intrathoracic pressure related to coughing, sneezing, or vomiting, forceful flushing or energetic movements of the upper extremity by the patient
  - □ symptoms include
    - ▽ inability or resistance when flushing or lack of a blood return
    - ▽ inability to infuse or withdraw
    - ▽ increased length of external catheter
    - ▽ patient reports arm/shoulder pain, back discomfort, chest pain, arrhythmias, or swelling
  - □ management includes
    - ▽ confirmation of placement with chest x-ray or venogram
    - ▽ flush catheter rapidly (i.e., inject fluid rapidly through the catheter)
    - ▽ fluoroscopic catheter guidance
    - ▽ partial catheter withdrawal or guidewire exchange
    - ▽ removal of catheter
- occlusion: can be caused by migration/malposition, which compresses the catheter, fibrin/blood in lumen or extraluminal fibrin sheath, precipitates, lipid deposits
  - □ symptoms indicating a partial occlusion include
    - ▽ inability to withdraw but having the ability to infuse
    - ▽ difficulty withdrawing and infusing
    - ▽ ability to withdraw/infuse can be dependent on position of the patient
  - □ symptoms indicating a total occlusion include
    - ▽ inability to withdraw or infuse
  - □ management of compression
    - ▽ obtain an x-ray to detect malposition or compression. Catheter removal is critical in preventing catheter fracture
  - □ management of intraluminal clot, precipitates, or lipid deposits; use a thrombolytic agent of choice
- infection
  - □ local Infection: drainage, erythema, local warmth, pain/tenderness, at catheter exit site
    - ▽ culture drainage and apply daily sterile gauze and tape dressing
    - ▽ apply antibiotic ointment
    - ▽ apply warm compress to the area
    - ▽ begin po/IV antibiotics as ordered for 10–14 days
    - ▽ if symptoms do not resolve within 48–72 hrs after initiating antibiotics, PICC should be removed
  - □ systemic infection: fever/chills/diaphoresis, flulike symptoms, positive blood cultures from lumen and/or peripheral site
    - ▽ administer antibiotics per orders
    - ▽ antibiotics can be locked in the device with heparin or saline to deliver higher antibiotic concentrations to an infected catheter
    - ▽ if a double-lumen catheter, rotate antibiotic administration to ensure all lumens are treated
    - ▽ if symptoms do not resolve within 24–48 hrs after initiating antibiotics, PICC should be removed
- thrombosis
  - □ symptoms may include edema of neck, face, shoulder/arm, neck/back, pain, skin color or temperature change
  - □ management with anticoagulants or thrombolytic agents (heparin) as continuous infusion followed by administration of low-dose warfarin
  - □ if thrombus-related infection, consider thrombolytic or anticoagulant therapy concurrently with antibiotics
  - □ catheter may need to be removed
- catheter removal
  - □ verify order for removal and indication
  - □ note length of catheter (refer to records indicating initial length of the catheter at the time of insertion)
  - □ measure circumference of upper arm
  - □ inspect condition of catheter, observe site for any swelling, redness, or other problems
  - □ put on gloves, grasp hub of VAD, and gently and steadily retract catheter until completely removed
  - □ apply pressure to exit site until bleeding stops or longer if platelets are decreased
  - □ apply occlusive dressing
  - □ inspect catheter integrity after it has been removed and document any abnormalities
  - □ if the catheter is removed due to infection, send catheter tip for culture

■ Special considerations
- lumen gauge is an indicator of how well catheter will withdraw and infuse blood
- local phlebitis may develop along the vein and may be treated with hot packs four times a day or antibiotics
- prophylactic coumadin may be ordered to begin at the time of catheter placement

■ Document procedure, findings, and interventions

ISSUES FOR PATIENT AND FAMILY TEACHING

■ Name of device: PICC (peripherally inserted central catheter)

■ Frequency and procedure for flushing and dressing changes

■ Report difficulty in flushing, pain/redness, discharge at site, neck/back/shoulder pain or swelling on the side where the catheter is placed

■ If catheter becomes wet or soiled, change dressing immediately

■ Activity/weight lifting restrictions apply to the arm with the catheter

■ When showering completely cover exit site and catheter with occlusive dressing

■ Routine assessment of compliance with recommendations for care

KEY REFERENCES

Access Device Guidelines: Recommendations for Nursing Practice and Education, D Camp-Sorrell (ed). Pittsburgh: Oncology Nursing Society, n.d.

Berg D: Drug delivery system. In *Cancer Chemotherapy: A Nursing Process Approach* (2nd ed., pp. 561–95), M Burke, G Wilkes, K Ingwersen (eds). London: Jones and Bartlett, 1996

Macklin D: How to manage PICCs [published erratum appears in Am J Nurs 1998; 98(1):27] Professional Learning System, Inc., Marietta, GA; Am J Nurs 1997; 97(9):26–32

Martin V: Delivery of cancer chemotherapy. In *Cancer Nursing: A Comprehensive Textbook* (2nd ed., pp. 395–433), R McCorkle, M Grant, M Frank-Stromborg, et al. (eds). Philadelphia: WB Saunders, 1996

Reyman P: Chemotherapy: practice and principles. In *Cancer Nursing Principles and Practice* (3rd ed., pp. 293–330), S Groenwald, M Frogge, M Goodman, et al. (eds). London: Jones and Bartlett, 1993

Smith J, Friedell M, Cheatham M, et al.: Peripherally inserted central catheters revisited. Am J Surg 1998; 176(2):208–11

Device: Port-A-Cath

Patricia A. Sorokin

Portal Location

In response to implantation and patient preferences, both chest- and arm-placed systems are available. The P.A.S. PORT® peripheral access systems are designed specifically for arm placement. PORT-A-CATH® Low Profile™ single- and dual-lumen systems are also appropriate for arm placement in large or obese patients. Peripheral placement is a convenient and cosmetically attractive option for many patients[1] and allows for a less traumatic outpatient implantation procedure and a minimized risk of immediate insertion complications.[2]

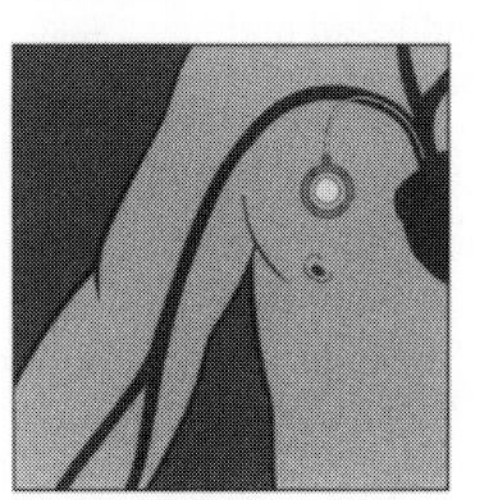

Chest placement
with the PORT-A-CATH® system

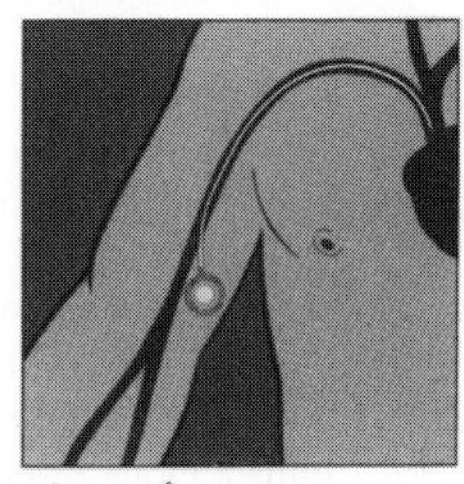

Arm placement
with the PORT-A-CATH® Low Profile™ system

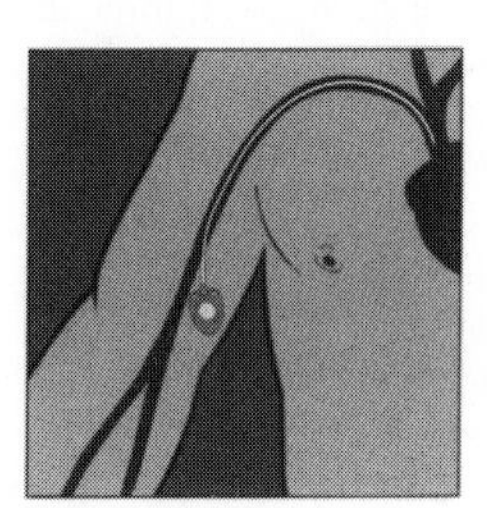

Arm placement
with the P.A.S. PORT® T2 system

Reproduced courtesy of SIMS Deltec, Inc., St. Paul, Minnesota

MULTIPLE MANUFACTURERS: BARD ACCESS SYSTEMS, COOK INC., SIMS DELTEC, INC.

TYPE: MAY HAVE SINGLE- OR DOUBLE-LUMEN PORTS: PERIPHERAL P.A.S. PORTS

■ Description: all ports have a basic design of a portal body, septum, reservoir, and catheter. This type of catheter is placed in the SubQ tissue adjacent to the venous insertion site and anchored to the underlying fascia. Port housings are made of titanium or plastic and have compressed silicone septum, which can withstand up to 2,000 punctures. The catheters are designed to withstand repeated punctures with a noncoring Huber needle and provide stability when accessed. A smaller septum, such as an antecubital port, can withstand up to 100–500 punctures. The use of larger needle gauges may affect the integrity of the septum and decrease the number of punctures the catheter can sustain. Port housings are designed to provide minimal distortion artifact on MRI or CT scanning

■ Indications for use: VADs are best used for patients receiving bolus injections of chemotherapy as an outpatient on an intermittent basis. Chest placement is not recommended for obese patients, on postradiated chest, or at mastectomy sites. Peripheral port should not be placed on the same side as the mastectomy site. May be in place months to years

■ Advantages: may be used immediately upon placement and does not require site care or maintenance. Good cosmetic appearance, no constant reminder of the device, and no limitations on activities. They may remain in place for years

RISKS/DISADVANTAGES

■ Cost of insertion because surgery is required to place the catheter and remove it. It requires flushing by a certified individual when not in use

SURGICAL CONSIDERATIONS

Mohamed Yassine

■ Preoperation
  - provide patient and relatives with information on the procedure, maintenance care, and expected outcome
  - involve the patient in the decision making. This facilitates the learning process and adaptation to the device after surgery
  - discuss different insertion site options, so the convenience and quality of life is minimally affected

■ Postoperation
  - obtain an x-ray study or a perfusion scan to confirm placement
  - observe for bleeding or drainage at the operation site
  - assess for the development of a hematoma or hygroma
  - apply cold packs or pressure to reduce postoperative discomfort and edema
  - the implanted port could be used 24 hrs postinsertion if no swelling is present (some surgeons prefer accessing the port several days after placement)
  - strict aseptic technique should be used to access the port
  - notify the physician if there is palpable movement of the implanted port
  - observe for any signs of resistance or occlusion
  - instruct the patient to monitor for any signs of swelling, pain, or drainage
  - showering is restricted until wound is healed

CLINICAL ASSESSMENT/ INTERVENTIONS/IMPLICATIONS

■ Patient assessment: includes examination of port site to check for swelling/redness/hematoma
  - assess the patient for pain/tenderness
  - after accessing the port, assess the flow (resistance) when flushing and for blood return when pulling back on the syringe
  - should the patient have fever or chills not related to therapy within 24 hrs of accessing, blood cultures should be obtained from port (both lumens if patient has 2) and peripherally
  - assess patient for side effects related to drug administered

■ Maintenance: Flushing
  - flush catheter with 5,000–10,000 units/ml of heparin sodium q4–6wks
  - use a noncoring needle when accessing the port
  - flush after each use or q4–6wks when not in use
  - flush all VADs vigorously with 10–20 ml of normal saline after infusing or withdrawing blood followed by heparin
  - never use excessive force when flushing; avoid using syringes < 3 ml in size to decrease the pressure on the catheter

- prophylactic coumadin may be ordered to begin at the time of catheter placement

- Catheter care/dressing requirements
  - prime needle and extension tubing with normal saline using sterile technique
  - cleanse skin with appropriate preparation: when using skin-cleansing agents (alcohol, iodophor) begin at the insertion site and cleanse outward in a circular motion, using care not to return to a clean area with the same sponge or swab
  - stabilize the port, and firmly insert needle, perpendicular to the skin, through the skin and septum until needle touches port backing
  - aspirate blood to verify placement, and flush with the normal saline to verify patency and to cleanse port
  - cleanse injection luer with cleansing agent before accessing port for continuous or bolus infusions
  - gauze/tape dressing: mesh material used for dressing that provides no occlusive barrier should be secured in place with clean or sterile tape and changed q48hrs
  - transparent dressing: allows for visualization of the exit site and acts as a barrier to extrinsic liquid and microorganisms. This dressing should be changed q5–7days or more often if indicated
  - when gauze is placed under a transparent dressing, it is considered the same as a gauze and tape dressing
  - change the cap when any of the following occur
    - □ cap is removed
    - □ cap has not been changed in 7 days
    - □ blood cannot be completely flushed from the cap
    - □ signs of blood, precipitates, cracks, leaks, or other defects are noted
  - when decanulating the port, maintain positive pressure on the syringe to prevent reflux of blood to the catheter
  - the needle should not be left in place for > 7 days
- Management of complications
  - occlusion: occurs because of fibrin sheath, thrombosis, lipid/precipitate deposits
    - □ partial occlusion: symptoms include inability to withdraw but ability to infuse; difficulty withdrawing but can infuse; ability to withdraw/infuse is dependent on patient position
    - □ total occlusion: symptoms include inability to withdraw or infuse
  - management of occlusion
    - □ reaccess port if the needle is not in the reservoir. Reposition the patient, have patient cough/deep-breathe as catheter may be positional
    - □ chest x-ray/dye study may be required to check catheter placement, clot formation, malposition, or compression
  - management of clot, precipitates, or lipid deposits use a thrombolytic agent of choice
  - infection
    - □ local infection: signs and symptoms may include drainage, erythema, local warmth, pain/tenderness at port site
      - ▽ do not access port if infection is suspected as it may introduce microorganisms into the bloodstream
      - ▽ culture the drainage and begin oral and IV antibiotics as ordered for 10–14 days
      - ▽ apply daily sterile gauze and tape dressing. Apply antibiotic ointment
      - ▽ apply warm compress to area
      - ▽ if symptoms do not resolve within 48–72 hrs after initiating antibiotics, port should be removed
    - □ systemic infection: signs and symptoms include fever/chills/diaphoresis, flulike symptoms, positive blood cultures from port and/or peripheral site
      - ▽ administer IV antibiotics per orders
      - ▽ antibiotics can be locked in device with heparin or saline to deliver higher antibiotic concentrations
      - ▽ if a double port, rotate the lumens for antibiotic administration to ensure all the lumens are treated
      - ▽ if symptoms do not resolve within 24–48 hrs after initiating antibiotics, port should be removed
  - thrombosis: signs and symptoms may include edema of neck, face, shoulder or arm, neck/shoulder/back pain, skin color or temperature changes
    - □ management of thrombosis
      - ▽ anticoagulants or thrombolytic agents (heparin) are given as a continuous infusion
      - ▽ can be followed with prophylactic administration of low-dose warfarin, if ordered
      - ▽ in cases of a thrombus-related infection, thrombolytic or anticoagulant therapy concurrently with antibiotics can be considered
  - other complications can include
    - □ a kinked, separated, or compressed catheter, which may result in extravasation if the port is used
    - □ if not adequately sutured in place, the port can malposition, in which case the nurse will be unable to insert the needle. If this occurs, notify the physician immediately so the port can be repositioned
    - □ *do not use device if function is questionable*
- Document procedure, findings, and interventions

ISSUES FOR PATIENT AND FAMILY TEACHING

- Name of device: port or vascular access device
- Must be flushed when not in use by a trained individual q4–6 wks
- If the needle is left in place, instruct patient to keep the VAD site dry. Dressings should be changed *immediately* if they become wet, soiled, or contaminated
- Notify nurse or physician if any of the following are noted: pain, redness, drainage, fever, flulike symptoms, bleeding, or pain/swelling at port site, neck, shoulder, or back
- Provide the patient with names and number of physician and nurse
- Provide written documentation regarding the device for the patient to carry. This will minimize risk of inappropriate use
- Routine assessment of compliance with recommendations for care

KEY REFERENCES

Access Device Guidelines: Recommendations for Nursing Practice and Education, D Camp-Sorrell (ed). Pittsburgh: Oncology Nursing Society, n.d.

Andrews JC, Walker-Andres SC, Ensminger WD: Long-term central venous access with a peripherally placed subcutaneous infusion port: initial results. Radiology 1993; 176(1):45–7

Baranowski L: Central venous access devises: current technologies, uses, and management strategies. J Intraven Nurs 1993; 16:167–94

Berg D: Drug delivery system. In *Cancer Chemotherapy: A Nursing Process Approach* (2nd ed., pp. 561–95), M Burke, G Wilkes, K Ingwersen (eds). London: Jones and Bartlett, 1996

Camp-Sorrell D: Implantable ports: Everything you always wanted to know. J Intraven Nurs 1992; 15:262–71

Cowan C: Antibiotic lock technique. J Intraven Nurs 1992; 15:283–7

Cunningham R, Bonam-Crawford D: The role of fibrinolytic agents in the management of thrombotic complications associated with vascular access devices. Nurs Clin North Am 1993; 28:899–907

Ensminger W: Regional chemotherapy. Sem Oncol 1993; 20:3–11

Gross J, Johnson R: *Handbook of Oncology Nursing.* London, Jones and Bartlett, 1994

Krzywada E, Andris D, Edmiston C, et al.: Treatment of Hickman catheter sepsis using antibiotics lock technique. Infect Control and Hospital Epidemiol 1995; 16(1):596–8

LaQuaglia M, Caldwell C, Lucas A, et al.: A prospective randomized double-blind trial of bolus urokinase in the treatment of established Hickman catheter sepsis in children. J Ped Surg 1994; 29:742–5

Lewis J, LaFrance R, Bower R: Treatment of an infected silicone eight atrial catheter with combined fibrinolytic and antibiotic therapy: Case report and review of the literature. J Parenteral and Enteral Nutr 1989; 13:92–8

Martin V: Delivery of cancer chemotherapy. In *Cancer Nursing: A Comprehensive Textbook* (2nd ed., pp. 395–433), R McCorkle, M Grant, M Frank-Stromborg, et al. (eds). Philadelphia: WB Saunders, 1996

McKee J: Future dimensions in vascular access: peripheral implantable ports. J Intraven Nurs 1991; 14:387–93

Petrosino B, Becker H, Christian B: Infection rates in central venous catheter dressings. Oncol Nurs Forum 1988; 15:709–17

Pizzo P: Management of fever in patients with cancer and treatment-induced neutropenia. New Engl J Med 1993; 328:1323–32

Raad I, Luna M, Kahil S, et al.: The relationship between the thrombotic and infectious complications of central venous catheters. JAMA 1994; 271:1014–19

Rumsey K, Richardson D: Management of infection and occlusion associated with vascular access devices. Sem Oncol Nurs 1995; 91:22–6

Shivan J, McGuire D, Freedman S, et al.: A comparison of transparent adherent and dry gauze dressings for long-term central catheters in patients undergoing bone marrow transplants. Oncol Nurs Forum 1991; 18:1349–55

Device: Ventricular Reservoir

Corinne Haviley

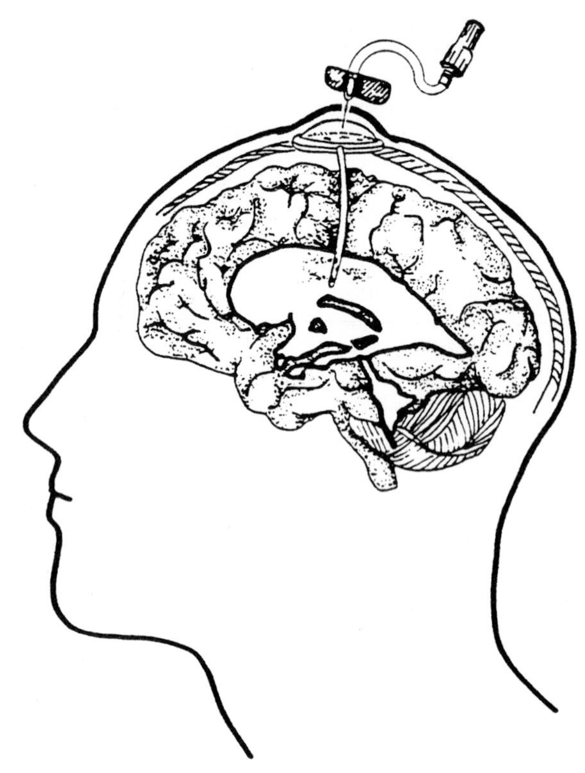

Cerebrospinal fluid reservoir and mode of use. From Regmann PE: Chemotherapy: Principles of administration. In *Cancer Nursing: Principles and Practice,* 3rd ed. Edited by Groenwald SL, Frogge MH, Goodman M, Yarbro CH. London: Jones and Bartlett, 1996, p. 311. Reprinted by permission.

TYPE: IMPLANTED DEVICE

■ Description: a ventricular reservoir is an implantable device that facilitates access to the intracranial ventricles or the lumbar subarachnoid space. The device is commonly referred to as the Ommaya reservoir. Configured similar to a mushroom, the silicone dome-shaped superior portion measures ~3.4 cm in diameter. It is connected to a side catheter attachment. The catheter length is ~7.25 cm and is manufactured in a variety of sizes to accommodate anatomic differences for pediatric and adult populations. The dome-shaped portion, resembling a disc, is self-sealing, which allows for repeated percutaneous access. Under local or general anesthetic, the dome is surgically implanted SubQ, generally above the nondominant area of the frontal parietal lobe. Via a burr hole, the catheter is threaded into the lateral ventricle. Access is achieved by inserting a small-gauged (e.g., 25 g) needle into the dome portion of the device

- Indications for use
  - administration of antineoplastic agents (e.g., cytarabine, methotrexate)
  - antibiotic instillation (e.g., amphotericin B, especially effective in the treatment of fungal brain lesions/abscesses and meningitis)
  - analgesic administration: intractable pain can be successfully managed through the administration of preservative-free narcotics (e.g., morphine). Percutaneous injection into the CSF bypasses the circulatory system and travels directly to the opiod receptors. Since morphine has poor lipid solubility the drug is retained in the CNS, which delays excretion in the urine; hence there is an extension in drug duration of action
  - intracranial pressure monitoring
  - removal of CSF for diagnostic purposes, to decrease intracranial pressure, or for analysis related to infection

■ Advantages: Ommaya reservoirs are convenient systems for administering intraventricular chemotherapy. Since the majority of antineoplastic agents do not cross the blood-brain barrier, this device allows for drug distribution directly into the ventricles with more predictable drug concentration and distribution. When an alternative procedure such as a lumbar puncture technique is used for drug instillation, commonly the medications do not ascend into the cranium. The pain perception both in the pediatric and adult population is reportedly decreased with the use of this device versus a lumbar puncture. The reservoir is not associated with a high rejection rate because of the inert material that contributes to its construction

RISKS/DISADVANTAGES

■ Requires operative procedure, which increases cost. Device access is associated with needle puncture into the scalp, risk of infection, and exacerbation of neurologic symptoms. Side effects can be minimized by appropriate patient selection, preoperative CT scan, precise surgical technique, perioperative prophylactic antibiotics, and meticulous procedure during use of reservoir. Complications can include aseptic chemical meningitis and catheter-related infections, which can be managed medically

SURGICAL CONSIDERATIONS

Mohamed Yassine

- Preoperation
  - overall patient fitness must be assessed and the ability to withstand anesthesia or sedation should be considered
  - involve the patient in the decision making. This facilitates the learning process and adaptation to the device
  - alleviate the patient's anxiety, increase compliance, and reduce complication by
    - □ use of a demonstration model for reinforcement of catheter teaching
    - □ informing patient of potential postinsertion complications
- Postoperation
  - confirm placement of catheter by a skull x-ray. A CT scan may further confirm appropriate placement
  - pressure and/or sterile dressings are applied over the insertion site for 24 hrs postoperatively
  - dressings should be changed 24–48 hrs after placement and then no dressing is required
  - the catheter is generally not used for 24 hrs postinsertion
  - monitor the patient for signs and symptoms of infection, bleeding, and neurologic changes. Do not handle catheter if patient is neurologically unstable
  - if resistance is encountered when using catheter, *do not* continue to access or use the device
  - sutures are generally removed within 1 wk

CLINICAL ASSESSMENT/ INTERVENTIONS/IMPLICATIONS

- Equipment
  - sterile gloves
  - 2 × 2 or 4 × 4 gauze pads
  - povidone-iodine swabs (3)
  - alcohol wipes or swabs (3)
  - 23 or 25 gauge butterfly needle or 5/8 inch straight needle
  - two-way or three-way stopcock
  - syringes (3, 5, or 10 cc) for CSF fluid removal or drug administration
  - premixed drugs (preservative free)

  - shaving or preparation kit, if applicable
  - equipment for specimen collection if necessary: 3 cc syringe(s) and collection tubes
- Patient assessment: prior to access, check the treatment parameters that are typically evaluated before specific drug administration occurs (e.g., CBC, BUN, vital signs, neurologic status, etc.)
  - ensure that premedication orders are carried out. If ordered, antipyretics, antihistamines, or antiemetics are generally delivered 15–30 min prior to access
  - explain the procedure to the patient/family and validate understanding
  - position patient preferably in a semirecumbent position, and support head with a pillow
  - wash hands
  - determine if hair removal is necessary. Hair should be removed in the approximate area of the dome, generally 3 cm in diameter. Shave if appropriate using a customary procedure
  - palpate the insertion site to locate the reservoir; examine for signs of infection, bleeding, and appropriate placement
  - verify that the device is functioning properly, using index finger and pressing down gently on the dome of the reservoir and release. The dome should easily fill with CSF fluid
  - assess patient for side effects related to drug administered
- Device care
  - use aseptic technique
  - cleanse the scalp using the povidone-iodine swabs: use a circular motion, moving from the center to the peripheral area of the scalp covering the dome. Allow enough time for the iodine to dry. Repeat the procedure using alcohol. Some centers recommend swabbing with alcohol followed by povidone-iodine. Refer to institutional policies
  - organize all supplies; draw up medications to be administered and label syringe appropriately; and place on a clean/sterile field
  - attach the stopcock and syringe to the butterfly or straight needle and place on clean/sterile field
  - wash hands again and don sterile gloves
  - insert the needle perpendicular to the dome of the device. An oblique angle is an acceptable approach if the perpendicular angle does not achieve successful insertion. The stopcock should be closed. Brace heel of the same hand being used for needle insertion against the patient's head for support and to stabilize the needle during the entire procedure. Use the opposite hand to hold the syringe(s). Open the stopcock. CSF fluid should freely flow upon gentle aspiration. If fluid cannot be withdrawn, needle placement can be changed. If fluid cannot be obtained after a second needle insertion attempt, pursue radiography studies to determine device patency and/or appropriate placement
  - a volume of CSF equal to that of the medication to be injected is removed. If the physician has not specified an order, remove 1–3 cc of CSF fluid volume. Close the stopcock
  - remove the collection syringe. Set the syringe filled with CSF fluid aside so it can be used for reinstallation, if ordered, after drug administration. Or remove the volume of fluid necessary for laboratory studies. Close the stopcock and set the syringe aside
  - normally, CSF fluid is clear and colorless. If the CSF fluid is blood tinged or cloudy, save the fluid for further testing and notify physician. *Do not* inject the medication until investigation occurs regarding the status of the patient's fluid
  - attach the medication syringe, open the stopcock, and inject the drug slowly over 3–10 min, pending the volume, patient's ventricular size and response, and/or physician's order. Slow administration is used to avoid meningeal irritation and to ensure optimum drug distribution. Do not inject air. Close the stopcock
  - attach the syringe containing the CSF fluid, open the stopcock and slowly (over 1–3 min) inject the fluid into the reservoir
  - note: some centers recommend manually compressing the dome of the device after drug administration to mix the medication with the CSF. Refer to institutional policy
  - remove the needle. Apply a sterile 2 × 2 or 4 × 4 gauze pad to the access site using light compression to stop any bleeding. Wipe with an alcohol swab
  - instruct the patient to lie supine for 30 min postprocedure to enhance drug distribution and to avoid neurologic symptoms (e.g., headaches)
  - evaluate the patient postaccess for signs of infection, bleeding, or neurologic changes (e.g., tinnitus, neck rigidity or pain, nausea and/or vomiting, respiratory difficulty or depression)
  - postprocedure, document date, time, drug dose, admixture, and volume at instillation. Document ease of drug administration and/or fluid removal, assessment of access site, drug assessment parameters, patient's response and understanding of the experience, and recommendations for future practice
  - heparinization and/or intermittent flushing is not necessary because CSF flows freely through the device
- Management of complications
  - infection: patients who are immunocompromised are highly susceptible to infection. Symptoms include tenderness, redness, swelling, heat, and drainage at the injection site. Additionally, fever of 101° F, elevated WBC, nuchal rigidity, nausea and/or vomiting, headache, and photophobia are contributing signs. CSF infection can occur as a result of residual infection or related to device usage. Obtain CSF for analysis: cytology, glucose, protein, LDH, cell count, bacterial culture, and gram stain. Appropriate administration technique including drug mixing is paramount to preventing infection. Treatment usually requires antibiotic therapy with device removal should therapy not be successful
  - reservoir failure: a blocked or kinked catheter can cause a malfunction. Device displacement can occur evidenced by lack of response to therapy (e.g., pain management). To assess for system function, pump the dome gently by compressing the dome and releasing it a few times. If the CSF fluid refills the dome, it can be felt with the finger. If the patient is neurologically unstable, however, this procedure should not be instituted. A CT or skull x-ray can verify the placement and function of the catheter
  - bleeding: intraventricular bleeding, subarachnoid hematoma, or subdural hematoma can occur. Assess for neurologic changes and sensory and motor deficits
  - shelf life or life span of the reservoir: in general, 200 needle punctures can be performed using the device before evidence of leakage occurs. Assessment for leakage at the injection site is important to identify early signs of fluid/drug loss
  - medication side effects: the drugs administered through the ventricular reservoir used for treatment of infection, cancer, or pain continue to have associated side effects consistent with systemic infusion. In some cases, the side effects can have greater toxicity due to the route of administration. Hence management of side effects needs similar treatment as with other routes of administration
  - neurologic changes: meticulous assessment of patient's neurologic status is essential, since the device is associated with the risk of developing disseminating necrotizing leukoencephalopathy, hemiparesis, and tissue damage. Standard neurologic assessments are appropriate. Symptoms include change in level of consciousness, confusion, seizures, spasticity, somnolence, ataxia, etc., in addition to the aforementioned signs and symptoms
  - document procedure, findings, and interventions

ISSUES FOR PATIENT TEACHING

- Name of device: ventricular reservoir
- Care of device/patient: observe the device for infection and bleeding. Avoid bumping, pushing, or twiddling with the insertion site
- Instruct the patient or family to report neurologic changes such as change in behavior, vision, ability to ambulate, memory, stiff neck, headache, or fever, chills, pain, drainage swelling/bruising at the insertion site
- Patients should be encouraged to allow caregivers to remove hair when necessary to prevent skin trauma
- Patients may shower and bathe normally postinsertion, pending physician recommendations
- Provide telephone numbers of health care providers and next appointment
- Routine assessment of compliance with recommendations for care

KEY REFERENCES

Access Device Guidelines: Recommendations for Nursing Practice and Education, D Camp-Sorrell (ed). Pittsburgh: Oncology Nursing Society, n.d.

Berg D: Drug delivery system. In *Cancer Chemotherapy: A Nursing Process Approach* (2nd ed., pp. 561–95), M Burke, G Wilkes, K Ingwersen (eds). London: Jones and Bartlett, 1996

Goodman M: Cancer nursing. In *Chemoterapy: Principles of Administration,* S Baird, R McCorkle, M Grant (eds): pp. 317–84. Philadelphia: WB Saunders, 1991

Chamberlin MC, Kormanik PA, Barba D: Complications associated with intraventricular chemotherapy in patients with leptomeningeal metastasis. J Neurosurg 1997; 87(5):694–9

Cornwell C: The Ommaya reservoir: implications for pediatric oncology. Pediatr Nurs 1990; 16(3):249–51

Esparza D, Weyland J: Nursing care for the patient with an Ommaya reservoir. Oncol Nurs Forum 1982; 9(4):17–20

Holmes B: Administration of cancer chemotherapy agents. In *Cancer Chemotherapy Handbook* (2nd ed., pp. 72–3, 98), R Dorr, D Von Hoff (eds). East Norwalk, CT: Appleton and Lange, 1994

LePage E: Using a ventricular reservoir to instill amphotericin B. J Neuroscience Nurs 1993; 25(4):212–17

Lishner M, Perrin RG, Feld R, et al.: Complications associated with Ommaya reservoirs in patients with cancer. The Princess Margaret hospital experience and a review of the literature. Department of Medicine, Ontario Cancer Institute, Toronto; Arch Intern Med 1990; 150(1):173–6

Martin V: Delivery of cancer chemotherapy. In *Cancer Nursing: A Comprehensive Textbook* (2nd ed., pp. 395–433), R McCorkle, M Grant, M Frank-Stromborg, et al. (eds). Philadelphia: WB Saunders, 1996

Oncology for the house officer: In J O'Donnell, C Coughlin, P LeMarbre (eds), pp. 211–213 Baltimore: Williams and Wilkins, 1992

Perrin RG, Liskner M, Guha A, et al.: Experience with Ommaya reservoir in 120 consecutive patients with meningeal malignancy. Can J Neurol Sci 1990; 17(2):190–2

Rahr V: Giving intrathecal drugs. Am J Nurs 1986; 86-T:829–31

Raney J, Kirk E: The use of an Ommaya reservoir for administration of morphine sulphate to control pain in select cancer patients. J Neurosci Nurs 1998; 20(1):23–8

Reyman P: Chemotherapy: practice and principles. In *Cancer Nursing Principles and Practice* (3rd ed., pp. 293–330), S Groenwald, M Frogge, M Goodman, et al. (eds). London: Jones and Bartlett, 1993

Device: Intraperitoneal: Tenckhoff Catheter

Susan C. Budds

MANUFACTURERS: BARD ACCESS SYSTEMS, PHARMACIA DELTEC, STRATO/INFUSAID MEDICAL

TYPE: SEMIPERMANENT INDWELLING TUNNELED EXTERNAL CATHETER

- Description: a soft flexible silicone or polyurethane catheter with one or two Dacron felt cuffs. This varies with manufacturer (Almadrones, Campana, & Dantis, 1995). It is placed either during a surgical procedure or as a sterile bedside procedure. It is inserted percutaneously below the umbilicus into the peritoneal cavity and threaded through a SubQ tunnel. The cuff(s) is then tunneled into SubQ tissue, and the proximal portion is externalized through a stab incision so it protrudes through the abdominal wall onto the skin. The cuff(s) adheres to the abdominal cavity wall in 1–2 wks, to lessen the chance of bacterial infection. The catheter should be anchored to prevent dislodgement and leakage of peritoneal fluid (Zook-Enck, 1990)
- Indications for use: administration of chemotherapy or biotherapy into the peritoneal cavity. Drainage of peritoneal fluid in patients experiencing ascites. Collection of peritoneal fluid for cytologic washings, when several months of therapy are planned
- Advantages: it is safe and medications can be easily instilled by trained oncology nurses and physicians in an outpatient setting. The large diameter of the catheter allows for rapid flow rate; capability to drain large volumes of fluid and manipulate the catheter with irrigation or increased force. It can remain in place for months. Surgery is not required to remove the catheter (Phillips, 1993)

RISKS/DISADVANTAGES

- There is an increased risk of bowel or visceral perforation during placement as compared to an implanted port. There is an increased risk of infection resulting from the external portion of the catheter and leakage around the catheter. Sterile technique is required for care. The external portion of catheter poses limitations in activity. A compliant patient or patient with strong caregiver support is required for external catheter site care (Phillips, 1993)

SURGICAL CONSIDERATIONS

Mohamed Yassine

- Preoperation
  - overall patient fitness must be assessed and the ability to withstand anesthesia or sedation should be considered
  - involve the patient in the decision making. This facilitates the learning process and adaptation to the device
  - discuss insertion site options, so the convenience and quality of life is minimally affected
  - alleviate patient's anxiety, increase compliance, and reduce complication by
    - □ use of a demonstration model for reinforcement of catheter teaching
    - □ informing patient of potential postinsertion complications
- Postoperation
  - monitor the patient's vital signs for 24 hrs
  - observe for signs of abdominal distention and pain
  - assess for leakage of fluid around the device and for signs of obstruction (most common complication)
  - evaluate patient for signs of bowel or visceral perforation
  - keep the site of insertion clean and comply with sterile technique when handling the catheter
  - use and handle the catheter only when needed to minimize potential infection (second most common complication)

CLINICAL ASSESSMENT/ INTERVENTIONS/IMPLICATIONS

- Patient assessment: involves assessment of the patient, catheter, and catheter site
  - therapy should be administered after the patient has emptied bladder to facilitate comfort
  - assess patient for side effects related to drug administered
- Infection: assess for signs and symptoms of local or systemic infection: temperature, redness and/or warmth, drainage, swelling, or pain around the catheter
- Peritonitis: may be due to infection or chemical irritation. Assess for fever, abdominal pain or tenderness, cloudy peritoneal fluid, ascites, abdominal distention, or increased white blood cell count
- Occlusion: assess catheter for leakage, rate of inflow or outflow, kinks in the tubing, height of administration or drainage bag, and ability to flush or aspirate
- increased intra-abdominal pressure: assess for discomfort, shortness of breath, gastrointestinal reflux, loss of appetite, diarrhea, constipation, nausea, and vomiting
- Treatment toxicities: assess according to the agent being administered. Toxicities are related to systemic absorption of the chemotherapy drug
- Management of complications
  - site infection: often caused by contamination of normal skin flora. Common intervention
    - □ culturing the exit site, cleansing with betadine or other prescribed antimicrobial agent
    - □ applying antimicrobial ointment
    - □ performing frequent dressing changes, maintaining sterile technique during site care
    - □ reassessing caregiver ability to perform site care
    - □ monitoring and documenting site condition
    - □ administration or monitoring of systemic antibiotics
  - peritonitis: may be caused by chemical irritation from drugs administered or bacterial contamination of the catheter. General interventions include
    - □ assessment of pain and pain control, administration of pain medication
    - □ monitoring of temperature and vital signs
    - □ documentation of peritoneal fluid and lab values
    - □ administration of antibiotics
    - □ warming intraperitoneal fluids/medications prior to administration to decrease discomfort
  - occlusion: occlusion may be caused by formation of fibrous sheaths or fibrin clots, plugs inside the catheter or around the catheter tip, formation of adhesions within the peritoneal space, catheter migration or displacement of the catheter. Universal interventions include
    - □ repositioning of the patient
    - □ milking of the tubing
    - □ vigorous flushing of the catheter with saline
    - □ radiologic study to confirm placement
    - □ increasing height of administration bag or lowering height of drainage bag
    - □ preparing patient for procedure to remove the catheter
  - increased intra-abdominal pressure: increased intra-abdominal pressure may result from administration of infusate or infection
    - □ mild analgesics or warm packs may be utilized for discomfort
    - □ oxygen may be indicated for shortness of breath
    - □ small frequent meals and elevating the head of the bed after meals are common interventions for GI reflux and loss of appetite
    - □ diarrhea may be treated with antidiarrhea medications
    - □ constipation can be prevented with increasing daily intake of fiber, monitoring daily bowel movements, and administration of stool softeners
    - □ termination of the infusion and/or drainage of peritoneal fluid may be required
  - treatment toxicities: treatment toxicities are related to systemic absorption of chemotherapy drugs. Assess according to the agent being administered. For example, if interleukins are being administered, presence of fever may be related to

the drug and not to infection. If cisplatin is being administered, careful observation of urine output may be indicated
- maintenance: use strict aseptic technique
- flushing: use 5–10 ml heparinized saline per physician, agency, or institution protocol after every use. Routine flushing not necessary, since it will be used frequently for treatments (Otto, 1995)
- catheter care/dressing requirements: frequency may vary depending on the physician, agency, or institution. Basic principles are to use sterile technique, avoid opening the system unnecessarily, use betadine to clean the site, and apply sterile dressing (Zook-Enck, 1990)
- home infusions: apply same principles of sterile technique in the home as in the hospital or outpatient/ambulatory environment. Planning and preparation is required to ensure all needed supplies are in the home if administration of medications is to occur there. Inspect home environment for potential sources of infection such as pets. Home environment should also be inspected for safety hazards such as throw rugs and excessive clutter where patients may fall causing dislodgment of the catheter
- special considerations: if patency of catheter is questionable, administration should be held until consultation with physician

■ Document procedure, findings, and interventions

ISSUES FOR PATIENT AND FAMILY TEACHING

■ Name of device: Tenckhoff catheter

■ Assessment of the patient/caregiver ability to care for catheter should include their ability to understand instructions, their ability to demonstrate correct technique, willingness to perform the care, and cleanliness of surroundings where care will take place

■ Patient should be provided with names and numbers of their physician and nurse

■ Routine assessment of compliance with recommendations for care

KEY REFERENCES

Access Device Guidelines: Recommendations for Nursing Practice and Education, D Camp-Sorrell (ed). Pittsburgh: Oncology Nursing Society, n.d.

Almodrones L, Campana P, Dantis E: Arterial, peritoneal and intraventricular access devices. Sem Oncol Nurs 1995; 11(3): 194–202

Berg D: Drug delivery system. In *Cancer Chemotherapy: A Nursing Process Approach* (2nd ed., pp. 561–95), M Burke, G Wilkes, K Ingwersen (eds). London: Jones and Bartlett, 1996

Martin V: Delivery of cancer chemotherapy. In *Cancer Nursing: A Comprehensive Textbook* (2nd ed., pp. 395–433), R McCorkle, M Grant, M Frank-Stromborg, et al. (eds). Philadelphia: WB Saunders, 1996

Otto S: Advanced concepts in chemotherapy drug delivery. J Intraven Nurs 1995; 18(4):170–6

Phillips L: *Manual of IV Therapeutics.* Philadelphia: FA Davis, 1993

Twardowski ZJ: Peritoneal catheter development. Currently used catheters—advantages/disadvantages/complication, and catheter tunnel morphology in humans. Department of Medicine, University of Missouri, Harry S. Truman Veterans Administration Hospital, Dalton Research Center, Columbia. ASAIO Trans 1988; 34(4):937–40

Zook-Enck D: Intraperitoneal therapy via the Tenckhoff catheter. J Intraven Nurs 1990; 13(6):375–82

Device: Intraperitoneal: Implanted Ports

Susan C. Budds

MULTIPLE MANUFACTURERS: SIMS DELTEC, STRATO/INFUSAID, BARD ACCESS SYSTEMS

TYPE: PERMANENT IMPLANTED CATHETER WITHOUT EXTERNAL PARTS

- Description: an implanted port is a permanent catheter made of two parts. The description may vary with the manufacturer. The portal body is made of titanium or polysulfone with a self-sealing silicone septum in the center. A radiopaque polyurethane or silicone catheter with a Dacron cuff protrudes from the side of the portal body. The portal body is inserted in a SubQ pocket and secured to the fascia muscles overlying an anatomic area that provides support and stability, usually the lower rib cage below the breast. The catheter is tunneled SubQ into the peritoneal space. It is placed in surgery with IV sedation. The catheter is accessed using sterile technique with a special noncoring Huber needle through the skin into the portal septum (Almadrones & Yerys, 1990)
- Indications for use: administration of chemotherapy or biotherapy into the peritoneal cavity. Drainage of peritoneal fluid in patients experiencing ascites. Collection of peritoneal fluid for cytologic washings
- Advantages: the implanted port has the advantage of the absence of external parts, decreases the risk of infection, lowers maintenance costs, and reduces body image concerns. It requires no care from the patient. There is a decreased risk of visceral or bowel perforation when placed during laparotomy

RISKS/DISADVANTAGES

- Surgery is required for placement and removal. Needle sticks are required to access the system. High pressure, forced irrigation, or manipulation to dislodge or loosen fibrin clots is not possible due to the portal body. Sterile technique is required when accessing port

SURGICAL CONSIDERATIONS

Mohamed Yassine

- Preoperation
  - provide patient and relatives with information on the procedure, maintenance care, and expected outcome
  - involve patient in decision making. This facilitates the learning process and adaptation to the device after surgery
  - discuss insertion site options, so convenience and quality of life is minimally affected
- Postoperation
  - x-ray study or a perfusion scan is useful to confirm placement
  - observe for bleeding or drainage at the operation site and pain
  - assess for the development of a hematoma or hygroma
  - prevent "flip-flop syndrome" (inability to locate the septum) from occurring by observing for seroma
  - apply cold packs or pressure to reduce postoperative discomfort and edema
  - the implanted port can be used 24 hrs postinsertion (avoid chemotherapy for 5–7 days)
  - strict aseptic technique should be used to access the port
  - observe for any signs of resistance or occlusion
  - patient may not shower until wound is healed

CLINICAL ASSESSMENT/INTERVENTIONS/IMPLICATIONS

- Patient assessment: includes assessment of the patient and catheter site
  - therapy should be administered after the patient has emptied bladder to facilitate comfort
  - assess patient for side effects related to drug administered
- Infection: assess for signs and symptoms of local or systemic infection: temperature, redness and/or warmth over the implanted port or abdomen, drainage, swelling, or pain around the port site or abdomen
- Peritonitis: can be due to infection or chemical irritation. Assess for fever, abdominal pain, tenderness or rigidity in the abdomen, cloudy peritoneal fluid, increased amount of peritoneal fluid, ascites, abdominal distention, or increased white blood cell count
- Occlusion: assess inflow and outflow, height of administration of drainage bag, and ability to flush or aspirate
- Increased intra-abdominal pressure: assess for discomfort, shortness of breath, gastrointestinal reflux, loss of appetite, diarrhea, constipation, nausea, and vomiting
- Treatment toxicities: treatment toxicities are related to systemic absorption of chemotherapy drugs. Assess according to the agent being administered
- Management of complications
  - infection: although the infection rate with implanted ports is less when compared to the Tenckhoff catheter, when it does occur, it is often caused by contamination of normal skin flora. Maintaining sterile technique during access is important. Common interventions include
    - □ cleansing with betadine or another prescribed antimicrobial agent
    - □ applying antimicrobial ointment
    - □ performing frequent dressing changes
    - □ reassessing caregiver's ability to perform site care
    - □ administration and monitoring of systemic antibiotics
    - □ monitor and document the condition of the catheter site regularly
  - peritonitis: may be caused by chemical irritation from drugs administered or bacterial contamination of the catheter. General interventions include
    - □ assessment of pain and pain control; administration of pain medication
    - □ monitoring of temperature and vital signs
    - □ documentation of peritoneal fluid and lab values
    - □ administration of antibiotics
    - □ warming intraperitoneal fluids/medications prior to administration to decrease discomfort
  - occlusion: occlusion may be caused by formation of fibrous sheaths or fibrin clots, plugs inside the catheter or around the catheter tip, formation of adhesions within the peritoneal space, catheter migration, or displacement of the catheter. Universal interventions include
    - □ checking for kinks or occlusions along the tubing
    - □ repositioning of the patient
    - □ milking of the tubing
    - □ vigorous flushing of the catheter with saline
    - □ radiologic study to confirm placement
    - □ increasing the height of the administration bag or lowering height of drainage bag
    - □ often this results in the ability to infuse and inability to aspirate
    - □ if placement is confirmed, then administration of chemotherapy may be continued
    - □ catheter removal is not necessary for partial occlusions of this type
    - □ removal is indicated if inflow is blocked
  - increased intra-abdominal pressure: increased intra-abdominal pressure may result from administration of infusate or infection
    - □ mild analgesics or warm packs may be utilized for discomfort
    - □ oxygen may be indicated for shortness of breath
    - □ small frequent meals and elevating the head of bed after meals are common interventions for GI reflux and loss of appetite
    - □ diarrhea may be treated with antidiarrhea medications
    - □ constipation can be prevented with increasing daily intake of fiber, monitoring daily bowel movements, and stool softeners
    - □ nausea and vomiting are treated with administration of medications
    - □ termination of the infusion and/or drainage of peritoneal fluid may be required

- treatment toxicities: caused by systemic absorption of medications administered. Need to assess for side effects related to specific drug administered. For example, if interleukins are being administered, presence of fever may be related to the drug and not to infection. If cisplatin is being administered, careful observation of urine output is indicated

■ Maintenance: Flushing: strict aseptic technique should be used when accessing the port. When not in use, the implanted port requires flushing with 5–10 ml of 100 units/ml heparinized saline q3–4wks (Otto, 1995; Booker & Ignatavicius, 1996)

■ Catheter care/dressing requirements: since there are no external parts to this catheter, no daily catheter or dressing care is required. When the catheter is accessed, cleansing with betadine using sterile technique is required

■ Home infusions: apply the same principles of sterile technique in the home as in the hospital or outpatient/ambulatory setting. Planning and preparation is required to ensure all needed supplies are in the home if administration of medications is to occur there. Inspect the home environment for potential sources of infection such as pets or excessive garbage

■ Special considerations: patients with implantable ports may be receiving continuous infusion chemotherapy via ambulatory pump; additional assessments are related to the type of pump being used. When receiving continuous infusion therapy, monitoring for extravasation is indicated due to the potential for the needle to become dislodged during administration

■ Document procedure, findings, and interventions

ISSUES FOR PATIENT AND FAMILY TEACHING

■ Name of device: intraperitoneal implanted port

■ Patient and family teaching needs are reduced with the implanted port and should focus on treatment side effects and emergency care for continuous infusions

■ Instruct patient to report signs of swelling, pain, or drainage

■ Patient should be provided with names and numbers of physician and nurse

■ Routine assessment of compliance with recommendations for care

KEY REFERENCES

Access Device Guidelines: Recommendations for Nursing Practice and Education, D Camp-Sorrell (ed). Pittsburgh: Oncology Nursing Society, n.d.

Almadrones L, Yerys C: Problems associated with the administration of intraperitoneal therapy using the Port-A-Cath system. Oncol Nurs Forum 1990; 17(1):75–80

Berg D: Drug delivery system. In *Cancer Chemotherapy: A Nursing Process Approach* (2nd ed., pp. 561–95), M Burke, G Wilkes, K Ingwersen (eds). London: Jones and Bartlett, 1996

Booker MF, Ignatavicius D (eds): *Infusion Therapy Techniques & Medications.* Philadelphia: WB Saunders, 1996

Doane LS: Administering intraperitoneal chemotherapy using a peritoneal port. Nurs Clin North Am 1993; 28(4):885–97

Gullo SM: Implanted ports. Technologic advances and nursing care issues. Cleveland Clinic Foundation, Ohio. Nurs Clin North Am 1993; 28(4);859–71

Johnson GB: Nursing care of patients with implanted pumps. Patient Services, Bethesda Hospitals, Inc., Ohio. Nurs Clin North Am 1993; 28(4):873–83

Martin V: Delivery of cancer chemotherapy. In *Cancer Nursing: A Comprehensive Textbook* (2nd ed., pp. 395–433), R McCorkle, M Grant, Frank-Stromborg, et al. (eds). Philadelphia: WB Saunders, 1996

Otto SE: Advanced concepts in chemotherapy drug delivery: regional therapy. J Intraven Nurs 1995; 18(4):170–6

Adjuvant Devices for the Management of Advanced Thoracic Malignancies

J. Heidi Downey

INTRODUCTION

■ As treatment options for advanced thoracic malignancies continue to evolve, so has the surgical management of the patients with these devices. Chest tube drainage is still considered paramount in the management of the patient with a symptomatic malignant effusion. Bedside tube thoracostomy remains suitable for drainage of effusions with subsequent pleurodesis with talc or sclerosing agents. In many institutions, the preferable management of a malignant effusion is drainage via a video-assisted thoracoscopy (VAT) approach. This procedure involves a local or general anesthetic and is undertaken in the operative suite. Drainage of the effusion through a thoracoscope is accomplished; mechanical and/or talc pleurodesis may be performed and chest tubes placed. This approach can also be used to obtain biopsies or perform decortication, if necessary

■ Occasionally, a pleuroperitoneal shunt or pleural catheter may be used for patients with symptomatic pleural effusions recalcitrant to the methods mentioned above. The pleural shunt allows for fluid to be drained from the pleural space to the peritoneal space. Disadvantages with the shunt include potential for infection and risk of obstruction secondary to high protein content of the malignant fluid. More commonly used today are intrapleural implantable ports. These catheters are similar to the intraperitoneal ports currently marketed by a variety of manufacturers. The insertion of a small bore percutaneously placed catheter or implantable port under local anesthetic allows for repeated thoracentesis on an as needed basis and permits patients to remain at home during their care

KEY REFERENCES

Andrews CO, Gora MA: Pleural effusions: pathophysiology and management. Ann Pharmacother 1994; 28:894–901

Kennedy L, Rusch VW, et al.: Pleurodesis using talc slurry. Chest 1994; 106:243–6

Device: Thoracic Drainage Tubes/Chest Tubes

J. Heidi Downey

MULTIPLE MANUFACTURERS

TYPE: INTRAPLEURAL DEVICE

- Description: silicone or polyvinylchloride tube with radiopaque strips for radiologic identification. Typically placed for temporary measures of drainage and sclerosis, but may remain in place for days to weeks. Available in sizes ranging from 12–42F
- Indications for uses: in the oncologic setting, chest tubes are used for drainage of malignant pleural effusions, and/or chemical and talc pleurodesis. Large-bore tubes (26–40F) are placed for drainage of viscous fluids including hemothorax or infection
- Advantages: immediate symptomatic relief; enables subsequent sclerotherapy with relative ease

RISKS/DISADVANTAGES

- Requires hospitalization for placement. There is an increased potential for infection with long-term use. Risk of pneumothorax, which can also be related to rapid removal of fluid from a relatively stiff noncompliant lung

SURGICAL CONSIDERATIONS

Mohamed Yassine

- Preprocedure
  - provide patient with information on procedure, maintenance, and expected outcome
  - involve the patient with the decision making to facilitate learning process and adaptation to the device
  - a CT scan and needle aspiration is suggested prior to tube placement if the effusion is complicated
  - examine chest tube for possible defects prior to placement
  - tube is usually aimed posteriorly and inferiorly via the sixth or seventh interspace in uncomplicated effusions
- Postprocedure
  - the tube is secured in place with silk sutures, a Vaseline coated gauze, and a pressure dressing prior to connecting it to a suction device
  - confirm chest tube placement by PA and lateral chest x-ray
  - ensure tube patency and correct intrapleural positioning by observing the water level in the water-seal chamber fluctuate with respirations while the suction is turned off
  - check for air leaks by looking for bubbles in the air leak chamber in the absence of suction

CLINICAL ASSESSMENT/ INTERVENTIONS/IMPLICATIONS

- Patient assessment
  - examine insertion site for drainage, erythema, or edema
  - inspect tubing at connections and at drainage collection system for visible or audible air leak
  - monitor temperature
  - assess for pain at insertion site
- Maintenance
  - collection system
    - assess collection system for visible air leak within the water-seal chamber; if present, resecure all connections and document
    - assess and document that suction chamber is set on appropriate negative pressure, if ordered
    - record amount and characteristics of initial and subsequent drainage from collection system at every nursing shift
  - chest tubes/dressing requirements
    - auscultate breath sounds
    - inspect tubing for kinking and patency; milk gently if necessary
    - assess chest tube placement by chest x-ray (PA and lateral)
    - dressing change requires sterile technique; change daily or whenever it becomes soiled or saturated
    - apply Vaseline gauze directly to insertion site; cover with additional gauze pads and tape occlusively
    - secure tube(s) at patient's side to protect from inadvertent pulling/disconnection
- Management of complications
  - if the chest tube is inadvertently removed while the patient is in the hospital: immediately occlude chest tube site by placing a Vaseline gauze and gauze pads over the site and tape to seal securely. Physician should be notified and a chest x-ray obtained
  - if the chest tube is inadvertently disconnected from the drainage system, clamp the chest tube with rubber-shod hemostat or with your hand until the tip can be cleansed quickly with an alcohol pad. Reconnect tubing to drainage system and check for an air leak
  - tubing obstruction: chest tubes may be gently "milked" for obstruction due to thick, viscous fluids or hemothorax. If a clot is suspected observe the water-seal chamber for tidaling
  - infection: can occasionally occur at the insertion site, in the tubing (tunnel), and systematically. Signs and symptoms include erythema and drainage at site with fever and malaise. Management includes obtaining cultures of the tubing site and initiating antibiotic treatment

SPECIAL CONSIDERATIONS FOR BEDSIDE PLEURODESIS/SCLEROSIS

- This procedure is used in the management of pleural effusions. The given dose of medication or talc is mixed with 30–50 cc of normal saline. Instillation of these agents is often painful; premedicate patient with parenteral opiates and/or intrapleural lidocaine
- Following instillation of the sclerosing agent, an additional 10–20 cc of saline solution is flushed through the tubing. The chest tube is immediately clamped and the sclerosing agent is left in the chest cavity from 30 min–6 hrs. While the chest tube is clamped, the nurse is often responsible for repositioning the patient (supine, prone, sitting, left, and right lateral decubitus) to allow for adequate distribution of the agent to all pleural surfaces
- Fever following talc pleurodesis is common. Notify physician immediately of reactions including fever, arrhythmias, acute respiratory distress, and dyspnea
- Document procedure, findings, and interventions

ISSUES FOR PATIENT TEACHING

- Name of device: chest tube
- Frequency and procedure for dressing changes; using clean technique cover with gauze pad and tape occlusively
- Report fever, redness, swelling, or drainage at insertion site, pain, or difficulty breathing
- Provide instruction sheet regarding care of chest tube with appropriate emergency numbers of physician and nurse
- Routine assessment of compliance with recommendations for care

KEY REFERENCES

Access Device Guidelines: Recommendations for Nursing Practice and Education, D Camp-Sorrell (ed). Pittsburgh: Oncology Nursing Society, n.d.

Andrews CO, Gora MA: Pleural effusions: pathophysiology and management. Ann Pharmacother 1994; 28:894–901

Berg D: Drug delivery system. In *Cancer Chemotherapy: A Nursing Process Approach* (2nd ed., pp. 561–95), M Burke, G Wilkes, K Ingwersen (eds). London: Jones and Bartlett, 1996

Chang YC, Patz EF, Goodman PC: Pneumothorax after a small-bore catheter placement for malignant pleural effusions. AJR Am J Roentgenal 1996; 166(5):1049–51

Martin V: Delivery of cancer chemotherapy. In *Cancer Nursing: A Comprehensive Textbook* (2nd ed., pp. 395–433), R McCorkle, M Grant, M Frank-Stromborg, et al. (eds). Philadelphia: WB Saunders, 1996

Quigley RL: Thoracentesis and chest tube drainage. Crit Care Clin 1995; 11(1):111–26

Device: Pleuroperitoneal Shunt

J. Heidi Downey

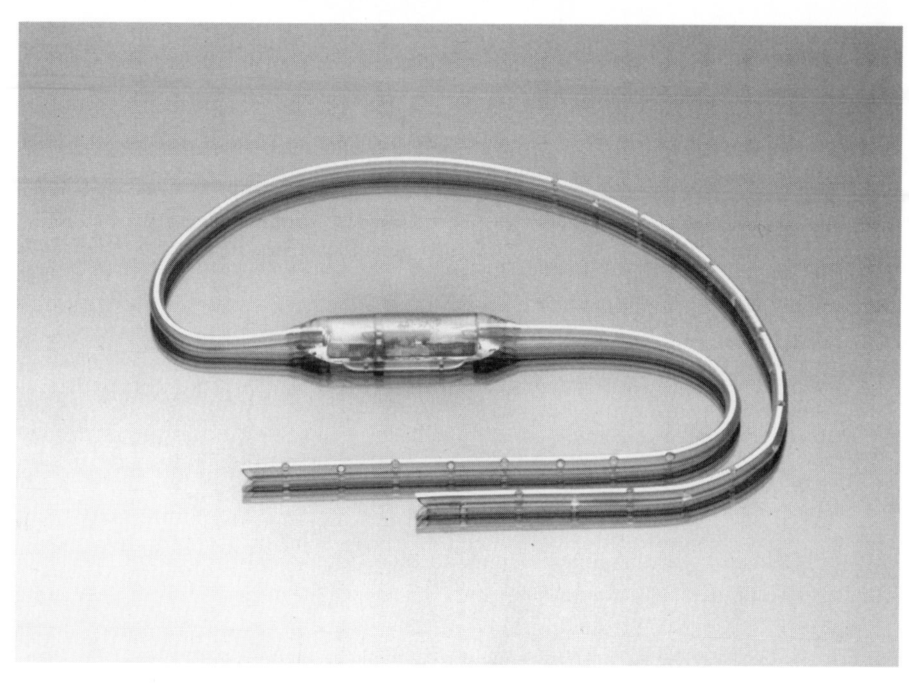

Reproduced by permission of Denver Biomedical, Inc.

VARIOUS MANUFACTURES; DENVER BIOMEDICAL, INC.

TYPE: INTRAPLEURAL DEVICE

■ Description: silicone catheter with single or dual valve chambers. One-way valve(s) promotes transfer of pleural fluid into the peritoneal cavity. The transfer of fluid is achieved by repeatedly compressing (pumping) and releasing the shunt's pump chamber. Currently, both implanted and external pump chambers are available

■ Indications for use: pleuroperitoneal shunts are indicated for the management of intractable malignant effusions and chylothorax when conventional methods have failed. Provides an alternative drainage method via chest tube placement with chemical or talc pleurodesis. Management of patients who are unable to achieve pleurodesis due to trapped lung (restrictive malignant cortex)

■ Advantages: provides immediate relief of dyspnea. Reduces patient trauma/discomfort and avoids repeated thoracentesis. Allows the patient to be home for treatment, reducing hospital costs

RISKS/DISADVANTAGES

■ Typically requires general anesthesia and limited hospitalization for placement

■ Shunts with external pump chambers have potential for topical infection

■ Potential for pump chamber occlusion

SURGICAL CONSIDERATIONS

Mohamed Yassine

- Preoperation
  - overall patient fitness must be assessed and the ability to withstand anesthesia or sedation should be considered
  - provide the patient with information regarding procedure, maintenance, and expected outcomes
  - involve the patient in the decision making to facilitate learning process and adaptation to the device
  - discuss insertion site options, so the convenience and quality of life is minimally affected
  - alleviate patient's anxiety, increase compliance, and reduce complication by
    - □ use of a demonstration model for reinforcement of catheter teaching
    - □ informing patient of potential postinsertion complications
- Postoperation
  - obtain chest x-ray to confirm placement
  - monitor patient vital signs for 24 hrs
  - observe for signs of chest discomfort and pain
  - assess for leakage of fluid and air around the device
  - assess the device for any signs of obstruction
  - use the pump every hour, at first, to ensure shunt patency
  - evaluate patient's pumping schedule
  - keep the site of insertion clean and comply with sterile technique

CLINICAL ASSESSMENT/ INTERVENTIONS/IMPLICATIONS

- Patient assessment
  - examine insertion site for drainage, erythema, or edema
  - for external pump chamber devices, inspect chamber for visible cracks or defects
  - monitor temperature
  - assess for pain at insertion site
- Maintenance
  - care and maintenance of the shunt whether the valve chamber is implanted or external is similar. The first 24 hrs is critical to ensure shunt patency. For the first few hours, the pump chamber should be compressed 25–30 times hourly. Pumping should then follow a routine of 25–30 times at least q3–4hrs. With each compression of the pump chamber, the transfer of 1.5–2.0 ml of fluid will occur
  - adjustments to this pumping schedule will be made based on the patient's clinical picture and chest x-rays. The number of pumps per day prescribed for the individual patient is determined by the physician and is based on an estimate of daily fluid accumulation
    - □ dressing requirements for external pump chambers: currently, manufactured shunts with external pump chambers (Denver Biomedical) provide polyester cuffs ~15 cm from the pump chamber, which are designed to permit tissue ingrowth into the cuff material. Following placement, a dressing may be used for the first few days and then discontinued
- Management of complications
  - shunt occlusion
    - □ place the patient in the supine position
    - □ firmly compress the pump chamber
    - □ if the chamber fails to reexpand after compression, the pleural catheter may be occluded. If the chamber is firm and meets with resistance with compression, there may be an occlusion within the pump chamber or in the peritoneal chamber. Pump chamber occlusion warrants notifying a surgeon immediately
  - infection
    - □ occurs occasionally at the insertion site and systematically
    - □ signs and symptoms include erythema and drainage at the insertion site, fever, and malaise. Management includes obtaining cultures of the site and initiating antibiotic treatment
- Document procedure, findings, and interventions

ISSUES FOR PATIENT TEACHING

- Name of device: pleuroperitoneal shunt
- Manual compression of chamber (pumping) and frequency
- Care of the device to patient and family
- Instruct patient to report fever, redness, swelling, drainage at the insertion site or possible occlusion
- Provide instructions for catheter care when showering and bathing
- Provide patient with names and numbers of physician and nurse
- Routine assessment of compliance with recommendations for care

KEY REFERENCES

Petrou M, Kaplan D: Management of recurrent malignant pleural effusions. Cancer 1995; 75:801–5

Pleural Effusion Shunt. Catalog No. 42-9000. Denver Biomedical. Inc.

Ponn RB, Blancaflor J: Pleuroperitoneal shunting for intractable pleural effusions. Ann Thorac Surg 1991; 51:605–9

Device: Pleural Access Port: Pleurx Pleural Catheter

J. Heidi Downey

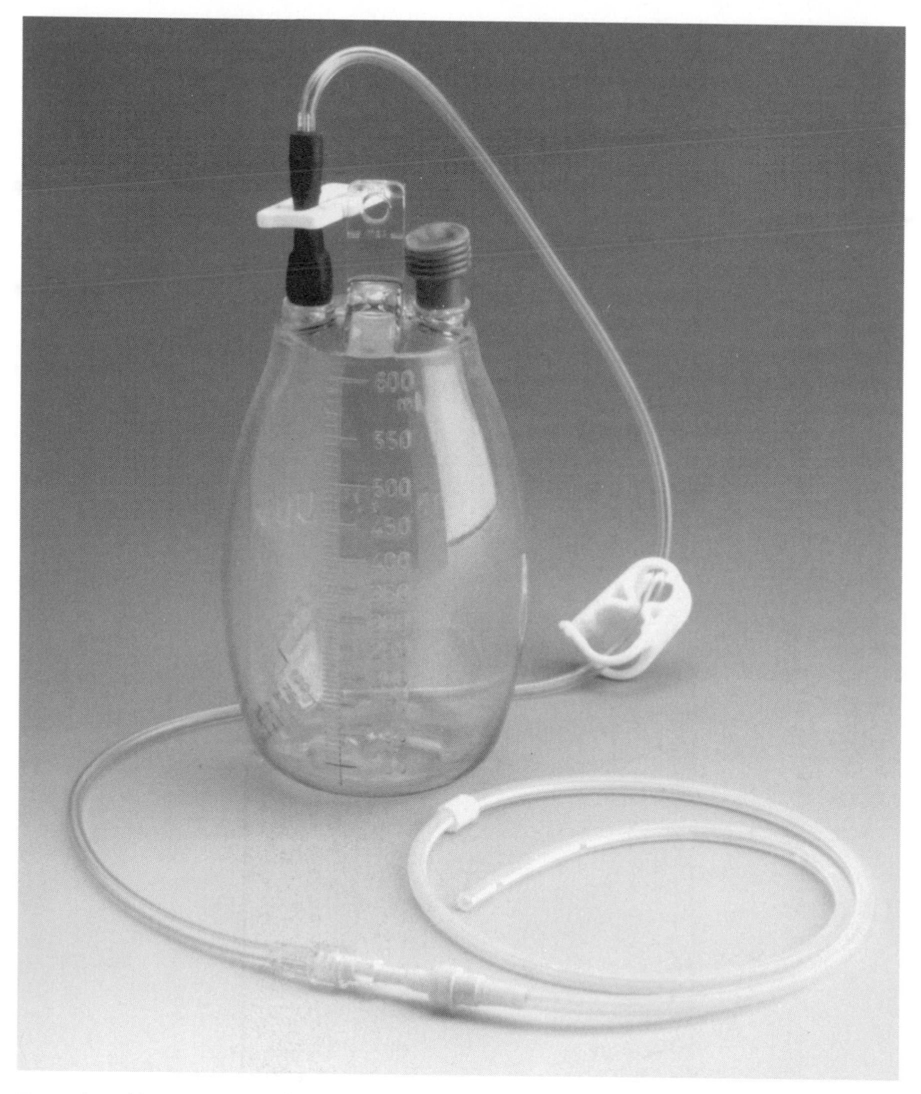

Reproduced by permission of Denver Biomedical Inc.

MANUFACTURER: DENVER BIOMATERIALS, INC.

TYPE: INTRAPLEURAL DEVICE

- Description: fenestrated silicone catheter with a polyester cuff and natural latex rubber safety valve. The cuff, which is ~1 cm from the incision, becomes enmeshed with scar tissue, which secures the catheter in place, reducing the risk of infection. The valve is designed to prevent the passage of air or fluid in either direction unless accessed with the proper drainage line
- Indications for use: this device is indicated for the palliation of dyspnea due to malignant effusion and provides pleurodesis (resolution of the malignant pleural effusion). Contraindicated in patients that exhibit a shift >2 cm in the mediastinum toward the ipsilateral side of the effusion; where the pleural space is multiloculated, and the drainage of a single loculation would not provide relief of dyspnea; when there is coagulopathy; if the pleural space is infected; and when the effusion is known to be chylous
- Advantages: provides relief of dyspnea. Allows for patient to be home for treatment. Placement of device can be performed in an outpatient setting

RISKS/DISADVANTAGES

- There is potential for topical or systemic infection. Care must be taken when inserting needle to avoid puncturing the lung or the liver. Drainage kits are expensive

SURGICAL CONSIDERATIONS

Mohamed Yassine

- Preoperation
  - overall patient fitness must be assessed and the ability to withstand anesthesia or sedation should be considered
  - provide patient with information regarding the procedure, maintenance, and expected outcome
  - involve patient in decision making to facilitate learning process and adaptation to the device
  - discuss insertion site options, so convenience and quality of life is minimally affected
  - alleviate patient's anxiety, increase compliance, and reduce complication by
    - □ use of a demonstration model for reinforcement of catheter teaching
    - □ informing patient of potential postinsertion complications
- Postoperation
  - monitor patient vital signs—up to 8° or until release
  - observe for signs of chest discomfort and pain
  - assess for leakage of fluid and air around the device
  - assess the device for any signs of obstruction
  - evaluate patient for signs of pain while draining fluids; if this happens reduce the rate of fluid removal
  - keep insertion site clean and comply with sterile technique when handling the catheter
  - use and handle the catheter only when needed to minimize potential infection

CLINICAL ASSESSMENT/ INTERVENTIONS/IMPLICATIONS

- Patient assessment
  - examine insertion site for drainage, erythema, or edema
  - inspect lumen for visible or audible air leak, cracks or defects in line
  - monitor temperature
  - assess for pain at insertion site
- Maintenance
  - drainage procedure: drainage of the effusion requires assessment of the volume of pleural fluid and the patient's individual status. In a single drainage, no more than ~1,000 ml should be removed. This drainage can be accomplished with either vacuum bottle or wall suction. Each drainage kit includes the drainage bottle, drainage setup equipment, and step-by-step instructions for draining the Pleurx catheter under sterile technique. Following the completion of the drainage process, the end of the valve should be wiped with a povidone-iodine swab. Do not try to push the swab through the valve because damage to the valve may occur
  - dressing requirements
    - □ dressing change requires sterile technique and should be changed whenever the drainage procedure is performed
    - □ cleanse exit site and surrounding tissue with a povidone-iodine swab stick

beginning at the exit site and with a spiral motion work outwardly
  - □ apply the provided soft foam catheter pad around the catheter on the patient's chest; wind the catheter into loops and cover with gauze pads; secure this dressing to the patient in an occlusive fashion
- Management of complications
  - if the patient experiences pain associated with drainage, use the clamp to slow down the fluid removal rate
  - reexpansion pulmonary edema may occur if *too* much fluid is removed too rapidly. Therefore, it is recommended to limit a single drainage to no more than ~ 1,000 ml
  - infection can occur at the insertion site, in the tubing tunnel, and systemically. Signs and symptoms include erythema and drainage at the insertion site, fever, and malaise. Management includes obtaining cultures of the tubing site and initiating antibiotic treatment
- Catheter removal procedure: removal of catheter may be necessary if after three successive attempts to drain fluid result is < 15 cc of fluid. This may indicate that pleurodesis has been achieved, the catheter is loculated away from the fluid, or the catheter is occluded. Physician should be notified
- Document procedure, findings, and interventions

ISSUES FOR PATIENT TEACHING

- Name of device: Pleurx Pleural Catheter manufactured by Denver Biomedical, Inc.
- Sterile technique for drainage procedure and dressing changes
- Frequency of drainage and the procedure to use in the event that more than one drainage bottle is required
- Instruct patient to report fever, redness, swelling, drainage at the insertion site, a change in the appearance of the fluid, or questions regarding drainage procedure
- Provide instructions regarding the use of self-adhesive dressings when showering and bathing
- Provide patient with names and numbers of physician and nurse
- Routine assessment of compliance with recommendations for care

KEY REFERENCES

Blendowski CB, Haapoja IS: Pleural access port: a creative alternative to repeated thoracentesis. Dev Support Cancer Care 1998; 2:41–4

Pleurx Drainage Kit. Catalog No. 50-7500. Denver Biomedical, Inc.

Putnam JB, Ponn R, et al.: A Phase III trial of treatment for malignant pleural effusions: Pleurx: Pleural Catheter (PC) versus chest tube + doxycycline sclerosis (CT-S). Chest 1997 (suppl); 112:26S

Rodriguez RL, Putnam JB, et al.: Predicting spontaneous pleurodesis in patients with malignant pleural effusion treated with an indwelling catheter. Respir Crit Care Med J 1998; 157:3

Device: SynchroMed Implanted Pump

Hollie Devine

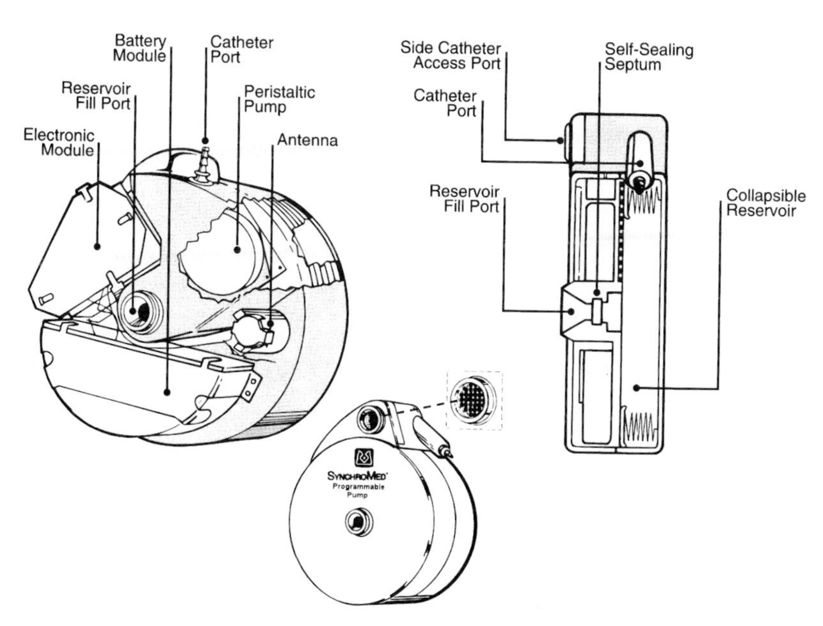

Courtesy of Medtronic Inc., Minneapolis, Minnesota.

MANUFACTURER: MEDTRONIC, INC.

TYPE: SINGLE LUMEN FOR INTRA-ARTERIAL DRUG ADMINISTRATION

■ Description: the only commercially implantable pump that can be programmed from outside the body via telemetry. It is utilized to provide long-term ambulatory therapy and includes various program options including constant flow continuous infusion; complex variable flow infusion; single time-qualified bolus infusion; and repeatable time-delayed bolus infusion. It is implanted SubQ in the subclavian fossa with the catheter tip in the superior vena cava. It may be noninvasively programmed (rate and time adjusted) through the use of an external computer and a handheld electronic wand, which transfers signals from the Medtronic desktop computer to the internal microprocessor. The pump contains either a 10 ml or an 18 ml refillable drug reservoir with a self-sealing fill port, a microprocessor powered by a lithium battery, and a peristaltic-type roller pump. An onboard alarm system is included that alerts one of a low reservoir condition, status of the microprocessor memory, and an end-of-life indicator for the power source. A trained clinician refills the pump by using a needle and syringe to inject the drug through the skin into the drug reservoir

■ Indications for use: can be used in the delivery of treatment for the following diseases: renal carcinoma, metastatic colorectal carcinoma, malignant/nonmalignant pain management, cerebral palsy, brain injury, severe spasticity associated with multiple sclerosis, and chronic muscle stiffness. Other potential uses include chronic pain, Alzheimer's disease, amylotrophic lateral sclerosis, and Huntington's disease

■ Advantages: using the pump achieves a constant drug administration. The drug dose can be precise to meet the needs of the patient by simply adjusting the medication flow rate and time of delivery. Appropriate for long-term use. It is totally implanted under the skin and is therefore unobtrusive. Enhances patient mobility and poses no restrictions on activities such as contact sports or swimming. It requires no self-care. Poses no maintenance cost and potentially decreases occurrence of infection

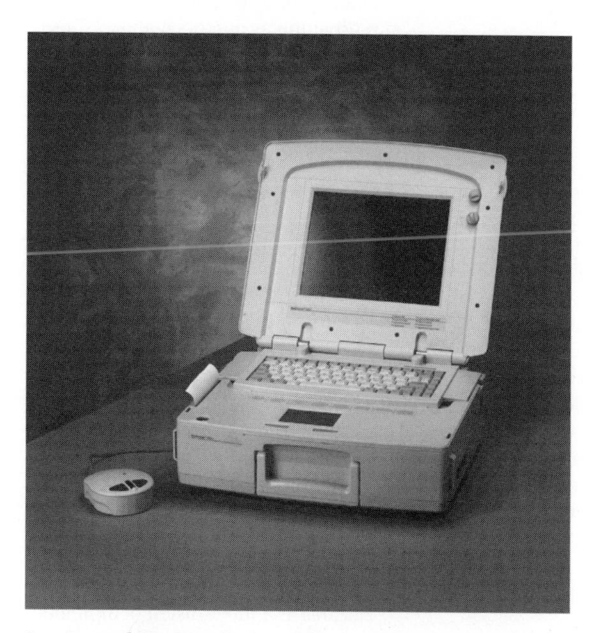

Courtesy of Medtronic, Inc., Minneapolis, Minnesota.

RISKS/DISADVANTAGES

■ Surgery is required for placement and removal. Cost of port insertion/removal, operating room, anesthesia, surgeon, and recovery room increase overall hospital cost. Discomfort may be associated with skin puncture at time of access. May interfere with CT scan, MRI procedures, radiation therapy. Special noncoring needles must be used to access port to prevent damage to the septum. Limited volume for infusions. To replace the battery, the entire pump must be removed surgically

SURGICAL CONSIDERATIONS

Mohamed Yassine

- Preoperation
  - overall patient fitness must be assessed and the ability to withstand anesthesia or sedation should be considered
  - involve the patient in the decision making and provide information regarding the procedure
  - discuss insertion site options, so convenience and quality of life is minimally affected
  - alleviate patient's anxiety, increase compliance, and reduce complications by
    - □ use of a demonstration model for teaching reinforcement
    - □ informing patient of potential postinsertion complications
- Postoperation
  - x-ray or perfusion scan should be done to confirm placement of catheter tip and visualize the area of perfusion

- observe for bleeding or drainage at the operation site
- assess for the development of a hematoma or hygroma
- prevent "flip-flop syndrome" (inability to locate the septum) from occurring by observing for seroma
- apply cold packs or pressure to reduce postoperative discomfort and edema
- the implanted port could be used 24 hrs postinsertion
- strict aseptic technique should be used to access the port
- notify the physician if there is palpable movement of the implanted port
- observe for any signs of resistance or occlusion
- instruct the patient to report signs of swelling, pain, or drainage
- showering is restricted until wound is healed

CLINICAL ASSESSMENT/ INTERVENTIONS/IMPLICATIONS

- ■ Patient assessment: observe for signs/symptoms of infection: erythema, tenderness, induration, or purulence
- ■ Pump assessment
  - excess mobility of implanted pump under the skin
  - development of erosion, seroma, or hygroma around the pump site
  - unusual resistance or occlusions of the catheter when accessing port
  - confirm drug stability for the length of infusion time in pump
  - plan refill schedule, taking into account office hours, patient vacations, and holidays. Pump usually requires refill q2wks
  - overfilling pump reservoir or injecting fluid too rapidly may damage the pump or affect infusion accuracy
  - refill interval calculation
    - □ pump reservoir volume (ml) ÷ pump flow rate (ml/day) = maximum refill interval (days)
- ■ Pump maintenance
  - battery needs to be exchanged q3–4yrs
  - SynchroMed supply kit obtained from the manufacturer includes 20 ml syringe, pressure monitor with stopcock, extension tubing set with clamp (160 mcg volume), 22 gauge noncoring needle, 0.22 micron filter, template (optional), fenestrated drape (optional). Not included in the kit: SynchroMed Programmer (if pump is to be programmed), 4 × 4 gauze pads, site prep materials, syringe containing 10 ml or 18 ml of prescribed drug (depending on the reservoir size), sterile gloves, adhesive bandage
  - accessing SynchroMed pump
    - □ identify pump model and reservoir volume size
    - □ confirm that refill volume of prescribed drug in syringe does not exceed the reservoir size of pump
    - □ prepare the site. Place fenestrated drape over pump site (optional). Assemble noncoring needle, tubing set, and an empty 20 ml syringe
    - □ position template over pump (optional). Locate center of pump
    - □ insert needle through template center hole and into the pump's septum until the needle touches the needle stop
    - □ open tubing clamp. Withdraw the fluid from the reservoir using gentle, negative pressure. Empty the reservoir completely. The amount withdrawn should approximately equal the calculated residual volume
    - □ close the clamp and remove the 20 ml syringe
    - □ attach the filter to the syringe containing the prescribed fluid and attach the pressure monitor to the filter
    - □ turn the pressure monitor to block the monitor tubing and purge all air from the filter/pressure monitor pathway
    - □ attach the syringe/filter/pressure monitor to the extension tubing set
    - □ open the clamp and slowly (1 ml per 3 sec) inject fluid into the reservoir. *Do not force* injection
    - □ maintain pressure on syringe and turn pressure monitor stopcock to *syringe off* position
    - □ release syringe plunger pressure and check position of fluid meniscus in the pressure monitor. Use the top of the fluid level, not the bubble area. The meniscus must not go beyond the marked area of the pressure monitor, filter, and syringe from tubing. Reattach an empty syringe to tubing and empty pump completely
    - □ refill pump as described above. Close tube clamp and carefully remove the needle from the pump septum
    - □ apply pressure to needle site, remove povidone-iodine if present, and apply adhesive bandage
    - □ to maintain pump and port patency, pump is emptied of remaining drug. For the 2 wk rest period, pump may be refilled with 10,000 units of heparinized saline, enough to make a 50 ml solution. For more long-term patency, 50 ml of 50% glycerol may also be used (lasts 5–6 wks)
- ■ Management of complications
  - infection
    - □ if an infection is suspected, do not access port because of the possibility of tracking infection into the bloodstream
    - □ if the port has already been accessed, the needle should be left in place for cultures and the infusion of antibiotics
    - □ if the infection does not resolve, port removal may be indicated
  - occlusion
    - □ to prevent occlusion, consider prophylactic use of daily low-dose warfarin
    - □ confirm that the needle has fully penetrated the septum and is not occluded by the silicone
    - □ reaccess port to ensure correct placement of the needle
    - □ attempt clearing the port with a 10 ml syringe and normal saline, using an "aspiration-flush" technique to loosen and aspirate the source of the block
    - □ agents such as hydrochloric acid may be utilized to restore patency
    - □ two noncoring needle/syringe method
      - ▽ 2 noncoring needles are used to access the port with syringes attached
      - ▽ one syringe should be empty with the plunger down to act as a vent
      - ▽ the second syringe should be filled with saline or thrombolytic agent
      - ▽ while pushing down on the fluid-filled syringe, the plunger of the other syringe will be forced back rinsing the reservoir
    - □ radionuclear scan to evaluate occlusion
  - extravasation
    - □ refer to manufacturer's guidelines and institutional policies and procedures
    - □ if an extravasation is suspected, stop the infusion and remove the IV tubing from the needle extension
    - □ connect a syringe to the needle extension and aspirate any trace of the drug left in the port reservoir
    - □ if applicable, inject the appropriate antidote through the needle extension tubing and around the needle injection site
    - □ remove the needle; apply a sterile dressing and cold/hot compresses
    - □ notify physician and document extravasation, describing site; obtain baseline measurements
  - malfunction: if fluid is not obtained after accessing the port
    - □ verify that the needle is through the septum
    - □ disconnect the syringe from the needle/extension set and attach a 10 ml saline syringe; inject 5 ml of saline, and allow solution to return or withdraw solution. If 5 ml returns, pump is empty. If there is no fluid return, verify the needle position
    - □ if the septum cannot be located, notify physician. Inserting needle under fluoroscopy is suggested
    - □ equipment problems: confer with the company technical support staff at 7000 Central Avenue NE, Minneapolis, MN 55432. Telephone: 763-514-4000. Fax: 763-514-4879. Toll free: 1-800-328-2518

- Special considerations
  - not recommended for obtaining laboratory data or withdrawing of blood samples because of high-pressure system within the artery and an increased rate of clot formation
- Document procedure, findings, and interventions

ISSUES FOR PATIENT TEACHING

- Name of device: SynchroMed implanted pump
- Provide patient and local physician with video, literature, and hands-on demonstration with the SynchroMed implanted infusion pump
- Implanted pump is a mode of delivering therapy, not a treatment itself
- Encourage patient to obtain medic alert emblem and pump identification card; device triggers metal detectors
- Instruct patient to report
  - prolonged fevers
  - redness, swelling, drainage at insertion of implanted infusion pump
  - excess mobility of implanted pump underneath the skin
  - development of erosion, seroma, or hygroma around the implanted pump site
- Provide patient with names and numbers of physician and nurse
- Routine assessment of compliance with recommendations for care

KEY REFERENCES

Access Device Guidelines: Recommendations for Nursing Practice and Education, D Camp-Sorrell (ed). Pittsburgh: Oncology Nursing Society, n.d.

Berg D: Drug delivery system. In *Cancer Chemotherapy: A Nursing Process Approach* (2nd ed., pp. 561–95), M Burke, G Wilkes, K Ingwersen (eds). London: Jones and Bartlett, 1996

Camp-Sorrell D: Implantable ports: Everything you always wanted to know. J Intraven Nurs 1992; 15(5):262–73

Gullo SM: Implanted ports. Technologic advances and nursing care issues. Cleveland Clinic Foundation, Ohio. Nurs Clin North Am 1993; 28(4):859–71

Johnson GB: Nursing care of patients with implanted pumps. Patient Services, Bethesda Hospitals, Inc., Ohio. Nurs Clin North Am 1993; 28(4):873–83

Lanning RM, von Roemeling R, Hrushesky W: Circadian-based infusional FUDR therapy. Oncol Nurs Forum 1990; 17(1):49–56

Martin V: Delivery of cancer chemotherapy. In *Cancer Nursing: A Comprehensive Textbook* (2nd ed., pp. 395–433), R McCorkle, M Grant, M Frank-Stromborg, et al. (eds). Philadelphia: WB Saunders, 1996

Medtronic, Inc. http://www.medtronic.com

Reyman P: Chemotherapy: practice and principles. In *Cancer Nursing Principles and Practice* (3rd ed., pp. 293–330), S Groenwald, M Frogge, M Goodman, et al. (eds). London: Jones and Bartlett, 1993

Device: Implantable Infusion Pumps

Hollie Devine

MANUFACTURER

- Infusaid Pump (formerly Strato/Infusaid, Inc) (No longer manufactured. Refill kits available by Arrow International, Inc)
- Model 3000 Series Constant Flow Implantable Pumps (Arrow International, Inc.)

TYPES: INFUSAID 400 PUMP: MODEL 3000 SERIES CONSTANT FLOW IMPLANTABLE PUMPS

- Description: Disc-shaped pump divided into two chambers by a bellow. Main (inner) chamber of the pump has a needle-access port and contains a drug chamber where the fluid is to be infused. Second (outer) chamber has an internal non-replaceable power source chamber that contains a propellant. The temperature of the body warms the propellant, which expands and exerts pressure on the bellow. This, in turn, forces the medication through a filter into an outlet catheter, which is positioned into the appropriate artery, vein, or anatomic space. The refilling action of the main (inner) chamber is the "power source." These pumps are utilized for continuous or bolus means to increase the concentration of the drug to known areas of tumor and decrease the systemic drug concentration and thus the side effects. The Infusaid pump holds up to 50 ml of fluid and contains a second port of entry. This side port bypasses the chamber pumping mechanism, allowing for bolus injections of medications, as well as for perfusion studies and catheter flushing. The Model 3000 Series pumps are available in three different reservoir sizes (16 ml, 30 ml, and 50 ml) and in three flow ranges (low, medium, and high) depending on the pump indication and the time interval for pump refills. These pumps can also be utilized for percutaneous bolus injections and contain a safety valve in-line with the bolus pathway to ensure that a bolus procedure can be performed only when using the appropriate needle. These infusion pumps are implanted into a surgically constructed subcutaneous pocket in the abdominal wall. For analgesic indications, a catheter may be placed in a lateral ventricle for access to cerebrospinal fluid or the epidural space at the appropriate vertebral levels and then connected to the pumping device, which is usually implanted in the chest cavity
- Indications for use: Metastatic colorectal cancer, liver metastases or primary liver disease, malignant and chronic pain management, severe spasticity secondary to multiple sclerosis or spinal cord injuries, and thromboembolic disease
- Advantages: Using the pump achieves a constant drug administration. Appropriate for long-term use. It is totally implanted under the skin and therefore unobtrusive. Enhances patient mobility; poses no restrictions on activities such as contact sports or swimming. It requires no self-care. Poses no maintenance cost and potentially decreases occurrence of infection

RISKS/DISADVANTAGES

- Requires surgical procedure for placement and removal. Cost of port insertion/removal, operating room, anesthesia, surgeon, and recovery room increases overall cost. Discomfort may be associated with skin puncture for access. May interfere with CT scan, MRI procedures, and radiation therapy. Limited volume for infusions

SURGICAL CONSIDERATIONS

MOHAMED YASSINE

- Preoperation
  - overall patient fitness must be assessed and the ability to withstand anesthesia or sedation should be considered
  - involve patient in decision making and provide information regarding the procedure
  - discuss insertion site options, so convenience and quality of life is minimally affected
  - alleviate patient's anxiety, increase compliance, and reduce complication by
    - use of a demonstration model for reinforcement of catheter teaching
    - informing patient of potential postinsertion complications
- Postoperation
  - x-ray or perfusion study should be done to confirm placement of catheter tip and visualize the area of perfusion
  - observe for bleeding or drainage at the operation site
  - assess for the development of a hematoma or hygroma
  - prevent "flip-flop syndrome" (inability to locate the septum) from occurring by observing for seroma
  - apply cold packs or pressure to reduce postoperative discomfort and edema
  - the implanted port can be used 24 hrs postinsertion
  - use strict aseptic technique when accessing the port
  - notify the physician if there is palpable movement of the implanted port
  - observe for any signs of resistance or occlusion
  - instruct the patient to monitor for any signs of swelling, pain, or drainage
  - showering is restricted until wound is healed

CLINICAL ASSESSMENT/ INTERVENTIONS/IMPLICATIONS

- Patient assessment
  - observe for signs/symptoms of infection: erythema, tenderness, induration, or purulence
  - assess patient for side effects related to drug administered
- Pump assessment
  - excess mobility of implanted pump under the skin
  - development of erosion, seroma, or hygroma around implanted pump site
  - unusual resistance or occlusions of catheter when accessing port
  - drug must be stable for length of infusion time in pump
  - plan refill schedule, taking into account office hours, patient vacations, and holidays. Pump refill depends on reservoir volume and flow range (varies from 10 days to 3 months)
  - overfilling pump reservoir or injecting fluid too rapidly may damage pump or affect infusion accuracy
- Pump maintenance: Infusaid and Model 3000 Series refill supply kits may be obtained from Arrow International, Inc. Kits include syringe, tubing set with stopcock, 22 gauge needles (different access needles for Model 3000 Series and Infusaid pump), alcohol, iodine, gauze, pump templates, fenestrated drape, data sticker, adhesive bandages, refill worksheet, instructions for use, and instruction posters. Not included are sterile gloves and infusate
- Access pump, utilizing sterile technique
  - locate port. Cleanse skin. Attach empty syringe barrel to stopcock, which attaches to tubing and then to needle. Close stopcock
  - stabilize port. Access with a 22 gauge needle provided in kit for reservoir refill firmly through center septum of pump until needle stop is felt. If needle is not properly positioned, drug extravasation may occur. Open stopcock and allow pump to empty. Close stopcock. Remove syringe barrel and stopcock from tubing. Note the returned volume (ml) and record on the data sticker provided
  - refill calculation for Infusaid:
    - pump reservoir volume (ml) ÷ pump flow rate (ml/day) = maximum refill interval (days)
    - Infusaid pump reservoir volume used should be 4 ml less than reservoir capacity to ensure pump does not empty completely
  - refill calculation for Model 3000 Series pumps
    - *note:* after emptying pump, approximately 1.5 ml of fluid from previous refill will remain in pump
    - subtract volume at last refill (depending on reservoir volume) from volume returned when emptying pump. Then divide volume infused by number of days from last refill to determine the flow rate in ml/day
  - attach syringe of infusate to tubing. Using both hands, inject 5 ml of infusate into pump. Release pressure on plunger

and allow small amount of fluid to return to syringe. This reconfirms correct positioning of the needle. Continue to inject and check needle placement at 5 ml increments until syringe is empty
- in Model 3000 Series, when the system is flushed with saline between therapies, patient will receive a bolus of drug equal to the volume of drug contained in the internal bolus pathway of the pump, plus the volume of drug in the catheter. Refer to the manufacturer's guidelines to calculate volume in the bolus pathway and catheter because it varies according to pump size utilized
- after injecting appropriate infusate, close the clamp on the tubing set and pull needle out of the septum. Apply adhesive bandage to site

■ When patient is between therapies, to maintain pump and port patency, empty pump of remaining drug. For Infusaid pump, 10,000 units of heparinized saline, enough to make a 50 ml solution, is recommended for short-term patency. For long-term patency, 50 ml of 50% glycerol may also be used (lasts 5–6 weeks). For Model 3000 Series, a heparinized saline should be utilized. Heparin strength and saline mixing recommendations should be followed according to manufacturer's guidelines. *Note:* Volume of heparin and saline will vary depending on reservoir volume of pump

■ Bolus access and pump refills: bolus procedures are performed percutaneously through the septum of the Model 3000 Series utilizing the Arrow Special Bolus Needle or the side port of the Infusaid pump. Never attempt to refill the Model 3000 Series using a Special Bolus Needle. This will result in giving the patient a bolus injection and may cause a fatal overdose

■ Management of complications
- infection
  - □ if an infection is suspected, do not access port because of the possibility of tracking infection into bloodstream
  - □ if port is already accessed, needle should be left in place for cultures and infusion of antibiotics
  - □ if infection does not resolve, port removal may be indicated
- occlusion
  - □ to prevent occlusion, consider prophylactic use of daily low-dose warfarin
  - □ evaluate if needle has fully penetrated septum and is not occluded by the silicone
  - □ reaccess port to ensure correct placement of needle
  - □ attempt clearing the port with a 10 ml syringe and normal saline, using an aspiration-flush technique to loosen and aspirate the source of the block
  - □ two needle method:
    - ▽ two 22 gauge needles are used to access the port with syringes attached
    - ▽ one syringe should be empty, with the plunger down to act as a vent
    - ▽ other syringe is filled with saline or thrombolytic agent
    - ▽ while pushing down on the fluid-filled syringe, the plunger of the other syringe will be forced back, rinsing the reservoir
  - □ radionuclear scan to evaluate occlusion
- extravasation
  - □ refer to manufacturer's guidelines and institutional policies and procedures
  - □ stop infusion and remove the IV tubing from needle extension
  - □ connect a syringe to the 22 gauge needle extension and aspirate any trace of the drug left in port reservoir
  - □ if applicable, inject appropriate antidote through needle extension tubing and around needle injection site
  - □ remove needle; apply sterile dressing and cold/hot compresses
  - □ notify physician and document extravasation, describing site; obtain measurements for baseline monitoring
- malfunction
  - □ if fluid is not obtained after accessing the port:
    - ▽ verify that needle is through the septum
    - ▽ disconnect syringe from needle/extension set and attach a 10 ml saline syringe; inject 5 ml of saline and allow solution to return, or withdraw solution. If 5 ml returns, pump is empty. If no fluid returns, verify needle position
    - ▽ if septum cannot be located, notify physician; inserting needle under fluoroscopy may be warranted
  - □ equipment problems/technical support staff/ordering supplies: 2400 Bernville Rd., Reading, PA 19605. Telephone: 610-378-0131; toll free: 800-523-8446; web site: www.arrowintl.com; fax: 610-478-3199. Orders only toll free fax: 800-343-2935

■ Special considerations
- not recommended for obtaining laboratory data or withdrawing blood samples because of high-pressure system within the artery and an increased rate of clot formation
- only 22 gauge Arrow Huber Point (noncoring) needles can be used with Model 3000 Series implantable pumps. Arrow International, Inc. also supplies Infusaid pump refill kits, which contain 22 gauge Infusaid needles. Pump-specific needles are utilized to access the pump to prevent damage to septum

■ Document procedure, findings, and interventions

ISSUES FOR PATIENT AND FAMILY TEACHING

■ Name of implantable infusion pump

■ Implanted pump is a mode of delivering therapy, not a treatment itself

■ Inform patient of date, time, and place of next pump refill

■ Encourage patient to obtain medic alert emblem and pump identification card; device may trigger metal detectors

■ Avoid sports or activities that may cause injury or dislodgement of pump

■ Premature emptying can result in pump occlusion; therefore, instruct patient that changes in altitude (deep sea and scuba diving, diving) or body temperature can alter flow rate

■ Avoid activities that increase body temperature such as hot baths and placing heating pads, blankets, and heat-producing ointments directly over pump site

■ Notify physician or nurse of:
- prolonged fevers
- flying, traveling to different altitudes, scuba diving, and mountain climbing. Medication may need to be adjusted

■ Provide patient with names and numbers of physician and nurse

■ Routine assessment of compliance with recommendations for care

KEY REFERENCES

Access Device Guidelines: Recommendations for Nursing Practice and Education, D Camp-Sorrell (ed). Pittsburgh: Oncology Nursing Society, 1996

Buchwald H, Rohde TD: Implantable pumps: Recent progress and anticipated future advances. ASAIO 1992; 38:772–78

Cozzi E, Hagle M, McGregor ML, Woodhouse D: Nursing management of patients receiving hepatic arterial chemotherapy through an implanted infusion pump. Cancer Nurs 1984; 7(3):229–34

Johnson GB: Nursing care of patients with implanted pumps. Nurs Clin North Am 1993; 28(4):873–83

Reyman P: Chemotherapy: Practice and principles. In *Cancer Nursing Principles and Practice* (3rd ed., pp. 293–330), S Groenwald, M Frogge, M Goodman, et al. (eds). London: Jones & Bartlett, 1993

Sheldon P, Bender M: High-technology in home care: An overview of intravenous therapy. Nurs Clin North Am 1994; 29(3): 507–19

Device: Urinary Catheter

Sheila M. O'Brien

MULTIPLE MANUFACTURERS FOR ADMINISTRATION OF INTRAVESICAL CHEMOTHERAPY

TYPE: A CATHETER (TYPICALLY A SINGLE-USE OR AN INDWELLING CATHETER WITH BALLOON)

■ Description: the catheter is inserted temporarily into the urinary bladder. This technique allows a high concentration of the antineoplastic agent to come into contact with the urothelium over a relatively long period of time

■ Indication for use: this catheter is used to instill intravesical chemotherapy for superficial bladder carcinoma in order to prevent or delay tumor recurrence or progression after a transurethral resection of the bladder (TURB). This technique is thought to have the ability to irradicate residual disease not removed or removable via TURB. Intravesicular chemotherapy became popular in the early 1960s, when investigators demonstrated that instillation of thiotepa could reduce tumor recurrence and eradicate about one-third of papillary tumors. Unfortunately, evidence suggests that neither long-term recurrence nor progression is reduced with current intravesical chemotherapy protocols. Response to intravesicular chemotherapy is proportional to the concentration rather than the dose of the drug and is also related to duration of exposure. The chemotherapy is usually retained in the bladder for 1–3 hrs after instillation with the patient repositioned at 15 min intervals to ensure bladder exposure. A course of therapy usually consists of a number of weekly (6–10) instillations. Chemotherapeutic agents commonly used for intravesical therapy include thiotepa, doxorubicin, mitomycin-C, ethoglucid, cisplatin, epirubicin, mitoxantrone, and BCG

■ Advantages: safe and simple method that allows direct contact of bladder urothelium and/or tumor with the chemotherapeutic agent with minimal to no systemic uptake of the drug. As a result, the toxic effects seen with this therapy are minimal, and urinary and sexual functions are preserved

RISKS/DISADVANTAGES

■ Local complications of catheterization include
- trauma to urethra or bladder
- systemic complications: urinary tract infection
- complications due to installation of chemotherapy: chemical cystitis, bladder spasms, dysuria, hematuria, and polyuria
- agents being instilled may cause other side effects: myelosuppression (thiotepa); contact dermatitis (mitomycin-C)
- uncommon complications include allergic reactions, bladder wall calcifications, and reduced bladder capacity

SURGICAL CONSIDERATIONS

Mohamed Yassine

■ Preoperation
- provide patient with information on the procedure, maintenance care, and expected outcome
- involve patient in decision making to facilitate the learning process and adaptation to the device
- assess for the presence of urinary abnormalities (e.g., strictures, benign prostatic hyperplasia [BPH]), which could make catheterization more difficult
- use a small-caliber catheter in patients with strictures
- use a large-caliber catheter in patients with BPH
- use a coudé catheter for a difficult catheterization in males
- lubricate the urethra, not just the catheter

■ Postoperation
- confirm catheter location by observing for urine flow
- irrigate with 30–60 ml of sterile water or saline and observe if flow is absent
- avoid inflammation of the prostatic fossa by inserting the catheter far enough that the balloon can set at the bladder neck
- use sterile water, not normal saline, to inflate the balloon of an indwelling catheter. This prevents the risk of crystallization over long periods of use and allows for subsequent balloon deflation
- tape the catheter in men to the anterior abdominal wall and in women to the thigh to prevent dislodgment or urethral pressure necrosis
- minimize the dilution of the chemotherapy by instructing the patient to limit or stop water intake for a few hours before administering the desired treatment

CLINICAL ASSESSMENT/ INTERVENTIONS/IMPLICATIONS

■ Patient assessment
- assess patient for symptoms of infection: fever, hematuria, dysuria, urinary frequency or urgency
- obtain urine specimen for urinalysis/culture per institutional policy/procedure

■ Method
- the patient should urinate immediately prior to the catheter insertion
- use aseptic technique
- insert urinary catheter per institutional policies. A catheter is never forced; it is maneuvered during insertion as patient coughs or bears down
- check for proper catheter placement and urine outflow; if evidence of traumatic catheterization (e.g., hematuria) withhold chemotherapy
- instill 5–10 cc of sterile water to test patency of catheter prior to instilling chemotherapy
- instill chemotherapy per institutional policy/procedure, either by slow push or by drip
- patient should retain chemotherapy for 1–3 hrs; refer to institutional policies and procedures
- patients should change positions (e.g., prone, supine, lying on left and right sides, and sitting upright) q15min while the chemotherapy is in the bladder to ensure maximum contact of the drug with the urothelium
- the drug should be kept in bladder *only* for the prescribed time; increased exposure can result in cystitis and excessive exfoliation of the bladder epithelium

■ Maintenance
- catheter care
  - □ as the catheter is usually removed immediately after chemotherapy is instilled, there is no catheter care
  - □ if the catheter must remain in place for several hours, it should be secured with tape laterally to the thigh to avoid trauma or tension of the balloon and compression at the penoscrotal angle in males

■ Management of complications
- infection/cystitis
  - □ assess patient for signs and symptoms of infection or cystitis: fever, chills, myalgias, dysuria, hematuria, increased frequency/urgency. If present, withhold chemotherapy for 1 wk
- traumatic catheterization
  - □ avoid traumatic catheterization because the chemotherapeutic agent could be systemically absorbed if the urothelium is damaged; if present, withhold chemotherapy

■ Document procedure, findings, and interventions

ISSUES FOR PATIENT AND FAMILY TEACHING

■ Name of the device: urinary catheter commonly referred as a Foley catheter

■ Instruct patient on the name and potential side effects of each chemotherapy drug received, the schedule of administration, and length of treatment plan

■ Instruct patient to limit or stop taking fluids for several hours prior to the instillation of chemotherapy (to minimize dilution of the drug in the bladder)

- Some institutions instruct patients to do the following for 6 hrs after the first postchemotherapy void: after urinating, pour 2 cups of household bleach into toilet and let stand for 15 min before flushing. Wash hands and genitals thoroughly after each urination to minimize/prevent contact dermatitis. Refer to institutional policies and procedures
- Men should sit when urinating to avoid splashing of urine
- Provide written instructions in addition to verbal instructions
- Instruct patient to report fevers, chills, myalgias, dysuria, hematuria, increased frequency/urgency of urination, or difficulty in voiding
- Provide telephone numbers of office, physician, and nurse
- Routine assessment of compliance with recommendations for care

KEY REFERENCES

Access Device Guidelines: Recommendations for Nursing Practice and Education, D Camp-Sorrell (ed). Pittsburgh: Oncology Nursing Society, n.d.

Berg D: Drug delivery system. In *Cancer Chemotherapy: A Nursing Process Approach* (2nd ed., pp. 561–95), M Burke, G Wilkes, K Ingwersen (eds). London: Jones and Bartlett, 1996

Cancio LC, Sabanegh ES Jr, Thompson IM: Managing the Foley catheter. Brooke Army Medical Center, Fort Sam Houston, Texas. Am Fam Physician 1993; 48(50):829–36

Goodman M: Delivery of cancer chemotherapy. In *Cancer Nursing* (p. 17), R McCorkle, M Grand (eds). Philadelphia: WB Saunders, 1994

Holmes BC: Administration of cancer chemotherapy agents. *Cancer Chemotherapy Handbook* (2nd ed., p. 73), R Dorr, D Von Hoff (eds). East Norwalk, CT: Appleton and Lange, 1994

Lamm D, Riggs D, Traynelis C, et al.: Apparent failure of current intravesicle chemotherapy prophylaxis to influence the long term course of superficial transitional cell carcinoma of the bladder. J Urol 1995; 153: 1444–50

Martin V: Delivery of cancer chemotherapy. In *Cancer Nursing: A Comprehensive Textbook* (2nd ed., pp. 395–433), R McCorkle, M Grant, M Frank-Stromborg, et al. (eds). Philadelphia: WB Saunders, 1996

Soloway M: Introduction and overview of intravesical therapy for superficial bladder cancer. Urology (suppl) 1988; 31(3):5–16

Thrasher J, Crawford E: Complications of intravesical chemotherapy. Urol Clin North Am 1992; 19(3):529–39

Witjies J, Oosterhof G, Debruyne F: Management of superficial bladder cancer Ta/T1/TIS: intravesical chemotherapy. In *Comprehensive Textbook of Genitourinary Oncology* (pp. 416–27), N Vogelzang et al. (eds). Baltimore: Williams and Wilkins, 1996

Ambulatory Pumps: Introduction

Sandra Purl, Susan C. Budds, and Paula O. Goldfarb

- Pump technology is expanding rapidly. With the economic shift of health care delivery to the outpatient and home care settings, ambulatory infusion pumps have become an important and increasingly more common means of drug delivery in cancer therapy. By facilitating delivery of therapy out of the hospital setting, ambulatory infusion pumps have decreased costs and have offered patients more control and flexibility of their lifestyles while on treatment
- In general, ambulatory infusion pumps can be classified into patient-worn (external) devices and totally implantable devices. Health care members are challenged to remain current with the diversity and the advances made with these pumps. Familiarity will help make the selection of the most appropriate pump to meet patient needs and desired therapy. Some considerations for selection include the following
  - therapy to be administered: considerations should include drug dose, stability, frequency, accuracy, and drug compatibility with pump reservoir
  - type/location of infusion site access
  - available support systems (i.e., family, health care member, pump manufacturer)
  - patient safety and protection features
  - cost and reimbursement issues

EXTERNAL AMBULATORY PUMPS

- External ambulatory infusion pumps can be classified into 3 groups based on mechanism of operation: syringe driven, peristaltic, and elastomeric balloon. All devices can be used for all types of infusional therapy ranging over a period of several minutes to multiple days. In oncology, external ambulatory pumps allow the feasibility of therapies such as prolonged chemotherapy, hydration, total parenteral nutrition (TPN), narcotic administration, anticoagulation, and antibiotics to be delivered via the IV, intra-arterial, SubQ, and epidural routes
- The electronic infusion pumps can be programmed to deliver several types of clinical applications including cyclical flow, circadian flow, and patient-controlled analgesia (PCA)
  - *cyclical flow:* delivery of drug at a controlled rate. The two modes of delivery are continuous flat rate and intermittent (which allows drug delivery at regular preset intervals). Continuous flat rate delivery reduces the peak and valley effects of bolus injections and helps maintain therapeutic drug levels in the bloodstream; its use can reduce drug toxicities thereby lowering the incidence of side effects. The intermittent mode is useful for delivery of drugs that require infusion at preset intervals such as antibiotic therapy. Additional features can include a taper program for infusion as used with TPN or a delayed start/auto program used when hookup of the pump occurs before the infusion start time
  - *circadian flow:* delivery of medication according to the body's natural metabolic clock (sleep-wake cycle). Circadian flow is indicated for treatment regimens employing single or multiple drugs to be delivered over variable time phases according to circadian scheduling. These pumps have the ability to deliver a drug(s) over 12 variable time phases in a 24 hr period. Time phases can be programmed by percentages, rates, or doses. With some neoplastic agents, circadian programming delivers more dose-intensive treatment with increased tumor cell kill and decreased toxicity
  - *patient-controlled analgesia (PCA):* delivery of a bolus dose of medication (i.e., analgesia) intended to be used by patients for relief of symptoms (i.e., pain) as needed. The prescriber sets the bolus dose. Additional features may include a basal dose rate and a lockout period between doses to prevent overdosing of medication
- Ambulatory infusion pumps are supplied with carrying cases or halters that fit onto a belt or are worn in a pouch on a shoulder

Device: Syringe-driven Ambulatory Pump

Sandra Purl and Susan Budds

MULTIPLE MANUFACTURERS; MOST COMMON: AUTO SYRINGE, BAXTER HEALTHCARE CORPORATION; GRASEBY, GRASEBY MEDICAL INC.

- Description
  - programmable infusion pump that utilizes a disposable syringe to deliver a controlled rate of infusion. The plunger of the syringe is progressively driven forward by means of a motor-driven screw
  - the delivery rate is directly related to the diameter of the syringe barrel and drive speed of the plunger
- Reservoir/accessories/maintenance
  - disposable syringes (most brands) 1–60 ml
  - customized tubing attaches syringe to patient infusion site access
  - syringes are changed daily to weekly depending on the length of treatment
- Power source
  - battery: 9 volt
  - rechargeable batteries or AC power adapter available on some pump models
  - battery life varies with the rate of infusion
- Rates/range of infusion
  - pump is intended for low-volume infusions (up to 100 ml) to be delivered at low flow rates (0.1–99 ml/hr) with high accuracy
  - minimum/maximum dose and delivery depends on syringe size and pump setting selected

CLINICAL ASSESSMENT/ INTERVENTIONS/IMPLICATIONS

- Alarms/safety mechanisms
  - alarms vary with the model of pump—common alarms available include low battery, low reservoir, high-pressure occlusion, near-end alert
  - alarms are both audible (beeping or whistling sounds) and visual (flashing light)
- Program modes
  - continuous or timed infusion modes (i.e., single dose, manual, or auto schedule)
  - accuracy varies with each pump, and manufacturers provide an acceptable margin of error
- Management of complications
  - pump malfunctions: check with pump manufacturer or rental company technical support staff; many have available 24 hr assistance
  - troubleshooting guidelines are provided in the manufacturer's operation manual
  - always check catheter function as well as pump function. Pumps may continue to operate despite catheter malfunction or dislodgement resulting in extravasation or infiltration of drug
- Advantages
  - reliable and affordable
  - cost effective—utilizes low-cost generic syringes and tubing
  - easy to visualize actual drug delivery
  - accurate volume infusion; greater accuracy at low flow rates over short intervals of time than other pumps
  - ideal for antibiotics and pain management
- Disadvantages
  - infusion volume limited due to size of syringe
  - not recommended for large-volume infusions (i.e., TPN)
  - plastic tip of syringe breakable
  - requires good vision and manual dexterity to program (small numbers and dials)
  - some devices can be bulky
- Special considerations
  - insurance precertification is necessary to ensure optimal reimbursement for the medication and infusion pump
  - current Medicare guidelines will not reimburse for certain IV medications given on a continuous infusion outpatient basis
  - pumps may be purchased or rented. Rental agreements vary from daily to monthly and may include cost of supplies
  - need for appropriate infusion site access device for type of therapy to be delivered
  - drug stability varies. Be sure to check drug stability to determine frequency of syringe changes

ISSUES FOR PATIENT AND FAMILY TEACHING

- Name of the pump
- Hands-on training regarding pump operation is required of the patient or caregiver
- Availability of written and/or audiovisual patient education materials
- Specific instructions for safe handling of pump in the home
- Ability of patient/caregiver to assess side effects and complications of therapy
- Discussion of lifestyle adjustments during infusional therapy including wearing of loose-fitting clothing to conceal pump, avoidance of strenuous activity while wearing pump, protection of pump during showering, bathing, and sleeping
- Provision of telephone numbers for troubleshooting: physician, nurse, 24 hr assistance
- Routine assessment of compliance with recommendations for care

KEY REFERENCES

Access Device Guidelines: Recommendations for Nursing Practice and Education, D Camp-Sorrell (ed). Pittsburgh: Oncology Nursing Society, n.d.

Lefever J: Infusion pumps. Professional Nurse 1998; 13(9):621–8

Rapsilber L, Camp-Sorrell D: Ambulatory infusion pumps: application to oncology. Sem Oncol Nurs 1995; 11(3):213–20

Schleis T, Tice A: Selecting infusion devices for use in ambulatory care. Am J Health-Syst Pharm 1996; 53:868–77

Device: Peristaltic Ambulatory Pump

Sandra Purl and Susan C. Budds

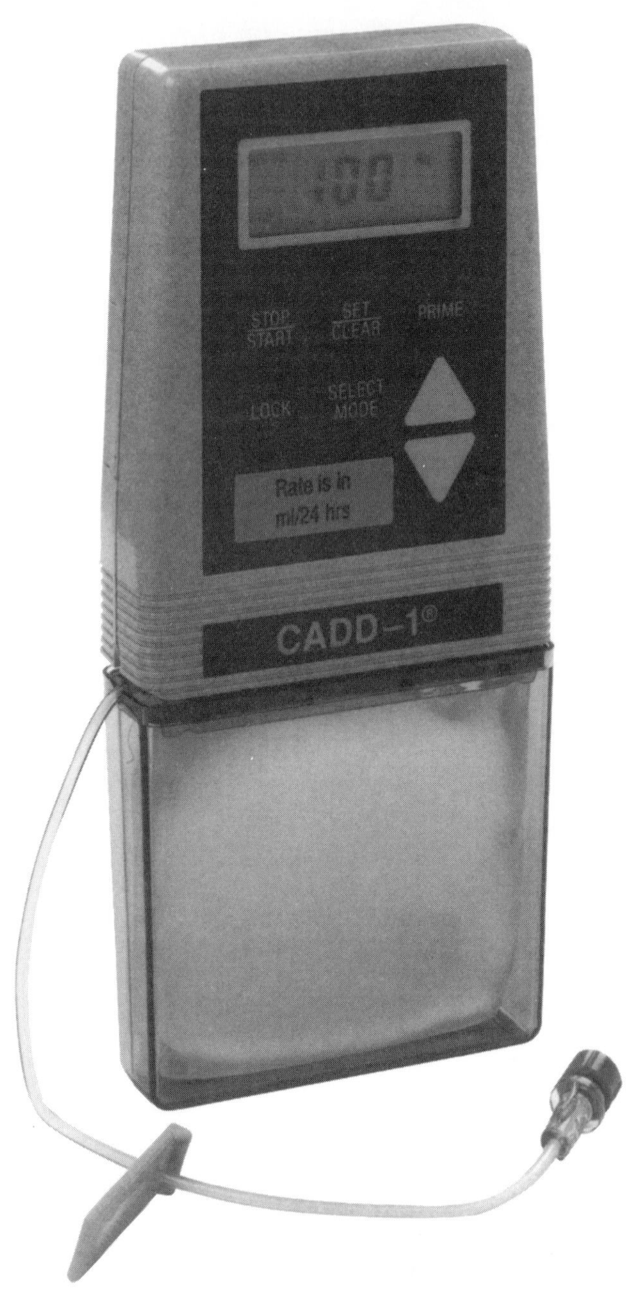

Reproduced courtesy of SIMS Deltec, Inc., St. Paul, Minnesota

MULTIPLE MANUFACTURERS; MOST COMMON: ABBOTT LABORATORIES; PHARMACIA DELTEC; MCKINLEY, INC.

- Description: peristaltic pumps work electronically utilizing varied pumping mechanisms. The three basic pump mechanisms are
  - rotating peristaltic: AimPlus
  - linear peristaltic: Walkmed
  - alternating pressure: CADD
- Reservoir/accessories/maintenance: most require custom tubing that includes a section which fits into the pumping mechanism
  - reservoir bags may be custom fitted (i.e., cassette with the CADD pump) or standard IV bags that are disposable
  - bags and tubing are changed daily to weekly depending on the type of treatment. For example, TPN requires daily bag and tubing changes
  - flushing requirements vary with the type of line and the rate of the infusion. Most intermittent programs have a KVO (keep vein open) rate. Continuous infusions require no flushing
- Power source
  - battery—varying in type from 9 volt to AA to AAA
  - rechargeable batteries or AC power adapter available on some pump models
  - battery life varies with the rate of infusion. Larger volumes with short infusion rates result in a shorter battery life. Battery backups are usually available
- Rates/range of infusions
  - pump models vary from .02–400 ml/hr

CLINICAL ASSESSMENT/ INTERVENTIONS/IMPLICATIONS

- Alarms/safety mechanisms
  - audible alarms such as beeping or whistling sounds are common
  - visual alarms include flashing lights or a digital readout
  - alarms vary with the model; most have both audible and visual alarms
  - most common alarms include volume infused, error in loading mechanism, infusion complete, check line, check system, occlusion, air in line, low battery, low reservoir, and malfunction
- Program modes
  - include continuous, taper, circadian, intermittent, delayed start/auto, and PCA
  - most pumps have one to several program modes; some manufacturers utilize a specific pump model for each type of program
  - some pumps feature a memory capacity to record programs for repeated use. This feature is useful for patients who receive multiple cycles of the same therapy regimen; complete reprogramming of the pump is not necessary, only review
  - other pump features, which vary with the model, include printing capability, patient lockout, alarm logs, and displays in languages other than English
  - programming is done using the keypad on the pump; prompts are displayed for easy programming
  - many of the keypads are color coded and marked to identify their function. Hourly rates may be programmed in mg or ml depending on the type of pump
  - accuracy varies with each pump, and manufacturers provide a range of error
- Management of complications
  - pump malfunctions: check with pump manufacturer or rental company technical support staff—many have available 24 hr assistance
  - troubleshooting guidelines are provided in the manufacturer's operational manual
  - always check catheter function as well as pump function. Pumps may continue to operate despite catheter malfunction or dislodgement resulting in extravasation or infiltration of drug
- Advantages
  - reliable and affordable

- controlled infusion rates
- availability of alarm systems for malfunctions
- flexible programming for all types of infusional therapy

- Disadvantages
  - complexity of programming on some pumps may be labor intensive to staff and patient
  - custom supplies can be expensive
  - the weight of larger infusions or weight of some infusion pumps may make ambulation difficult for patients
- Special considerations
  - insurance precertification is necessary to ensure optimal reimbursement for the medication and infusion pump
  - current Medicare guidelines will not reimburse for certain IV medications given on a continuous infusion outpatient basis
  - pumps may be purchased or rented. Rental agreements vary from daily to monthly and may include cost of supplies
  - need for appropriate infusion site access device for type of therapy to be delivered
  - drug stability varies with concentration of the drug. Need to check drug stability to determine frequency of bag changes. Stability of some drugs may require frequent bag changes
  - remote access and telephone program capability available on some peristaltic pumps

ISSUES FOR PATIENT/ FAMILY TEACHING

- Name of pump
- Hands-on training regarding pump operation is required of the patient or caregiver
- Availability of written and/or audiovisual patient education materials
- Specific instructions for safe handling of pump in the home
- Ability of patient/caregiver to assess side effects and complications of therapy
- Discussion of lifestyle adjustments during infusional therapy including wearing of loose-fitting clothing to conceal pump, avoidance of strenuous activity while wearing pump, protection of pump during showering, bathing, and sleeping
- Provision of telephone numbers for troubleshooting: physician, nurse, 24 hr assistance
- Routine assessment of compliance with recommendations for care

KEY REFERENCES

Abbott Lefever J: Infusion pumps. Professional Nurse 1998; 13(9):621–8

Rapsilber L, Camp-Sorrell D: Ambulatory infusion pumps: application to oncology. Sem Oncol Nurs 1995; 11(3):213–20

Schleis T, Tice A: Selecting infusion devices for use in ambulatory care. Am J Health-Syst Pharm 1996; 53:868–77

Device: Elastomeric "Balloon" Ambulatory Pump

Sandra Purl and Susan C. Budds

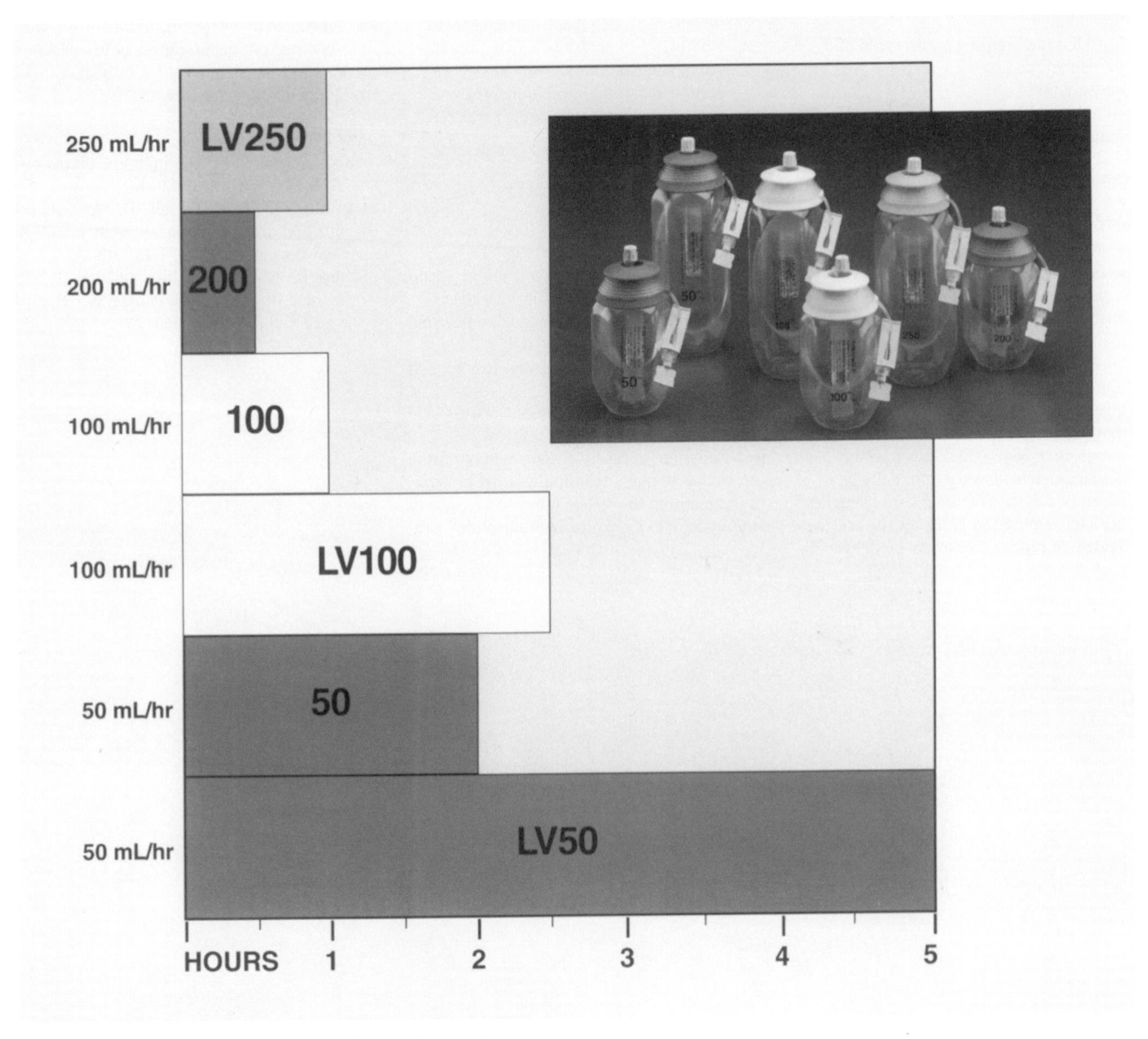

Reproduced by permission of Baxter Healthcare Corporation.

MULTIPLE MANUFACTURERS; MOST COMMON: INFUSOR, BAXTER HEALTHCARE CORPORATION; HOMEPUMP "C" SERIES, I FLOW CORPORATION

- Description
  - a lightweight fixed-rate pump, which uses a balloonlike reservoir to infuse medication
  - when filled, the elasticity of the balloon exerts a constant internal pressure on the fluid within. The fluid is forced through a filter and a flow restrictor controlling the rate of infusion
  - the predetermined rate cannot be altered
- Reservoir/accessories/maintenance
  - disposable elastomeric balloonlike reservoir encased in a protective soft/hard plastic outer shell
  - reservoir capacity is variable ranging from 50–500 ml depending on manufacturer
- Power source: none
- Rates/range of infusion: a variety of drug delivery duration times range from 30 min–10 days depending on manufacturer

CLINICAL ASSESSMENT/ INTERVENTIONS/IMPLICATIONS

- Alarms/safety mechanisms
  - no alarms available
  - built-in flow regulators decrease risk of runaway infusions; closed system decreases risk of contamination
- Program modes
  - continuous infusion
- Management of complications
  - pump malfunctions: check with pump manufacturer
  - troubleshooting guidelines are provided by manufacturer

Device: Elastomeric "Balloon" Ambulatory Pump *(Continued)*

- always check catheter function as well as pump function. Pumps may continue to operate despite catheter malfunction or dislodgement resulting in extravasation or infiltration of drug

- ■ Advantages
  - compact, lightweight
  - requires no batteries or programming
  - ideal for antibiotic therapy and single/multiple-day chemotherapy infusions
  - simple to use, requiring minimal patient education and responsibilities
  - disposable; no pump maintenance
  - convenience: tubing is preattached; device is self-priming
  - ease of patient training
- ■ Disadvantages
  - expensive, particularly for multiple days of long-term therapies
  - infusion rate limited and cannot be changed (not ideal for large-volume infusions)
  - some drugs incompatible with elastic material of reservoir
  - more pharmacy time to prepare than minibags or syringes
  - patient movement and temperature of solution may alter infusion time
  - lack of audible or visual alarms to indicate malfunctioning
- ■ Special considerations
  - reimbursement—current Medicare guidelines will not reimburse for disposable balloon pumps
  - drug must be stable for duration of infusion
  - need for appropriate infusion site access device for type of therapy to be delivered
  - ongoing upgrades make pumps easier for patients and staff to use

ISSUES FOR PATIENT/ FAMILY TEACHING

- ■ Name of the pump
- ■ Hands-on training regarding pump operation is required
- ■ Availability of written and/or audiovisual patient education materials
- ■ Specific instructions for safe handling and disposal of pump in the home
- ■ Ability of patient/caregiver to assess side effects and complications of therapy
- ■ Discussion of lifestyle adjustments during infusional therapy including wearing of loose-fitting clothing to conceal pump, avoidance of strenuous activity while wearing pump, protection of pump during showering, bathing, and sleeping
- ■ Provision of telephone numbers for troubleshooting: physician, nurse, 24 hr assistance
- ■ Routine assessment of compliance with recommendations for care

KEY REFERENCES

Access Device Guidelines: Recommendations for Nursing Practice and Education, D Camp-Sorrell (ed). Pittsburgh: Oncology Nursing Society, n.d.

Lefever J: Infusion pumps. Professional Nurse 1998; 13(9):621–8

Rapsilber L, Camp-Sorrell D: Ambulatory infusion pumps: application to oncology. Sem Oncol Nurs 1995; 11(3):213–20

Schleis T, Tice A: Selecting infusion devices for use in ambulatory care. Am J Health-Syst Pharm 1996; 53:868–77

Appendix A

CONSIDERATIONS FOR HEALTH PROFESSIONALS

Extravasation

Catherine Kefer

DEFINITION AND CAUSES

- Extravasation is the infiltration or leakage of an intravenous (IV) chemotherapeutic agent or other drug into the surrounding tissues which results in local tissue damage; may occur when administering drugs peripherally or through a central venous access device (VAD)
- In patients with VADs, extravasation may result from improper Huber needle placement, separation of the port and catheter, dislodgment of catheter, or thrombus formation
- Drugs associated with severe necrosis when extravasated are known as *vesicants:*
  - a vesicant is a medication that has the potential to cause cellular damage or tissue destruction if leakage into SubQ tissue occurs; sloughing of tissue, prolonged pain, infection, and/or loss of mobility are potential injuries that can result from an extravasation
- Drugs associated with less severe burning or inflammation are known as *irritants:*
  - irritants may produce pain and inflammation at the site of administration or along the path of the vein by which it is administered
  - irritants such as carmustine, dacarbazine, and etoposide usually do not cause blisters, ulcerations, or skin burns
  - reaction caused by an irritant is often classified as a *flare reaction;* a flare is a raised, red streak along the course of a vein, which may be mistaken for extravasation

SIGNS AND SYMPTOMS

- Degree of tissue damage varies depending on the drug, drug concentration, total amount extravasated; early recognition and intervention will affect the clinical course of tissue destruction
- Onset of symptoms may occur immediately or several days to weeks following the incident
- Tissue damage may initially appear minimal as a result of the indolent course of most extravasations; the actual extent of damage is usually evident with ulceration, demarcation, and eschar formation within 12–14 days
- Treatment management of extravasations continues to be controversial, although there is consensus that early recognition and intervention are key
- Nursing management should consist of prevention and providing supportive measures once extravasation has occurred
- Knowledge regarding the agents true (vesicants and/or irritants) will better prepare the nurse in evaluating patients receiving chemotherapy

FACTORS THAT AFFECT AND INFLUENCE THE RISK OF EXTRAVASATION

- The skill of the practitioner
- The condition of the vein
- The site chosen for venous access
- Administration technique
- The order of drug administration
- The use of a preexisting IV line

GENERAL GUIDELINES FOR DRUG ADMINISTRATION

- Evaluate potential sites to access: never use veins in areas of compromised circulation (lower extremities, a mastectomy site, areas of phlebitis, lymphedema, or hematomas). Avoid the antecubital fossa. Use hand to forearm rule
- Begin a new infusion for drug administration. Avoid use of preexisting IV lines unless their patency can be confirmed (e.g., time of insertion, flow of fluid, condition/location of the vein, and blood return)
- Secure needle/catheter site to be visible at all times
- Infuse an adequate amount of normal saline (10–20 ml) to test vein patency
- With IV fluid running slowly, inject vesicant into IV line slowly and check frequently for patency by allowing IV fluid to flow freely or withdraw blood (avoid pinching the line while administering drug because this could cause increased pressure in the vein)
- Assess for blood return every 1–2 ml of injection
- Continuously observe for signs of infiltration
- Instruct the patient to report changes in sensation immediately (particularly pain, burning, or stinging) during drug administration and after treatment

MANAGEMENT OF EXTRAVASATION

- If an extravasation has occurred, immediately stop administration of the agent
- Leave needle in place and aspirate any residual agent and blood from the IV tubing, needle, and suspected infiltration site. If unable to aspirate residual agent from the IV tubing, *do not* instill the antidote through the needle
- Inform the physician and initiate appropriate treatment measures. Refer to institutional policies and procedures
- Document the date and time of the initial incident. Using a daily flow sheet, record changes in the skin, mobility, and color of the infiltration every other day for the first 2 wks, then weekly for 6 wks. Documentation records for venipuncture sites and reactions provide valuable information and legal protection
- For monitoring purposes, take a baseline photograph with periodic photographs thereafter
- Obtain an early consultation with a plastic surgeon and a physical therapist, if symptoms are present
- A standard plan for follow-up of the patient should be in place and initiated with each suspected or actual extravasation
- Patients should receive written information regarding home care of the infiltration and should be provided with contact names and numbers of their physician and nurse should questions and problems arise

Extravasation *(Continued)*

Common chemotherapy agents and antidotes

Agent	Antidote
Nitrogen mustard Cisplatin Dactinomycin Mechlorethamine Mithramycin Mitomycin-C	Sodium thiosulfate (see preparation below)
Carmustine Daunomycin Doxorubicin Epirubicin hydrochloride Mitoxantrone Vinblastine	Sodium bicarbonate Topical cooling
Dactinomycin Mitomycin-C	Vitamin C
Vincristine Vindesine Teniposide (VM-26) Taxanes Etoposide (VP-16)	Hyaluronidase (Wydase) (see preparation below)
Doxorubicin Daunomycin Mitomycin-C Mechlorethamine	Dimethylsulfoxide (DMSO) (see preparation below)

General antidotes: cold, corticosteroids, lidocaine HCL (Xylocaine), isoproterenol HCL (Isuprel), EDTA

PREPARATION OF ANTIDOTES

- Sodium thiosulfate 1/6 molar solution
  - sodium thiosulfate solution 10%: mix 4–8 ml with 6 ml of sterile water and immediately inject through IV cannula (inject 2 ml for every milligram of mechlorethamine extravasated or for every 100 mg of cisplatin extravasated)
  - sodium thiosulfate solution 25%: mix 1.6 ml with 8.4 ml of sterile water
  - remove needle
  - inject antidote into SubQ tissue following institutional policy. The needle should be changed with each injection
  - heat or cold has not proven effective
- Hyaluronidase
  - vinca alkaloids: mix 150 units of hyaluronidase with 1–3 ml saline
    - □ inject into IV line (1 ml for each 1 ml infiltrated). If IV has been removed inject SubQ. The needle should be changed with each injection
    - □ apply warm compresses for 30–60 min, then alternate off/on q15–20min for at least 24–48 hrs, elevate extremity
  - taxanes: mix 300 units of hyaluronidase with 3 ml saline
    - □ inject into IV line (1 ml for each 1 ml infiltrated). If IV has been removed inject SubQ. The needle should be changed with each injection
    - □ apply ice packs for 15 min at least 4 times/day for 24 hrs
    - □ if chemotherapy extravasation occurred in a peripheral line, elevate extremity
- Dimethylsulfoxide (DMSO)
  - doxorubicin
    - □ a recent study with 20 patients demonstrated that local applications of 1.5 ml of DMSO q6hrs for 14 days was effective in preventing severe skin damage in patients with extravasations with doxorubicin
    - □ current data supports the immediate application of cold packs with circulating ice water or ice packs for 24 hrs as an effective intervention
    - □ protect site from light and heat
    - □ avoid applying pressure to the suspected area of infiltration
    - □ cover lightly with an occlusive sterile dressing. Instruct the patient in the care and follow-up of the site
    - □ instruct patient to rest and elevate site for at least 48 hrs, and then resume normal activity

KEY REFERENCES

Access device guidelines: recommendations for nursing practice and education: In D Camp-Sorrell (ed): Oncology Nursing Society. Pittsburgh: 1997

Berg D: Drug delivery system. In *Cancer Chemotherapy: A Nursing Process Approach* (2nd ed., pp. 561–95), M Burke, G Wilkes, K Ingwersen (eds). London: Jones and Bartlett, 1996

Chabner B, Longo D: Chemoterapy administration; practical guidelines. In *Cancer Chemotherapy & Biotherapy: Principles & Practice* (2nd ed.), A Galassi, S Hubbard, HR Alexander, et al. (eds). Philadelphia: Lippincott-Raven, 1996

Holmes BC: Administration of cancer chemotherapy agents. In *Cancer Chemotherapy Handbook* (2nd ed., pp. 109–18), R Dorr, D Von Hoff (eds). East Norwalk, CT: Appleton and Lange, 1994

Martin V: Delivery of cancer chemotherapy. In *Cancer Nursing: A Comprehensive Textbook* (2nd ed., pp. 395–433), R McCorkle, M Grant, M Frank-Stromberg (eds.). Philadelphia: WB Saunders, 1996

Oliver IN, Aisner J, Hament A, et al.: A prospective study of topical demethyl sulfoxide for treating anthracycline extravasations. J Clin Oncol 1998; 6(11):1732–5

Appendix B

SAFETY PRECAUTIONS DURING CHEMOTHERAPY ADMINISTRATION

From Oncology Nursing Society: *Cancer Chemotherapy Guidelines and Recommendations for Practice,* 1996

CANCER CHEMOTHERAPY GUIDELINES AND RECOMMENDATIONS FOR PRACTICE

Editor: Lorrie L. Powel, RN, MS, OCN

Contributing Editors: Maryanne Fishman, RN, MS; Mary Mrozek-Orlowski, RN, MSN, AOCN

Writers: Jeannine Brant, RN, MS, AOCN; Aurelie Cormier, RN, CS, MS, OCN; Rebecca Hawkins, RN, MN, ANP, AOCN; Cindy Johnson, RN; Pamela Kennedy, RN, OCN; Maureen O'Rourke, RN, MN, OCN; Mary Beth Riley, RN, MSN, OCN; Deborah Rust, RN, MSN, OCN; Charleen Sakuri, RN

Reviewers: 1993–1994 Clinical Practice Committee; 1994–1995 Clinical Practice Committee; Margaret Barton-Burke, RN, MS; Robert Dorr, PhD, RPH; Nancy A. Hayes, RN, MS, OCN; Robert J. Ignoffo, PharmD, FASHP; Tish Knobf, RN, MSN; Connie Leek, RNC, MSN, OCN; Barbara Livingston, RN, OCN; Rita Wickham, RN, MS, AOCN; Gail Wilkes, RNC, MS, ANP, AOCN

ONS Staff: Linda M. Worrall, RN, BSN, OCN, Director of Education, ONS

G. Safety precautions during chemotherapy administration
   1. Administer drugs in a safe, unhurried environment.
   2. Wear protective apparel, including a gown and disposable, powder-free, surgical latex gloves. People with latex allergies can use hypoallergenic latex products or polyvinylchloride gloves (Lavaud et al., 1995). Face shields/eye protection should be worn if there is a danger of spraying or splashing.
   3. Place a disposable, absorbent pad under the area where the drug is being administered.
   4. Observe precautions when working with chemotherapy agents.
      a) Wash hands before and after handling the drug, avoid touching the drug, and always wear gloves when handling it.
      b) Wash surfaces that came in contact with the drug with soap and water, and dispose of toweling in a chemotherapy waste receptacle.

H. Disposal, accidental exposure, and spills
   1. Handling body fluids after chemotherapy administration
      a) Institute universal precautions when handling blood, vomitus, or excreta of patients who have received chemotherapy within the past 48 hours. Wear a gown and goggles when appropriate and if expecting splashing.
      b) Provide a urinal with a tight-fitting lid for male patients (Gullo, 1988).
      c) For children in diapers or incontinent adults, apply a protective ointment to the diaper area to avoid painful chemical burns when voiding. Clean the skin well with each diaper change, and change diapers frequently (Meeske & Ruccione, 1987).
      d) Flush the toilet twice after disposing of body excreta from patients who have received chemotherapy within the past 48 hours.
   2. Linen
      a) Institute universal precautions when handling linen soiled with blood or body fluids.
      b) Linens contaminated with chemotherapy or excreta from patients who have received chemotherapy within the past 48 hours should be contained in specially marked impervious bags. Linens should be prewashed and then added to the hospital or industry laundry for a second wash (OSHA, 1995).
      c) In the home, wear gloves when handling bed linens or clothing contaminated with chemotherapy or patient excreta within 48 hours of chemotherapy administration. Place linens in a separate, washable pillow case. Wash soiled linens twice in hot water with regular detergent in a washing machine. Do not wash with other household items (Gullo, 1988).
      d) Discard disposable diapers with other hazardous wastes in plastic bags intended for hazardous waste disposal. Cloth diapers should be laundered twice, as should other chemotherapy- or fluid-soiled linens.
      e) After use, discard gloves and gown (if disposable) in a hazardous waste container.
      f) For further information, see *Safe Handling of Cytotoxic Agents: An Independent Study Module,* ONS (1989), *ASHP Technical Assistance Bulletin on Handling Cytotoxic and Hazardous Drugs,* American Society of Hospital Pharmacists (ASHP) (1990), and *Controlled Occupational Exposure to Hazardous Drugs,* OSHA (1995).
   3. Disposal (Dunne, 1989; Hoffman, 1980; OSHA, 1995)
      a) Identify antineoplastic waste products by using leak-proof, sealable, plastic bags or other appropriate containers with brightly colored

labels designating the hazardous nature of the contents.

b) Use puncture-proof containers for sharp or breakable items.

c) Only those housekeeping personnel who have previously received instruction in safe-handling procedures should handle waste containers. Personnel should be properly dressed in gowns with cuffs and back closure and should wear latex rubber or polyvinylchloride disposable gloves.

d) Place all supplies used in home chemotherapy administration in an appropriate leak-proof container, and remove from the home to a designated area for appropriate disposal by a nurse, patient, or significant other. Make arrangements with the physician's office, hospital, or private waste-management firm for proper disposal (Blecke, 1989; Gullo, 1988; Sansivero & Murray, 1989). Check county and state regulations regarding the handling of biohazardous wastes.

4. Accidental exposure
   a) Appropriate personal protective equipment (e.g., gown, gloves, eye protection, masks) should be worn when participating in the following.
      (1) Withdrawing needles from vials
      (2) Transferring drugs using needles or syringes
      (3) Opening ampules
      (4) Expelling air from a drug-filled syringe
      (5) Injecting the drug
      (6) Changing IV bags or tubing of continuous infusion therapy
      (7) Being exposed to inadvertent puncture of a closed system
      (8) Printing IV tubing
      (9) Handling leakage from the tubing, syringe, and connection site
   b) Improper technique, faulty equipment, or negligence in hood operation can lead to increased exposure (OSHA, 1995).
5. Spills
   a) Spills and breakage should be immediately cleaned up by a trained and protected person (Harrison, 1992).
   b) Spills should be immediately identified with a warning sign so others in the vicinity will not be contaminated (Gullo, 1988).
   c) Chemical inactivators, with the exception of sodium thiosulfate (for use with mechlorethamine/nitrogen mustard), should not be used to absorb drug spills because potentially dangerous byproducts may be produced (Harrison, 1992).
   d) All spills should be wiped up with the absorbent toweling available in spill kits.
   e) If spills occur on a carpeted surface, absorb the spill as much as possible with absorbent toweling. Then, clean the surface three times with soap and water. Do not use carpet cleaners on spills because they may trigger a chemical reaction (ASHP, 1990; OSHA, 1995).
   f) All contaminated surfaces should be cleaned thoroughly with a detergent solution and wiped clean with water. Contaminated absorbents and other soiled materials should be disposed of in a hazardous-drug disposal bag (ASHP, 1990).
   g) If a spill occurs inside a BSC and the high-efficiency particulate air filter of the hood is contaminated, the unit must be labeled "DO NOT USE—Contaminated" and the filter must be changed and disposed of properly as soon as possible by personnel wearing protective equipment. Decontamination of all hood surfaces is necessary before the hood can be used (Harrison, 1992).
   h) Each time a spill of more than 5 ml occurs, a complete record of the spill should be sent to the safety director or a designee of the agency (Cloak et al., 1985; Harrison, 1992).
   i) If an oral chemotherapeutic drug bottle is broken, double bag all of its contents and return them to the manufacturer (Anderson et al., 1993).
   j) For spills at home, see Appendix C.

I. Institutional considerations
   1. Handling
      a) Agencies must have policies and procedures that protect employees, patients, customers, and the environment from exposure to hazardous agents.
      b) Agencies must have policies and procedures that ensure safe storage, transport, administration, and disposal of hazardous agents.
      c) Training programs must be available to all employees involved in the handling of hazardous agents.
      d) Agencies should have written policies and procedures related to the medical surveillance of employees involved in the handling of hazardous agents.
      e) All employees handling chemotherapy drugs should wear protective clothing, which includes disposable gloves, a gown, and eye protection. All equipment should be removed, and hands should be washed, before leaving the work area.
   2. Preparation and administration
      a) Obtain and maintain a BSC, class II, type B, for the preparation of chemotherapy agents. The BSC should be vented outside with a blower in constant operation (Harrison, 1992; OSHA, 1995; Tenenbaum, 1992).
      b) Implement policies and procedures that require personnel who may be exposed to airborne particles or aerosols of chemotherapy generated during handling to wear a National Institute of Occupational Safety and Health–approved dust/mist respirator or face mask unless proper ventilation (i.e., class II BSC) is available.
      c) Implement policies that prohibit eating, drinking, smoking, chewing of gum or tobacco, applying cosmetics, and storing food in areas where chemotherapy is used.
      d) Train all employees who will prepare or administer chemotherapy in the proper safety procedures, and document the occurrence of such training programs.
      e) Include compliance with chemotherapy policy and procedures as part of the quality-improvement program (Tenenbaum, 1992).
      f) Distribute chemotherapy drug work loads among the trained personnel to minimize daily exposure (Harrison, 1992).
      g) Although no information is available on the reproductive risks of handling chemotherapy drugs in workers who use a BSC and wear protective clothing, employees who are pregnant, planning a pregnancy (male or female), or breast-feeding or who have other medical reasons prohibiting exposure to chemotherapy may elect to refrain from preparing or administering these agents or caring for patients during their treatment (up to 48 hours after completion of therapy) (Harrison, 1992; OSHA, 1995). Institutional policies and procedures that support this practice should be in place.

Safety Precautions During Chemotherapy Administration *(Continued)*

3. Spills
   a) Spill kits should be available in all areas where chemotherapy is stored, transported, prepared, or administered. All employees who work in these areas should be trained regarding safe containment of spills.
   b) Advise employees to report all spills, exposures, or unsafe conditions to their supervisors.
   c) Prohibit wet mopping or sweeping in areas where spills have occurred until spills have been contained (Harrison, 1992).
   d) Once spills have been contained, cleaning should proceed from the least to most contaminated areas. All materials used in the cleaning process should be disposed of as hazardous drugs according to federal, state, and local laws (OSHA, 1995).

Appendix C

SPILL KIT PROCEDURE FOR HOME USE

(PLEASE REVIEW THIS PROCEDURE WITH YOUR NURSE.)

1. Do not touch the spill with unprotected hands.
2. Open the spill kit and put on both pairs of gloves. If the bag or syringe with chemotherapy drugs has been broken or is leaking, and you have a catheter or Port-a-Cath® in place, first disconnect the catheter from the tubing and rinse and cap according to normal procedure before cleaning the spill.
3. Put on the gown (closes in back), splash goggles, respirator.
4. Use spill pillows to contain spill—put around puddle to form a V.
5. Use the absorbent sheets to blot up as much of the drug as possible.
6. Put contaminated clean-up materials directly into the plastic bag contained in the kit. Do not lay them on unprotected surfaces.
7. Use the scoop and brush to collect any broken glass, sweeping toward the V'd spill pillows, and dispose of the glass in the box of the kit.
8. While still wearing the protective gear, wash the area with dishwashing or laundry detergent and warm water using disposable rags or paper towels and put them in the plastic bag with other waste. Rinse the area with clean water and dispose of the towels in the same plastic bag.
9. Remove gloves, goggles, respirator, and gown and place in plastic bag. Put all contaminated materials, including the spill kit box, into the second large plastic bag and label with the hazardous waste label in the kit.
10. Wash your hands with soap and water.
11. Call the home health nurse, clinic, or doctor's office promptly to report the spill. Plans need to be made to replace the spilled chemotherapy so the treatment can be completed. Arrangements will be made to have the waste material picked up or have you bring it to the hospital for proper disposal.
12. If upholstered or carpeted area is contaminated, follow the above procedure—blot as much of the solution as possible with the absorbent sheets, wash the area with detergent, and follow with a clean water rinse. Do not use chemical spot removers or upholstery dry cleaners as they may cause a chemical reaction with the drug.
13. If the spill occurs on sheets or clothing, wash in hot water separately from the other wash. Wash clothing or bed linen contaminated with body wastes in the same manner.
14. Patients on 24-hour infusions should use a plastic-backed mattress pad to protect the mattress from contamination.

Following these procedures prevents undue exposure and assures your safety. Call your nurse if you have any questions. Thank you.

INDEX

Note: Page numbers in *italic* indicate illustrations; those followed by t refer to tables.

I

J

K

L

M

N

O

P

Q

R

S

T

U

V

X

Z